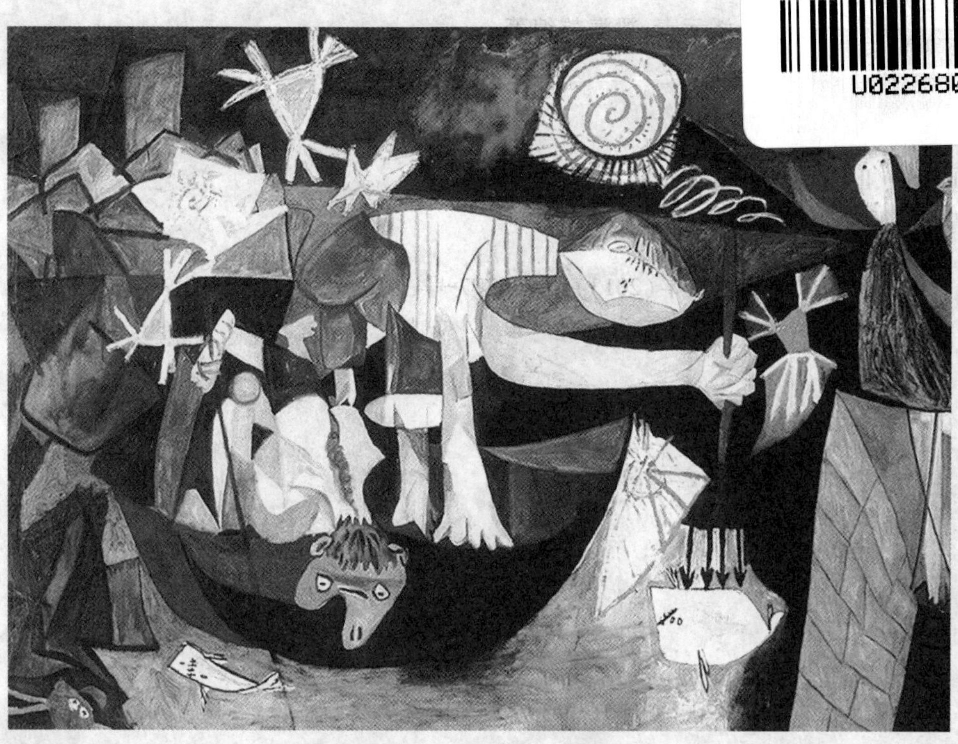

学心理与精神障碍

Medical Psychology and Mental Disorders

蘭州大學出版社

图书在版编目(CIP)数据

医学心理与精神障碍 / 潘元青,梁海乾编著. —兰州:兰州大学出版社,2013.10

ISBN 978-7-311-04280-6

Ⅰ.①医… Ⅱ.①潘… ②梁… Ⅲ.①医学心理学—研究 ②精神障碍—研究 Ⅳ.①R395.1 ②R749

中国版本图书馆 CIP 数据核字(2013)第 246707 号

策划编辑 陈红升
责任编辑 郝可伟
封面设计 李鹏远 潘元青

书　　名 医学心理与精神障碍
作　　者 潘元青 梁海乾 编著
出版发行 兰州大学出版社 (地址:兰州市天水南路 222 号 730000)
电　　话 0931-8912613(总编办公室) 0931-8617156(营销中心)
　　　　 0931-8914298(读者服务部)
网　　址 http://www.onbook.com.cn
电子信箱 press@lzu.edu.cn
印　　刷 兰德辉印刷有限责任公司
开　　本 787 mm×1092 mm 1/16
印　　张 33.25
字　　数 885 千
版　　次 2013 年 11 月第 1 版
印　　次 2013 年 11 月第 1 次印刷
书　　号 ISBN 978-7-311-04280-6
定　　价 68.00 元

Preface

The volume sets forth the basic principles and the clinical practice of psychology as a true science of medical psychology and mental disorders. This book is to be viewed benefit from a better understanding of the causes of behavior as we go through life trying to make sense of our own behavior. In Section Ⅰ, which is written by Pan Yuanqing, it is focused on simply enhancing the quality of life and our ability to function in a wide variety of circumstances (education, work, relationships, etc.). We will explore what psychology is, how psychology originated as a science, what clinical psychologists do, and what contents do medical psychology study. In Section Ⅱ, which is written by Liang Haiqian, it aims to understanding how can we distinguish normal from abnormal behavior, what are the major perspectives on mental disorders used by mental health professionals. In Section Ⅱ, it introduces a wide range of mental disorders, covering epidemiology, clinical features, and both psychosocial and somatic therapies.

Contents

Section I

Chapter 1 Introduction — The Science of Psychology ········ 003
Chapter 2 Research Methods in Psychology ········ 022
Chapter 3 Brain and Behavior ········ 049
Chapter 4 Sensation and Perception ········ 080
Chapter 5 Memory and Intelligence ········ 106
Chapter 6 Motivation, Emotion and Personality ········ 134
Chapter 7 Child, Adolescent and Adult Development ········ 164

Section II

Chapter 1 Dementia, Delirium and Amnestic Disorders ········ 207
Chapter 2 Anxiety and Mood Disorder ········ 236
Chapter 3 Personality Disorders ········ 291
Chapter 4 Eating Disorders ········ 319
Chapter 5 Sexual Dysfunction, Gender Identity Disorders and Paraphilias ········ 340
Chapter 6 Childhood Mental Disorders ········ 369
Chapter 7 Introduction to Psychiatric Treatment ········ 408
Chapter 8 Psychotherapy ········ 421
Chapter 9 Psychology Care for the Chronically Ill and Dying Patient ········ 465
Chapter 10 Forensic Psychiatry ········ 487

References ········ 508

Section I

Psychology can be focused on the study of the human mind and behavior. It involves a comprehensive understanding of emotional issues at the deep root level which brings about health, happiness and functionality in the client, and it is a systematic approach to the understanding of people, their thoughts, emotions and behaviors. The study of psychology allows one to appreciate the relationship between thoughts, emotions and the resulting behavior. Research in psychology seeks to understand and explain how we think, act and feel. Applications for psychology include mental health treatment, performance enhancement, self-help, ergonomics and many other areas affecting health and daily life. We can benefit from a better understanding of the causes of behavior as we go through life trying to make sense of our own behavior or that of friends, family, lovers, co-workers, politicians. Everyone needs to be able to critically evaluate the claims concerning behavior that are so much a part of news reports, commercials, and conversation. This course will help you with each of these. Many of you, raising children — now or in the future, will be better prepared with some understanding of developmental psychology. And all of you, in one way or another, will cross paths with someone in psychology or related fields. Perhaps you already have, in school (counselors, school psychologists). Recent statistics suggest that 1 out of 2 Chinese suffer from some sort of psychological disorder in their lifetime. You or someone you care about may seek out some type of mental health treatment or advice, or you may hear testimony from someone in this field while on jury duty. This course will help you understand the qualifications of and differences among professionals in the field. In addition, about 1 out of 5 Americans will have some kind of nervous system disorder or disease which affects behavior. Biopsychology, the study of brain-behavior relationships, can help you understand what is happening when someone you know is affected by autism or Alzheimer's disease or other neurological problem. But psychology is not only concerned with treating behavioral problems. A good part of it is focused on simply enhancing the quality of life and our ability to function in a wide variety of circumstances (education, work, relationships, etc.). You can use what you learn to improve your life!

Our aims is written in a conversational style that is easy to understand. You are responsible for that reading! Attending class is important — sometimes what we cover in class will not be covered in the textbook. But attending class is only part of what's involved in becoming an educated person. Do set aside time for that reading, preferably before or while we are covering that topic in class — it is key to your success.

In this topic, we will explore what psychology is, what psychologists do, and how psychology originated as a science. As you read the material in this topic, you should find the answers to the following questions.

Chapter 1 Introduction — The Science of Psychology

What is Psychology?

There are many ways to find out about ourselves and the world in which we live. Some of our beliefs are a matter of faith. Such faith - based beliefs require no empirical evidence — evidence gathered through direct sensory experience or observation. Some beliefs come through tradition, passed on from one generation to the next, accepted simply because "they said it is so". Some beliefs are credited to common sense (for example, beat a dog often enough and sooner or later it will get mean). Some of the insights we have about the human condition are taken from art literature, poetry, and drama. For example, some of our ideas about romantic love may have roots in literature, such as Shakespeare's *Romeo and Juliet*. Although all of these ways of learning about ourselves and the world have value in certain contexts, psychologists maintain that there is a better way: applying the values and methods of science.

When psychologists try to learn about behavior and mental processes, they avoid faith - based and common sense explanations. Instead, they approach problems from a scientific perspective. This involves: 1) attempting to isolate the factors that contribute to behavior; 2) developing theories and laws to account for the behavior of interest.

Psychology is the science of behavior and mental processes. It will be worth our time to take a few minutes now to dissect this definition to look at its component parts.

First and foremost, the definition tells us that psychology is a science, just like biology, physics, and chemistry. As a science, psychology approaches its subject matter from a scientific perspective. This means that psychologists use accepted scientific techniques to build a body of knowledge about behavior and mental processes. Second, the definition tells us that psychologists have an interest in both humans and animals. We'll see many examples of psychological research that uses animals in an effort to help us understand human behaviors and mental processes. On the other hand, some psychologists study the behaviors and mental activity on non - human animals simply because they find them interesting and worthy of study in their own right. Finally, our definition suggests that psychologists study both behavior and mental processes.

Psychology meets the second requirement of a science because what is known in psychology has been learned mostly through the application of the scientific method. The scientific method is a method of acquiring knowledge by observing a phenomenon, formulating hypotheses, further observing and experimenting, and refining and re - testing hypotheses.

Scientific methods reflect an attitude or an approach to problem solving. It is a process of inquiry, a particular way of thinking, rather than a special set of procedures that must be followed rigorously.

There may not be specific rules to follow in doing science, but there are guidelines. The basic process goes like this: The scientist (psychologist) makes observations about his or her subject matter. For example, he or she notices that when there are several bystanders to an emergency, help is less likely to be given than if there is only one bystander. On the basis of such preliminary observations, the scientist develops a hypothesis. A hypothesis is a tentative explanation of some phenomenon that can be tested and then either supported or rejected; it is an educated guess about one's subject matter. It links together two things: factors believed to control behavior and the behavior itself. In our example, the scientist might hypothesize that as the number of bystanders to an emergency increases, the likelihood of the person in need receiving help decreases. In this hypothesis, a causal factor (number of bystanders) is tentatively linked to behavior (helping or lack of helping).

Hypotheses are logically deduced from preliminary observations and from their reading of existing scientific literature. Hypotheses, although they may sound intuitively obvious, are not accepted as the final explanation for behavior. Instead, the scientist proceeds by systematically testing his or her hypothesis with empirical research, making careful observations of behavior (this time under specified and controlled conditions). For example, the psychologist could test the hypothesis linking the number of bystanders and helping behavior by designing a study in which she systematically increases the number of bystanders to a staged emergency and observes the bystanders' behaviors. These new observations would then be analyzed to see if they confirm the previously stated hypothesis.

Psychological Approaches Past and Present

In this section, we add to our definition of psychology by considering some of the major perspectives or approaches, that have been developed throughout psychology's history.

Psychology's Roots in Philosophy

Psychology did not suddenly appear as the productive scientific enterprise we know today. The roots of psychology are found in philosophy and science.

We credit philosophers for first suggesting that it is reasonable and potentially profitable to seek explanations of human behaviors at a human level. Early explanations tended to be at the level of God — or the gods. If someone suffered from fits of terrible depression, for example, it was believed that person had offended the gods. A few philosophers successfully argued that they might be able to explain why people behave, feel, and think as they do, without constant reference to God's intentions in the matter.

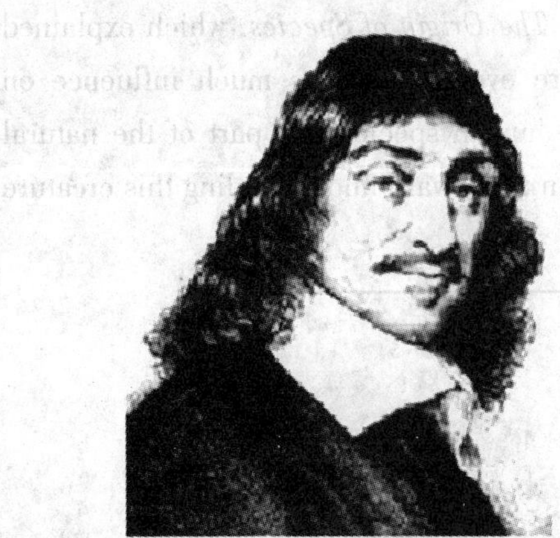

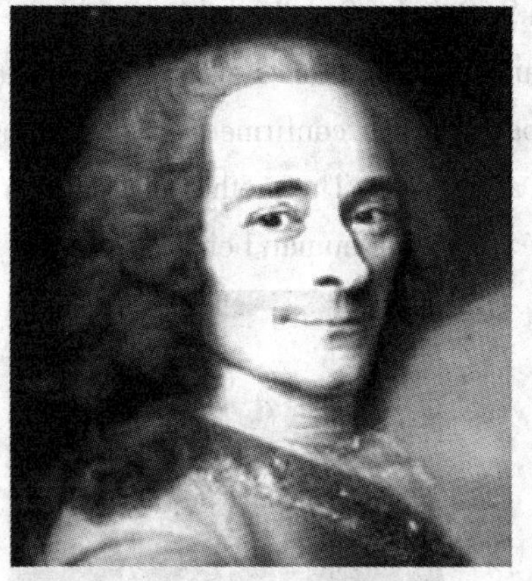

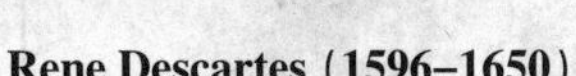

Rene Descartes (1596–1650) **John Locke (1632–1704)**

The French philosopher Rene Descartes (1596–1650) is a good example of such a philosopher. He pondered how the human body and mind produced the very process he was then engaged in — thinking. Descartes envisioned the human body as a piece of machinery: intricate and complicated. Descartes went further. According to the doctrine of dualism, human process more than just a body: They have minds. It is likely, thought Descartes that the mind similarly function through the action of knowable law, but getting those laws would sure be more difficult. Here's where Descartes had a truly important insight. We can learn about the mind because the mind and the body interact with each other. That interaction takes place in the brain. In these matters, Descartes' position is called interactive dualism; dualism because the mind and the body are separate entities, and interactive because they influence each other. Thus, we have with Rene Descartes the real possibility of understanding the human mind and how it works.

Nearly a hundred years later, a group of British thinkers brought that part of philosophy concerned with the workings of the human mind very close to what was soon to become psychology. This group got its start from the writings of John Locke (1632–1704). Locke was sitting with friends after dinner one evening discussing philosophical issues when it became clear that no one in the group really understood how the human mind understands anything, much less complex philosophical issues. Locke announced that within a week he could provide the group with a short explanation of the nature of human understanding. What was to have been a simple exercise took Locke many years to finish, but it gave philosophers a new set of ideas to ponder.

Psychology's Roots in Science

Philosophers had gone nearly to the brink. They had raised intriguing questions about the mind, how it worked, where its contents (ideas) came from, how ideas could be manipulated, and how the mind and body might influence each other. Could the methods of science provide answers to any of the philosophers' questions? A few natural scientists and physiologists believed that they could.

During the nineteenth century, natural science was making progress on every front. Charles Darwin (1809–1882) was a naturalist biologist. In 1859, just back from a lengthy sea voyage on the H.M.S. Beagle, Darwin published his revolutionary *The Origin of Species*, which explained the details of evolution. Few non - psychologists were ever to have as much influence on psychology. Darwin confirmed for psychology that the human species was part of the natural world of animal life. The methods of science could be turned toward understanding this creature of nature called the human being.

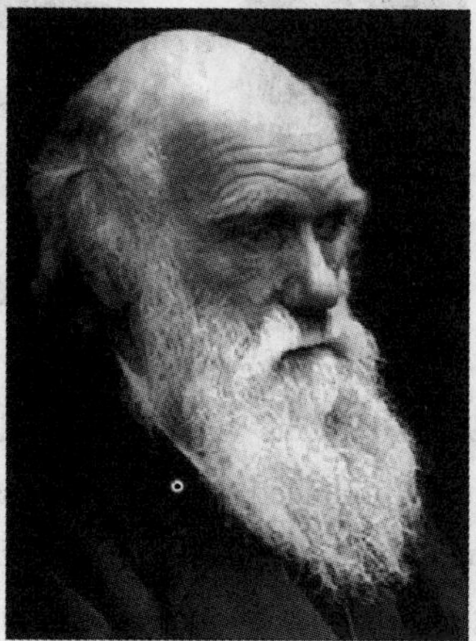

Charles Darwin (1809–1882)

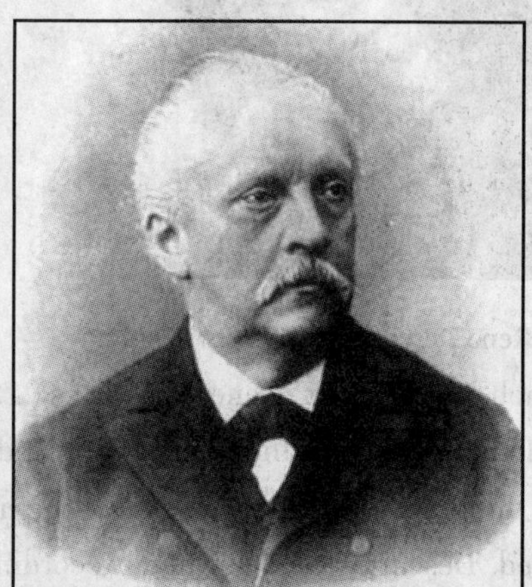

Hermann von Helmholtz (1821–1894)

Darwin made it clear that all species of this planet are, in a nearly infinite number of ways, related to one another. The impact of this observation, of course, is that what scientists discover about the sloth, the ground squirrel, or the rhesus monkey may enlighten them about the human race. Another concept that Darwin emphasized was adaptation. Species will survive and thrive only to the extent that they can, over the years, adapt to their environments. Psychologists were quick to realize that adaptation to one's environment was often a mental as well as a physical process.

The mid - 1800s also found physiologists better understanding how the human body functions. By then it was known that nerves carried electrical messages to and from various parts of the body, that nerves serving vision are different from those serving hearing and the other senses, and are also different from those that activate muscles and glands. Of all the biologists and physiologists of the nineteenth century, the one whose work is most relevant to psychology is Hermann von Helmholtz (1821–1894). In the physiology laboratory, Helmholtz performed experiments and developed theories on how long it takes the nervous system to react to stimuli, how we process information through our senses, and how we experience color. These are psychological issues, but in the mid- 1800s there was no recognized science of psychology as we know it today.

The Early Years: Structuralism

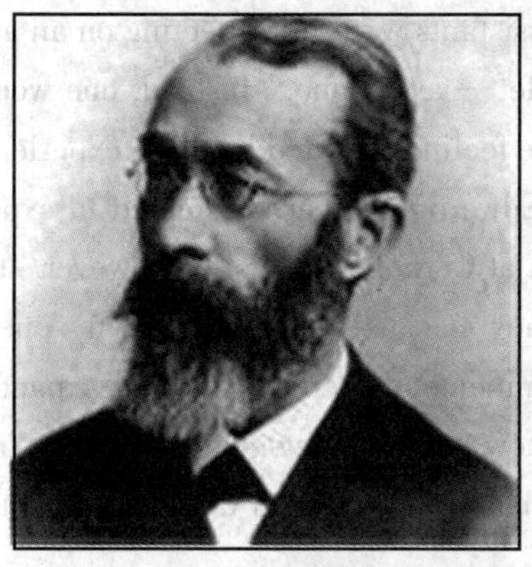

Wilhelm Wundt (1832–1920)

It is often claimed that, as a science, psychology began in 1879, when Wilhelm Wundt (1832–1920) opened his laboratory at the University of Leipzig. Wundt had been trained to practice medicine, had studied physiology, and had served as a laboratory assistant to the great Helmholtz. He also held an academic position in philosophy. Wundt was a scientist-philosopher with an interest in such psychological processes as sensation, perception, attention, word associations, and emotions.

Although others might be credited with founding psychology, Wundt receives credit for getting psychology recognized as a separate science. Wundt wrote in the preface of the first edition of his *Principles of Physiological Psychology*, "The work I here present is an attempt to mark out a new domain of science." Clearly, Wundt's intention was to define the parameters of a new science.

It is no accident that psychology began in Germany. Toward the end of the nineteenth century, the zeitgeist (loosely translated as the intellectual "spirit of the times") in Germany favored the emergence of a new science. Experimental physiology was well established in Germany, which was not the case in France or England. Biology and physiology were stressed in Germany, while physics and chemistry were stressed in France and England. In short, the climate was perfect in Germany for the emergence of the new science of psychology.

For Wundt, psychology was the scientific study of the mind. Under carefully controlled laboratory conditions, Wundt and his assistants tested and re-tested his hypotheses. The work performed in Wundt's laboratory focused on the discovery of basic elements of thought. Beyond that, Wundt wanted to see how elements of thought were related to one another and to events in the physical environment the latter notion picked up from the work of Fechner. Wundt wanted to systematically describe the basic elements of mental life. Because the psychologists in Wundt's laboratory were mostly interested in describing the structure of the mind and its operations, Wundt's approach to psychology is referred to as structuralism.

Along with the careful observation and experimentation, an important method used to dissect mental activity into its component parts was introspection. Introspection required a great deal of training as individuals were asked to describe in great detail their basic sensations, thoughts and feelings of conscious experience when presented with a particular stimulus. For example, if one of Wundt's assistants were introspecting on an apple, it would not be enough to say, "Oh yes, that's an apple — a red one." Instead, one would have to describe the actual sensations experienced and the feelings elicited by those experiences.

A student of Wundt's, Edward Titchner, attempted to export structuralism to the United States when he took a position at Cornell University. However, structuralism never caught on in America as it had in Germany because the zeitgeist in America was much different than Germany's. America in the nineteenth century was an expanding nation. People were most concerned about adapting to new environments. Quite simply, Americans were not interested in a psychology that focused so much attention on dissecting mental activity into components, or elements.

As Wundt's new laboratory was flourishing in Germany, an American philosopher at Harvard University, William James(1842–1910), was opposed to the type of psychology that was being studied in Leipzig. James agreed that psychology should study consciousness and should use scientific methods to do so. He defined psychology as "the science of mental life", a definition very similar to Wundt's. Still, he thought the German — trained psychologists were off base trying to discover the contents and structure of the human mind. James argued instead that consciousness could not be broken down into elements. He believed consciousness to be dynamic, a stream of events, personal, changing, and continuous. According to James, psychology should therefore be concerned not with the structure of the mind but with its function. The focus of psychology should be on the practical uses of mental life. In this regard, James was responding to Darwin's lead. To survive requires that a species adapt to its environment. How does the mind function to help organisms adapt and survive in the world?

James's practical approach to psychology found favor in North America, and a new type of psychology emerged, largely at the University of Chicago. Psychologists there continued to focus on the mind, but emphasized its adaptive functions. This approach is known as functionalism. Functionalists still relied on experimental methods and introduced the study of animals to psychology, again reflecting Darwin's influence. One of the most popular textbooks of this era was *The Animal Mind* by Margaret Floy Washburn (1871–1939), the first woman to be awarded a Ph. D. in psychology. She addressed questions of animal consciousness and intelligence. One of the characteristics of functionalism was its willingness to be open to a wide range of topics — as long as they related in some way to mental life, adaptation, and practical application. The origins of child, abnormal, educational, social, and industrial psychology can be traced to this approach.

In the early days of American psychology, societal pressure was such that earning agraduate-level education, or any academic appointment, was exceedingly difficult for women, no matter how capable. Still, one woman, Mary Calkins (1863–1930), so impressed William James that he allowed her into his classes, although Harvard would not allow her to enroll formally (nor would Harvard award her a Ph. D., for which she had met all academic requirements). Mary Calkins went on to do significant experimental work on human learning and memory and, in 1905, was the first woman elected president of the American Psychological Association (Madigan & O'Hara, 1992). Christine Ladd-Franklin (1847–1930) did receive a Ph.D., but not until 40 years after it was earned and Johns Hopkins University lifted its ban on awarding advanced degrees to women. In the interim, she authored an influential theory on how humans perceive color.

Behaviorism

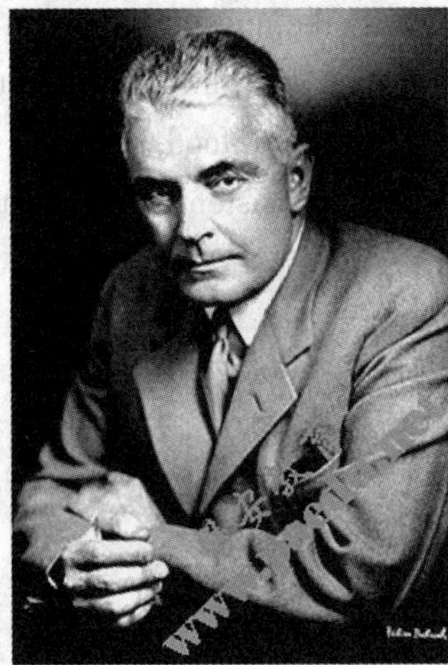

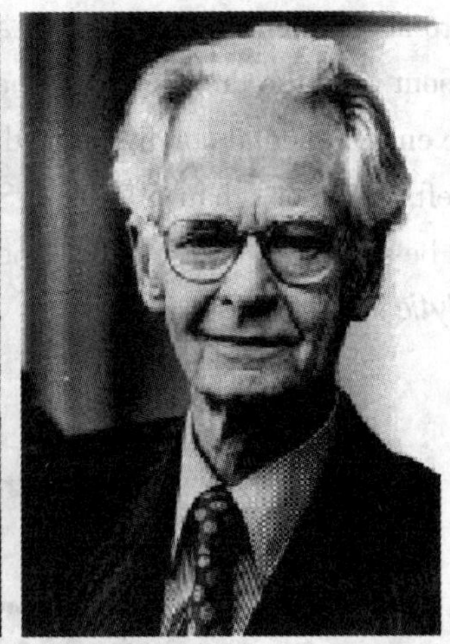

While John B. Watson (1878–1958)　　B. F. Skinner (1904–1990)

While John B. Watson (1878–1958) was a student at Furman University, his mother died, thus relieving one of the pressures he felt to enter the ministry. He enrolled instead as a graduate student in psychology at the University of Chicago. As an undergraduate, he had read about the new science of psychology, and he thought Chicago, where many leading functionalists were, would be the best place to study. However, he was soon disappointed. It turned out he had little sympathy or talent for attempts to study mental processes with scientific methods. He was not very good at giving introspective reports and failed to see how they could be useful. Even so, he stayed on at the university as a psychology major, studying the behavior of animals.

With his new Ph. D. in hand, Watson went to Johns Hopkins University, where, almost single-handedly, he changed both the focus and the definition of psychology. Watson argued that if psychology was to become a mature, productive science, it had to give up the preoccupation with consciousness and mental life that characterized functionalism and concentrate instead on events that can be observed and measured. He felt psychology should give up the study of the mind and study behavior. The new approach became known as behaviorism.

Neither Watson nor the behaviorists who followed him claimed that people do not think or have ideas. What Watson did say was that such processes were not the proper subjects of scientific investigation. After all, no one else can share the thoughts or feelings of the next person. Watson argued that the study of psychology should leave private, mental events to the philosophers and theologians and instead make psychology as rigorously scientific as possible.

Watson once referred to behaviorism as common sense grown articulate. Behaviorism is a study of what people do.

No one has epitomized the behaviorist approach to psychology more than B.F. Skinner (1904–1990). Skinner took Watson's ideas and spent a long and productive career in psychology trying to demonstrate that the behaviors of organisms can be predicted and controlled by studying relationships between their observable responses and the circumstances under which those responses occur. What mattered for Skinner is how behaviors are modified by events in the environment. Behaviorists did not address the question of why a rat turns left in a maze by talking about what the rat wanted or what the rat was thinking at the time. Rather, they tried to specify the environmental conditions (the presence of food, perhaps) under which a rat is likely to turn left. For more than 50 years, Skinner consistently held to the argument that psychology should be defined as the science of behavior.

Psychoanalytic Psychology

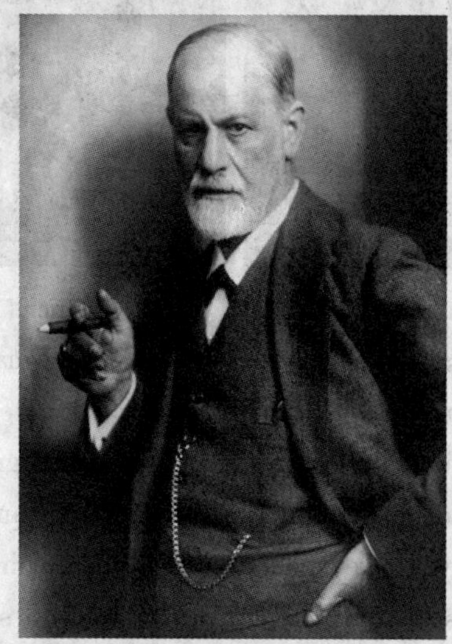

Sigmund Freud (1856–1939)

Sigmund Freud, the father of psychoanalysis, was a physiologist, medical doctor, psychologist and influential thinker of the early twentieth century. Working initially in close collaboration with Joseph Breuer, Freud elaborated the theory that the mind is a complex energy-system, the structural investigation of which is the proper province of psychology. He articulated and refined the concepts of the unconscious, infantile sexuality and repression, and he proposed a tripartite account of the mind's structure — all as part of a radically new conceptual and therapeutic frame of reference for the understanding of human psychological development and the treatment of abnormal mental conditions. Notwithstanding the multiple manifestations of psychoanalysis as it exists today, it can in almost all fundamental respects be traced directly back to Freud's original work.

Freud's innovative treatment of human actions, dreams, and indeed of cultural artifacts as invariably possessing implicit symbolic significance has proven to be extraordinarily fruitful, and has had massive implications for a wide variety of fields including psychology, anthropology, semiotics, and artistic creativity and appreciation. However, Freud's most important and frequently re-iterated claim, that with psychoanalysis he had invented a successful science of the mind, remains the subject of much critical debate and controversy. It is famous for the ideas and theory from him: The Theory of the Unconscious. Infantile Sexuality, Neuroses and The Structure of the Mind and Psychoanalysis as a Therapy.

Critical Evaluation of Freud Early in the twentieth century, Sigmund Freud (1856–1939), a practicing physician in Vienna, became intrigued with what were then called "nervous disorders". He was struck by how little was known about these disorders and, as a result, he chose to specialize in identifying and treating "nervous disorders", a discipline now called psychiatry.

Freud was not a laboratory scientist. Most of his insights about the mind came from his careful observations of his patients and himself. Freud's works were particularly perplexing to the behaviorists. Just as they were arguing against a psychology that concerned itself with consciousness, here came Freud declaring that we are often subject to forces of which we are not aware. Our feelings, actions, and thoughts (A, B, and C) are often under the influence of the unconscious mind, wrote Freud, and many of our behaviors are expressions of instinctive strivings. Freud's views were clearly at odds with Watson's. We call the approach that traces its origin to Sigmund Freud and that emphasizes innate strivings and the unconscious mind psychoanalytic psychology. Psychoanalytic psychology can be viewed as the beginning of modern clinical psychology.

Humanistic Psychology

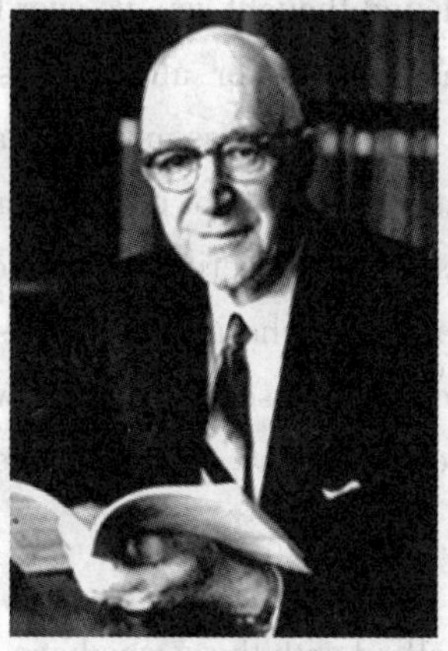

Carl Rogers (1902–1987)

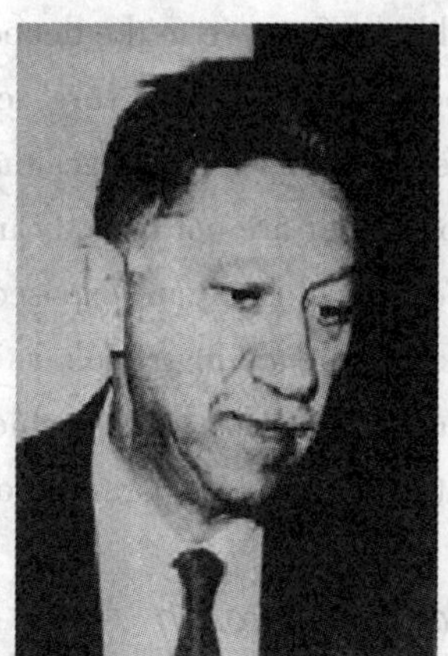

Abraham Maslow (1908–1970)

In many respects, the approach we call humanistic psychology arose as a reaction against behaviorism and psychoanalysis. The leaders of this approach were Carl Rogers (1902–1987) and Abraham Maslow (1908–1970). Humanistic psychology takes the position that the individual, or the self, should be the central concern of psychology. If psychologists concern themselves only with stimuli in the environment and observable responses to those stimuli, they leave the person out of the middle; that's dehumanizing.

Such matters as caring, intention, concern, will, love, and hate are real phenomena and worthy of scientific investigation whether they can be directly observed or not. Attempts to understand people without considering such processes are doomed. To the humanistic psychologists, the Freudian reliance on instincts was too controlling. Our biology: not withstanding, we are — or can be — in control of our destinies. Rogers, Maslow, and their intellectual heirs emphasized the possibility of personal growth and achievement. This approach led Rogers to develop a system of psychotherapy, and Maslow to develop theory of human motivation.

Contemporary Approaches to Psychology

Psychology has come a long way since those few students gathered around Wilhelm Wundt in his laboratory at Leipzig back in the late 1800s. There are more than 500,000 psychologists at work today. The American Psychological Association(APA) claims more than 159,000 members and list over 50 divisions areas of specialization to which its members belong.

Here we review some of the more common perspectives or points of view that guide psychologists in their work. Some have a history dating back to psychology's early days, while some are much more contemporary in origin.

The Biological Approach

Underlying all of our thoughts, feelings, and behaviors is a living biological organism, filled with tissue, fibers, nerves, and chemicals. Psychologists who take a biological perspective seek to explain psychological functioning in terms of genetics and the operation of the nervous system, the brain in particular. Their argument is that, ultimately, every single thing you do, from the simplest blink of an eye to the deepest, most profound thought you've ever had, can be explained by biochemistry. To be sure, experience may modify or alter one's biological structure. Must there not be some changes that take place in our brains as memories are formed? Even most types of cancer are not directly inherited. That is, they do not come from our genes, but from substances to which we are exposed. Psychologists who subscribe to a biological point of view might look at violence in schools as a reflection of some inherited predisposition, some hormonal imbalance, or, perhaps, some problem with the activity of a section of the lower brain — a section deep in the center of the brain known to be involved in raw, primitive emotions, such as fear and rage.

The Evolutionary Approach

Yes, psychologists with this point of view are closely allied with those who have a biological perspective. However, they take a broader, long - range view of human and animal behaviors. Although this tradition can trace its roots to Darwin, it is one of the newer perspectives in psychology. Here, the argument is that we should, explain behaviors and mental processes in terms of how they promote the species' survival and help members of the species adapt to their environments. It is something of an oversimplification, but the point is that we do what we do in order to pass our genes along to those who will survive us. We help others on the chance that they will help us later or that they will assist our offspring if they should need help. An evolutionary approach may suggest that members of the human race are becoming more aggressive (even violent), because in the long run, more aggressive behaviors are adaptive.

The Psychodynamic, or Psychoanalytic Approach

As you might have guessed, this approach is one of psychology's oldest, originating with Sigmund Freud and his students. Psychoanalysis as Freud practiced it is not as common today as it was 50 years ago, but many psychologists approach their subject matter with many Freudian notions in mind. What are some of the basic premises of this approach today? Much of one's behavior as an adult has its roots or foundation in early childhood experiences. Behaviors and mental processes often reflect an interaction, or downright conflict, among unconscious urges, drives, instincts, and the perceptions of societal pressures. As an adolescent, one's body and hormones provide a message ("having sex is a good thing") while parents and society are telling them something else ("sex is dirty, bad, and sinful"). School violence might be at least partially explained interns of inadequate nurturing in young childhood and feelings of isolation turned outward.

The Behavioral Approach

John B. Watson first brought behaviorism to psychology and B. F. Skinner championed it. Their approach to psychology no longer dominates (as it did from, roughly, 1920 to 1970), but focusing one's study on observable behavior is still a popular point of view. A basic premise of this perspective is that who we are, what we do, think, and feel is the result of our unique experiences in the world. Yes, we maybe born with certain inherited predispositions, but to try to explain what we do in terms of evolution or biology or any sort of inner consciousness is silly. We do not need "theories of personality"; we need only a better understanding of learning. If you want people to stop littering, don't try to make them feel guilty or threaten them, but reinforce their appropriate behaviors. Behavior - based psychotherapy takes the position that if one can change unfortunate behaviors, unpleasant feelings and disruptive thoughts will change as well. On the other hand, people, even high school students, can learn to react to upsetting events in their lives with aggression, horrific, openly violent, aggression.

The Cognitive Approach

We have seen that cognitions include such mental contents as ideas, beliefs, knowledge, and understanding. Those psychologists who favor a cognitive approach argue that the focus of our attention should be on how an organism processes information about itself and the world in which it lives. Just what do we believe? Where did these beliefs come from? Why are we able to remember some things, yet forget others? How are perceptions turned into memories? How do existing memories affect what we perceive? How do we make decisions? How do we solve problems? Are there better ways to make decisions or to solve problems? How do humans acquire their language, and once acquired, how do we produce language utterances in order to communicate with others? Why do French children acquire their language so easily, while I struggle so to learn it? What is intelligence? Are there different ways to be intelligent ? Might people become depressed because they believe things that are not true? Might young high school boys turn to violence if they come to believe that no one likes them and that there is no other way to gain the attention of others? Now that's quite a list of questions, and it only scratches the surface of the sorts of issues that cognitive psychologists pursue. As a subfield of psychology, cognitive is one of the fastest growing.

The Cross-Cultural Approach

If psychologists understood all there was to know about the affects, behaviors, and cognitions of young, white, middle-class, American males, they would know a lot — surely a lot more than they know now. However, wouldn't we still have to ask: But what about females? What about the elderly? What about the poor? What about African-Americans or Cuban-Americans? What about Mexicans or Australians-Germans? Do we have any reason to believe that what is true of young, middle-class American males is also true of elderly, poor, Jordanian women?

Even very basic psychological issues, such as what an individual finds reinforcing or what motivates an individual to action, vary enormously from culture to culture. How East Asians and Americans perceive and account for cause-and-effect relationships maybe significantly different. How members of different cultures define mental illness and the treatment/therapy options that are available are significantly different from one culture to another. Please understand: Psychologists have always been aware of cultural differences. It has only been recently, however, that so many others have recognized the value of taking a cross-cultural perspective to the study of psychology.

An Emerging Approach: Positive Psychology

Only recently have two psychologists, Martin Seligman and Mihaly Csikszentmihayi introduced an approach to psychology that is qualitatively quite different from those we've mentioned so far. They, and a growing group of colleagues, call their new perspective "positive psychology". On the surface, the approach seems simple. For too long, psychologists followed the medical model (or perspective) of flocking to fix that which is wrong. Instead of a focus on stress and mental illness, we should focus on mental health. Instead of trying to understand depression, we seek an understanding of happiness. What leads to well-being, to enjoyment, to individuals and communities that thrive? Positive psychology asks about the kinds of families who produce children who flourish, the kinds of work situations that lead to productivity and worker satisfaction. Seligman says that there are three pillars to positive psychology, "First, the study of subjective well-being-life satisfaction and contentment when about the past; happiness, joy, and exuberance when about the present; and optimism, faith and hope when about the future ... The second pillar is the study of positive individual traits — intimacy, integrity, leadership, altruism, vocation and wisdom, for example. Third, the study of positive institutions." Those who are comfortable with a positive approach to psychology would not say that we should ignore the causes of violence in public schools. They would only argue that we spend equal effort, time, and money investigating why so many school youngsters are not violent and contribute to their school environments in positive and healthy ways.

This is, no doubt, quite enough for now. You get the point: There are many ways to approach the scientific study of behavior and mental processes. No one way is best. And few psychologists adhere to only one perspective. Most psychologists understand the benefits that each of these approaches can bring to our understanding. You shall encounter these approaches as you continue your study of psychology.

What is Health Psychology?

Health psychology is a recent development within psychology. Pitts and Phillips (1991) trace this development back to 1978/1979 with the setting up of Health Psychology section of the American Psychological Association (APA). Subsequently the British Psychological Association (BPA) set up their own Health Psychology section in 1986. The emergence of health psychology, can be understood in terms of what it was a response to and critique of, namely the biomedical model. Broome and Lewelyn (1995) propose the following factors may have been contributing factors in awakening interest in health psychology.

Identification of epidemiological and social factors that relate certain behaviors to increased risks of serious disease. (eg, smoking, alcohol/drug misuse etc.)

An increase in chronic disease as a proportion of total illness suffered.

Escalating costs of health care, and the need to contain demand for services.

A growing public awareness of complementary/holistic methods of treatment, and the desire for self-care and self-control methods of treatment.

The growth in psychological research and effective psychological therapy.

Significant developments in psychosomatic research, leading to the identification of psychosocial factors in the vulnerability to and maintenance of health problems.

Dissatisfaction with medical care and an increasing awareness of iatrogenic problems.

Ogden (1996) suggests that the emergence of health psychology can be viewed as an evolutionary phenomenon that developed over the twentieth century. Namely the following were benchmarks in this process.

Psychosomatic Medicine

This challenged the medical model's assumption that only organic changes in (or to) the body were responsible for disease and illness. Freud described the term "hysterical paralysis", whereby patients would develop paralysis of the limbs, in the absence of any organic cause. Freud argued this was the result of the individual's state of mind.

Behavioral Health

Behavioral health was concerned with the maintenance of health and the prevention of disease. Early attempts of health education to change behavior and lifestyle, can be seen as a challenge to the hegemony over health matters created by the medical professional.

Behavioral Medicine

This can be described as a combination of therapies to change behavior that resulted in improved health (eg, behavior modification, person centred counselling). The implication being that psychological/behavioral dysfunction could result in exacerbated health problems. This was not just the domain of psychiatry, but other disciplines such as cardiology acknowledged the importance of psychological/behavioral factors in the treatment of disease.

The Biomedical Model

It is argued that the biomedical model has been dominant in shaping our understanding of andattitude towards health and illness. The biomedical model is premised upon the assumption that mind and body are separate from each other (Cartesian Dualism). McClelland (1985) describes the biomedical model as a mechanistic model where the body is treated like a machine, which one can repair or replace with new parts. Questions from the biomedical model is as following.

What causes illness? Disease comes from within or from outside the body. Disease invades the body and causes physical changes. Diseases are caused by a number of factors such as bacteria, viruses, chemical imbalance, genetic predisposition, etc.

Who is responsible for illness? Because diseases are seen as arising from biological changes, individuals are not generally seen as being responsible for their condition. They are generally seen as victims of the disease they are suffering from.

How should illness be treated? Disease is generally treated by vaccination, surgery, chemotherapy and radiotherapy.

Who is responsible for treatment? The medical profession.

What is the relationship between health and illness? Health and illness are quite separate. You are either ill or you are not.

What is the relationship between mind and body? Mind and body function separately from each other. Mind consists of abstract entities such as feelings and thoughts. The body is made up of material properties such as skin, tissues, and organs. Changes in physical matter are regarded as independent of changes in the state of one's "psychological" make up.

What is the role of psychology in health and illness? Illness may have psychological consequences, but not psychological causes.

The biomedical model of illness and healing focuses on purely biological factors, and excludes psychological, environmental, and social influences. This is considered to be the dominant, modern way for health care professionals to diagnose and treat a condition in most Western countries. Most health care professionals do not first ask for a psychological or social history of a patient; instead, they tend to analyze and look for biophysical or genetic malfunctions. The focus is on objective laboratory tests rather than the subjective feelings or history of the patient.

According to this model, good health is the freedom from pain, disease, or defect. It focuses on physical processes that affect health, such as the biochemistry, physiology, and pathology of a condition. It does not account for social or psychological factors that could have a role in the illness. In this model, each illness has one underlying cause, and once that cause is removed, the patient will be healthy again.

Biopsychosocial Model

In 1977, a psychiatrist called George Engel proposed the biopsychosocial model as a challenge to the predominant medical model. His intention was to provide a framework whereby biological, psychological and sociological factors could be integrated. Essentially the biopsychosocial model is based upon systems theory, which proposes that any change with the "system" will result in reciprocal changes taking place in other parts of the system. For example if a person experiences organic pain, this will result in the person becoming more anxious, changes in health beliefs, and changes in social interaction. This model has been widely accepted and welcomed by professions allied to medicine, who have to care for the "whole person" and by social scientists as it highlighted the importance of social factors in health and disease.

Bio	Psycho	Social
Viruses	Behavior	Class
Bacteria	Beliefs	Economics
Chemical changes	Stress & coping	Ethnicity
Trauma	Pain	Politics
Genetics	Anxiety	Social support
	Personality	

Figure 1 The biopsychosocial model

Questions from the Biopsychosocial Model

What causes illness? Illness is caused by a number of interconnecting variables. It is not usually caused by one single entity. The biopsychosocial model (Engel 1977) presents an integrated model of causes, whereby the "bio" related to factors including bacteria, viruses, chemical changes etc. The "psycho" relates to aspects such as cognitions (beliefs/perceptions), affections (fears, attitudes) and behaviors (eg, smoking, exercise, diet etc.). The "social" relates to social norms of behavior (eg, cultural aspects of health and illness) and to relationships (eg, social support available) and larger macro socio - economic factors (eg, whether one is in a poor or rich nation etc.)

Who is responsible for illness? Because there are a number of interconnecting factors causing ill health. An individual can no longer be regarded as a passive victim. There is therefore a responsibility placed on the individual to adopt behaviors that are less risky in terms of illness and disease.

How should illness be treated? The whole person should be treated. Attention should not be directed solely at the physical changes.

Who is responsible for treatment? Because the whole person is treated the individual is partly responsible for their treatment. They must take responsibility to take medication, adopt healthier lifestyle changes etc.

What is the relationship between health and illness? Health and illness are not qualitatively different. They are not two states; rather they are part of a dynamic continuum.

What is the relationship between mind and body? The shift towards an holistic approach suggests that mind and body interact. Debate surrounds the nature of the relationship between mind and body. One position states that mind and body are essentially separate, but interact and influence each other. The other position states that mind and body are indivisible, and are part of each other.

What is the role of psychology in health and illness? Illness has psychological consequences, but also it may have psychological causes.

Proponents of the biopsychosocial model argue that the biomedical model alone does not take into account all of the factors that have an impact on a patient's health. Biological issues, as well as psychological factors such as a patient's mood, intelligence, memory, and perceptions are all considered when making a diagnosis. The biomedical approach may not, for example, take into account the role sociological factors like family, social class, or a patient's environment may have on causing a health condition, and thus offer little insight into how illness may be prevented. A patient who complains of symptoms that have no obvious objective cause might also be dismissed as not being ill, despite the very real affect those symptoms may have on the patient's daily life.

Many scholars in disability studies describe a medical model of disability that is part of the general biomedical approach. In this model, disability is an entirely physical occurrence, and being disabled is a negative that can only be made better if the disability is cured and the person is made "normal". Many disability rights advocates reject this, and promote a social model in which disability is a difference — neither a good nor bad trait. Proponents of the social model see disability as a cultural construct. They point out that how a person experiences his or her disability can vary based on environmental and societal changes, and that someone who is considered disabled can often be healthy and prosperous without the intervention of a professional or the disability being cured.

Counseling is another field that often uses a more holistic approach to healing. Proponents of this framework note that, in the biomedical model, a patient looks to an expert for a specific diagnosis and treatment. Many counselors often try not to label patients with a specific condition, and instead help them recognize their strengths and build on their positive traits. The relationship is far more collaborative than in the biomedical model where a health care professional instructs a patient to follow medical orders so he or she can be cured.

Ethics in Psychological Research

The goals of science are more often than not, noble: finding a cure for cancer, developing programs to help disadvantaged children in school, or finding a way to effectively treat schizophrenia, for example. However, does having a noble goal justify any research practice? Are there ethical boundaries that should not be crossed in the quest for scientific knowledge and practical applications of that knowledge? As you continue reading, you will find the answer to be a resounding "yes". Researchers in psychology must adhere to a strict code of ethics when conducting research. These ethical codes are designed research subjects from potentially harmful experiments and ensure the well-being of the subjects.

Psychology has something of a unique problem with regard to ethics. To be sure, ethical matters are important in the application of psychological knowledge, be it in diagnosis, therapy, counseling, or training. But in psychology, concerns about ethics are crucial in the gathering of information. After all, the objects of psychological research are living organisms. Their physical and psychological welfare must be protected as their behaviors and mental processes are being investigated.

Psychologists have long been concerned with the ethical implications of their work. Since 1953, the American Psychological Association has regularly revised *Ethical Principles of Psychologists* for practitioners and researchers (APA, 1992, 2001). In fact, concern over how humans are treated in research predates the APA's involvement. Concern over how subjects in experiments are treated can be traced back to the Nuremberg Code developed after the Nuremberg war-crime trials that followed World War II. During the war, the Nazis conducted many medical "experiments" on unwilling inmates in concentration and death camps. For example, research was conducted to find the best way to sterilize "inferior races" through surgery done without anesthetic. Josef Mengle conducted a series of sadistic experiments using twin children as subjects. Once the news of these research abuses came to light, the Nuremberg code was put into place. The code of ethics eventually adopted by the APA and other professional organizations closely followed the guidelines set down in the Nuremberg Code.

Making Sense Out of Psychology Research

Psychological research can produce results that are fascinating to consider and sometimes difficult to understand. A few traps should be avoided as you read about the research in the remainder of this book. Let's take a look at three such traps.

That Can't Be Right; I Would Never Do That

Imagine you are in class and your professor is lecturing on helping behavior. He tells you about the "bystander effect" that involves less help given to a person in need when many, as opposed to few, bystanders are present. He tells you that when there are many bystanders, individuals tend not to help. You are sitting there thinking to yourself, "That's not right. I remember I helped once when there were loads of bystanders around!" Does your experience mean that the research on the bystander effect is invalid? No. Here's why.

When you read about research, or when your professor talks about it in class, keep in mind that the differences we are talking about are average differences across groups and not individual behaviors within a group. For example, let's say you run a bystander-helping experiment with two groups. In Group One, you approach a person walking alone and drop some papers in front of him or her. In Group Two, you approach a person walking near five others and do the same thing. Count the number of people who help you pick up the papers. Let's say in Group One, 80 percent (eight out of ten) stop and help and in Group Two, only 30 percent (three out of ten) stop and help. You conclude that helping is more likely to occur when there is only one bystander than if there are six. Notice, however, that not all participants in Group One helped and not all participants in Group Two failed to help. So, it is entirely possible that for you the bystander effect doesn't apply all the time. But on average, we would still expect more people to help if they were the only bystander as opposed to being with several other bystanders.

The Hindsight Bias

Another trap to avoid when considering the results of psychological research is the hindsight bias, also known as the "I knew it all along" effect. Sometimes the results from psychological research might seem so obvious that you say to yourself, "Why did they bother doing an experiment on that? I knew that all along." This is a strong tendency, mainly because psychology deals with topics and issues with which we are all familiar. However, keep this fact in mind: If a person is told how a study came out, the results might not seem surprising. However, if the person is told how an experiment was conducted and then asked to predict how it came out, the results can be predicted no better than a guess. You can demonstrate this for yourself using ten friends. Give half of them the following statement:

"Psychological research has shown that the old adage 'birds of a feather flock together' is true. Do you agree or disagree with this statement?"

Give the other half the following statement:

"Psychological research has shown that the old adage 'opposites attract' is true. Do you agree or disagree with this statement?"

Most of your friends in each group will probably agree with the statement given, even though they diametrically oppose each other.

Avoiding Circular Explanations

As noted, the goal of the science of psychology is to provide explanations for behavior such as why people fail to help when bystanders are present or why people commit suicide. After years of research in psychology, psychologists have at least partial explanations for these and other psychological events. However, sometimes when an explanation is offered, it is not a true explanation at all. Rather, what is offered is a circular explanation (also known as a pseudoexplanation). A circular explanation does nothing more than provide a new label for some observed behavior. For example, Sigmund Freud gave some ideas about why a person might commit suicide. Freud proposed that much of behavior is instinctive. He proposed that there are two major instincts: the life instinct and the death instinct. The life instinct impels us toward self-preserving behaviors, such as eating and drinking. On the other hand, the death instincts cause us to engage in self-destructive behaviors like smoking and suicide. So, Freud would say that suicide is caused by an activation of the death instinct.

Although instincts were a popular "explanatory" concept in the nineteenth and early twentieth centuries, they are not true explanations. Rather, they are circular. Let's see why. The death instinct is used to explain suicide. So far, so good. But something is a miss: when we ask the question of how we know that there is a death instinct, suicide is used to verify the existence of the death instinct. Whenever a situation arises in which the behavior that you are trying to explain is used as evidence for the existence of the underlying explanation, the result is a circular explanation. A similar relationship exists with concepts like explaining hallucinations with a label like schizophrenia. Why do people hallucinate? They are schizophrenic. How do you know the person is schizophrenic? Because they hallucinate. Round and round we go.

To avoid the trap of circular explanations, independent operational definitions for the explanatory concept and the behavior being explained are needed. For example, we could explain hallucinations by postulating that an overabundance of a certain brain chemical triggers hallucinations. We could measure the concentration of this chemical independently from the frequency or seriousness of hallucinations. If we show that increases in the chemical are associated with increased hallucinations, then we have a true explanation for hallucinations that does not merely reliable the behavior we are trying to explain.

Chapter 2 Research Methods in Psychology

Psychology is, like any science, a branch of knowledge that deals with a body of facts systematically arranged and shows the operation of general laws.

In all sciences, including psychology, a special procedure, the scientific method, must be used to collect data to answer a question or to solve a problem. The scientific method not only answers the question at hand but also is used to construct scientific theories. A theory is systematically organized knowledge applicable in a wide variety of circumstances. (The amount of information available in any science is too vast to be useful unless it is organized through the use of theories.) Theories are also used to predict events or to answer questions in a specific scientific discipline. In psychology, theories are used to organize and predict behavior and mental processes. The findings of a particular study may support or lead to the alteration of a theory. While the scientific method doesn't provide a step - by - step recipe for dealing with specific circumstances, it does provide general guidelines for the following procedures in any scientific data collection, research path show as following(Figure 2.1):

· Formulation of the problem;
· Design of the study;
· Collection of data;
· Analysis of data;
· Conclusions drawn from data.

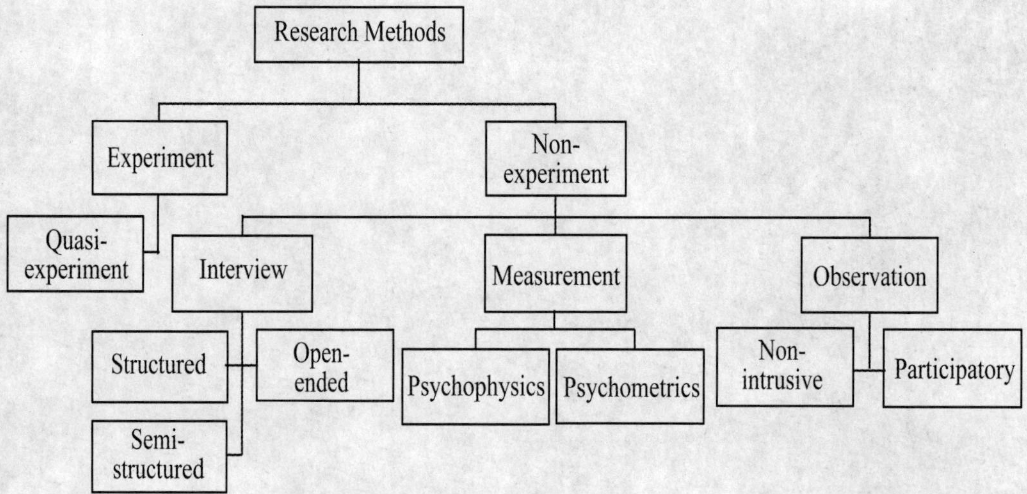

Figure 2.1 Research path in Psychology

The description of a study, its procedures, and its conclusions is frequently published as an article in a scientific journal. Careful attention to following the scientific method allows a second investigator to replicate or refute the findings of a study. For ease of replication, the variables (items under consideration in a study that can change or vary during the course of the study) in a study are defined in terms of observable operations called operational definitions.

Research psychology encompasses the study of behavior for use in academic settings, and contains numerous areas. It contains the areas of abnormal psychology, biological psychology, cognitive psychology, comparative psychology, developmental psychology, personality psychology, social psychology and others. All branches of psychology can have a research component to them. Research psychology is contrasted with applied psychology.

Research in psychology is conducted in broad accord with the standards of the scientific method, encompassing both qualitative ethological and quantitative statistical modalities to generate and evaluate explanatory hypotheses with regard to psychological phenomena. Where research ethics and the state of development in a given research domain permits, investigation may be pursued by experimental protocols. Psychology tends to be eclectic, drawing on scientific knowledge from other fields to help explain and understand psychological phenomena. Qualitative psychological research utilizes a broad spectrum of observational methods, including action research, ethography, exploratory statistics, structured interviews, and participant observation, to enable the gathering of rich information unattainable by classical experimentation. Research in humanistic psychology is more typically pursued by ethnographic, historical, and historiographic methods.

The testing of different aspects of psychological function is a significant area of contemporary psychology. Psychometric and statistical methods predominate, including various well-known standardized tests as well as those created as the situation or experiment requires.

Academic psychologists may focus purely on research and psychological theory, aiming to further psychological understanding in a particular area, while other psychologists may work in applied psychology to deploy such knowledge for immediate and practical benefit. However, these approaches are not mutually exclusive and most psychologists will be involved in both researching and applying psychology at some point during their career. Clinical psychology, among many of the various disciplines of psychology, aims at developing in practicing psychologists knowledge of and experience with research and experimental methods which they will continue to build up as well as employ as they treat individuals with psychological issues or use psychology to help others.

When an area of interest requires specific training and specialist knowledge, especially in applied areas, psychological associations normally establish a governing body to manage training requirements. Similarly, requirements may be laid down for university degrees in psychology, so that students acquire an adequate knowledge in a number of areas. Additionally, areas of practical psychology, where psychologists offer treatment to others, may require that psychologists be licensed by government regulatory bodies as well.

Quantitative psychology involves the application of statistical analysis to psychological research, and the development of novel statistical approaches for measuring and explaining human behavior. It is a young field (only recently have Ph.D. programs in quantitative psychology been formed), and it is loosely comprised of the subfields psychometrics and mathematical psychology.

Psychometrics is the field of psychology concerned with the theory and technique of psychological measurement, which includes the measurement of knowledge, abilities, attitudes, interests, achievement in particular degree or course, and personality traits. Measurement of these unobservable phenomena is difficult, and much of the research and accumulated knowledge in this discipline has been developed in an attempt to properly define and quantify such phenomena. Psychometric research typically involves two major research tasks, namely: the construction of instruments and procedures for measurement and the development and refinement of theoretical approaches to measurement.

Descriptive/Correlational Research

Any scientific process begins with description, based on observation, of an event or events, from which theories may later be developed to explain the observations. In psychology, techniques used to describe behavior include case studies, surveys, naturalistic observation, and psychological tests.

Case Studies

A case study is a method of obtaining information from the detailed observation of an individual or individuals. Much information about behavior and mental processes has been obtained through such studies of individual clinical cases. (Sigmund Freud, for example, formulated psychoanalytic theory after many years of treating and studying patients with emotional problems.) Although valuable information about certain types of problems may be obtained by this method, the procedure is time consuming, and it is difficult to obtain data from a broad sampling of people.

Case studies are in - depth investigations of a single person, group, event or community. Typically data are gathered from a variety of sources and by using several different methods (eg, observations & interviews). The case study research method originated in clinical medicine (the case history, ie, the patient's personal history — idiographic method).

The case study method often involves simply observing what happens to, or reconstructing "the case history" of a single participant or group of individuals (such as a school class or a specific social group), ie, the idiographic approach. Case studies allow a researcher to investigate a topic in far more detail than might be possible if they were trying to deal with a large number of research participants (nomothetic approach) with the aim of "averaging".

The case study is not itself a research method, but researchers select methods of data collection and analysis that will generate material suitable for case studies such as qualitative techniques (semi - structured interviews, participant observation, diaries), personal notes (eg, letters, photographs, notes) or official document (eg, case notes, clinical notes, appraisal reports). The data collected can be analyzed using different theories (eg, grounded theory, interpretative phenomenological analysis, text interpretation (eg, thematic coding) etc. All the approaches mentioned here use preconceived categories in the analysis and they are ideographic in their approach, ie, they focus on the individual case without reference to a comparison group.

Case studies are widely used in psychology and amongst the best known were the ones carried out by Sigmund Freud. He conducted very detailed investigations into the private lives of his patients in an attempt to both understand and help them overcome their illnesses. Freud's most famous case studies include *Little Hans* and *The Rat Man*. Even today case histories are one of the main methods of investigation in abnormal psychology and psychiatry. For students of these disciplines they can give a vivid insight into what those who suffer from mental illness often have to endure.

Case studies are often conducted in clinical medicine and involve collecting and reporting descriptive information about a particular person or specific environment, such as a school. In psychology, case studies are often confined to the study of a particular individual. The information is mainly biographical and relates to events in the individual's past (ie, retrospective), as well as to significant events which are currently occurring in his or her everyday life. In order to produce a fairly detailed and comprehensive profile of the person, the psychologist may use various types of accessible data, such as medical records, employer's reports, school reports or psychological test results. The interview is also an extremely effective procedure for obtaining information about an individual, and it may be used to collect comments from the person's friends, parents, employer, workmates and others who have a good knowledge of the person, as well as to obtain facts from the person him or herself.

This makes it clear that the case study is a method that should only be used by a psychologist, therapist or psychiatrist, ie, someone with a professional qualification. There is an ethical issue of competence. Only someone qualified to diagnose and treat a person can conduct a formal case study relating to atypical (ie, abnormal) behavior or atypical development. The procedure used in a case study means that the researcher provides a description of the behavior. This comes from interviews and other sources, such as observation. The client also reports detail of events from his or her point of view. The researcher then writes up the information from both sources above as the case study, and interprets the information. Interpreting the information means the researcher decides what to include or leave out. A good case study should always make clear which information is factual description and which is inference or the opinion of the researcher.

Strengths of Case Studies

Case studies give psychological researchers the possibility to investigate cases, which could not possibly be engineered in research laboratories. For example, the Money Case Study.

Case studies are often used in exploratory research. They can help us generate new ideas (that might be tested by other methods). They are an important way of illustrating theories and can help show how different aspects of a person's life are related to each other. The method is therefore important for psychologists who adopt a holistic point of view (ie, humanistic psychologists).

Limitations of Case Studies

Because a case study deals with only one person/event/group we can never be sure whether conclusions drawn from this particular case apply elsewhere. The results of the study are not generalizable because we can never know whether the case we have investigated is representative of the wider body of "similar" instances.

Because they are based on the analysis of qualitative (ie, descriptive) data a lot depends on the interpretation the psychologist places on the information she has acquired. This means that there is a lot of scope for observer bias and it could be that the subjective opinions of the psychologist intrude in the assessment of what the data means. For example, Freud has been criticized for producing case studies in which the information was sometimes distorted to fit the particular theories about behavior (eg, *Little Hans*). This is also true of Money's interpretation of the Bruce/Brenda case study when he ignored evidence that went against his theory.

Surveys

In a survey, people from a wide sample are asked questions about the topic of concern. The Kinsey survey on sexual behavior is a well-known example. Surveys can supply useful information, but they have their problems and limitations. For example, the people who respond may not be representative of the population in general, or those polled may be reluctant to respond to questionnaires or to answer them accurately.

Naturalistic Observation

In another approach to gathering information, naturalistic observation, people or animals are observed in their everyday behaviors, and their behaviors of interest are documented. For example, valuable information on wild animals, such as lions, has come from studying them in their natural habitats as opposed to observing them in a zoo because their zoo behavior may be quite different from their natural behavior. Similarly, the behavior of a human in a home environment may differ considerably from that in a laboratory.

Psychological Testing

Many standardized procedures (tests) have been developed to measure specific behaviors or characteristics of organisms. Most of us have been subjected to such tests — for example, the intelligence, aptitude, and achievement tests used to predict behaviors. To be useful, tests must be both reliable and valid.

Correlation

Correlation, a statistical measure of a relationship between two or more variables, gives an indication of how one variable may predict another. The descriptive techniques discussed above permit a statement, in the form of correlations, about that relationship. However, correlation does not imply causation; that is, simply because two events are in some way correlated (related) does not mean that one necessarily causes the other. For example, some test data indicate that boys receive higher math-aptitude scores on college entrance exams than girls, indicating a correlation of gender with mathematical ability. But before concluding that gender determines mathematics aptitude, one must demonstrate that both the boys and the girls in the study have had the same mathematics background. Some studies have shown that girls are discouraged from taking or at least not encouraged to take more than the minimum mathematics requirements. Such discrepancies in mathematical accomplishment may also arise in the home — for example, from a parental belief that a girl does not need much mathematical training to be a good wife and mother.

Experimental Research

If researchers intend to make cause-and-effect statements, they typically use experimental research, which is usually, but not always, conducted in a laboratory. The laboratory environment allows the experimenter to make controlled observations using the steps of the scientific method.

Formulation of the Problem

In formulating the problem in a psychological study, the researcher raises a question about behavior or mental processes. Perhaps the investigator wonders whether certain environmental conditions improve or adversely affect motor performance. The investigator might operationally define the environmental condition of interest as "background music" and the motor performance as "typing speed". Next, the investigator proposes an answer to the research question "What is the relationship between typing speed and background noise?", an answer called a hypothesis. A hypothesis postulates a relationship between two variables, an independent variable (that which the experimenter manipulates — in this case, the background music) and a dependent variable (that which changes as a consequence of manipulation of the independent variable — in this case, the typing speed). The experimenter hypothesizes that "an increase in loudness of background music will produce a decrease in typing speed".

The key features are control over variables, careful measurement, and establishing cause and effect relationships. An experiment is an investigation in which the independent variable is manipulated (or changed) in order to cause a change in the dependent variable.

There are three types of experiments you need to know:

Laboratory / Controlled Experiments

This type of experiment is conducted in a well-controlled environment — not necessarily a laboratory — and therefore accurate measurements are possible. The researcher decides where the experiment will take place, at what time, with which participants, in what circumstances and using a standardised procedure. Participants are randomly allocated to each independent variable group. An example is Milgram's experiment on obedience.

Pro: It is easier to replicate (ie, copy) a laboratory experiment.

Pro: They allow for precise control of extraneous and independent variables.

Pro: They allow cause and effect relationships to be established.

Con: The artificiality of the setting may produce unnatural behavior that does not reflect real life, ie, low ecological validity.

Con: Demand characteristics or experimenter effects may bias the results and become confounding variables.

Field Experiments

Field Experiments are done in the everyday (ie, real life) environment of the participants. The experimenter still manipulates the IV, but in a real-life setting (so cannot really control extraneous variables), eg, Holfing's Hospital Study on Obedience.

Behavior in a field experiment is more likely to reflect life real because of its natural setting, ie, higher ecological validity than a lab experiment.

There is less likelihood of demand characteristics affecting the results, as participants may not know they are being studied.

There is less control over extraneous variables that might bias the results. This in turn makes the experiment harder to replicate.

They are more difficult to replicate compared to lab experiments.

Natural Experiments

Natural Experiments are conducted in the everyday (ie, real life) environment of the participants but here the experimenter has no control over the IV as it occurs naturally in real life, eg, Hodges and Tizard's attachment research (1989) which compared the long term development of children who have been adopted, fostered or returned to their mothers with a control group of children who had spent all their lives in their biological families.

Behavior in a natural experiment is more likely to reflect life real because of it natural setting, ie, very high ecological validity.

There is less likelihood of demand characteristics affecting the results, as participants may not know they are being studied.

It can be used in situations in which it would be ethically unacceptable to manipulate the independent variable.

They may be more expensive and time consuming than lab experiments.

Experiment Definitions

Ecological Validity

The degree to which an investigation represents real-life experiences.

Experimenter Effects

These are the ways that the experimenter can accidentally influence the participant through their appearance or behavior.

Demand Characteristics

The clues in an experiment that lead the participants to think they know what the researcher is looking for (eg, experimenter's body language).

Independent Variable (**IV**)

Variable the experimenter manipulates (ie, changes) – assumed to have a direct effect on the dependent variable.

Dependent Variable (DV)

Variable the experimenter measures.

Extraneous Variables (EV)

All variables, which are not the independent variable, but could affect the results (DV) of the experiment. EVs should be controlled were possible.

Confounding Variables

Variable(s) that have effected the results (DV), apart from the IV. A confounding variable could be an extraneous variable that has not been controlled.

Design of the Study

Once the problem to be investigated has been selected, the experimenter must decide how to conduct the study. Much of the information used in psychology and other sciences has been collected in laboratory situations because they facilitate the use of many controls during data collection. In the background music/typing speed study, for example, all subjects would be taken to a laboratory for testing and would use the same typewriters to take the typing tests. The experimenter would have to decide whether to use two groups of subjects with comparable typing skills and expose one group to a music loudness level different from that used with the other (a between-subjects design) or sequentially expose the same subjects to music of two loudness levels (a within-subjects design). Each procedure has advantages and disadvantages. (Decisions concerning the procedure to use depend on many factors, which are studied in experimental design courses.)

Collection of Data

The experimenter collects data (typing speed at different loudness levels) to test the hypothesis according to the selected experimental design.

Analysis of Data

The data are analyzed by appropriate statistical methods. In this case, mean scores of the two sets of typing speed/loudness level data would be compared to see if differences are significant or could be due to chance.

Conclusions Drawn from the Data

Based on analysis of data, conclusions may be drawn about the hypothesized relationship between the independent and dependent variables. The hypothesis, that "an increase in loudness of background music will produce a decrease in typing speed," may be supported by the data (the increase in loudness of background music — manipulation of the independent variable — did produce a decrease in typing speed — the dependent variable) or may not be supported by the data (the increase in loudness did not produce a decrease in typing speed).

Reporting Results

The process used in and the results obtained from the study are gathered and written. If the study results are of sufficient significance, they may be published in a scientific journal (as mentioned above, allowing the study to be replicated or refuted by another researcher) and may eventually be used quite pragmatically. For example, if a study determines that background music (or perhaps background music of a certain loudness level) improves typing performance, certain employers would be likely to make use of the findings in their businesses. Scientific knowledge in all sciences grows as a result of information collected through the scientific method.

Basic and Applied Research

The goal of basic research in psychology is primarily to describe and understand behavior and mental processes without immediate concern for a practical use. Such research, usually conducted in university settings, is essential to the expansion of scientific knowledge and the development of theories. Applied research uses scientific studies to solve problems of everyday life.

In reality, there is crossover between the two types of research. For example, after conducting basic science experiments to delineate the neural mechanisms associated with Parkinson's disease, the same researcher might then undertake an applied project by continuing the study to find a therapeutic drug that alters the functioning of identified neural mechanisms of the disorder and thereby relieves the symptoms.

Validity

When designing a study you must always keep the validity of your study in the back of your mind. Validity concerns whether the conclusions that you want to draw from your study are appropriate or not. Aspects of your study that might potentially make your study invalid are called threats to validity. Issues of validity are of concern to both experiments and surveys.

Validity is specically tied to the conclusions being drawn from a study. For any given study there are a set of valid conclusions and a set of invalid conclusions that may be drawn. The important question is whether the design of the study allows the conclusions stated by the researcher. Therefore, before designing a study you should explicitly decide what conclusions you wish to make so you can spot potential threats to the validity of your study.

Construct Validity

Construct validity concerns the extent to which the variables in your experiment accurately and exclusively represent the corresponding theoretical constructs. When assessing the construct validity of a variable you should consider both convergent validity and divergent validity. A variable with convergent validity shows relationships with other variables that should be related to the theoretical construct of interest. A variable with divergent validity has no relationships with other variables that are theoretically unrelated to the construct of interest. Manipulations lack construct validity either when they fail to alter the theoretical construct of interest or when outside variables are inadvertently changed along with the construct of interest. Measurements lack construct validity either when changes in the construct of interest fail to cause changes in the measure or when changes in outside variables can cause changes in the measure when the construct of interest is held constant. Here are some questions that you can ask about a study to assess its construct validity.

Do the manipulations applied in the study actually change what they are supposed to?

Is anything influenced by manipulations in the study other than the construct of interest?

Do the measures in the study accurately reflect what they are designed to measure?

Can different responses on measures be caused by anything else other than changes in the construct of interest?

Below are descriptions of some specific threats to construct validity.

Mono-method Bias

Sometimes a study (or an entire field of research) consistently manipulates a variable in a single fashion, or uses a single way to measure a variable. Any single method is necessarily going to contain idiosyncratic elements that are not truly part of the theoretical construct of interest. When you use a single method to examine a variable you cannot separate the theoretical construct of interest from irrelevant characteristics of the method. It is therefore best to demonstrate relationships using multiple ways of manipulating or measuring the constructs of interest.

Hypothesis Guessing

People have a natural tendency to try to figure out what is going on around them. When placed in an study they will try to make some guesses as to what it is about. Their actions will sometimes be influenced by these beliefs, causing them to behave in a way that is unnatural. Sometimes this simply contributes random noise to your data, but other times (such as when people are able to accurately guess your hypotheses) this can systematically affects your results. It is therefore important to keep your hypotheses hidden from your participants, and to try to reduce hypothesis - guessing tendencies in general. One way of accomplishing the latter is to provide reasons (though not necessarily accurate ones) for each task that participants perform. People are less likely to try to come up with their own explanations if you give one to them first. It can also be useful to ask participants afterwards what they thought the study was about. If people seem to be able to regularly guess the purpose of your study then you know you may need to worry about hypothesis-guessing biases.

Administrator Expectations

Studies have shown that the beliefs of research administrators can have profound influences on the data they collect, even when they are making supposedly objective measurements. The responses then reflect the behavior of the researchers instead of the behavior of the participants. The easiest way to prevent this problem is to minimize the role of the administrator in the study. Try to use standardized methods of manipulating and measuring your variables. If your study requires that the administrator be more deeply involved then you should try to use administrators who are unaware of the research hypotheses.

Evaluation Apprehension

People are generally concerned whenever they are being evaluated by someone they perceive to be an authority. They will therefore do their best to present themselves in a way that makes them appear competent and psychologically healthy. You must consider whether your manipulations are inducing a desire in your participants to be perceived favorably in addition to (or instead of) causing changes in the construct of interest. You should also examine your response items to make sure that they are not simply reflecting participants' attempts to create favorable impressions.

Placebo/Hawthorne Effects

The mere presence of an experimental environment can sometimes cause changes in participants. It is well known, for example, that the mere expectation that they are receiving medical care can sometimes cause improvement in people's health, even if they actually receive no medical treatment. This can obscure the effect of any manipulations you wish to perform. When designing your study you should include control groups of people who are placed in similar circumstances.

Order Effects

Sometimes one part of your study can influence the way that people perform in another part. For example, if you have people perform a difficult arithmetic task it might make them feel dejected, causing them to put less effort into their responses on later tasks. You should therefore try to put important tasks, as well as tasks that might be sensitive to order effects, early in your study.

Internal Validity

Internal validity concerns the plausibility of alternative causal explanations for the results of a study. If a study is not attempting to demonstrate any causal relationships then internal validity is not a concern. The first thing that you need to consider when a study proposes a causal relationship is whether the direction of causation is correct. This will not be an issue if the predictor is manipulated but may be difficult to demonstrate when both the predictor and the response variable are measured.

Even when you manipulate your predictor variable you must be concerned with potential confounding variables. A confounding variable is an outside variable (one not examined in your experiment) that covaries with your predictors and could potentially influence your response variable. If a predictor covaries with a confounding variable then you cannot conclude that the predictor causes the response. The confound always provides a possible alternative explanation for your results.

While people assessing internal validity are typically interested in confounding variables that might have produced the observed relationships between variables, it is also possible for a confounding variable to obscure a relationship between two variables. For example, people who know that they are in a more difficult level of a factor may try to work harder than those in an easier level. This confound would reduce the difference between these groups.

Most threats to internal validity can be avoided if you randomly assign participants to the different between-subject conditions in your study. On average every outside variable should be evenly distributed throughout the different conditions of your study, removing most potential threats to validity. To properly randomize the assignment of participants to conditions you must choose a method that makes each participant equally likely to be in each level of your between-subject variable.

It is important that you use the same recruitment procedures for participants in every condition of an experiment. If the different levels of a between - subject manipulation have different requirements then participants recruited for the experiment should all meet the requirements of every condition. Similarly, if different conditions take different amounts of time then all participants should be recruited expecting that they may be in the longest condition. People willing to be in a longer experiment may be different from people who are not.

It is better if you assign the level of your between-subject conditions on a participant-by-participant basis than to entire groups of participants. For example, it is a bad idea for you to assign the first level of a variable to the first 10 participants and the second level to the next 10 participants. This confounds your manipulation with the order of recruitment, and possibly with the time of day the study was conducted. Sometimes you must run people in groups, such as when the manipulation is a film clip seen by participants. If you have multiple participants in each session of your experiment it may not be practical to try to show them each a movie individually. In this case you should randomly determine which groups are exposed to each level of your between-subjects variable. Having multiple sessions for each level (so the conditions are at least somewhat dispersed) can also reduce the potential for a confound.

There are some threats that neither matching nor randomization will be able to prevent. Specifically, if a confound is in some way created by your manipulation then randomization will not help. For example, a manipulation that withholds rewards from some participants may inspire resentment, a potential alternative explanation for your results. Additionally, if the influence of an outside factor would be different for different levels of a predictor (ie, the confound interacts with the predictor variable) its influence will also not be removed by randomization. For example, consider a study trying to determine whether taking school trips to a museum influences school performance. One potential confound is the SES of the student, since wealthier students might be more likely to go to museums on their own. This confound also may interact with the condition, because wealthy students who don't go on school trips may go on their own while wealthy students who do go during school may not go on if your two groups are equally wealthy there will still be differences in the behaviors of the groups.

If you cannot remove the potential influence of a confounding variable through randomization then you will need to include extra measurements or control groups in your design to test for the influence of the potential confound on your response variables.

Here are some questions that you can ask about a study to assess its internal validity.

Is the direction of causality clearly established?

Could the observed relationships have been created by unaccounted outside influences?

Could some outside influence be obscuring the true relationships between the variables?

Is the assignment of participants to between-subjects conditions properly randomized?

Below are descriptions of some specific threats to internal validity.

History

If your study takes place over an extended period of time there is a possibility that some unusual event might take place during the course of your study that might affect your results. In this case you cannot be sure whether you would have obtained the same results in the absence of the event.

Testing

Participants who are asked to fill out a questionnaire or perform a test more than a single time may use their past performance to guide their behavior on later tests. They may remember specific responses and just recall them instead of regenerating their response. If you are specifically investigating memory then this is not a problem, but most often you want the tests to reflect changes caused by some other variable. In this case their experience acts as a confound. To get around this you can design parallel versions of the tests and use a different version at each test session.

Maturation

If your study takes place over an extended period you need to take into account that people grow and change over time. It is possible that any differences that you see over the course of treatment are due to natural development instead of your manipulation. This is especially important to consider when using younger participants.

Regression toward the Mean

If you administer a test to a sample at one point in time you will naturally observe that some people will score high and some will score low. Any form of measurement, however, naturally involves some amount of random error. So if you were to administer the same test again you would observe some differences in the scores, even if there were no actual change. You would also see that those who scored high on the first test will tend to score lower on the second, while those who scored low on the first test will tend to score higher on the second. This is because if a person received a high score, they are more likely to have had random factors working to their benefit. In a sense, they are toward the high end of the possible values they might obtain on the test. If they took the test again they would be more likely to have a lower score. Similarly, people with low scores are more likely to have had random factors working against them, so later tests are likely to provide higher results.

This can be a problem if you put people into different groups based on a pretest score and then you want to observe the effect of a manipulation with a posttest. Even without the influence of any other factors, regression toward the mean will cause the high group to have lower scores and the low group to have higher scores at a posttest. To minimize the influence of this threat you should choose measures with as little random error as possible.

Selection

This is a threat when you have different types of people in different levels of a between-subjects manipulation. In this case you can't be certain whether the effects you observe are caused by the manipulation or the individual differences. Random assignment to conditions can usually remove threats of selection.

Mortality

If you conduct a study that occurs for a long period of time it is common to have a certain percentage of your participants drop out before the study is completed. Sometimes this dropout creates differences between the people in your different conditions.

External Validity

External validity concerns the ability to apply inferences drawn from a study to other populations, environments, and times. The more reliant a study's results are on the specific features present in the original study the less external validity is possessed by the study.

To assess external validity you must first determine the real-life circumstance to which the researcher wants to generalize their conclusions. You then consider what characteristics of the study were important for obtaining the results related to that conclusion. If these characteristics are not likely to be present in the real-life circumstance then you have reason to question the external validity of the results.

External validity is not equally important for all types of studies. It is very important for studies whose aim is to describe the relationships between variables in a particular target population. However, it is much less important for studies whose goal is to test some aspect of a theory. For example, a theory might predict that a particular pair of variables should be related. This relationship should be present in any particular sample your might draw. If you conducted a study and found no relationship this would be evidence against the theory even if the study had low external validity. Even studies testing theories can benefit from having external validity. Externally valid tests of a theory provide more general (and thus stronger) evidence for or against the theory. For example, contradictory findings with low external validity may be dismissed by supporters of the theory as unimportant exceptions. Contradictory findings with high external validity, on the other hand, are much more difficult to ignore.

A study can provide conclusions that may be validly generalized to one population but which do not validly apply to another. For example, a study providing information about shopping preferences may provide valid conclusions for the community in which the study was conducted but might be invalid for understanding the preferences of a different community in another part of the country.

Not all differences between samples and target populations create external validity problems. In order for a difference to be a threat to external validity there must be a reason to suspect that the difference would influence the results of the study.

When conducting your own study the key to establishing external validity is to make the important characteristics of your research environment match those of the real-world situation to which you wish to generalize your findings.

Here are some questions that you can ask about a study to assess its external validity.

Is the purpose of a study to test a theory or to provide a description of a target population?

What differences are there between the people, time, and setting of the study and the target situation?

Could these differences conceivably have influenced the results?

Below are descriptions of some specific threats to external validity.

Unrepresentitive Sample

If the type of people that you select for your study are affected by your treatment differently than would the average person that makes up your target population then the results of your study cannot be properly generalized to the population of interest. This is why it is best to draw a sample that is truly representative of the target population.

Unrepresentative Setting

Similarly, if the environment in which you conduct your study is very different from that to which you would like to generalize your results then your conclusions may not be valid. It is usually more important to consider what is present in your study environment than what is absent. You do not necessarily need to replicate all of the different things that you feel would be present in real life. However, you should be fairly certain that the results you obtained were not caused by some peculiarity of your study environment.

Progress of the Research Methods in Cognitive Psychology

FMRI and PET

Functional magnetic resonance imaging, or FMRI, is a technique for measuring brain activity. It works by detecting the changes in blood oxygenation and flow that occur in response to neural activity — when a brain area is more active it consumes more oxygen and to meet this increased demand blood flow increases to the active area. FMRI can be used to produce activation maps showing which parts of the brain are involved in a particular mental process (Shengyong, 2012).

The cylindrical tube of an MRI scanner houses a very powerful electro-magnet. A typical research scanner (such as the FMRIB Centre scanner) has a field strength of 3 teslas (T), about 50,000 times greater than the Earth's field. The magnetic field inside the scanner affects the magnetic nuclei of atoms. Normally atomic nuclei are randomly oriented but under the influence of a magnetic field the nuclei become aligned with the direction of the field. The stronger the field the greater the degree of alignment. When pointing in the same direction, the tiny magnetic signals from individual nuclei add up coherently resulting in a signal that is large enough to measure. In FMRI it is the magnetic signal from hydrogen nuclei in water (H_2O) that is detected (Andreas, 2012).

The key to MRI is that the signal from hydrogen nuclei varies in strength depending on the surroundings. This provides a means of discriminating between grey matter, white matter and cerebral spinal fluid in structural images of the brain.

The image shown is the result of the simplest kind of FMRI experiment. While lying in the MRI scanner the subject watched a screen which alternated between showing a visual stimulus and being dark every 30 second. Meanwhile the MRI scanner tracked the signal throughout the brain. In brain areas responding to the visual stimulus you would expect the signal to go up and down as the stimulus is turned on and off, albeit blurred slightly by the delay in the blood flow response. The "activity" in a voxel is defined as how closely the time-course of the signal from that voxel matches the expected time-course. Voxels whose signal corresponds tightly are given a high activation score, voxels showing no correlation have a low score and voxels showing the opposite (deactivation) are given a negative score. These can then be translated into activation maps (I. Bojak, 2012).

Physicians use fMRI to assess how risky brain surgery or similar invasive treatment is for a patient and to learn how a normal, diseased or injured brain is functioning. They map the brain with FMRI to identify regions linked to critical functions such as speaking, moving, sensing, or planning. This is useful to plan for surgery and radiation therapy of the brain. Clinicians also use FMRI to anatomically map the brain and detect the effects of tumors, stroke, head and brain injury, or diseases such as Alzheimer's (Keith, 2012).

Clinical use of FMRI still lags behind research use. Patients with brain pathologies are more difficult to scan with FMRI than are young healthy volunteers, the typical research-subject population. Tumors and lesions can change the blood flow in ways not related to neural activity, masking the neural HDR. Drugs such as antihistamines and even caffeine can affect HDR. Some patients may be suffering from disorders such as compulsive lying, which makes certain studies impossible. It is harder for those with clinical problems to stay still for long. Using head restraints or bite bars may injure epileptics who have a seizure inside the scanner; bite bars may also discomfit those with dental prostheses (Aini, 2012 & Ratha, 2010).

Despite these difficulties, FMRI has been used clinically to map functional areas, check left-right hemispherical asymmetry in language and memory regions, check the neural correlates of a seizure, study how the brain recovers partially from a stroke, test how well a drug or behavioral therapy works, detect the onset of Alzheimer's, and note the presence of disorders like depression. Mapping of functional areas and understanding lateralization of language and memory help surgeons avoid removing critical brain regions when they have to operate and remove brain tissue. This is of particular importance in removing tumors and in patients who have intractable temporal lobe epilepsy. Lesioning tumors requires presurgical planning to ensure no functionally useful tissue is removed needlessly. Recovered depressed patients have shown altered FMRI activity in the cerebellum, and this may indicate a tendency to relapse. Pharmacological FMRI, assaying brain activity after drugs are administered, can be used to check how much a drug penetrates the blood-brain barrier and dose vs effect information of the medication(Gary H, 2011).

Recent advances in positron emission tomography (PET) and functional magnetic resonance imaging (FMRI), now routinely applied to the mapping of cognitive systems in the brain, have generated an explosion of activity in numerous research centres around the world. The potential of this new method for assessing brain activation in relation to cognitive tasks has great interest and appeal. There is the hope and indeed the widely held expectation, that these major developments will ultimately add important insights on brain behavior relationships that may not be accomplished using other existing techniques. For cognitive neuropsychologists and cognitive scientists such insights concern the nature of the functional architecture mediating basic abilities like single word comprehension and production, reading single words, identifying objects and face recognition, and recollection of personal or factual events. The question from this perspective is: What has been learned so far by the numerous studies in functional imaging as regards the modular organization of the cognitive system? Does this research qualify or extend the conclusions derived from the analysis of brain - damaged cases with specific functional deficits or the performance of normal individuals? What new directions or theoretical possibilities are suggested by the evidence obtained thus far? Cognitive scientists are markedly divided on the immediate potential of functional imaging as a means of answering these questions. For example, in a recent discussion of the role of phonology in word recognition, Nicole (2011) asks whether functional imaging could possibly shed any light on the controversy in the immediate future.

To what extent, then, can questions regarding the functional organisation of cognitive systems be informed by studies that rely on PET and FMRI ? Are there any clear examples in the literature that would demonstrate the usefulness of brain mapping as an important source of relevant evidence? The book *Human Brain Function* is the outcome of a joint venture between two major centres in functional imaging, and it represents a comprehensive summary of work accomplished in these two laboratories over the last decade. The volume is divided into three sections, the first dealing with general statistical methods and image analysis, while the second summarises empirical work in a variety of domains. The third section looks to the future and speculates on new directions and developments in the field. The purpose of the book is to provide a general synthesis of the available knowledge in functional imaging that encompasses all aspects of the process of constructing are presentation of brain activation from them measurement of regional blood flow. There are formidable technical challenges that must be met in this regard. The dynamic changes in a very large number of correlated intracerebral voxels must be transformed into a meaningful statistical description that includes a spatial representation of the inappropriate location in the brain (Robert, 2012 & Tracy, 2010).

It is clear that just as the methods of PET and FMRI impose novel demands at the level of data analysis, so do they present a unique challenge when we seek to formulate a clear argument or proof in testing a theoretical claim about the cognitive architecture. We cannot simply apply existing methodological principles to the data for an umber of important reasons. Cognitive neuropsychology has relied primarily on the logic of dissociations and double dissociations between elementary tasks to draw inferences about the underlying architecture. Generally, the tasks being compared differ in numerous ways, only a small subset of which are theoretically relevant, so that a variety of constraining facts must accumulate before it is possible to meaningfully interpret a dissociation in performance. For example, repetition of a sequence of digits requires, in addition to the short-term retention of auditory forms, some kind of acoustic segmentation, encoding of word identity, and organization of speech out put, as well as specific executive functions by which the participant mobilises whatever general procedures are needed to carryout the task. A great deal of background observation, much of which is implicit, lies behind any attempt to locate the functional deficit at the relevant point in the cognitive architecture. For claims about the distinction between auditory short-term memory and long-term memory, the majority of cognitive processes involved in serial recall must be ruled out, either explicitly or tacitly, as an account of the patient's failure to repeat a phonological sequence, in order to obtain evidence for the hypothesis under investigation. The dissociation between two tasks, say digit span versus learning 10 words over reiterated trials, is actually situated within a complex of other facts that define the nature of the comparison, limiting it to are stricted part of the phonological system (Jon,2007).

MEG and EEG

Magnetoencephalography (MEG) is a non-invasive technique used to measure magnetic fields generated by small intracellular electrical currents in neurons of the brain. Thus MEG provides direct information about the the dynanamics of evoked and spontaneous neural activity and the location of their sources in the brain.

MEG and EEG are closely related, the latter detecting the electric potentials generated by neural currents instead of the corresponding magnetic fields. However, it turns out that the task of inferring the sites of brain activation is often more straightforward from MEG than from EEG. This is due to the electric and magnetic properties of the tissues in the cranium and also to the fact that MEG is selectively sensitive to currents flowing tangential to the scalp, corresponding to sulcal activations. On the other hand, the interpretation of EEG is often complicated by the simultaneous presense of both sulcal and gyral sources, the latter as exemplified by this special issue on open-source analysis toolboxes, many software solutions exist to suit a variety of experimental goals and level of end-user programming experience, including the option to mix and match toolboxes for different stages of processing. However, a decade ago, few options existed for analyzing magnetoencephalography (MEG) data with noncommercial open-source software, especially for more sophisticated inverse algorithms or with a graphical interface to navigate results (Deng, 2012).

Synchronized neuronal currents induce weak magnetic fields. At 10 femtotesla (fT) for cortical activity and 10^3 fT for the human alpha rhythm, the brain's magnetic field is considerably smaller than the ambient magnetic noise in an urban environment, which is on the order of 10^8 fT. The essential problem of biomagnetism is thus the weakness of the signal relative to the sensitivity of the detectors, and to the competing environmental noise (Roozbeh, 2011).

Electroencephalogram (EEG) is a test used to detect abnormalities related to electrical activity of the brain. This procedure tracks and records brain wave patterns. Small metal discs with thin wires (electrodes) are placed on the scalp, and then send signals to a computer to record the results. Normal electrical activity in the brain makes a recognizable pattern. Through an EEG, doctors can look for abnormal patterns that indicate seizures and other problems.

EEG has several strong points as a tool for exploring brain activity. EEG's can detect changes over milliseconds, which is excellent considering an action potential takes approximately 0.5 - 130 milliseconds to propagate across a single neuron, depending on the type of neuron. Other methods of looking at brain activity, such as PET and FMRI have time resolution between seconds and minutes. EEG measures the brain's electrical activity directly, while other methods record changes in blood flow (eg, SPECT, FMRI) or metabolic activity (eg, PET, NIRS), which are indirect markers of brain electrical activity. EEG can be used simultaneously with FMRI so that high - temporal - resolution data can be recorded at the same time as high - spatial - resolution data, however, since the data derived from each occurs over a different time course, the data sets do not necessarily represent exactly the same brain activity. There are technical difficulties associated with combining these two modalities, including the need to remove the MRI gradient artifact present during MRI acquisition and the ballistocardiographic artifact (resulting from the pulsatile motion of blood and tissue) from the EEG. Furthermore, currents can be induced in moving EEG electrode wires due to the magnetic field of the MRI. EEG can be used simultaneously with NIRS without major technical difficulties. There is no influence of these modalities on each other and a combined measurement can give useful information about electrical activity as well as local hemodynamics (Cathy, 2012).

EEG reflects correlated synaptic activity caused by post - synaptic potentials of cortical neurons. The ionic currents involved in the generation of fast action potentials may not contribute greatly to the averaged field potentials representing the EEG. More specifically, the scalp electrical potentials that produce EEG are generally thought to be caused by the extracellular ionic currents caused by dendritic electrical activity, whereas the fields producing magnetoencephalographic signals are associated with intracellular ionic currents. EEG can be recorded at the same time as MEG so that data from these complementary high - time - resolution techniques can be combined.

The electric current also produces the EEG signal. The MEG (and EEG) signals derive from the net effect of ionic currents flowing in the dendrites of neurons during synaptic transmission. In accordance with Maxwell's equations, any electrical current will produce an orthogonally oriented magnetic field. It is this field which is measured. The net currents can be thought of as electric dipoles, ie, currents with a position, orientation, and magnitude, but no spatial extent. According to the right - hand rule, a current dipole gives rise to a magnetic field that flows around the axis of its vector component.

To generate a signal that is detectable, approximately 50,000 active neurons are needed. Since current dipoles must have similar orientations to generate magnetic fields that reinforce each other, it is often the layer of pyramidal cells, which are situated perpendicular to the cortical surface, that give rise to measurable magnetic fields. Bundles of these neurons that are orientated tangentially to the scalp surface project measurable portions of their magnetic fields outside of the head, and these bundles are typically located in the sulci. Researchers are experimenting with various signal processing methods in the search for methods that detect deep brain (ie, non-cortical) signal, but no clinically useful method is currently available.

It is worth noting that action potentials do not usually produce an observable field, mainly because the currents associated with action potentials flow in opposite directions and the magnetic fields cancel out. However, action fields have been measured from peripheral nerves.

In order to estimate the locations of activated brain areas from the measured data a suitable source model is employed. Many primary sensory responses can be adequately accounted for with a dipole model which relies on the assumption that the extent of the activity is sufficiently small to appear as a point source at a typical measurement distance of at least three centimeters. Single time instant or a whole epoch of data is then employed in the estimation of the locations and timecourses of one or more dipole sources. Since MEG does not provide anatomical information, the locations of the sources are displayed in the anatomical MRI data of the subject or patient, which are coregistered with the MEG coordinate frame using fiducial marker locations and the overall shape of the scalp.

Electroencephalography (EEG) analysis and corresponding software packages are dominated by sensor level processing, such as topography, evoked responses, and ICA. Source localization is more feasible with MEG data; however, many commercial packages offer only one of several basic inverse methods (dipole fitting, beamforming, and minimum-norm). Within open-source options available at present, Brain Storm and MNESuite offer similar source localization options; Field Trip additionally offers beamforming, and SPM 8 offers an advanced Bayesian source estimation method. However, to date, other packages do not provide a whole suite of reconstruction algorithms ranging from the simple to the complex powerful ones that have been recently published.

In 2003, the seeds of NUTMEG (Neurodynamic Utility Toolbox for Magnetoencephalo- and Electroencephalo-Graphy) were planted at the University of California, San Francisco (UCSF), with the motivation to meet several research goals, including implementation of experimental source localization algorithms and general independence from commercially provided software, as well as user extensibility for custom analyses. Specific strengths of NUTMEG include: (1) choice of several inverse algorithms, including variants of popular beamforming, minimum-norm, and Bayesian inference techniques, (2) intuitive viewing and navigation of results, (3) both GUI and command-line batch use, and (4) several methods of source space functional connectivity analysis.

NUTMEG can be downloaded from http://nutmeg.berkeley.edu/. Documentation and a user's wiki are also located at this website, and users can subscribe to a mailing list which is intended as a general forum for questions related to the software itself or analysis procedures.

NUTMEG is primarily written in MATLAB (MathWorks, Natick, MA, USA). The MATLAB Signal Processing Toolbox is required for digital filter operations, and the Image Processing Toolbox is needed for (optional) graphical volume-of-interest (VOI) selection. A link with SPM8 allows activations to be overlaid onto standard orthogonal magnetic resonance imaging (MRI) slices or a rendered 3D brain volume; at present, SPM8's data analysis engine is not used. Via SPM8, activations may also be spatially normalized and displayed on an MNI template brain. Visualization tools in Python are under development and will be made available in future versions (Sarang, 2011 & Seppo, 2010).

Other functional neuroimaging modalities such as FMRI benefit from a relatively established stream of standard processing steps that facilitate learning by beginners and batch processing by more experienced users. However, with MEG and EEG, it sometimes seems that there can be as many ways of analyzing the data as there are datasets, as appropriate analyses can vary considerably according to the paradigm and the types of responses. A useful software package needs to be flexible enough to introduce the various analysis streams as they are developed and straightforward to use for routine analysis.

Experiment types that have been successfully processed with NUTMEG include (1) evoked paradigms, for example, auditory stimulation in healthy subjects, verbal stimulation compared between healthy subjects and schizophrenia patients, perturbation of self - speech perception, and somatosensory stimulation in humans and monkeys, (2) time - frequency analysis, for example, finger movements, visual stimulation, decision making, discrimination of tone rate modulation, and visually guided behavior, and (3) resting state and task - induced connectivity. Data types supported in NUTMEG include MEG, EEG, and intracranial EEG. The future of NUTMEG is influenced by both the research priorities of the developers as well as requests from users (Sarang, 2011).

At present, we intend to create more formal links with SPM8, FieldTrip, and Brainstorm. Specifically, as methods developers, we would like to import, view, and directly compare the Multiple Sparse Priors from SPM8 with other source estimation methods included in NUTMEG; further, we would like to enable direct comparison within NUTMEG of Dynamic Causal Modelling (DCM) for M/EEG with other metrics for functional connectivity. The advanced time - frequency analysis and viewing tools for sensor level data within FieldTrip can be useful to NUTMEG users for planning of further analysis in source space. NUTMEG should be able to display source level results computed in FieldTrip. The cluster - based and permutation test statistics for sensor and source space results implemented in FieldTrip would also be of benefit to be more formally linked to the NUTMEG format. Sensor selection via visual inspection is a highly developed tool within Brainstorm, the output of which could be imported to NUTMEG. Brainstorm also contains useful GUIs for dataset, trial - condition selection, and batch processing setup, which could be linked to NUTMEG via a conversion of MATLAB data structures (Vladimir, 2011).

As several methods for connectivity analysis have recently become available within NUTMEG and additional methods are planned for inclusion, a means to visually browse the results is needed beyond a simple extension of the current source - space viewer. The eConnectome package already implements the computation and elaborate visualization of connectivity, to which we may link(Bin, 2011).

The fusion of multiple sensor types (MEG magnetometers and planar gradiometers, scalp EEG, and intracranial EEG) simultaneously recorded for source reconstruction is a compelling need, but is not yet considered directly straightforward or well established; NUTMEG and other open-source software packages would benefit greatly from further developments on this topic.

NUTMEG provides a full set of MATLAB-based open-source functions with which to compute neural source estimates and additional manipulations thereof, as well as a graphical interface to process and view results. It is linked (to varying degrees) to other open-source packages for processing steps which are better performed by those toolboxes. NUTMEG is flexible to inclusion of new methods at any stage and welcomes new users and developers.

Eye Movements

Eye movements as indicators of specific cognitive processes is one of the most well known, if controversial, discoveries of NLP, and potentially one of the most valuable. According to NLP, automatic, unconscious eye movements, or "eye accessing cues", often accompany particular thought processes, and indicate the access and use of particular representational systems.

Eyes are the visual organs that have the retina, a specialized type of brain tissue containing photoreceptors. These specialised cells convert light into electrochemical signals through the ganglion cell layer and travel along the optic nerve fibers to the brain.

Primates and many other invertebrates use three types of voluntary eye movement to track objects of interest: smooth pursuit, vergence shifts and saccades. These movements appear to be initiated by a small cortical region in the brain's frontal lobe. This is corroborated by removal of the frontal lobe. In this case, the reflexes (such as reflex shifting the eyes to a moving light) are intact, though the voluntary control is obliterated.

Eye movements are controlled by muscles innervated by cranial nerves Ⅲ, Ⅳ and Ⅵ. In this chapter, the testing of these cranial nerves will be discussed. The most common symptom of damage to these nerves is double vision. The oculomotor nerve has the additional function of control of the pupil and therefore this will be discussed here as well. Eye movements are carefully controlled by other systems. Some of these will be discussed here, while others, such as the vestibular system, will primarily be discussed in other chapters (Javier, 2010).

Central control of eye movement, on the other hand, is worthwhile at this point to review the anatomy of the central pathways of the oculomotor system and schematically outline the major central pathways that are important to conjugate lateral gaze, conjugate vertical gaze and convergence. Additionally, the deficits caused by destructive lesions in various parts of these systems are diagrammed.

The central control of eye movement can be distilled into the principle types of functions. These include voluntary, conjugate horizontal gaze (looking side-to-side); voluntary, conjugate vertical gaze (looking up and down); smoothly tracking objects; convergence; and eye movements resulting from head movements. These latter movements are part of the vestibular reflexes for eye stabilization and will be discussed with the vestibular nerve. The vestibular chapter is also where nystagmus (a to-and-fro movement of the eye) will be discussed (King, 2011).

All movements of the eyes that are produced by the central nervous system are conjugate (ie, both eyes moving in the same direction in order to keep the eyes focused on a target) except for convergence, which adducts the eyes to focus on near objects. Voluntary horizontal gaze in one direction begins with the contralateral frontal eye fields (located in the premotor cortex of the frontal lobe). This region has upper motor neurons that project to the contralateral paramedian pontine reticular formation (PPRF), which is the organizing center for lateral gaze in the brain stem. The PPRF projects to the ipsilateral abducens nucleus (causing eye abduction on that side). There are fibers extending from the abducens nucleus, which is located in the caudal pons, to the contralateral oculomotor nucleus of the midbrain. The projection pathway is the medial longitudinal fasciculus (MLF). The oculomotor nucleus then activates the medial rectus, adducting the eye in order to follow the abducting eye. This is illustrated schematically for voluntary horizontal gaze to the left (Keller, 2011 & Bernard, 2010).

Damage to the frontal eye-fields will initially prevent voluntary gaze away from the injured frontal lobe. However, that improves with time. Damage to the PPRF will abolish the ability to look toward the side of the lesion. Damage to the MLF produces the curious finding of "internuclear ophthalmoplegia" in which the patient will be able to abduct the eye, but the adducting eye will not follow. Additionally, there will be some nystagmus in the abducting eye (Athena, 2011).

Vertical gaze does not have one center in the cerebral cortex. Diffuse degeneration of the cortex (such as with dementia) can diminish the ability to move the eyes vertically (particularly upward). There is a brain stem center for vertical gaze (in the midbrain, the rostral interstitial nucleus). Degeneration of this nucleus (such as can occur in rare conditions like progressive supranuclear palsy) can abolish the ability to look up or down. Additionally, there are connections between the two sides that traverse the posterior commissure. Pressure on the dorsum of the midbrain, such as by a pineal tumor, can interrupt these fibers and prevent upgaze, Parinaud syndrome (Michael, 2009).

Neural causes and consequences of small saccades, two new sets of neurophysiological investigations shed light on both the generation of microsaccades and their significance for vision. Microsaccades are generated by activity in the superior colliculus. Hafed, Goffart & Krauzlis (2009) performed a pioneering study of the neural origin of microsaccades. They studied responses of neurons in the deep layers of the rostral pole of the superior colliculus, an area that had been associated with the maintenance of fixation and inhibition of large saccades (Munoz & Wurtz, 1993). Previously, Hafed et al (2008) found that inactivation of the rostral region could produce systematic offsets in the preferred locus of fixation. Hafed et al (2009) found single neurons that fired before microsaccades, with neurons selective as to preferred direction and size. The neurons responded before or during saccades as small as 3 min arc, a microsaccade by anyone's definition. Some neurons also responded before or during saccades as large as 5 degrees. The neural activity associated with the saccades persisted in darkness.

Hafed et al(2009) proposed a model of microsaccade generation based on the idea that the function of the neurons in the rostral pole is to ensure accurate fixation. These neurons could do so, they suggested, by "monitoring" the mean activity level encoded by the neural population in the colliculus relative to a representation of the selected locus of fixation. Changes in the mean activity level of the population, which could be caused by any number of factors, then would evoke a microsaccade. While this model would seem to revive the original position-correcting-reflex model of microsaccade generation proposed by Cornsweet, and challenged by subsequent work, Hafed et al did not talk about fixation reflexes. Instead, they emphasized that by placing the control center in the colliculus, all sorts of higher level influences, from attention shifts to voluntary or task-based strategies (eg, Basso & Wurtz, 2010; McPeek & Keller, 2004; Krauzlis, Liston & Carello, 2004; Kustov & Robinson, 1996) could bias the population activity, and in so doing increase the probability of microsaccades. It is useful to note that in this model, microsaccades could also be evoked by noisy fluctuations in the neural population mean.

Saccades and microsaccades modulate neural firing in V1 and V4. The past 25 years of oculomotor research saw the emergence of a new, and technically challenging, endeavor, namely, the study of the response of visual neurons to the retinal image changes and motor commands produced by eye movements. This extends and develops the original findings of Wurtz (2011), who showed that neurons in V1 respond equivalently to image motion whether produced by saccades or by a rapid translation of the stimulus across the retina. Interest in recent years has turned to the neural effects associated with the smaller eye movements of fixation. Leopold & Logothetis (2009) reported that neurons in V1 responded with either suppressed (37%) or enhanced activity (17%) following saccades as small as 10', while V4 always showed enhancement. They speculated that these effects might mean that the saccade-linked signals could enhance temporal synchronization of visual activity. Martinez-Conde, Macknick & Hubel (2000) reported bursts in V1 following somewhat larger saccades, up to 2 degrees. Snodderly, Kagan & Gur (2008), on the other hand, found a more complex pattern: post-saccadic bursts in some cells, and sustained activity during the fixation pauses between saccades in others. Kagan, Gur & Snodderly (2008) confirmed and then extended these findings in two ways. First, they found that the responses of the saccade-linked burst cells could also be produced by high speed retinal image motion, even in the absence of saccades. Second, they found neurons that were sensitive to saccades in the dark, responding with a brief decrease, then an increase, in activity following the occurrence of a saccade (Rajkai, Lakatos, Chen, Pincze, Karmos & Schroeder, 2008, reported comparable patterns of activity in V1 following large saccades made in darkness). Taken together, these results show eye movement related modulation of neural activity with a variety of different patterns: post-saccadic enhancements, post-saccadic suppression, and drift-based modulations.

Using a somewhat different approach, Bosman, Womelsdorf, Desimone & Fries (2009) studied neural effects linked to saccades that occurred during intervals of fixation while the monkey was engaged in a task requiring attention to an eccentric grating pattern. They found that saccades during fixation (the population ranged in size from a few minutes of arc to 1 deg) modified the temporal synchronization of neural activity in V1 and V4, in support of the proposal by Leopold & Logothetis (2009) (see above). Bosman et al (2009) were particularly interested in evidence that the saccades modified the power of the local field potential in the 40–60 Hz frequency band (ie, gamma-band synchronization), which had previously been associated with modulations in the strength of attention (Womelsdorf et al, 2006). Bosman et al (2009) found that for an interval of about 200 ms following the saccades, the strength of the gamma-band synchronization decreased, and this decrease was associated with slightly slower responses in the psychophysical task

Eye movements during fixation result from activity of the visual and vestibular compensatory systems that function to keep gaze relatively stable in the face of movements of the head. The past 25 years has seen renewed interest in the eye movements during fixation and their effects on vision. The interest in the effects of eye movements of fixation on vision has centered around the role of retinal image motion. There continues to be broad agreement (going back to the original studies of vision with stabilized images) that retinal image motion during maintained fixation is critical for vision: too much image motion degrades resolution, and too little motion can lead to image fading. In natural situations, where the head is free to move, retinal image motion is provided by head movements, and thus the main task for compensatory eye movements is to prevent retinal motion from becoming too fast to allow clear vision.

Ethical Considerations

Ethical considerations are taken into account when an experiment is planned. In most academic institutions, the proposed experimental protocol is reviewed by an institutional review board to ensure that experimental procedures are appropriate (if they are not, federal funds will not be granted for the research). In dealing with human subjects, psychologists follow a code of ethical principles published by the American Psychological Association, which requires investigators to obtain informed consent from all subjects; protect subjects from harm and discomfort; treat all experimental data confidentially; explain the experiment and the results to the subjects afterward.

Similarly, when research is conducted with animals, the project is reviewed by an institutional animal care and use committee (IACUC) to be certain that it is necessary to use animals as subjects to test the hypotheses and that other procedures are not feasible. It also determines that appropriate sample sizes and procedures are used in the experiment and that animals will be given proper care. The IACUC also periodically visits all of the animal colonies to ensure that the research animals are appropriately cared for.

Ethics and Research with Human Participants

How are the current APA ethical guidelines applied to modern-day psychological research? In planning research, psychologists assess the degree to which participants will be put at risk. What are the potential dangers, physical or psychological, that might accompany participation? Even if potential risks are deemed slight, they need to be considered. Researcher Gregory Kimble put it this way: "Is it worth it? Do the potential benefits to science and eventually to animal and human lives justify the costs to be extracted here and now?" Seldom will any one psychologist have to make the ultimate decision about the potential benefits or risks of research. An institutional review board (IRB) typically reviews research proposals to ensure that all research meets the requirements of ethical research practice.

Here are some other ethical issues related to research in psychology:

1. Participants' confidentiality must be guaranteed. Often names are not used; instead, they are replaced with identification numbers. No matter what participants are asked to do or say, they should be confident that no one will have access to their responses but the researchers.

2. Participation in research should be voluntary. No one should feel coerced or compelled to participate in psychological research. For example, college students cannot be offered extra credit for participating in psychological research unless other options are available for earning the same amount of extra credit. Volunteers should be allowed the option of dropping out of any research project, even after it has begun.

3. Persons should be included in experiments only after they have given their consent. Participants must know the risks of participation, why a project is being done, and what is expected of them. For example, a participant in an experiment on the effects of punishment on learning must be told why the project is being done (to determine if punishment is an effective teaching tool), what they will be doing in the experiment (receiving a mild shock for an incorrect response), and potential risks (pain from the shocks). In some cases, it is not possible to fully disclose the true nature and purpose of a study to participants. Some small amount of deception may be required when doing experiments. In this case, the amount of deception needs to be balanced against the potential benefits of the research and justified to an institutional review board.

4. Particularly if participants have been deceived about the true nature of an experiment, and even if they haven't been, all participants should be debriefed after the experiment has been completed. That means that the project and its basic intent should be fully explained to all those who participated in it. Participants should also be provided with a copy of the results of the project when they are available.

What are some ethical questions raised by that experiment? Were the participants informed in advance of their participation? Did the participants have an opportunity for informed consent? Is it ethical to engage in clandestine observation of a private behavior? These and perhaps other questions must be considered when evaluating any research project, especially one done in the field.

Note that there are additional guidelines if children are used as participants in research or if other specialized populations are used (for example, mentally retarded individuals). These guidelines are enforced in addition to the normal APA guidelines.

Ethics and the Use of Animal Suspects in Research

Published ethical guidelines for the use of animals in research are also quite stringent, sometimes more stringent than those published for humans. Current APA ethical guide-lines for using animals in research include the following points:

1. Obtaining, caring for, using, and disposing of animals used in research must comply with all federal, state, and local laws, and be consistent with professional standards.

2. A psychologist trained in the care and use of animals must supervise any procedures involving animals and is ultimately responsible for the comfort, health, and human treatment of the animals.

3. The psychologist must ensure that all assistants are trained in research methods and the care, maintenance, and handling of the animal species being used.

4. Roles assigned to assistants must be consistent with their training.

5. Efforts must be made to minimize any discomfort, infection, illness, or pain of animal subjects.

6. Procedures that subject animals to pain, stress, or privation should only be used when no alter natives are available.

7. When an animal's life is to be terminated, it must be done rapidly with an effort to minimize pain.

8. Proper anesthesia must be used for all surgical procedures.

In addition to these guidelines established by the APA, government regulations must be followed. These government regulations not only specify how animals are to be treated in research, but also dictate minimum standards for housing and caring for animal research subjects.

Just like research using human participants, research using animal subjects must be screened for adherence to ethical guidelines before it can be done. Proposals for research using animal subjects must be reviewed by an institutional animal care and use committee (IACUC). The IACUC normally has the following make-up:

1. A veterinarian who is trained and has experience either with laboratory science or with the species being used.

2. At least one practicing scientist who has experience using animals in research.

3. At least one member of the public to represent the general community's attitudes about the care and use of animals in research. Public members must not be involved in animal research, be affiliated with the institution where the research is to be conducted, or be members of the immediate family of a person affiliated with the institution where the research is being done.

Chapter 3 Brain and Behavior

In this Topic we will explore how information is transmitted within your nervous system. While reading this Topic, find the answers to the following key questions:

The Nervous System and Behavior

Our behaviors, from simple to complex: every emotion you've ever experienced, from mild to extreme; all your thoughts, from the trivial to the profound — all of these can ultimately be reduced to molecules of chemicals racing in and out of the microscopically tiny cells that comprise your nervous systems. Regardless of the complexity of a stimulus or a behavior, there is a remarkable series of biochemical and physiological reactions that take place in your body. These reactions are the focus of this chapter.

Nerve Cells and How They Communicate

You are sitting in your room studying for an important exam while listening to a CD. When your favorite song comes on, you break from your studies and listen carefully to the music. On your desk a fragrant candle burns. As you pick it up to get a better smell, a drop of hot wax hits your hand, resulting in a small amount of pain. You utter a few colorful metaphors, nearly drop the candle, and abruptly put it down. Soon, you sense your stomach beginning to rumble and grab a bag of chips. With your hunger satisfied, you return to your studies.

Sequences like this occur each day. You are bombarded in sights, sounds, smells, tastes, and tactile stimuli. You enjoy listening to music and smelling the scent of some - thing fragrant, like a candle burning. You sense and satisfy hunger. These are things taken for granted. Have you considered how those notes wafting from your stereo's speakers get to your brain so that you can enjoy them? Or how your brain and nervous system operate to produce an emotional reaction to your favorite music? As you will see in this Topic, the process of getting information to and from the brain (and other parts of your body) involves a complex set of processes that take place on a cellular level.

The Neuron: The Basic Building Block of the Nervous System

Our exploration of the nervous system begins at the level of the nerve cell, or neuron, the small cell that transmits information — in the form of neural impulses — from one part of the body to another. Neurons were not recognized as separate structures until the turn of the century. To put things in perspective, there are approximately million specialized neurons that line the back of each human eye, and an estimated 100 billion neurons in the human brain (Hubel, 1979; Kolb, 1989).

Even though, much like snowflakes, no two neurons are exactly alike, there are some commonalities among neurons. Figure 3.1 illustrates these common features.

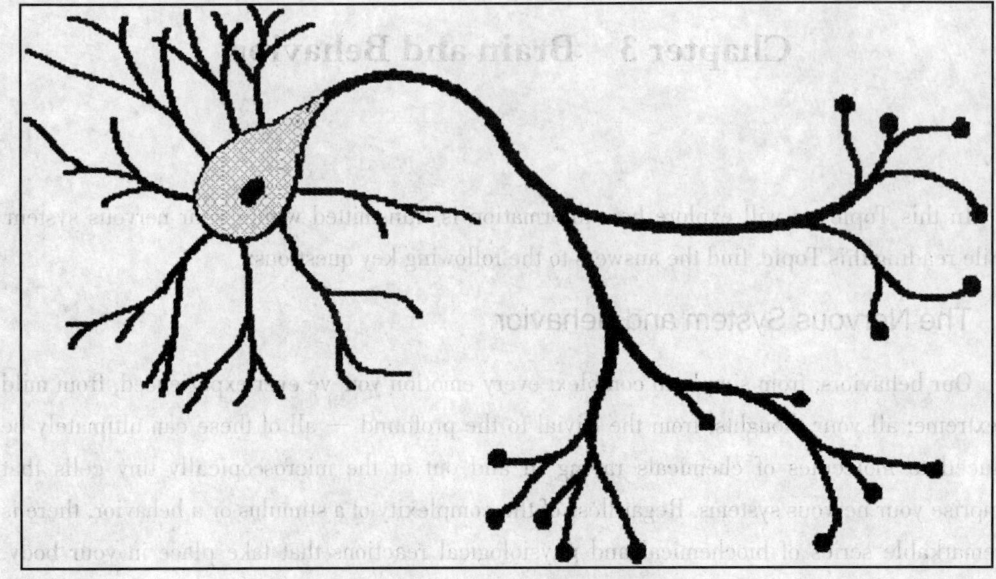

Figure 3.1 A typical nerve with its major structures

One structure that all neurons have is a cell body, the largest concentration of mass in the neuron. The cell body contains the nucleus of each cell. It is in the nucleus of any living cell that we find the genetic information that keeps the cell functioning as it should. Protruding from the cell body are several tentacle - like structures called dendrites, and one particularly long structure called the axon. Typically, dendrites reach out to receive messages, or neural impulses, from nearby neurons. These impulses are sent to the cell body and down the axon to other neurons, muscles, or glands. Some axons are quite long as much as two to three feet long in the spinal cord. Within a neuron, impulses travel from dendrite to cell body to axon, and most of the trip is made along the axon.

The neuron illustrated in Figure 3.1 has a feature not found on all neurons. The axon of this neuron has a cover, or sheath, of myelin. Myelin is a white substance composed of fat and protein found on about half the axons in an adult's nervous system. Myelin is produced by special glia cells and is not an outgrowth of the axon itself. Myelin covers an axon in segments, rather than in one continuous coating. Between each segment of myelin is an unmyelinated segment of axon called a node. It is the absence or presence of myelin that allows us to distinguish between the gray matter (dendrites, cell bodies, and unmyelinated axons) and white matter (myelinated axons) of nervous system tissue.

We tend to find myelin on axons that carry impulses relatively long distances. Neurons that carry messages up and down the spinal cord, for instance, have myelinated axons, whereas those that carry impulses back and forth across the spinal cord do not.

Myelin serves several functions. It protects the long, delicate axon. It also acts as an insulator, separating the activity of one neuron from those nearby. Myelin speeds impulses along the length of the axon. As we will see later in this chapter, this is because the neural impulse that travels down the axon can "jump" from node to node in a process called saltatory conduction. Because of this form of conduction, myelinated neurons carry impulses nearly ten times faster than unmyelinated ones (up to 120 meters per second).

Interestingly, myelin can be found only in vertebrate animals. Invertebrates (eg, worms) have neurons and axons, but no myelin. In order to speed neural impulses, invertebrates thinner vertebrate axons. Because they don't have myelin, the speed of impulse conduction in invertebrates is quite slow, thereby limiting the size of these organisms. Complex, coordinated behaviors are impossible if invertebrates become too large. Such complex behavior requires more rapid impulse transmission.

Whether myelinated or not, axons end in a branching series of bare end points called axon terminals. At the axon terminal, a neuron communicates with other neurons. To review, within a neuron, impulses travel from the dendrites to the cell body, to the axon (which may be myelinated), and then to axon terminals.

Very few new neurons are generated after birth. We are born with more neurons than we will ever have again. In fact, we are born with about twice as many neurons as we'll ever use. What happens to the rest? Those that are not strengthened by experience eventually die off. In normal development, the brain is "constructed" in a manner rather like that in which a statue is chipped away from a block of granite. Rather than building up the finished product one small piece at a time, more material than one needs is available. What is needed or used is retained, and the rest dies away. For example, a young infant (six to ten months old) has neural circuitry that allows him or her to distinguish between most human speech sounds. Experience with his or her native language environment strengthens those neurons that are important to the native language, whereas those that are not, die off. The result is that an infant that at six to ten months of age could discriminate between speech sounds from his or her non-native language can no longer do so at ten to twelve months of age. In a sense, we are born with a "generic brain" that, much like sculpture, is molded by experience. However, the sculpture analogy goes just so far. While it is true that unnecessary neurons die off, the inter-connections between neurons become more numerous and complex as the brain develops.

It is a related observation. To have billions of neurons in our brains at birth, brain cells must be generated at a rate of about 250,000 per minute while the brain is being formed.

In most cases, dead neurons are not replaced with new ones. We constantly make new blood cells to replace lost ones; if we didn't, we could never donate a pint of blood. Lost skin cells are rapidly replaced by new ones. You rinse away skin cells by the hundred seach time you wash your hands. Most neurons are different; once they're gone, they're gone forever. We're often in luck, however, because the functions of lost neurons can betaken over by other surviving neurons. There is also evidence that in the primate brain some new neurons are generated in adulthood through a process called neurogenesis. These new neurons are found predominately in those areas of the brain that only process incoming sensory information. There is also evidence that new nerve cell growth can be stimulated in rats with exposure to a chemical called "recombined human nerve growth factor," when it is give nearly in life. Rats exposed to the nerve growth factor showed better learning skills than did untreated rats, and this difference persisted into adulthood. Results like these suggest that the brain has the capacity to regenerate lost neurons, but certainly not at the rate that is seen in prenatal and early postnatal development. These new neurons end up in areas associated with higher cognitive functions and may relate to one's ability to continue to learn throughout life or after brain injury. Furthermore, exposure to the growth factor is not the only condition that can produce neurogenesis. Gould et al found that learning stimulated growth of new neurons in specific parts of the hippocampus of rats. There is also evidence that neurogenesis occurs in the adult human brain. Eriksson and his colleagues found clear evidence of new neuron production in the hippocampus, an area of the brain associated with memory. They concluded that neurogenesis occurs in this area of the brain throughout life.

The Function of Neurons

The function of a neuron is to transmit neural impulses from one place in the nervous system to another. Let's start with a definition. A neural impulse is a rapid, reversible change in the electrical charges within and outside a neuron. This change in electrical charge travels from the dendrites to the axon terminal when the neuron fires. Now let's see what all that means.

Neurons exist in a complex biological environment. As living cells, they are filled with and surrounded by fluids. Only a very thin membrane (like a skin) separates the fluids inside a neuron from those outside. These fluids contain chemical particles called ions. Chemical ions are particles that carry a small, measurable electrical charge that is either positive (+) or negative (-). Electrically charged ions float around in all the fluids of the body, but are heavily concentrated in and around the nervous system. If you examine the distribution of ions inside and outside the neuron, you find that the inside of the neuron has a more negative charge than the outside. What does this mean? There are more negative ions than positive ions inside the axon. Conversely, there are more positive ions outside the neuron than negative ions. At rest, the axonal membrane does not allow the negatively and positively charged ions to pass across the membrane. The physiology of the neuron keeps the inside of the axon negatively charged compared to the outside. A tension develops between the electrical charge of ions that have been trapped inside the neuron (predominantly negative ions) and the electrical charge of ions that have been trapped outside the neuron (predominantly positive ions). Positive and negative ions are attracted to each other; however, they cannot come into contact because the neuron's membrane separates them.

The tension that results from the positive and negative ions' attraction to each other is called a resting potential. The resting potential of a neuron is about -70 millivolts (mV), which makes each neuron rather like a small battery. A D-cell battery (the sort used in a flashlight) has two aspects (called poles): one positive and the other negative. The electrical charge possible with one of these batteries — its resting potential — is 1500 mV, much greater than that of a neuron. The resting potential of a neuron is negative 70 millivolts (- 70 mV) because we measure the inside of a neuron relative to the outside, and the negative ions are concentrated inside. At rest, the neuron is in a polarized state.

When a neuron is stimulated to fire, or produce an impulse, the electrical tension of the resting potential is released. Very quickly, the polarity of the nerve cell changes a process called depolarization. This occurs when the axon membrane suddenly allows positively charged sodium ions to flood into the interior of the axon, drastically changing the electrical potential of the axon. Then, the membrane allows positively charged potassium ions to exit the axon. For an instant (about one one-thousandth of a second), the electrical charge within the cell becomes more positive than the area outside the cell. This new charge is called the action potential, which is about +40 mV. The positive sign indicates that the inside of the neuron is now more positive than the outside (there are more positive ions inside than outside). In a fraction of a second, the neuron returns to its original state with the tension redeveloped, and after a few thousandths of a second it is ready to fire again (see Figure 3.2).

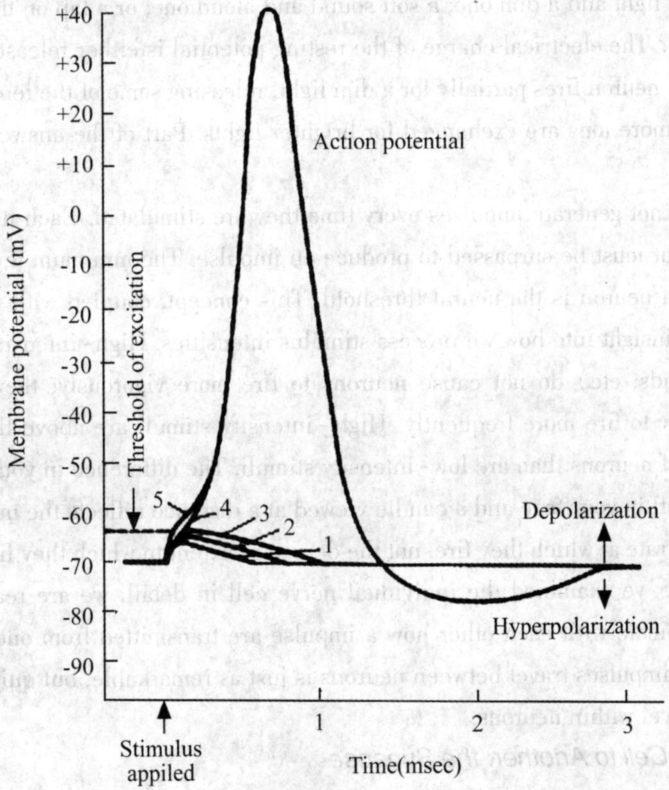

Figure 3.2 An Impulse "Travels Down a Neuron "

Before the neuron returns to its normal resting state, it actually becomes hyperpolarized — its negative charge is even more negative than the normal - 70mV. This occurs because the neuron's membrane allows too much potassium to leak out of the cell making the inside of the cell too negative. For a few thousandths of a second, there is a refractory period during which the neuron cannot fire. Eventually, the membrane returns to normal and the sodium - potassium pump restores the normal distribution of ions across the cell membrane.

To repeat, when a neuron is at rest, there is a difference between the electrical charges inside and outside the neuron (the inside is more negative). When the neuron is stimulated, the difference reverses, so that the inside becomes slightly positive. The tension of the resting potential then returns. When an impulse "travels down a neuron", nothing physically moves from one end of the neuron to the other. The only movement of physical particles is the movement of the electrically charged ions into and out of the neuron through its membrane.

When a neuron is stimulated by another neuron, it may or may not transmit a neural impulse. It either fires or it doesn't, a fact called the all - or - none principle. There is no such thing as a weak or strong neural impulse; the impulse is either there or it isn't. Based on your knowledge of the physiology of the neuron, you can see why this is so. The depolarization of the neuron during the action potential is an all - or - none proposition. When the membrane of the axon is depolarized, it cannot stop. This raises a psychological question: How does the nervous system react to differences in stimulus intensity? How do neurons react to the difference between a bright light and a dim one; a soft sound and aloud one; or a tap on the shoulder and a slap on the back? The electrical charge of the resting potential is either released or it isn't. We cannot say that a neuron fires partially for a dim light, releasing some of the tension of its resting potential, while more ions are exchanged for brighter lights. Part of the answer involves neural thresholds.

Neurons do not generate impulses every time they are stimulated. Each neuron has a level of stimulation that must be surpassed to produce an impulse. The minimum level of stimulation required to fire a neuron is the neural threshold. This concept, coupled with the all - or - none principle, lends insight into how we process stimulus intensities. High - intensity stimuli (bright lights, loud sounds, etc) do not cause neurons to fire more vigorously; they stimulate more neurons to fire or to fire more frequently. High - intensity stimuli are above the threshold of a greater number of neurons than are low - intensity stimuli. The difference in your experience of a flashbulb going off in your face and a candle viewed at a distance reflects the number of neurons involved and the rate at which they fire, not the degree or extent to which they fire.

Now that we've examined the individual nerve cell in detail, we are ready to learn how neurons communicate with each other how a impulse are transmitted from one cell to another. The story of how impulses travel between neurons is just as remarkable, but quite different from, how impulses travel within neurons.

From One Cell to Another: the Synapse

In your nervous system there are billions of points where neurons interact with one another. The location at which an impulse is relayed from one neuron to another is called the synapse. In the cerebral cortex of the human brain alone, there are billions of synaptic interconnections among neurons. At these synapses, neurons do not physically touch one another. Instead, there is a microscopic gap between the axon terminal of one neuron and another neuron terminals. There, new neurotransmitter chemicals are released from vesicles, which cross the synaptic cleft and stimulate the next neuron in the sequence. This is the case when the neurotransmitter excites and stimulates the next neuron to fire in a sequence. These neurotransmitters are referred to as excitatory. As it happens, there are many neurons throughout our nervous systems that hold neurotransmitters that have the opposite effect. When they are released, they flood across the synaptic cleft and prevent the next neuron from firing. We refer to these synapses as inhibitory (see Figure 3.3).

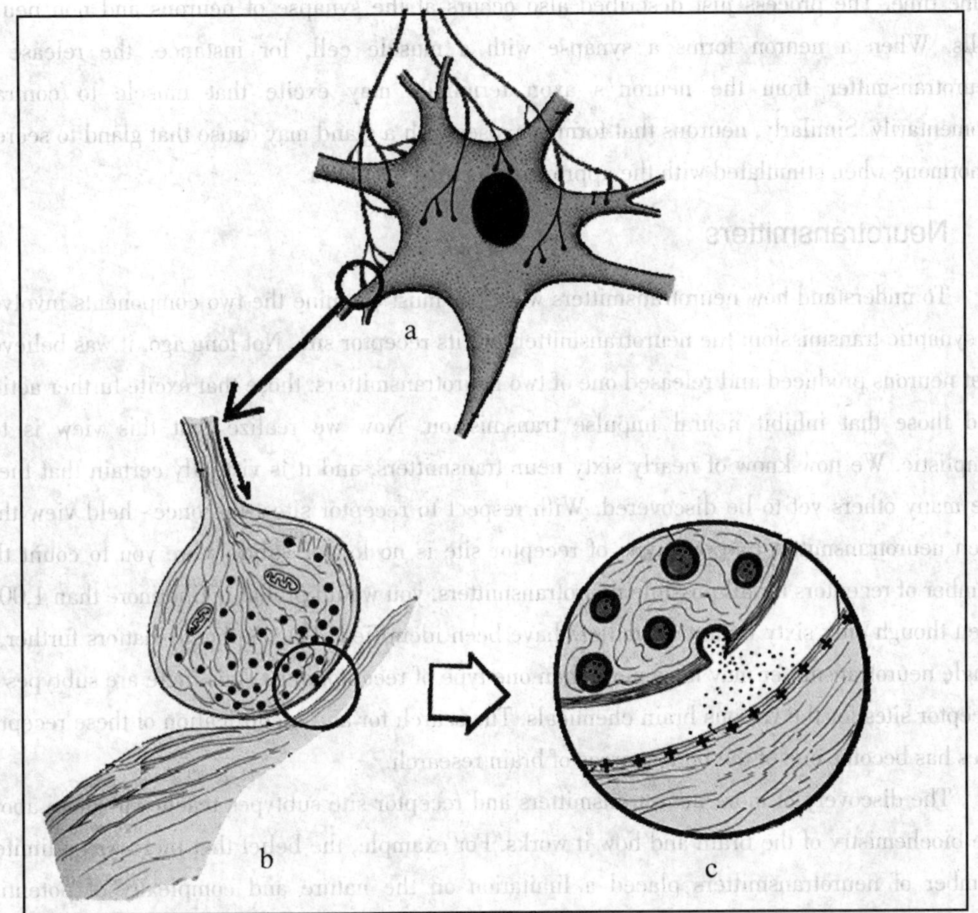

Figure 3.3 Synaptic Transmission

The final step in the process of synaptic transmission is the elimination of the neurotransmitter from the synaptic cleft. This is done in one of two ways: destruction by an enzyme or reuptake. Some neurotransmitters, such as acetylcholine, are broken down by special enzymes secreted into the synaptic cleft. In the case of acetylcholine the enzyme is acetylcholinesterase. Other neurotransmitters, such as serotonin, are reabsorbed by the presynaptic membrane (the membrane of the neuron, from which the neurotransmitters originated) through a process called reuptake. Many psychoactive drugs work by affecting the breakdown or reuptake of neurotranmitters. For example, Prozac (a popular rantidepressant drug) operates by inhibiting the reuptake of serotonin. Myasthenia Gravis, a disease relating to the under activity of acetylcholine is effectively treated with drugs that block acetylcholinesterase.

If you recall the last section in which we talked about neural thresholds, you may now appreciate how that concept works. Imagine a neuron's dendrite at rest, with many axon terminals (of many neurons) just across the synaptic cleft. For this neuron to begin a new impulse, it may require a greater amount of excitatory chemical than just one axon terminal can provide, particularly if nearby terminals are releasing inhibitory neurotransmitters at about the same time. The process just described also occurs at the synapse of neurons and non neural cells. When a neuron forms a synapse with a muscle cell, for instance, the release of neurotransmitter from the neuron's axon terminals may excite that muscle to contract momentarily. Similarly, neurons that form synapses with a gland may cause that gland to secrete a hormone when stimulated with the appropriate neurotransmitter.

Neurotransmitters

To understand how neurotransmitters work, we must examine the two components involved in synaptic transmission: the neurotransmitter and its receptor site. Not long ago, it was believed that neurons produced and released one of two neurotransmitters: those that excite further action and those that inhibit neural impulse transmission. Now we realize that this view is too simplistic. We now know of nearly sixty neurotransmitters, and it is virtually certain that there are many others yet to be discovered. With respect to receptor sites, the once - held view that each neurotransmitter had one type of receptor site is no longer valid. Were you to count the number of receptors for all possible neurotransmitters, you would probably find more than 1,000, even though only sixty neurotransmitters have been identified. To complicate matters further, a single neurotransmitter may have more than one type of receptor site. Thus there are subtypes of receptor sites for the various brain chemicals. The search for and identification of these receptor sites has become one of the hottest areas of brain research.

The discovery of more neurotransmitters and receptor site subtypes teaches us more about the biochemistry of the brain and how it works. For example, the belief that there was a limited number of neurotransmitters placed a limitation on the nature and complexity of potential synaptic communication. More neurotransmitters, receptor sites, and specialized sites indicates a potential for clearer and more complex communication within the nervous system. Imagine that a part of the brain receives separate signals indicating two different emotions (fear and surprise). Were only one neurotransmitter and receptor site involved, the different emotions could not be recognized. More neurotransmitters and receptor sites allow the independent signals to be separated, sorted, and more clearly recognized.

Despite the complexities involved in the biochemistry of the nervous system, we can provide a few details about the activity of some of the neurotransmitters that have been discovered. For now, let's briefly note five of the better- known neurotransmitters.

Acetylcholine, or ACh, is nervous system, where it acts as either an excitatory or inhibit depending on where it is found. It is a common neurotransmitter (in the 1920s). Not only is

ACh found in the brain, but it is common between neurons and muscle tissue cells. One form of food poisoning, botulism, blocks the release of acetylcholine at neuron - muscle cell synapses; this can paralysis of the respiratory system and may result in death unless an antitoxin is given. The poisonous drug curare works in much the same fashion. Some other poisons (eg, the venom of the black widow spider) have just the opposite effect, causing excess amounts of ACh to be released, resulting in muscle contractions or spasms so severe as to be deadly. Nicotine is a chemical that in small amounts tends to increase the normal functioning of ACh, but in large doses acts to override the normal action of acetylcholine — a reaction that can lead to muscle paralyzsed even death. Smoking or chewing tobacco seldom causes such adramatic effect because large amounts of nicotine first stimulate a brain center that causes vomiting before too much nicotine has been absorbed into one's system. Low levels of acetylcholine are associated with loss of cognitive functioning in patients with Alzheimer's disease. Two drugs that act on acetylcholine mechanisms are currently being used to treat Alzheimer's disease. One drug, tacrine, inhibits the action of acetylcholinesterase which breaks down acetylcholine after synaptic transmission. Use of this drug in patients with mild to moderate cases of Alzheimer's disease has led to slight memory enhancement. Unfortunately, prolonged use of this drug may lead to liver problems, so it is no longer a treatment of choice. The other drug, donepezil, is also an acetylcholinesterase inhibitor and has shown promise as a treatment for memory loss in Alzheimer's patients. It is necessary for the patient to remain on the drug in order for the memory improvement to persist. Finally, the link between nicotine and enhanced acetylocholine activity would suggest this drugs another treatment for Alzheimer's disease. Delagarza (1998) reported that nicotine is associated with some memory enhancement in Alzheimer's patients, but it is not now ended for treatment of the disease.

Norepinephrine is a common and important neurotransmitter that is associated with regulation. Norepinephrine is involved in the physiological reactions associated with high levels of emotional arousal, such as increased heart rate, perspiration, and blood pressure. When there is an abundance of norepinephrinein a person's brain or spinal cord, feelings of arousal, agitation, or anxiety may result. (Cocaine increases the release of norepinephrine leading to a state of agitation and a "high" mood state.) Too little norepinephrine in the brain and spinal cord is associated with feelings of depression.

Dopamine is also a common neurotransmitter associated with mood regulation. It has intrigued psychologists for some time. It is involved in a wide range of reactions. Either too much or too little dopamine within the nervous system seems to produce a number of effects, depending primarily on which system of nerve fibers in the brain is involved. Dopamine has been associated with the thought and mood disturbances of some psychological disorders. It is also associated with the impairment of movement: when there is not enough dopamine, we find difficulty in voluntary movement; too much and we find involuntary tremors.

Serotonin is another important neurotransmitter. Its action in the nervous system is quite complex and not completely understood. We do know, however, that serotonin is related to various behaviors. For example, serotonin is involved in the sleep/waking cycle. An increase in levels of serotonin in parts of the brain associated with sleep are related to sleep onset. Serotonin has also been found to play a role in depression. Depleted levels of serotonin are related to depressive symptoms. Drugs, like Prozac, that increase serotonin levels reduce depressive symptoms. Finally, low levels of serotonin have been implicated in aggressive behavior. In one study, for example, monkeys with low levels of serotonin tended to be much more aggressive and prone to risky behavior than monkeys with higher levels of serotonin. In fact, Higley, et al (1996) found that monkeys with low levels of serotonin — which made them more aggressive - were more likely to be dead four years after the study began, largely due to those monkeys attacking larger monkeys. In contrast, none of the high - level serotonin monkeys were dead.

Endorphins (there are several of them) are natural pain suppressors. The pain threshold — the ability to tolerate different levels of pain — is a function of endorphin production. With excess levels of endorphins, we feel little pain; a deficit results in an increased experience of pain. When we are under extreme physical stress, endorphin levels rise. Many long - distance runners, for instance, often report a near - euphoric "high" after they run great distances, as though endorphins have kicked into protect them against the pain of physical exhaustion.

We could easily continue this list, but for now our focus is on what neurotransmitters do: they are the agents that either excite or inhibit the transmission of neural impulses throughout the nervous system. That excitation or inhibition can have a consider able effect on our thoughts, feelings, and behavior.

So that a simplified description does not leave a false impression, neural impulse transmission is seldom a matter of one neuron stimulating another neuron in a chain reaction. Any neuron can nave hundreds or thousands of axon terminals and synapses. and has the potential for exciting or inhibiting (or being excited by or inhibited by) many other neurons.

The Human Nervous System: The Big Picture

Now that we know how neurons work individual and in combination, let's consider the context in which they function. Behaviors and mental activities require large numbers or integrated neurons working together in complex, organized systems. Figure 3.4 depicts these systems. We have also depicted the endocrine system in Figure 3.4. Although it is not composed of neurons, the endocrine system interacts with the nervous systems to control behaviors and mental processes.

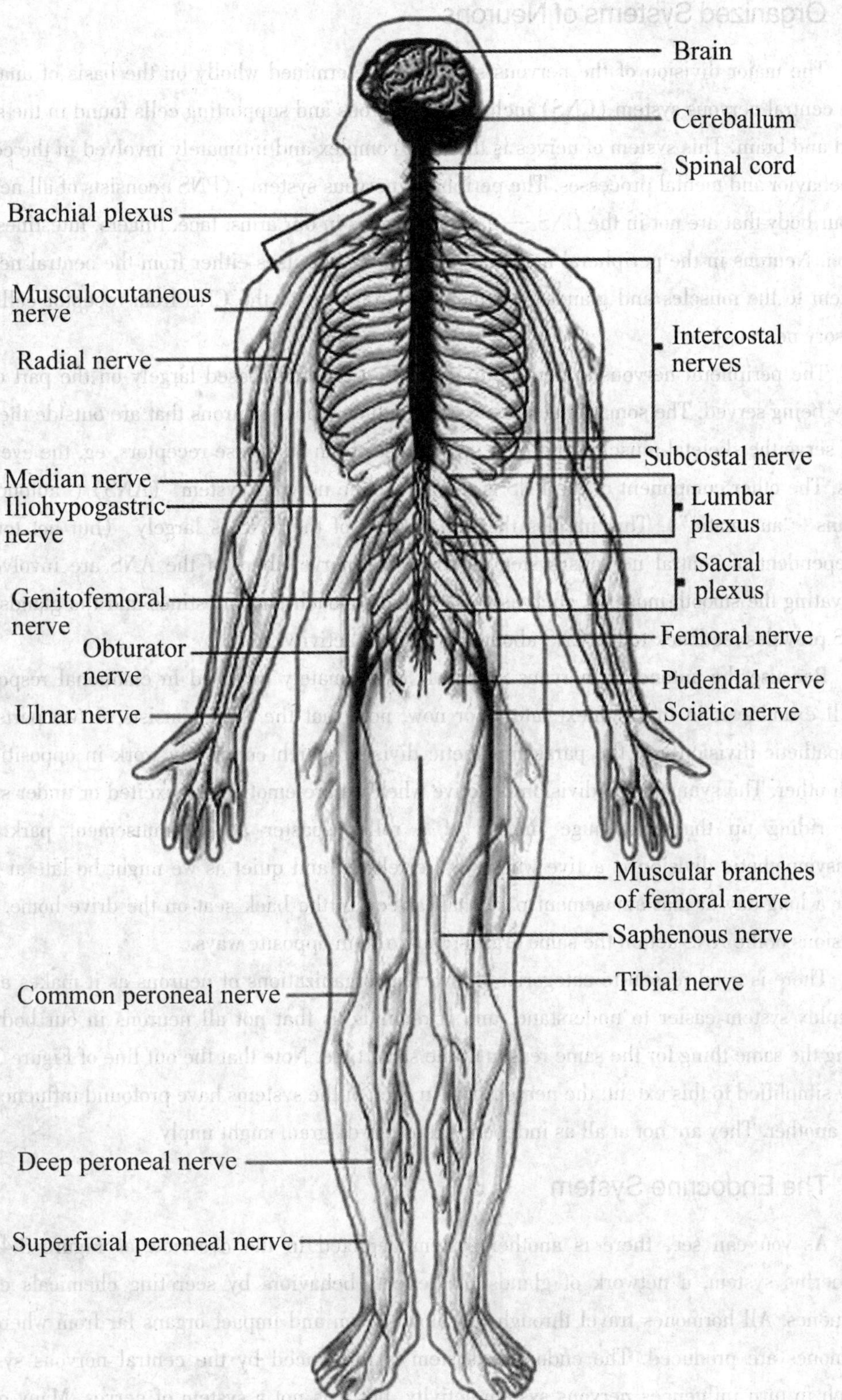

Figure 3.4 Organized Systems of Neurons

Organized Systems of Neurons

The major division of the nervous systems is determined wholly on the basis of anatomy. The central nervous system (CNS) includes all neurons and supporting cells found in the spinal cord and brain. This system of nerves is the most complex and intimately involved in the control of behavior and mental processes. The peripheral nervous system (PNS) consists of all neurons in our body that are not in the CNS — the nerve fibers in our arms, face, fingers, intestines, and so on. Neurons in the peripheral nervous system carry impulses either from the central nervous system to the muscles and glands (on motor neurons) or to the CNS from receptor cells (on sensory neurons).

The peripheral nervous system is divided into two parts, based largely on the part of the body being served. The somatic nervous system includes those neurons that are outside the CNS and serve the skeletal muscles and pick up impulses from our sense receptors, eg, the eyes and ears. The other component of the PNS is the autonomic nervous system (ANS) ("autonomic" means "automatic"). This implies that the activity of the ANS is largely (but not totally) independent of central nervous system control. The nerve fibers of the ANS are involved in activating the smooth muscles, such as those of the stomach and intestines and the glands. The ANS provides feedback to the CNS about this internal activity.

Because the autonomic nervous system is so intimately involved in emotional responses, we'll examine it in that context later. For now, note that the ANS consists of two parts: the sympathetic division and the parasympathetic division which commonly work in opposition to each other. The sympathetic division is active when we are emotionally excited or under stress, like riding up that first huge incline of a roller coaster at an amusement park. The parasympathetic division is active when we are relaxed and quiet as we might be late at night after a long day at that amusement park, half asleep in the back seat on the drive home. Both divisions of the ANS act on the same organs, but do so in opposite ways.

There is good reason to categorize the various organizations of neurons as it makes a very complex system easier to understand, and it reminds us that not all neurons in our body are doing the same thing for the same reason at the same time. Note that the out line of Figure 3.4 is very simplified to this extent: the nerve fibers in each of the systems have profound influences on one another. They are not at all as independent as our diagram might imply.

The Endocrine System

As you can see, there is another system depicted in the overview of Figure 3.4: the endocrine system, a network of glands that effects behaviors by secreting chemicals called hormones. All hormones travel through the bloodstream and impact organs far from where the hormones are produced. The endocrine system is influenced by the central nervous system, which in turn influences nervous system activity, but it is not a system of nerves. Many of the hormones produced by the glands of the endocrine system are chemically similar to neurotransmitters and have similar effects. The endocrine system's glands and hormones are controlled by both the brain of the central nervous system and the autonomic nervous system. We have included the endocrine system in this discussion for two reasons. First, its function is like that of the nervous system: to transmit information from one part of the body to another. Second, hormones exert a direct influence on behavior (see Figure 3.5).

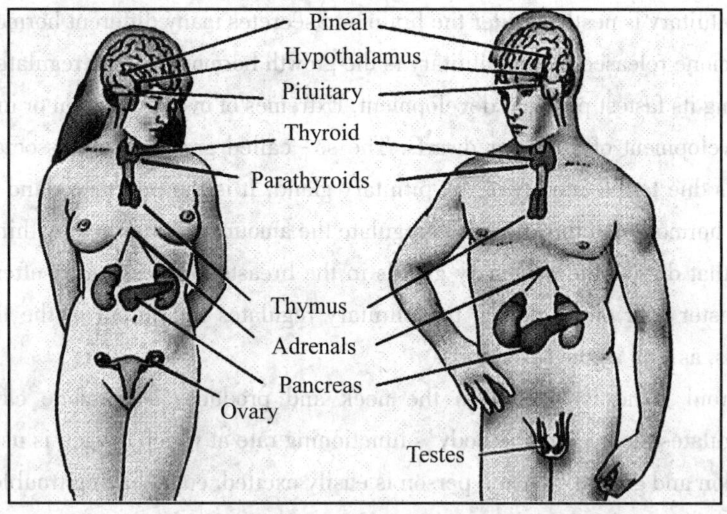

Figure 3.5 Endocrine System

Consider the male hormone testosterone secreted by the testes. High testosterone levels are associated with increased aggression; however, the relationship between testosterone and aggression is quite complex. Testosterone's impact is experienced most before birth (prenatally) and at puberty. During prenatal development, the male genetic code produces high levels of testosterone in the male brain, which causes the male brain to be wired for aggression. This is known as the organization function of testosterone. At puberty, testosterone serves an activation function for aggression. Generally, research on animal subjects has confirmed the organization and activation functions of testosterone levels.

Hormones alone don't drive aggressive behavior; however, testosterone levels tend to interact with environmental conditions to increase or decrease aggression. In an experiment male rats were castrated and implanted with a capsule. Half of the rats received empty capsules; however, the other capsules contained testosterone. The rats were housed in a cage with another rat under one of two conditions. In one condition, there was one feeding tube, creating competition for food. In the other condition, there were two feeding tubes, eliminating competition for food. The rats who had the testosterone capsules were tested for aggression. The results showed that only the testosterone-treated males housed in a cage with one feeding tube exhibited an increased level of aggression. So, testosterone levels interacted with the competitive/ noncompetitive environment to influence aggression.

Endocrine Glands

There are several endocrine glands throughout our bodies. We'll discuss the pituitary gland, the thyroid gland, and the adrenal gland to examine how this system works. The sex glands are part of this system, but we'll discuss their operation later. (Glands in our bodies that are not part of the endocrine system because their secretions do not enter the bloodstream are called exocrine glands. Tear glands and sweat glands are two examples.)

Perhaps the most important endocrine gland is the pituitary gland. It is often referred to as the master gland, reflecting its direct control over the activity of many other glands in the system. The pituitary is nestled under the brain and secretes many different hormones.

One hormone released by the pituitary is the growth hormone, which regulates the growth of the body during its fastest physical development. Extremes of overproduction or underproduction cause the development of giants or dwarfs. The so - called growth spurt associated with early adolescence is due to the activity of the pituitary gland. It is the pituitary gland that stimulates the release of hormones on the kidneys to regulate the amount of water held within the body. It is the pituitary that directs the mammary glands in the breasts to release milk after childbirth. In its role as master over other glands, the pituitary regulates the output of the thyroid and the adrenal glands, as well as the sex glands.

The thyroid gland is located in the neck and produces a hormone called thyroxine. Thyroxine regulates the pace of the body's functioning rate at which oxygen is used and the rate of body function and growth. When a person is easily excited, edgy, having trouble sleeping, and losing weight, he or she may have too much thyroxine in the system, a condition called hyperthyroidism. Too little thyroxine leads to a lack of energy, fatigue, and an inability to do much, a condition called hypothyroidism.

The adrenal glands, located on the kidneys, secrete a variety of hormones into the bloodstream. The hormone adrenaline (more often referred to as epinephrine) is very useful in times of stress, danger, or threat. Adrenaline quickens breathing, causes the heart to beat faster, directs the flow of blood away from the stomach and intestines to the limbs, dilates the pupils of the eyes, and increases perspiration. When our adrenal glands flood epinephrine into our system during a perceived emergency, we usually feel the resulting reactions; but, typical of endocrine system activity, these reactions may be delayed. For example, as you drive down a busy street, a child suddenly darts out in front of you from behind a parked car and races to the other side of the street. You slam on the brakes, twist the steering wheel, and swerve to avoid hitting the child. As the child scampers away, oblivious to the danger just past, you proceed down the street. Then, about half a block later, your hormone - induced reaction strikes. Your heart pounds, a lump forms in your throat, your mouth dries, and your palms sweat. Why now when the incident is past, the child is safely across the street, and you are no longer in danger? The reason is that your reaction is largely hormonal, involving the adrenal glands, and it takes that long for the epinephrine to get from those glands through the bloodstream.

The Central Nervous System

The Spinal Cord

As we have noted, the central nervous system consists of the brain and the spinal cord. In this section, we'll consider the structure and fiction of the spinal cord, reserving our disscussion of the brain for the next section.

The Structure of the Spinal Cord

The spinal cord is a mass of interconnected neurons within the spinal column, which looks rather like a section of rove or thick twine. It is surrounded and protected by hard bone and cartilage of the vertebrae. A cross - sectional view of the spinal column and the spinal cord is illustrated in Figure 3.6. A few structural details need to be mentioned. Note that the spinal cord is located in the middle of the spinal column, and extends from your lower back to high in your neck just below your brain. Then note that nerve fibers enter and leave the spinal cord from the side. Neurons that carry impulses toward the brain or spinal cord are called sensory neurons or sensory fibers, and the impulses they transmit enter the spinal cord on dorsal roots (dorsal means toward the back). Neurons and nerve fibers that carry impulses away from the spinal cord and brain to muscles and glands are called motor neurons or motor fibers. Impulses that leave the spinal cord on motor neurons do so on ventral roots (ventral means toward the front). Neurons within the central nervous system are called inter neurons(see Figure 3.6).

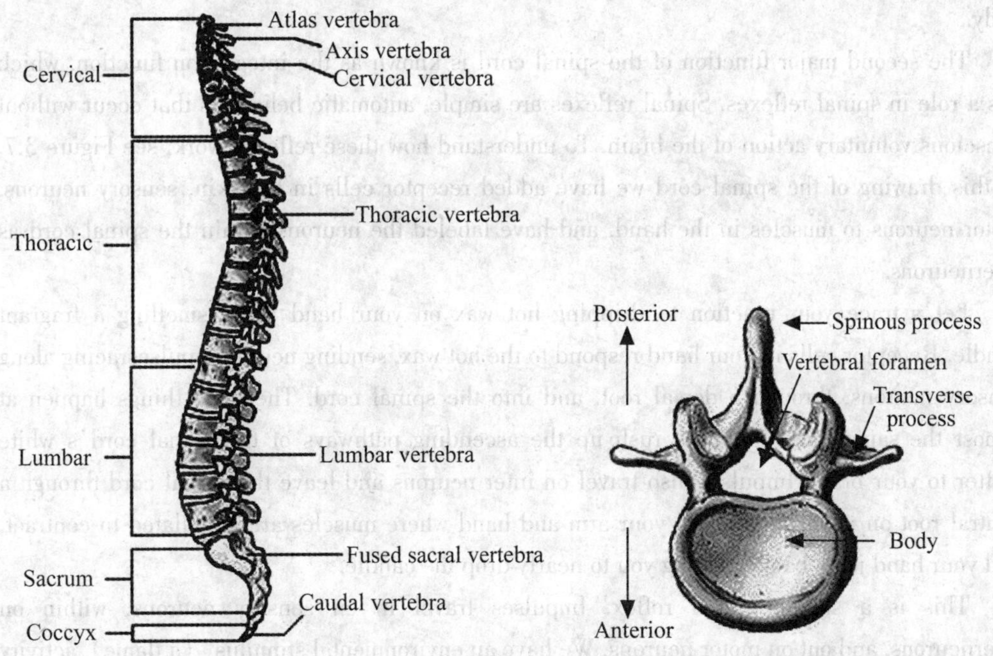

Figure 3.6 spinal cord

Also notice that the center area of the spinal cord consists of gray matter in the shape of a butterfly, while the outside area is light, white matter. This means that the center portion is filled with cell bodies, dendrites, and unmyelinated axons, while the outer section is filled with myelinated axons. Both of these observations about the structure of the spinal cord are key to understanding its functions.

The Functions of the Spinal Cord

The spinal cord has two major functions. The communication function of the spinal cord involves transmitting impulses rapidly to and from the brain. When sensory impulses originate in sense receptors below the neck and make their way to the brain, they do so through the spinal cord. When the brain transmits motor impulses to move or activate parts of the body below the neck, those impulses first travel down the spinal cord. For example, if you stub your toe, pain messages travel up the spinal cord and register in the brain. Motor impulses are then sent down your spinal cord causing you to lift your foot, grab it, and hop around.

Impulses to and from various parts of the body leave and enter the spinal cord at different points (impulses to and from the legs, for example, enter and leave at the very base of the spinal cord). If the spinal cord is damaged, the communication function may be disrupted. This is what happened to actor Christopher Reeves, who was thrown from his horse and severed his spine near his neck. The consequences of such an injury are disastrous, resulting in a loss of feeling from the part of the body severed and a loss of voluntary movement (paralysis) of the muscles in the region. The higher in the spinal cord that damage takes place, the greater the resulting losses. In Reeves' case his injury led to quadraplegia, or the loss of function of all four limbs, because his injury was so high on the spinal cord. Had his injury been closer to the base of his spine he would have had a condition called paraplegia, or loss of function in the legs and lower body.

The second major function of the spinal cord is known as the integration function, which has a role in spinal reflexes. Spinal reflexes are simple, automatic behaviors that occur without conscious voluntary action of the brain. To understand how these reflexes work, see Figure 3.7. In this drawing of the spinal cord we have added receptor cells in the skin, sensory neurons, motor neurons to muscles in the hand, and have labeled the neurons within the spinal cord as interneurons.

Let's trace your reaction to dripping hot wax on your hand while smelling a fragrant candle. Receptor cells in your hand respond to the hot wax, sending neural impulsesracing along sensory neurons, through a dorsal root, and into the spinal cord. Then two things happen at almost the same time. Impulses rush up the ascending pathways of the spinal cord's white matter to your brain. Impulses also travel on inter neurons and leave the spinal cord through a ventral root on motor neurons to your arm and hand where muscles are stimulated to contract, and your hand jerks back, causing you to nearly drop the candle.

This is a simple spinal reflex. Impulses travel in on sensory neurons, within on interneurons, and out on motor neurons. We have an environmental stimulus (a flame), activity in the central nervous system (neurons in the spinal cord), and an observable response (withdrawal of the hand).

There are a few observations we must make about the reflex of the type shown in Figure 3.7. First, the fact that impulses enter the spinal cord and immediately race to the brain is not indicated in the drawing. In a situation such as the candle example, you may jerk your hand back "without thinking about it", but very soon thereafter you are aware of what has happened. Awareness occurs in the brain, not in the spinal cord. It is also true that some reflexes are more simple. The reflex shown in Figure 3.7 involves three neurons: a sensory neuron, an interneuron, and a motor neuron. Other reflexes involve only a sensory and a motor neuron which synapse directly. The knee jerk reflex is an example of such a reflex where a sensory and motor peuronsynapse directly in the spinal cord with no interneuron.

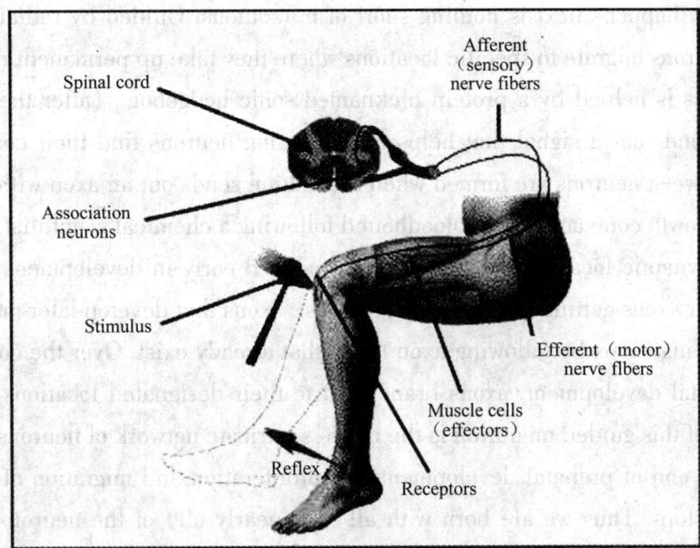

Figure 3.7 Spinal Reflex

The Brain

Perched atop your spinal cord, encased in bone, is a wonderful and mysterious organ: your brain. Your brain is a mass of neurons, glia cells and other supporting cells, blood vessels, and ventricles (hollow tubes and spaces containing fluid). Your brain accounts for a small fraction of your body weight, but due to its importance, it receives almost 20 percent of the blood in your body. It contains a storehouse of memories and is the seat of your emotions and your motivation. It regulates your breathing and the beating of your heart.

For convenience, we will divide the brain into two major categories of structures. We will first discuss the role of some of the "lower brain centers", which are involved in several important aspects of behavior. Then we will examine the role of the cerebral cortex, the largest structure in the brain. The cerebral cortex, generally speaking, is the part of the brain that controls higher mental functions. Before we look at how the brain is structured and how it functions, let's look at how the brain develops.

How Does the Brain Develop?

Your adult brain contains billions of neurons and connections, intricately woven together to give you the capabilities you have. The process by which this marvelous organ develops is fascinating and begins with the fertilization of an egg by a sperm. After fertilization, the zygote (the first new cell created after fertilization) begins to divide rapidly until it forms a hollow ball of cells that implants itself onto the uterine wall. Development now proceeds very rapidly. During the next phase, the period of the embryo which lasts for about two months, all of the major organ systems of the body are formed.

One of these systems is the central nervous system, which begins as a primitive neural tube that eventually becomes the spinal cord and brain. One end of the neural tube begins to swell. This swelling will eventually become the brain. Brain cells (neurons and glia cells) begin to proliferate. What happens next is nothing short of miraculous. Guided by radial glia cells, the proliferating neurons migrate to specific locations where they take up permanent residence.

This process is helped by a protein nicknamed sonic hedgehog (after the popular video game), which sends out a signal that helps the migrating neurons find their correct locations. Connections between neurons are formed when the neuron sends out an axon with a growth cone at its tip. This growth cone acts like a bloodhound following a chemical scent that helps the axon find its proper synaptic location. Axons that are produced early in development do not have to worry about other axons getting in the way. In contrast, axons that develop later must weave their way around existing axons by following axon tracts that already exist. Over the course of several months of prenatal development, axons branch out to their designated locations in waves. The net result of all of this guided migration is the brain's intricate network of neurons and synapses.

Toward the end of prenatal development, the proliferation and migration of neurons slows and eventually stops. Thus we are born with all (or nearly all) of the neurons we will have. Although few, if any, new neurons develop after birth, the brain still undergoes considerable development. Axons need to be myelinated, interconnections between neurons must form, and the various parts of the brain must mature. Take, for example, the visual system, which is underdeveloped at birth. During the first six months of life, the brain cells involved in vision mature and vision improves. Generally, the most rapid period of postnatal brain growth spans the first three years of life, during which time, the brain reaches about 80 percent of its adult size.

Two factors affect brain development. First, a genetic code directs the proliferation and migration of neurons and axonal connections. Second, environmental events also can influence brain development. For example, substances known as teratogens (substances that can cause malformations in an unborn child) can have profound effects on the wiring of the brain. One way this happens is by interrupting the normal operation of the sonic hedgehog signaling process sending neurons to the wrong place after migration. For example, alcohol (a powerful teratogen which crosses the placenta very easily) causes neurons to overshoot their destinations in the brain. This results in a jumble of neurons above where the normal surface of the brain should be. This abnormal cell migration is associated with reduced levels of intelligence in children with fetal alcohol syndrome. Other teratogens, for example radiation, cause neurons to undershoot their target locations which also results in mental retardation.

The brain that results from normal prenatal and postnatal development is a complex organ capable of many things. In the sections that follow, we will explore the regions of the brain and see what each of them does for you. We'll use a simple organizational scheme and divide the brain into two parts: the cerebral cortex and everything else, which we will refer to as lower brain centers.

The "Lower" Brain Centers

One morning Cheryl Jones woke up with a blinding headache, which went away almost as fast as it started. Her headache was followed by nausea, dizziness, and loss of motor coordination. On her way to the bathroom she stumbled. She woke her husband who rushed her to the hospital. A CT-scan (a sophisticated X-ray procedure that provides a detailed picture of the brain) quickly revealed that Cheryl had an aneurysm (a ballooning of a blood vessel) the size of a grape at the base of her brain. Without surgery, the aneurysm would surely burst, shutting down Cheryl's critical body functions (breathing and heartbeat) and she would die. Opting for surgery that put not only her life, but the life of her unborn baby at risk, Cheryl and the baby survived.

What could have been so important in the structures at the very base of Cheryl's brain that caused her to risk her life and the life of her child? As we will see, these "lower centers" of the brain contain vital structures involved in regulating crucial, involuntary functions like respiration and heartbeat. Though we call these structures "lower", they are by no means unimportant to an organism's functioning. Lower brain centers are "lower" in two ways. First, they are physically located beneath the cerebral cortex. Second, these brain structures develop first both in an evolutionary sense and within the developing human brain. They are the structures we most clearly share with other animals. In no way are these centers less important. As you will soon see, our very survival depends on them. Use Figure 3.8 as a guide to locate the various structures as we discuss them.

The Brain Stem

As you look at the spinal cord and brain, you cannot tell where one ends and the other begins. There is no abrupt division of these two aspects of the central nervous system. Just above the spinal cord there is a slight widening of the cord that suggests the transition to brain tissue. Here two important structures form the brain stem: the medulla and the pons.

The lowest structure in the brain is the medulla. In many ways, the medulla acts like the spinal cord in that its major functions involve involuntary reflexes. There are several small structures called nuclei (collections of neural cell bodies) in the medulla that control such functions as coughing, sneezing, tongue movements, and reflexive eye movements. You don't have to think about blinking your eye as something rushes toward it, for example; your medulla produces that eye blink reflexively.

The medulla also contains nuclei that control breathing reflexes and monitor the muscles of the heart to keep it beating rhythmically. We can exercise some voluntary control over the nuclei of the medulla, but only within limits. For example, the medulla controls our respiration (breathing), but we can override the medulla and hold our breath. We cannot, however, hold our breath until we die. We can hold our breath until we lose consciousness, which is to say until we give up voluntary control; then the medulla takes over and breathing continues.

At the level of the medulla, most nerve fibers to and from the brain cross from right to left and vice versa. Centers in the left side of the brain receive impulses from and send impulses to the right side of the body, although some are also sent to the left side. Similarly, the left side of the body sends impulses to, and receives messages from, the right side of the brain (which explains why electrically stimulating the correct area in the left side of the brain produces a movement in the right arm). This arrangement of fibers crossing from one side of the body to the opposite side of the brain is called cross laterality (also known as contralateral control, and it takes place in the brain stem). Note that there is some same-side control. The left side of the brain has some control over the left side of the body, and the right side of the brain has some control over the right side of the body. This control is known as ipsilateral control. Ipsilateral control is extremely limited.

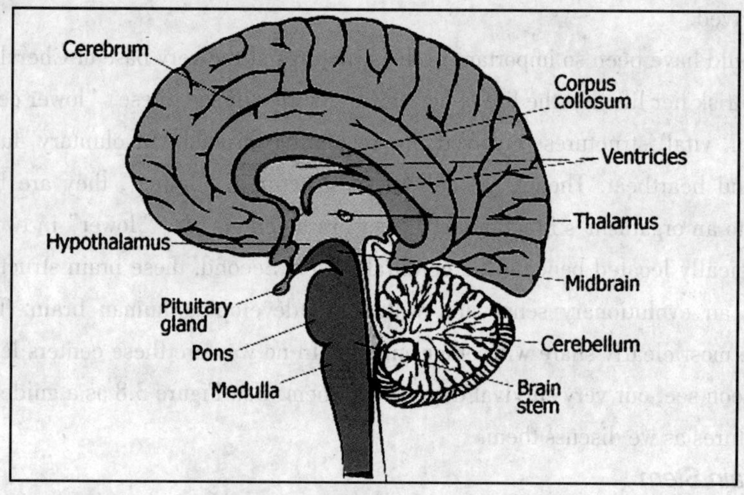

Figure 3.8 the Brain Stem

Just above the medulla is a structure called the pons. (The pons is one structure; there is no such thing as a "pon"). The pons serves as a relay station or bridge (which is what pons means), sorting out and relaying sensory messages from the spinal cord and the face up to higher brain centers and reversing the relay for motor impulses coming down from higher centers. The cross laterality that begins in the medulla continues in the pons.

Nuclei in the pons are also responsible, at least in part, for the rapid movement of our eyes that occurs when we dream. Other centers in the pons are involved in determining our cycles of being awake and being asleep.

The Cerebellum

The cerebellum sits behind your pons, tucked up under the base of your skull. Your cerebellum (literally, "small brain") is about the size of your closed fist and is the second largest part of your brain. Its outer region (its cortex) is convoluted — the tissue is folded in upon itself creating many deep crevices and lumps.

The major role of the cerebellum is to smooth and coordinate rapid body movements. Most intentional voluntary movements originate in higher brain centers (usually the motor area of the cerebral cortex) and are coordinated by the cerebellum. Because of the close relationship between body movement and vision, many eye movements originate in the cerebellum.

Our ability to stoop, pick a dime off the floor, and slip it into our pocket involves a complex series of movements made smooth and coordinated by our cerebellum. When athletes train a movement, such as a golf swing or a gymnastic routine, we may say that they are trying to "get into a groove", so that their trained movements can be made simply and smoothly. In a way, the athletes are training their cerebellums. In fact, the cerebellum plays an important role in making movements that are "ballistic", meaning they occur without any sensory feedback. Examples would be catching a fast line drive hit right to you, playing a well-practiced piano piece, or quickly reaching out to save a priceless vase you just knocked off a table with your elbow. The cerebellum learns to make such movements, and this process is the focus of research by psychobiologists interested in how learning experiences are represented in the brain.

Few of our behaviors are as well-coordinated or as well-learned as the rapid movements we need to speak. The next time you're talking to someone, focus on how quickly and effortlessly your lips, mouth, and tongue, are moving thanks to the cerebellum. Damage to the cerebellum slurs speech. In fact, damage to the cerebellum disrupts all coordinated movements. One may shake and stagger when walking. Someone with cerebellum damage may appear to be drunk. On what region of the brain do you suppose alcohol has a direct effect?

Damage to the cerebellum can disrupt motor activity in other ways. If the outer region of the cerebellum is damaged, tremors, involuntary trembling movements that occur when the person tries to move (called intention tremors) result. Damage to inner, deeper areas of the cerebellum leads to "tremors at rest", and the limbs or head may shake or twitch rhythmically even when the person tries to remain still.

The Reticular Formation

The reticular formation is hardly a brain structure at all. It is a complex network of nerve fibers that begins in the brain stem and works its way up through and around other structures to the top portions of the brain.

What the reticular formation does, and how it does so, remains something of a mystery; however, we do know that it is involved in determining our level of activationor arousal. It influences whether we are awake, asleep, or somewhere in between.

Electrical stimulation of the reticular formation can produce EEG patterns of brain activity associated with alertness. Classic research has shown that lesions of the reticular formation cause a state of constant sleep in laboratory animals. In a way, the reticular formation acts like a valve that either allows sensory messages to pass from lower centers up to the cerebral cortex or shuts them off, partially or totally. We don't know what stimulates the reticular formation to produce these effects.

The Basal Ganglia

A curious set of tissues is the basal ganglia. The basal ganglia are collections of small, loosely connected structures in front of the limbic system. Like the cerebellum, the basal ganglia primarily control motor responses. Unlike the cerebellum, the role of the basal ganglia is involved in the initiation and coordination of large, slow movements. Although the basal ganglia are clearly related to the movements of some of our body's larger muscles, there are no pathways that lead directly from the ganglia down the spinal cord and to those muscles.

Some functions of the basal ganglia have become clearer as we have come to understand Parkinson's disease, a disorder involving the basal ganglia in which the most noticeable symptoms are impairment of movement and involuntary tremors. At first there may be a tightness or stiffness in the fingers or limbs. As the disease progresses, it becomes difficult, if not impossible, to initiate bodily movements. Walking, once begun, involves a set of stiff, shuffling movements. In advanced cases, voluntary movement of the arms is nearly impossible. Parkinson's disease is more common with increasing age, afflicting approximately 1 percent of the population.

The neurotransmitter dopamine is usually found in great quantity in the basal ganglia. Indeed, the basal ganglia are the source of much of the brain's dopamine. In Parkinson's disease, the cells that produce dopamine die off, and levels of the neurotransmitter in the basal ganglia (and elsewhere) decline. As dopamine levels in the basal ganglia become in sufficient, behavioral consequences are noted as symptoms of the disease. Treatment, you might think, would be to inject dopamine back into the basal ganglia. Unfortunately, that isn't possible. There's simply no way to get the chemical in there so that it will stay. But another drug, L-dopa (in pill form), has the same effect. L-dopa increases dopamine availability in the basal ganglia, and as a result, the course of the disease is slowed.

One treatment for Parkinson's disease has received considerable attention in the 1900s: the transplantation of the brain cells from fetuses directly into the brain of someone suffering from the disease. After many studies demonstrated that cells from fetuses of rat could grow in the brain of adult and increase the amount of dopamine there, the procedure was tried with human. The result so far has been promising. Studies have shown that transplanting fetal brain cells into the brain of individuals with Parkinson's disease can reverse the course of the disease.

The Thalamus

The thalamus sits just below the cerebral cortex and is involved in its functioning. Like the pons, it is a relay station for impulses traveling to and from the cerebral cortex. Many impulses traveling from the cerebral cortex to lower brain structures, the spinal cord, and the peripheral nervous system pass through the thalamus. Overcoming the normal function of the medulla (eg, by voluntarily holding your breath) involves messages that pass through the thalamus. The major role of the thalamus, however, involves the processing of information from the senses.

In handling incoming sensory impulses, the thalamus collects, organizes, and then directs sensory messages to the appropriate areas of the cerebral cortex. Sensory messages from the lower body, eyes, and ears, (not the nose) pass through the thalamus. For example, at the thalamus, nerve fibers from an eye are spread out and projected onto the back of the cerebral cortex.

Because of its role in monitoring impulses to and from the cerebral cortex, the thalamus has long been suspected to be involved in the control of our sleep-wake cycle. Although the issue is not settled, some evidence suggests that nuclei in the thalamus (as well as the pons) do have a role in establishing a person's normal pattern of sleep and wakefulness.

The Limbic System

The limbic system is actually a collection of structures rather than a single unit. It is important in controlling the behaviors of animals which do not have the large, well-developed cerebral cortexes of humans. In humans, the limbic system controls many of the complex behavioral patterns considered instinctive. The limbic system is in the middle of the brain and comprises several structures including the amygdala, septum, hippocampus, hypothalamus, parts of the thalamus (anterior nuclei) and parts of the basal ganglia. Its major parts are shown in Figure 3.9. Within the human brain, parts of the limbic system are intimately involved in the display of emotional reactions. One structure in the limbic system, the amygdala, produces reactions of rage or aggression when stimulated, while another area, the septum has the opposite effect, reducing the intensity of emotional responses when it is stimulated. The influence of the amygdala and the septum on emotional responding is immediate and direct in nonhumans. In humans, it is more subtle, reflecting the influence of other brain centers. The amygdala also plays an important role in deciding whether a stimulus is dangerous or not.

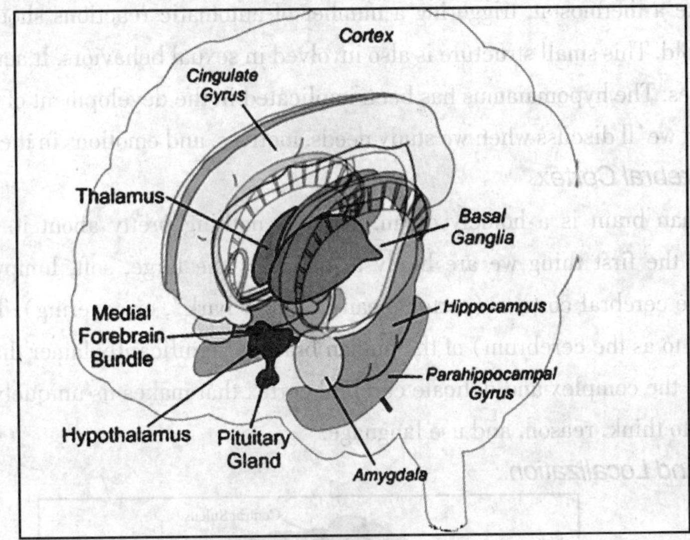

Figure 3.9 Limbic System

Another structure in the limbic system, called the hippocampus, is less involved in emotion and more involved with the formation of memories for experiences. People with a damaged hippocampus are often unable to "transfer" experiences (eg, a birthday party) into permanent memory storage. They may remember events for short periods and may be able to remember events from the distant past, but only if these events occurred before the hippocampus was damaged. Interestingly, hippocampal damage does not interfere significantly with verbal aspects of memory, for example, learning and remembering a list of words.

The hypothalamus is a structure that plays a complex role in motivational and emotional reactions. Among other things, it influences many of the functions of the endocrine system, which, as we have seen, is involved in emotional responding. Actually, the hypothalamus is not a unitary structure; instead it is a collection of smaller structures known as nuclei. Each nucleus plays a different role in the regulation of motivation and emotion.

The major responsibility of the hypothalamus is to monitor critical internal bodily functions. The ventromedial nucleus, for example, mediates feeding behaviors. Destruction of this nucleus in a rat results in a condition called hyperphagia which causes the animal to lose its ability to regulate food intake and become obese. Similarly, the anterior hypothalamus involves the detection of thirst and the regulation of fluid intake.

The hypothalamus also plays a role in aggression. Stimulation of the lateral nucleus in a produces aggression that looks much like predatory behavior. The cat is highly selective in what it attacks and stalks before pouncing. Stimulation of the medial nucleus results in an anger-based aggression. The cat shows the characteristic signs of anger (arched back, ears flattened, hissing and spitting) and will attack anything in its way. Interestingly, the role of the hypothalamus in hunger and aggression is not as simple as it may seem. For example, if you apply mild stimulation to the lateral nucleus, the cat shows signs of hunger (but not aggression). Increase the strength of the stimulation to the same site, and aggression is displayed. The hypomaiamus also acts something like a thermostat, triggering a number of automatic reactions should we become too warm or too cold. This small structure is also involved in sexual behaviors. It acts as a regulator for many hormones. The hypomaiamus has been implicated in the development of sexual orientation, an implication we'll discuss when we study needs, motives, and emotions in the later chapters.

The Cerebral Cortex

The human brain is a homely organ. There's nothing pretty about it. When we look at human brain, the first thing we are likely to notice is the large, soft, lumpy, creviced outer-covering of the cerebral cortex (cortex means "outer bark", or covering). The cerebralcortex (also referred to as the cerebrum) of the human brain is significantly lamer than any other brain structure. It is the complex and delicate cerebral cortex that makes us uniquely human by giving us our ability to think, reason, and use language.

Lobes and Localization

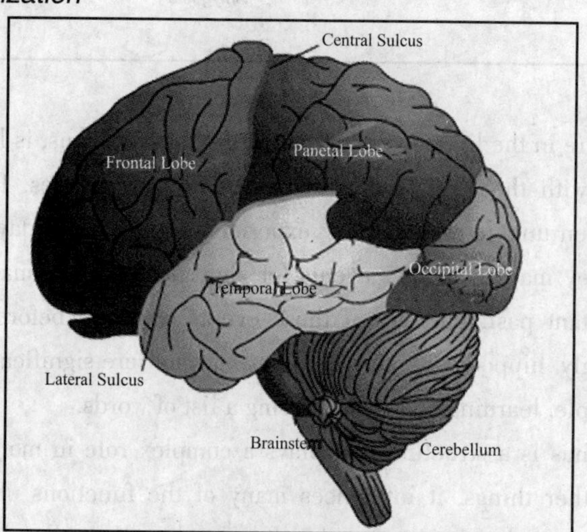

Figure 3.10 Lobes and Localization of Brain

Figure 3.10 presents two views of the cerebral cortex: a top view and a side view. You can see that the deep folds of tissue provide us with markers for dividing the cerebrum into major areas. The most noticeable division of the cortex can be seen in the top view. We clearly see the deep crevice that runs down the middle of the cerebral cortex from front to back, dividing it into the left and right cerebral hemispheres.

A side view of a hemisphere (Figure 3.10 shows us the left one) allows us to see the four major divisions of each hemisphere, called "lobes". The frontal lobes (plural because there is a left and a right) are the largest and are defined by two large crevices called the central fissure and the lateral fissure. The temporal lobes are located at the temples below the lateral fissure, with one on each side of the brain. The occipital lobes, at the back of the brain, are defined somewhat arbitrarily, with no large fissures setting them off, and the parietal lobes are wedged behind the frontal lobes and above the occipital and temporal lobes.

Researchers have learned much about what normally happens in the various regions of the cerebral cortex, but many of the details of cerebral function are yet to be understood. Three major areas have been mapped: sensory areas, where impulses from sense receptors are sent; motor areas, where most voluntary movements originate; and association areas, where sensory and motor functions are integrated, and where higher mental processes are thought to occur. We'll now review each of these in turn, referring to Figure3.10 as we go along.

Sensory Areas

Let's review for a minute. Receptor cells (specialized neurons) in our sense organs respond to stimulus energy from the environment. These cells then pass neural impulses along sensory nerve fibers, eventually to the cerebral cortex. Senses in our body below our neck first send impulses to the spinal cord. Then, it's up the spinal cord, through the brain stem, where they cross from left to right and from right to left, on up to the thalamus, and beyond to the cerebrum. After impulses from our senses leave the thalamus, they go to a sensory area, an area of the cerebral cortex that receives impulses from our senses. The sensory area involved depends on the sense that was activated.

Large areas of the cerebral cortex are involved with vision and hearing. Virtually the entire occipital lobe processes visual information (labeled "visual area" in Figure 3.11). Auditory (hearing) impulses take up large centers ("auditory areas") in the temporal lobes. In addition to being involved in hearing, the undersides of the temporal lobes have a curious function. If certain parts of the underside of the temporal lobes are damaged, a condition called prosopagnosia exists. In this curious disorder, a person loses the ability to recognize faces (but not voices). Remember the story about your friend who was in a motorcycle accident, with which we began this chapter? Where do you think he had brain damage?

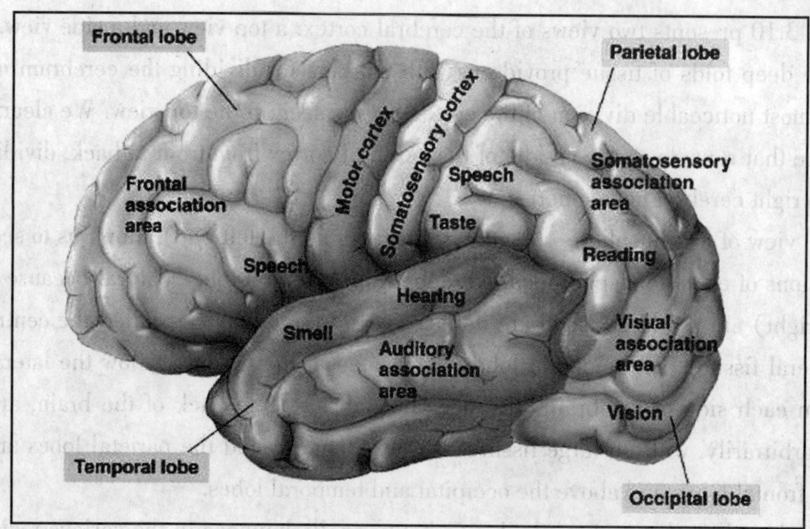

Figure 3.11 Sensory Areas of Brain

Our bodily senses (touch, pressure, pain, etc.) send impulses to a strip at the very front of the parietal lobe (labeled "body sense area" in Figure 3.11). In this area of the parietallobe, we can map out specific regions that correspond to various parts of the body. When we do so, we find that some body parts — the face, lips, and fingertips, for example are over represented in the body sense area of the cerebral cortex, reflecting their high sensitivity. In other words, some parts of the body, even some very small ones, are processed in larger areas of the cortex than are other parts.

Finally, let's remind ourselves of cross laterality, the crossing over of information from senses on the left side of the body to the right side of the brain, and vice versa, that occurs in the brain stem. When someone touches your right arm, that information ends up in your left parietal lobe. A tickle to your left foot is processed by the right side of your cerebral cortex.

Motor Areas

We have seen that some of our actions, at least very simple and reflexive ones, originate below the cerebral cortex. Although lower brain centers, such as the basal ganglia, maybe involved, most voluntary activity originates in the motor areas of the cerebral cortex in strips at the very back of our frontal lobes. These areas (remember, there are two of them, left and right) are directly across the central fissure from the body sense areas in the parietal lobe (see Figure 3.11). We need to make the disclaimer that the actual, thoughtful, decision-making process of whether one should move probably occurs elsewhere, almost certainly farther forward in the frontal lobes.

Electrical stimulation techniques have allowed us to map locations in the motor areas that correspond to, or control, specific muscles or muscle groups. As is the case for sensory processing, we find that some muscle groups (such as those that control movements of the hands and mouth) are represented by disproportionally larger areas of cerebral cortex.

We also find cross laterality at work with the motor area. It is your right hemisphere's motor area that controls movements of the left side of your body, and the left hemisphere's motor area that controls the right side. Someone who has suffered a cerebral stroke (a disruption of blood flow in the brain that results in the loss of neural tissue) in the left side of the brain will have impaired movement in the right side of his or her body.

Association Areas

Once we have located the areas of the cerebral cortex that process sensory information and originate motor responses, we still have a lot of cortex left. The remaining areas of the cerebral cortex are called association areas, which are areas of the cerebrum where sensory input is integrated with motor responses, and where cognitive functions such as problem solving, memory, and thinking occur. There are three association areas in each hemisphere: frontal, parietal, and temporal. The occipital lobe is so "filled" with visual processing, there is no room left over for an occipital association area.

There is considerable support for the idea that so-called higher mental processes occur in the association areas. Frontal association areas are involved in many such processes. For instance, more than a century ago, Pierre-Paul Broca (1824–1880) discovered that speech production and some other language behaviors are localized in the left frontal association area. Broca's conclusions were based on observations he made of human brains during autopsy. Persons with similar speech disorders commonly had noticeable damage in the very same region of the left hemisphere of the cerebral cortex. Logic led Broca to suspect that normal speech functions are controlled by this portion of the brain, which we now call Brocas area (see Figure 3.12). Broca's area controls the production of speech. That is, it coordinates the actual functions needed to express an idea. A person with damage to Broca's area shows an interesting pattern of speech defects. If asked a question, such as "Where is your car?" a person with Broca's area damage could communicate to you the location of his or her car, but only in broken, forced language. For example, the person might say, "Car ... lot ... parked by ... supermarket."

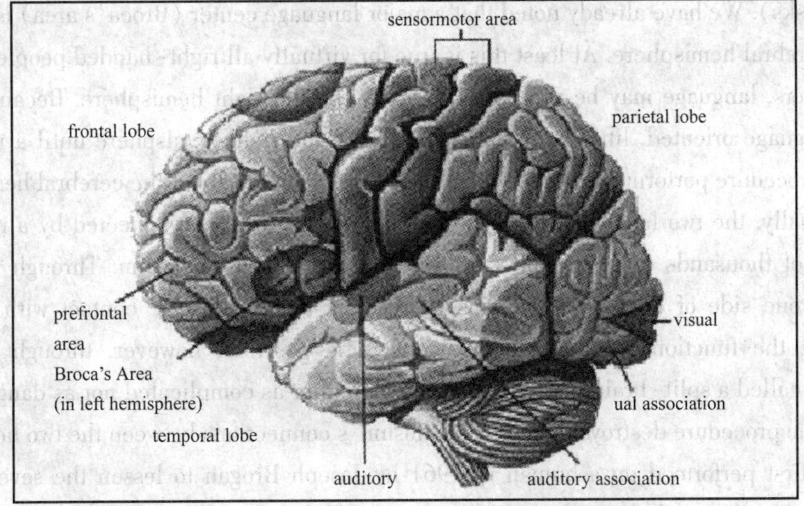

Figure 3.12 Broca Area

Another part of the brain involved in language and speech is Wernicke's area, which is involved in speech comprehension and organizing ideas. A bundle of nerve fibers connects Wemicke's and Broca's areas so that the language comprehended and organized in Wernicke's area is transmitted to Broca's area, which then coordinates the speech output. If Wemicke's area is damaged (or if the fibers connecting it to Broca's area are damaged), a different speech problem is manifested. If a person with Wernicke's area damage is asked where her car is parked the answer that comes out will be in beautiful, grammatically correct language. The only catch is that it will make no sense whatsoever. For example, the person might say, "Isn't the seashore beautiful this time of year?"

Damage to the very front of the right frontal lobe or to an area where the parietal and temporal lobes come together often interrupts or destroys the ability to plan ahead, to think quickly, or to think things through. Interestingly, these association areas of the brain involved in forethought and planning nearly cease to function when we are feeling particularly happy.

We should not get carried away with cerebral localization of function. Let's not fall into the trap of believing that separate parts of the cerebral cortex operate independently and have the sole responsibility for any one function. This will be particularly important to cerebral cortex. keep in mind as we look at the division of the cerebral cortex into right and left hemispheres.

The Two Cerebral Hemispheres: Splitting the Brain

The ancient Greeks knew that the cerebral cortex was divided into two major section, or hemispheres. That the cerebral cortex is divided in half seems quite natural. After all, we have two eyes, arms, legs, lungs, and so forth. Why not two division of the brain? In the last thirty years, interest in this division into hemispheres has heightened as scientists have accumulated evidence that suggests that each half of the cerebral cortex may have primary responsibility for its own set of mental functions.

In most humans, the left hemisphere is the larger of the two halves, contains a higher proportion of gray matter, and is considered the dominant hemisphere (active to a greater degree in more tasks). We have already noted that a major language center (Broca's area) is housed in the left cerebral hemisphere. At least this is true for virtually all right-handed people. For some left-handers, language may be processed primarily by the right hemisphere. Because humans are so language oriented, little attention was given to the right hemisphere until a remarkable surgical procedure performed in the 1960s gave us new insights about the cerebral hemispheres.

Normally, the two hemispheres of the cerebral cortex are interconnected by a net work of hundreds of thousands of fibers collectively called the corpus callosum. Through the corpus callosum, one side of our cortex remains in constant and immediate contact with the other. Separating the functions of the two hemispheres is possible, however, through a surgical technique called a split-brain procedure, which is neither as complicated nor as dangerous as it sounds. The procedure destroys the corpus callosum's connections between the two hemispheres and was, first performed on a human in 1961 by Joseph Brogan to lessen the severity of the symptoms of epilepsy. As an irreversible treatment of last resort, the split-brain procedure has been very successful.

Most of what we know about the activities of the cerebral hemispheres has been learned from split brain subjects, both human and animal. One of the things that makes this procedure remarkable is that under normal circumstances split - brain patients behave normally. Only in the laboratory using specially designed tasks can we see the results of independently functioning hemispheres of the cerebral cortex.

Experiments with split brain patients confirm that speech production is a left - hemisphere function in a majority of people. Imagine you have your hands behind your back. I place a house key in your left hand and ask you to tell me what it is. Your left hand feels the key. Impulses travel up your left arm, up your spinal cord, and cross over to your right cerebral hemisphere (remember cross laterality). You tell me that the object in your hand is a key because your brain is intact. Your right hemisphere passes information about the key to your left hemisphere, and your left hemisphere directs you to say, "It's a key."

Now suppose that you are a split - brain subject. You cannot answer my question even though you understand it perfectly. Why not? Your right brain knows that the object in your left hand is a key, but without an intact corpus callosum, it cannot inform the left hemisphere where speech production is located. Under the direction of the right cerebral hemisphere, you would be able to point out with your left hand the key from among other objects placed before you. Upon seeing this, your eyes would communicate that information to your left hemisphere.

A major task for the left hemisphere is the production of speech and processing of language. But, we must be cautious about making too much of the specialization of function. When the results of the original split - brain research were published, many drew faulty conclusions. We now know that virtually no behavior, or mental process, is the product of the operation of one hemisphere alone . For example, Gazzaniga reports that one split - brain patient learned to speak from the right hemisphere 13 years after surgery severing the corpus callosum. This individual can report on information verbally, regardless of which hemisphere receives the information. Further, although the left hemisphere is dominant for language, the right hemisphere does do some language processing even if full language functions are not present. For example, the right hemisphere is involved in processing common phrases and cliches, such as "have a nice day". Thus, it is more reasonable to say that one hemisphere is dominant with respect to a given task, or that one hemisphere may be better than the other at processing certain types of information.

Despite the early over interpretation of findings from split - brain research, most of the research conducted shows a remarkable amount of hemispheric specialization. Gazzaniga points out that split - brain research has led to the conclusion that brain modules develop in the brain. Each module is designed to carry out a specific function. When the brain is split, modules devoted to specific functions are not affected. So when the brain is split, the left hemisphere retains its superior linguistic ability, presumably because the modules needed for language processing are located in the left hemisphere. The information processing modules in the left hemisphere also function better with information that comes in serially, one piece at a time, although the data in this area are tenuous. Finally, the left hemisphere also has an interpreter mechanism that can create explanations for events presented to the right hemisphere in a split-brain patient. Gazzaniga and his colleagues selectively presented information to the right and left hemispheres. When tested, the right hand correctly identified the picture presented to the left hemisphere, and the left hand did the same for the information presented to the right hemisphere. However, when the patient was asked why the left hand was pointing to a given picture, the left hemisphere instantly made up an explanation to fit the situation.

What about the right hemisphere? The clearest evidence is that the right hemisphere dominates the processing of visually presented information. Putting together a jigsaw puzzle, for instance, uses the right hemisphere more than the left. Skill in the visual arts (eg, painting, drawing, and sculpting) is associated with the right hemisphere. It is involved in the interpretation of emotional stimuli and in the expression of emotions. While the left hemisphere is analytical and sequential, the right hemisphere is considered better able to grasp the big picture the overall view of things and tends to be somewhat creative.

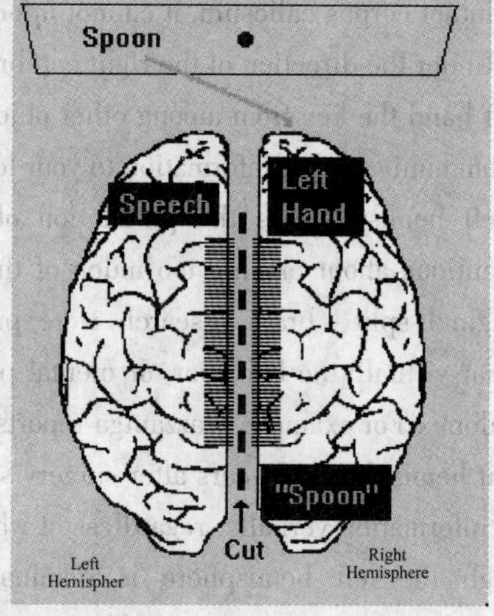

So, say a "typical" (language in the LEFT hemisphere) split-brain patient is sitting down, looking straight ahead and is focusing on a dot in the middle of a screen. Then a picture of a spoon is flashed to the right of the dot. The visual information about the spoon crosses in the optic chiasm and ends up in the LEFT HEMISPHERE. When the person is asked what the picture was, the person has no problem identifying the spoon and says "Spoon." However, if the spoon had been flashed to the left of the dot (see the picture), then the visual information would have traveled to the RIGHT HEMISPHERE. Now if the person is asked what the picture was, the person will say that nothing was seen!! But, when this same person is asked to pick out an object using only the LEFT hand, this person will correctly pick out the spoon. This is because touch information from the left hand crosses over to the right hemisphere — the side that "saw" the spoon. However, if the person is again asked what the object is, even when it is in the person's hand, the person will NOT be able to say what it is because the right hemisphere cannot "talk". So, the right hemisphere is not stupid, it just has little ability for language — it is

"*non-verbal*".

These possibilities are intriguing. While it seems that there are differences in the way the two sides of the cerebral cortex normally process information, these differences are slight and many are controversial. In fact, the more we study hemispheric differences, the more we discover similarities.

Chapter 4 Sensory and Perception

This Topic introduces you to sensory processes or sensation. Sensation is the process whereby your sense organs (eg, your eyes, ears, nose) detect external stimuli. Detection of external stimulation is crucial because only those stimuli that you detect can be transmitted to your brain for further processing and interpretation. As you will see in the sections that follow, sensory processes are more complex than meet the eye (no pun intended). We will explore all of your major senses and show how they respond to and transmit sensory information to your brain.

Sensation and Perception

Generally, we divide the initial stages of information processing into two subprocesses: sensation and perception. Sensation is the process of detecting external stimuli and changing those stimuli into nervous system activity. Sensation yields our immediate experience of the stimuli in our environment. The psychology of sensation deals with how our various senses do what they do. Sense receptors are the specialized neural cells in sense organs that change physical energy into neural impulses. In other words, each of our sense receptors is a transducer — a mechanism that converts energy from one form to another. A light bulb is a transducer. It converts electrical energy into light energy (and a little heat energy). Your eye is a sense organ that contains sense receptors that transducer light energy into neural energy. Your ear is a sense organ that contains sense receptors that transduce the mechanical energy of sound waves into neural energy.

Compared to sensation, perception is a more active, complex, even creative, process. It acts on stimulation received and recorded by the senses. Perception is a process that involves the selection, organization, and interpretation of stimuli. Perception is more cognitive and central process than sensation. We say that our senses present us with information about the world in which we live, whereas perception represent that information, often flavored by our motivational states, our expectation, and our past experience. In other words, we sense the presence of a stimulus, but we perceive what it is.

Sensory Processes

In this Topic, we explore how our senses detect and respond to external stimulation. However, before we get into the story of how each of our sense organs goes about transducing physical energy from the environment into neural energy, we'll consider a few concepts common to all of our senses.

Sensory Thresholds

Think about an electronic device that runs on a solar battery, for example, a calculator. If you use it in the dark, it will not work. In dim light, you might see some signs of life from the calculator. In bright light, the calculator functions fully: the display is bright and easy to read, and all of its features work properly. The calculator's power cell requires a minimum amount of light to power the calculator sufficiently. This is the threshold level of stimulation for that device. Light intensities below the threshold will not allow the electronics of the calculator to work. Light intensities at or above the threshold allow the calculator to operate properly.

Your sense organs operate in a manner similar to the photoelectric cell in the calculator. A minimum intensity of a stimulus must be present for the sense organ to transducer the external physical stimulus from the environment (for example, light, sound, pressure on your skin) into a neural impulse that your nervous system can interpret. This intensity is known as the sensory threshold, or the minimum intensity of a stimulus needed to operate your sense organs.

Physiologists and psychologists have studied sensory thresholds for over a century. This was one of the pioneering areas of research in the early days that led to psychology's emergence as a separate science. Psychophysics is the study of relationships between the physical attributes of stimuli and the psychological experiences they produce. It is one of the oldest subfields of psychology. Many methods of psychophysics were developed before Wundt opened his psychology laboratory in Leipzig in 1879.

There are two ways to think about psychophysics. First, at an applied level, we can say that the techniques of psychophysics are designed to assess the sensitivity of our senses providing answers to such questions as, "Just how good is your hearing after all these years of playing in a rock band?" Second, at a theoretical level, psychophysics provides a systematic means of relating the physical world to the psychological world. Now we might ask, "How much of a change in the physical intensity of this sound will it take for you to experience a difference in loudness?" Most psychophysical methods are designed to measure sensory thresholds, indicators of the sensitivity of our sense receptors. There are two types of sensory thresholds: absolute thresholds and difference thresholds.

Absolute Thresholds

Imagine the following experiment. You are seated in a dimly-lighted room staring at a small box. The side of the box facing you is covered by a sheet of plastic. Behind the plastic is a light bulb. The physical intensity of the light bulb can be decreased to the point where you cannot see it at all. The light's intensity can also be increased so that you can see it very clearly. There are many intensity settings between these extremes. At what point of physical intensity will the light first become visible to you? Common sense suggests that there should be a level of intensity below which you cannot see the light and above which you can. That level is your absolute threshold. In other words, sensory thresholds are inversely related to sensitivity. That is, as threshold values decrease, sensitivity increases. The lower the threshold of a sense receptor, the more sensitive it is.

Let's return to our imaginary experiment. The light's intensity is repeatedly varied, and you are asked to respond, "Yes, I see the light," or "No, I don't see the light." (In this experiment, you won't be allowed the luxury of saying you don't know or aren't sure.)

When this experiment is done, we discover something that seems strange. The intensity of the light can be reduced so low that you never report seeing it, and the light can be presented at intensities so high that you always say you see them. However, there are light intensities to which you sometimes respond "yes" and sometimes respond "no", even though the physical intensity of the light is constant.

In reality, there isn't much about absolute thresholds that is absolute. They change from moment to moment, reflecting subtle changes in the sensitivity of our senses. They also reflect such factors as momentary shifts in our ability to pay attention to the task at hand and the issue we'll get back to soon. Because there are no absolute measures of sensory sensitivity, psychologists use the following operational definition of absolute threshold: the physical intensity of a stimulus that a person reports detecting 50 percent of the time. In other words, Intensities below threshold are those detected less than 50 percent of the time, and intensities above threshold are those detected more than 50 percent of the time. This complication occurs for all of our senses, not dust vision.

What good is the concept of absolute threshold? Determining absolute thresholds is not just an academic exercise. Absolute threshold levels as a measure of sensitivity are used to determine if one's senses are operating properly and detecting low levels of stimulation (which is what happens when you have your hearing tested, for example). Engineers who design sound systems need to know about absolute thresholds; stereo speakers that do not reproduce sounds above threshold levels aren't of much use. Warning lights must be well above absolute threshold to be useful. How much perfume do you need to use for it to be noticed? How low must you whisper so as not to be overheard in a classroom?

Difference Thresholds

Imagine that one day a friend makes a claim that you just can't believe. She states that she can tell the difference between the tastes of the various colored candies. That is, she claims that she can tell the difference in taste between a red candies and a brown candies. Of course, you are skeptical and decide to test her amazing taste abilities. You setup an experiment. You blindfold your friend and feed her pairs of M&Ms, one at a time, giving her a small drink of water between each one. Sometimes you give her pairs of candies that have different colors, and other times you give her pairs of the same color. You keep track of the number of times she correctly discriminates between the pairs of candies. To your amazement, your friend can tell the difference between the differently colored candies!

The truth is, we don't often encounter situations that test our abilities to detect differences between or among very low-intensity stimuli as in our M&M test. However, we are often called upon to detect differences between or among stimuli that are above our absolute thresholds. The issue is not whether the stimuli can be detected, but whether they are in some way different from each other. So, a difference threshold is the smallest difference between stimulus attributes that can be detected. As you may have anticipated, we encounter the same complication as when we try to measure absolute thresholds. One's difference threshold for any stimulus attribute varies slightly from moment to moment. So, again we say that to be above one's difference threshold, differences between stimuli must be detected more than 50 percent of the time (see Figure 4.1).

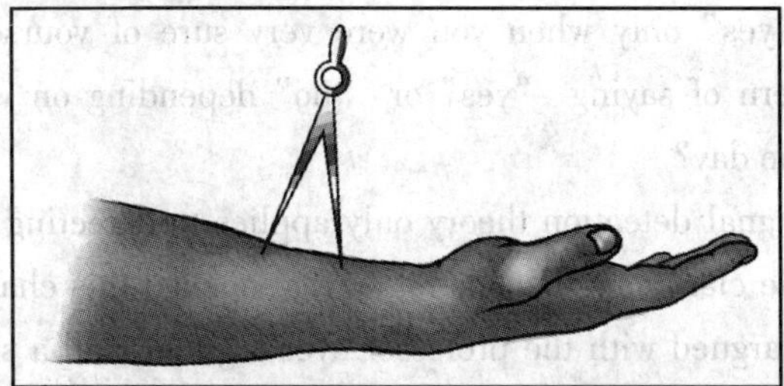

Figure 4.1 Difference Thresholds

Here's an example. You are presented with two tones. You hear them both (they are above your absolute threshold), and you report that they are equally loud. If I gradually increase the intensity of one of the tones, I will eventually reach a point at which you can just detect a difference in the loudness of the tones. This just noticeable difference, the amount of change in a stimulus that makes it just noticeably different from what it was.

The concept of just noticeable difference is relevant in many contexts. A parent tells a teenager to "turn down that stereo!" The teenager reduces the volume, but not by a noticeable difference from the parent's perspective, and trouble may be brewing. Does the color of the shoes match the color of the dress closely enough? Can anyone notice the difference between the expensive ingredients in the stew and the cheaper ones?

Signal Detection

When we are asked to determine if a stimulus has been presented, we are being asked to judge if we can detect a signal against a background of other stimuli and randomly changing neural activity called "noise". When we consider thresholds this way, we are using the basics of signal detection theory. Signal detection theory states that stimulus detection is a decision-making process of determining if a signal exists against a background of noise.

According to this point of view, one's absolute threshold is influenced by many factors in addition to the actual sensitivity of one's senses. Random nervous system activity has to be accounted for, as do the person's attention, expectations, and biases. For example, in experiments that determine one's absolute threshold, people are more likely to respond positively when asked if they can detect a stimulus. In other words, when in doubt, people simply have a tendency to say "yes" more often than "no".

Remember the absolute threshold study with which we began our discussion of psychophysics? The intensity of a light in a box changed and you were asked if you could notice. Your absolute threshold was the intensity of light to which you responded "yes" 50 percent of the time. Signal detection theory considers all of the factors that might have prompted you to say "yes" at any exposure to the light. What might some of these factors be? One might be the overall amount of light in the room. Wouldn't you be more likely to detect the signal of the light in a room that was totally dark as opposed to a room in which all of the lights were on? What if you were offered a $5 reward each time you detected the light? Wouldn't you tend to say "yes" more often, whether you were really sure of yourself or not? By the same token, if we were to fine you $1 for each time you said "yes" when the light was not really on, might you not become more conservative, saying "yes" only when you were very sure of yourself? Might we expect a difference in your pattern of saying "yes" or "no" depending on whether you were tested midmorning or late in the day?

If you think that signal detection theory only applies to detecting lights in boxes, you are wrong. Think back to the classroom demonstration that opened this chapter. An irate "student" came into a classroom, argued with the professor over a grade, and a shot was fired. Following the event, the professor asked the students to write down everything they had seen. As you may recall, the students' memories were not terribly accurate. Now, let's do things a bit differently. Instead of having the students recall what took place, ask them to pick the irate student out of a lineup. Let's say that a short time after the incident, six males are brought to the front of the room, and each student is asked if the irate student is present in the lineup. In this situation, we are asked to determine if the perpetrator (the irate student) is or is not in the lineup, which is a signal detection task.

Sensory Adaptation

Sensory adaptation occurs when our sensory experience decreases with continued exposure to a stimulus. There are many examples of sensory adaptation. When we jump into a pool or lake, the water feels very cold. After a few minutes, we adapt and are reassuring our friends to "Come on in; the water's fine." When we walk into a house in which cabbage is cooking, the odor is nearly overwhelming, but soon we adapt and do not notice it. When the compressor motor of the refrigerator turns on, it seems to make a terribly loud noise which we soon do not notice until the motor stops and silence returns to the kitchen.

There is an important psychological implication in these common examples of sensory adaptation: One's ability to detect the presence of a stimulus depends in large measure on the extent to which our sense receptors are being newly stimulated or have adapted. Our sense receptors respond best to changes in stimulation. The constant stimulation of a receptor leads to adaptation and less of a chance that the stimulation will be detected.

There is an exception to this use of the term adaptation. What happens when you move from a brightly lit area to a dimly lit one? You enter a darkened movie theater on a sunny afternoon. At first you can barely see, but in a few minutes, you see reasonably well. What happened? We say that your eyes have "adapted to the dark". Here we use the term adaptation differently. Dark adaptation refers to the process in which the visual receptors become more sensitive with time spent in the dark. There is also light adaptation which occurs when you move from a darkened area to a lighted one. For example, imagine you need to use the bathroom in the middle of the night. You stumble out of bed and head to the bathroom. Without thinking, you reach for the light switch and are nearly blinded by the light, which, as you know, can even be painful. After a short period of time, you adapt to the light and are no longer bothered by it. This occurs because while you are asleep, your eyes are maximally dark adapted (that is they are very sensitive to light). When you turn on the light, the visual sense receptors in your eyes fire all at once, flooding your brain with visual stimulation. It takes a shorter period of time for your eyes to light adapt than it takes then to dark adapt.

The Stimulus for Vision

The stimulus for vision is light, which travels in waves. The amplitude (wave height) is associated with the sensory experience of brightness; the wavelength determines the hue (color) of the light; and the wave purity (whether there is more than one type of wave) produces the psychological experience of saturation.

The Receptor for Vision: The Eye

Vision involves changing, or transducing, light wave energy into the neural energy of thenervous system, ie, causing neurons to transmit impulses to the brain. The sense receptorfor vision is the eye. The eye is a complex organ comprising several structures, most of which are involved in focusing light on the back of the eye where transduction of lightenergy into neural energy takes place.

Light travels to the eye and passes through the cornea, the pupil (regulated in size by the iris), and the lens and then moves to the retina, where it strikes the photoreceptors for vision, the cones and the rods. The cones, in the center (fovea) of the retina, are responsible for color vision, and operate best in intense illumination. The rods are important for night vision and peripheral vision and have a greater density at the edge of the retina. Visual information proceeds from the eye through optic nerves attached to the retina at the back of each eye; the optic nerves meet and then divide at the optic chiasm in the center of the brain (Figure 4.2). The lateral portion of each optic nerve travels from the optic chiasm to the lateral visual cortex on the same side of the brain (that is, the outside of the right nerve to right visual cortex and the outside of the left nerve to the left visual cortex). However, the medial portion of each nerve crosses over at the optic chiasm and goes to the medial visual cortex on the other side of the brain (medial right nerve to left medial visual cortex and medial left nerve to right medial visual cortex).

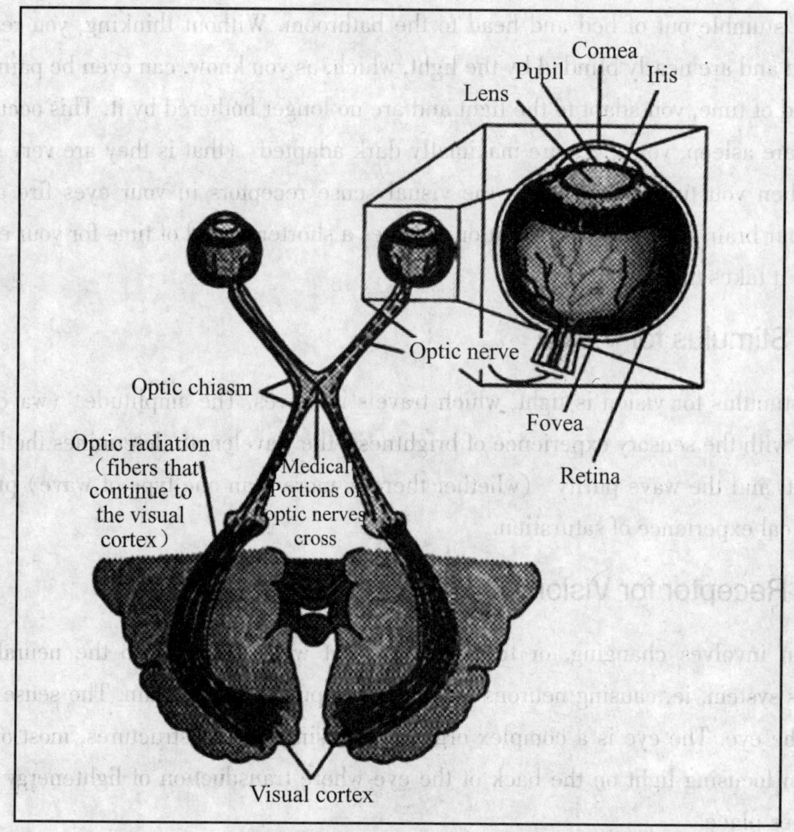

Figure 4.2 The Vision System

As we discussed in the previous section, sensation is the process of detecting various stimuli from the environment around us. The physical stimulus for vision is electromagnetic energy, or light waves, which are measured in nanometers (nm), or one billionth of a meter. Of the full spectrum of electromagnetic radiation, only the narrow band between 400 nm (blue-violet) and 700 nm (red) are visible to the human eye. Why is our visual spectrum so limited? The most likely answer is that our visual system evolved in the sun's light. Thus, our visual system is able to perceive the range of energy emitted by the sun, which by the time it reaches the earth is strongest in the 400–700 nanometer range, (Figure 4.3).

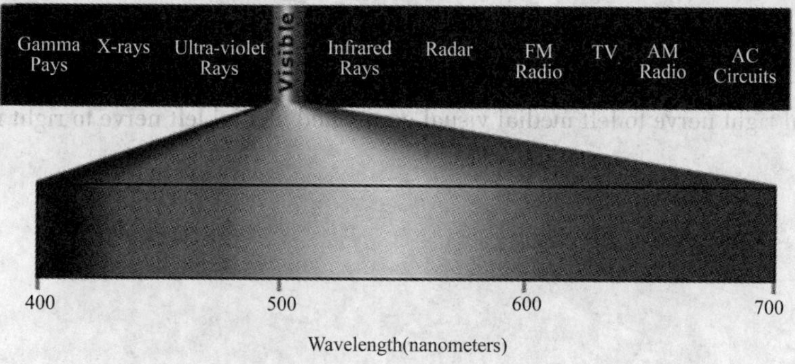

Figure 4.3 Spectrum of Electromagnetic Radiation

Light waves are usually defined by their wavelength or frequency (the distance from the peak of one wave to the peak of the next), their amplitude (ie, wave height), and their purity (ie, saturation). Shorter wavelengths are higher in frequency, as reflected in blue colors, and longer wavelengths are lower in frequency, as reflected in red colors. In addition, light waves of greater amplitude make up brighter light and light waves of shorter amplitude make up dimmer light.

Take a moment to explore this relationship in the below animation. Notice how the hue changes as the wavelength size increases and the intensity or brightness of the hues varies depending on the wave's amplitude.

Color Vision and Color Blindness

Explaining how the eye responds to various intensities of light is simple. High-intensity lights cause more rapid firings of neural impulses than do low-intensity lights, and high-intensity lights stimulate more cells to fire than do lights of low-intensity. How the eye responds to differing wavelengths of light to produce differing experiences of color, however, is another story. Here things are not simple at all. Two theories of color vision, proposed many years ago, have received research support. As is often the case with competing theories that explain the same phenomenon, both are probably partially correct.

The older of the two theories of color vision is the trichromatic theory. It was first proposed by Thomas Young early in the nineteenth century and was revised by Hermannvon Helmholtz, a noted physiologist, about 50 years later. As its name suggests, the trichromatic theory proposes that the eye contains three distinct receptors for color. Although there is some overlap, each receptor responds best to one of three primary hues of light: red, green, or blue. These hues are primary because the careful combination of the three produces all other colors. This happens every day on your TV screen because the picture consists of a pattern of very small red, green, or blue dots. From these three wavelengths, all other colors are constructed or integrated. (Don't confuse the three primary hues with the primary colors of pigment, which are red, blue, and yellow. The primary colors of paint, dye, pastel, etc., can be mixed together to form all other pigment colors. Our eyes respond to light, not pigment, and the three primary hues of light are red, green, and blue.)

Because the sensitivity of the three types of receptors overlaps, when our eyes are stimulated by a nonprimary color, for example, orange, the orange-hued light stimulates each receptor to varying degrees to produce the experience of orange. What gives this theory credibility is that there are such receptor cells in the human retina: cones, which are responsible for color vision. The relative sensitivity of these three cone systems is shown, see Figure 4.4.

Ewald Hering thought the Young-Helmholtz theory left a bit to be desired, and in 1870 he proposed the opponent-process theory. Hering believed there are three pairs of visual mechanisms that respond to different wavelengths of light: a blue-yellow processor, a red-green processor, and a black-white processor.

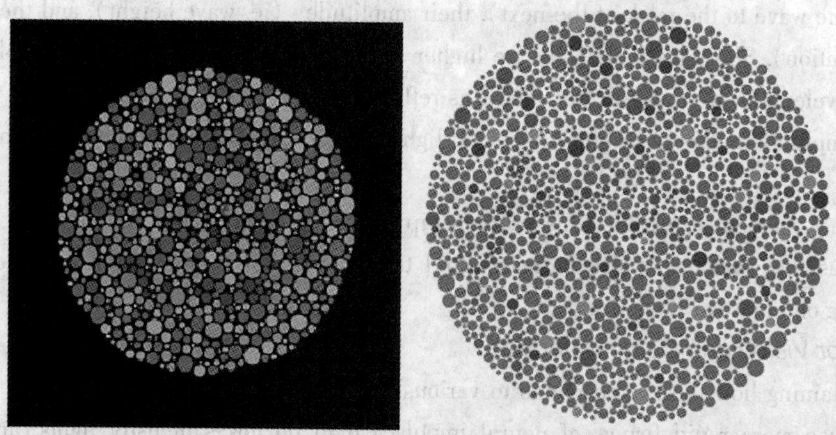

Figure 4.4 Color Blindness

Each mechanism is capable of responding to either of the two hues that give it its name, but not both. That is, the blue-yellow processor can respond to blue or to yellow, but cannot handle both simultaneously. The second mechanism responds to red or to green, but not both. The third mechanism codes brightness. Thus, the members of each pair work in opposition, hence the theory's name. If blue is excited, yellow is inhibited. If red is excited, green is inhibited. A light may appear to be a mixture of red and yellow, but it cannot be seen as a mixture of red and green because red and green cannot be excited at the same time. (It is difficult to imagine what "reddish green" or "bluish yellow" would look like. Can you picture a light that is bright and dim at the same time?

Although the opponent-process theory may seem complicated, there are some strong signs that Hering was on the right track. Excitatory-inhibitory mechanisms such as he proposed for red-green, blue-yellow, and black-white have been found. They are not at the level of rods and cones in the retina as Hering thought, but at the layer of the ganglion cells and in a small area of the thalamus.

Support for Hering's theory also comes from our experiences with negative afterimages. If you stare at a bright green figure for a few minutes and then shift your gaze to a white surface, you notice an image of a red figure. Where did that come from? While you stared at the green figure, the green component of the red-green process fatigued because of the stimulation it received. When you stared at the white surface, the red and green components were equally stimulated; but because the green component was fatigued, the red predominated and produced the image of a red figure.

Evidence supporting both theories of normal color vision comes from studies of persons with color vision defects. Defective color vision of some sort occurs in about 8 percent of males and slightly less than 0.5 percent of females. Most cases are genetic. It makes sense that if cones are our receptor cells for the discrimination of color, people with some deficiency in color perception would have a problem with their cones. This is consistent with the Young-Helmholtz theory. In fact, there is a noticeable lack of one particular type of cone in the most common of the color vision deficiencies (dichromatism); which type depends on the color that is "lost".

Those people who are red-green color-blind, for instance, have trouble distinguishing between red and green. People with this type of color blindness also have trouble distinguishing yellow from either red or green. The deficiency is not in actually seeing reds or greens. It is in distinguishing reds and greens from other colors. Put another way, someone who is red-green color-blind can clearly see a bright red apple; it just looks no different than a bright green apple. Some color vision defects can be traced to cones in the retina, but damage to cells higher in the visual pathway is implicated in some rare cases of color vision problems. When such problems do occur, there are losses for both red and green or both yellow and blue as predicted by the opponent-process theory.

The Receptor for Hearing: The ear

Sound, the stimulus for hearing, is made up of a series of pressures, usually of air, that can be represented as waves. Sound waves have three characteristics — amplitude, frequency, and purity — each of which is related to a psychological experience. Greater wave amplitudes are related to greater loudness; wave frequency is related to pitch; and wave purity is related to timbre.

The Hearing System

The outer ear, the pinna, collects sound waves and funnels them through the auditory canal to the eardrum (which separates the outer and middle ears) and causes it to vibrate (See Figure 4.5). The middle ear contains the malleus (hammer), incus (anvil), and stapes (stirrup), which move and transmit the sound to the oval window, which separates the middle ear from the inner ear. Beyond the oval window is the inner ear, whose main structure is the cochlea, a snail-like structure that has a membrane, the basilar membrane, stretched along its length. When the stapes vibrates against the oval window, the fluid in the cochlea moves and causes the basilar membrane to vibrate. The receptors for hearing, the hair cells, lie in the basilar membrane and convert the vibrations into neural impulses. The neural impulses, in turn, move along the auditory nerve to the lower brain stem and then ascend to the auditory part of the thalamus and on to the auditory cortex in the temporal lobe. Input from each ear is received on both sides of the brain.

Hearing is the process by which humans, using ears, detect and perceive sounds. Sounds are pressure waves transmitted through some medium, usually air or water. Sound waves are characterized by frequency (measured in cycles per second, cps, or hertz, Hz) and amplitude, the size of the waves. Low-frequency waves produce low-pitched sounds (such as the rumbling sounds of distant thunder) and high-frequency waves produce high-pitched sounds (such as a mouse squeak). Sounds audible to most humans range from as low as 20 Hz to as high as 20,000 Hz in a young child (the upper range especially decreases with age). Loudness is measured in decibels (dB), a measure of the energy content or power of the waves proportional to amplitude. The decibel scale begins at 0 for the lowest audible sound, and increases logarithmically, meaning that a sound of 80 db is not just twice as loud as a sound of 40 db, but has 10,000 times more power! Sounds of 100 db are so intense that they can severely damage the inner ear, as many jack-hammer operators and rock stars have discovered.

The ear is a complex sensory organ, divided into three parts: external (outer) ear, middle ear, and inner ear. The outer and middle ear help to protect and maintain optimal conditions for the hearing process and to direct the sound stimuli to the actual sensory receptors, hair cells, located in the cochlea of the inner ear.

Outer Ear and Middle Ear

The most visible part of the ear is the pinna, one of two external ear structures. Its elastic cartilage framework provides flexible protection while collecting sound waves from the air (much like a funnel or satellite dish); the intricate pattern of folds helps prevent the occasional flying insect or other particulate matter from entering the ear canal, the other external ear component. The ear (auditory) canal directs the sound to the delicate eardrum (tympanic membrane), the boundary between external and middle ear. The ear canal has many small hairs and is lined by cells that secrete ear wax (cerumen), another defense to keep the canal free of material that might block the sound or damage the delicate tympanic membrane.

The middle ear contains small bones (auditory ossicles) that transmit sound waves from the eardrum to the inner ear. When the sound causes the eardrum to vibrate, the malleus (hammer) on the inside of the eardrum moves accordingly, pushing on the incus (anvil), which sends the movements to the stapes (stirrup), which in turn pushes on fluid in the inner ear, through an opening in the cochlea called the oval window. Small muscles attached to these ossicles prevent their excessive vibration and protect the cochlea from damage when a loud sound is detected (or anticipated). Another important middle ear structure is the auditory (eustachian) tube, which connects the middle ear to the pharynx (throat). For hearing to work properly, the pressure on both sides of the eardrum must be equal; otherwise, the tight drum would not vibrate. Therefore, the middle ear must be connected to the outside.

Sometimes, when there are sudden changes in air pressure, the pressure difference impairs hearing and causes pain. In babies and many young people, fluid often builds up in the middle ear and pushes on the eardrum. The stagnant fluids can also promote a bacterial infection of the middle ear, called otitis media (OM). OM also occurs when upper respiratory infections (colds and sore throats) travel to the middle ear by way of the auditory tube. Sometimes the pressure can be relieved only by inserting drainage tubes in the eardrum.

Inner Ear

The inner ear contains the vestibule, for the sense of balance and equilibrium, and the cochlea, which converts the sound pressure waves to electrical impulses that are sent to the brain. The cochlea is divided into three chambers, or ducts. The cochlear duct contains the hair cells that detect sound. It is sandwiched between the tympanic and vestibular ducts, which are interconnected at the tip. These ducts form a spiral, giving the cochlea a snail shell appearance. Inside the cochlear duct, the hair cells are anchored on the basilar membrane, which forms the roof of the vestibular duct. The tips of the hair cells are in contact with the tectorial membrane, which forms a sort of awning. When the stapes pushes on the fluid of the inner ear, it creates pressure waves in the fluid of the tympanic and vestibular ducts (like kicking the side of a wading pool). These waves push the basilar membrane up and down, which then pushes the hair cells against the tectorial membrane, bending the "hairs" (stereocilia). When stereocilia are bent, the hair cell is excited, creating impulses that are transmitted to the brain.

How does the cochlea differentiate between sounds of different pitches and intensities? Pitch discrimination results from the fact that the basilar membrane has different vibrational properties along its length, such that the base (nearest the oval window) vibrates most strongly to high frequency sounds, and the tip to low frequencies. The hair cells along the length of the cochlea each make their own connection to the brain, just like the keys on an electric piano are each wired for a certain note. Loud (high-amplitude) sounds cause the basilar membrane to vibrate more vigorously than soft (low-amplitude) sounds. The brain thus distinguishes loud from soft sounds by differences in the intensity of nerve signaling from the cochlea.

Hair cells themselves do not make the impulses that are transmitted to the central nervous system (CNS); they stimulate nerve fibers to which they are connected. These nerve fibers form the cochlear branch of the eighth cranial (vestibulocochlear) nerve. In the CNS, the information is transmitted both to the brainstem, which controls reflex activity, and to the auditory cortex, where perception and interpretation of the sound occur. By comparing inputs from two ears, the brain can interpret the timing of sounds from right and left to determine the location of the sound source. This is called binaural hearing.

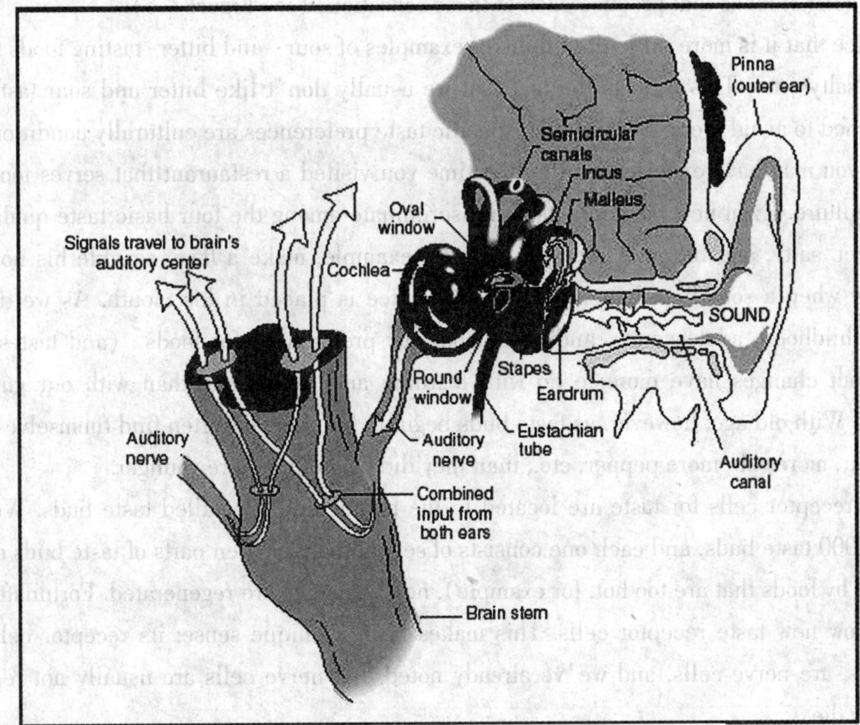

Figure 4.5 The Hearing System

The Chemical Sense

Taste and smell are referred to as chemical senses because the stimuli for both are molerules of chemical compounds. For taste, the chemicals are dissolved in liquid (usually the saliva in our mouths). For smell, they are dissolved in the air that reaches the smell receptors high inside our noses. The technical term for taste is gustation; for smell, it is olfaction.

If you have ever eaten while suffering from a head cold, you appreciate the extent to which our experiences of taste and smell are interrelated. Most foods seem to lose their taste when we cannot smell them. This is why we differentiate between the flavor off oods (which includes such qualities as odor and texture) and the taste of foods. A simple test demonstrates this point. While blindfolded, eat a small piece of peeled apple and a small piece of peeled potato. See if you can tell the difference between the two. You shouldn't have any trouble with this discrimination. Now hold your nose very tightly and try again. Without your sense of smell to help you, discrimination on the basis of taste alone is very difficult.

Taste (*Gustatioit*)

Our experience of the flavors of foods depends so heavily on our sense of smell, texture, and temperature that we sometimes have to wonder if there is truly a sense of taste. Well, there is. Even with odor and texture held constant, tastes can vary. Taste has four basic psychological qualities (and many combinations of these four): sweet, salt, sour, and bitter. Most foods derive their special taste from a unique combination of these four basic taste sensations. You can generate a list of foods that produce each of these sensations (see Figure 4.6).

Notice that it is more difficult to think of examples of sour- and bitter-tasting foods than of sweet or salty ones. This reflects the fact that we usually don't like bitter and sour tastes and have learned to avoid them. Beyond that, specific taste preferences are culturally conditioned — a reality you may have experienced the first time you visited a restaurant that serves food from another culture. Even new born infants can discriminate among the four basic taste qualities of sour, sweet, salty, and bitter. A newborn will, for example, make a face, wrinkle his nose and turn away when a sour liquid such as grapefruit juice is placed in his mouth. As we develop through childhood, adolescence, and adulthood, our preferences for foods (and tastes) may change, but changes have more to do with learning and experience than with our gustatory receptors. With old age, however, as taste buds begin to fail, persons often find themselves using more sugar, more salt, more pepper, etc., than they did when they were younger.

The receptor cells for taste are located in the tongue and are called taste buds. We have about 10,000 taste buds, and each one consists of several parts. When parts of taste buds die (or are killed by foods that are too hot, for example), new segments are regenerated. Fortunately, we always grow new taste receptor cells. This makes taste a unique sense: its receptor cells, the taste buds, are nerve cells, and we've already noted that nerve cells are usually not replaced when they die.

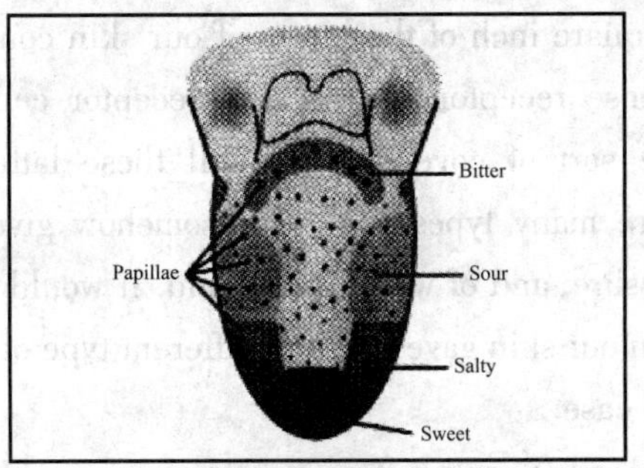

Figure 4.6 Taste Receptors

Taste buds respond primarily to chemicals that produce one of the four basic taste qualities. However, some receptor cells respond best to salts, whereas others respond primarily to sweet-producing chemicals, such as sugars. These receptors are not evenly distributed on the surface of the tongue; receptors for sweet tastes are concentrated at the tip of the tongue, for example. Nonetheless, all four qualities of taste can be detected at all locations of the tongue. Recent research provides evidence that in addition to responding to the various chemicals that we put in our mouths, our taste buds also respond to different temperatures. In fact, as many as half of the neurons in mammalian taste pathways — from the taste buds to the brain — respond to temperature. For example, warming the very tip of the tongue from a cold temperature gives rise to the experience of sweetness.

Smell (*Olfaction*)

Smell is a poorly understood sense. It often gives us great pleasure; think of the aroma of bacon frying over a wood fire or of freshly picked flowers. Smell can also produce considerable displeasure; consider the smell of a skunk, old garbage, or rotten eggs.

The sense of smell originates in hair cells located high in the nasal cavity, very close to the brain itself. We know that the pathway from these receptors to the brain is the most direct and shortest of all the senses. What we don't understand is how molecules suspended in air and gases stimulate the small hair cells of the olfactory receptors to fire neural impulses. The sense of smell is very important for many nonhumans. Many animals, including humans, emit chemicals called pheromones that produce distinctive odors. Sometimes pheromones are released by cells in the skin, sometimes in the urine, and occasionally from special glands (in some deer, this gland is located near the rear hoof). One purpose of pheromones is to mark territory. If you take a dog for a walk and discover that he wants to stop and deposit small amounts of urine on almost every signpost, he is leaving a pheromone message that says, "I have been here; this is my odor; this is my turf."

The Skin: Cutaneous Senses

Most of us take our skin for granted; we seldom think about it very much. We frequently abuse our skin by overexposing it to the sun's rays in summer and to excess cold in winter. We scratch it, cut it, scrape it, and wash away millions of its cells every time we shower or bathe.

Figure 4.7 is a diagram of some of the structures found in an area of skin from a hairy part of the human body. Each square inch of the layers of our skin contains nearly 20 million cells including many special sense receptors. Some skin receptor cells have free nerve endings, whereas others have some sort of covering. We call these latter cells encapsulated nerve endings, of which there are many types. Our skin somehow gives rise to our psychological experience of touch or pressure, and of warmth and cold. It would be convenient if each of the various receptor cells within our skin gave rise to a different type of psychological sensation, but this does not seem to be the case.

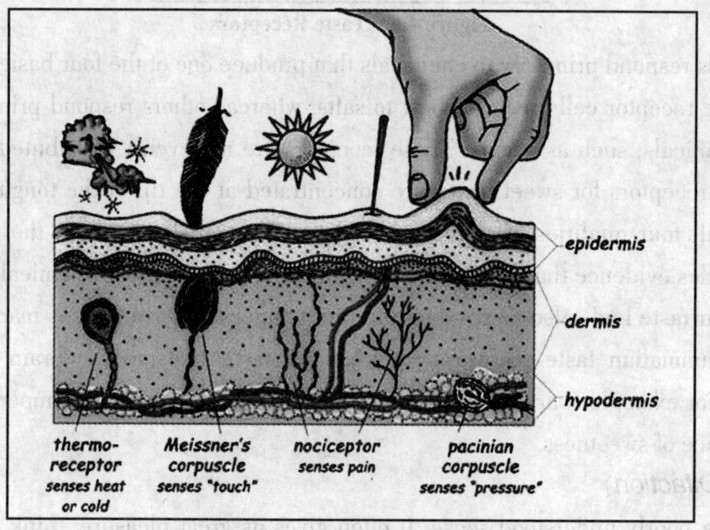

Fig 4.7 Special Senses in Skin

A more general special sense is all over the body in the skin. These "cutaneous sensory receptors" are actually part of the nervous system. Little nerve endings in our skin pick up on signals from the outside world, like heat, cold, pressure and pain. There are many kinds of receptors. Meissner's corpuscles are egg-shaped receptors found just below the top layer of the skin (in the epidermis). They pick up light touch. These receptors help us identify objects by touch. Close your eyes and have someone place an object in your hands, feel it with your fingers until you know what it is. Those are your Meissner's corpuscles at work! Deep in your skin (in the dermis) pacinian corpuscles feel deep pressure, like a painful squeeze. Free nerve endings sit just below the top layer of the skin (in the epidermis). They pick up heat, cold or pain. The receptors that pick up heat and cold are called thermoreceptors. The receptors that pick up pain are called nociceptors.

One of the problems in studying the cutaneous senses is trying to determine which cells in the skin give rise to different sensations of pressure and temperature. We can discriminate clearly between a light touch and a strong jab in the arm and between vibrations, tickles, and itches. A simple proposal is that there are different receptors in the skin responsible for each sensation, but this is not supported by facts. Although some types of receptor cells are more sensitive to some types of stimuli, current thinking is that ourability to discriminate among types of cutaneous sensation is due to the unique combination of responses the many receptor cells have to various types of stimulation.

As good as our cutaneous senses are, those of the common cockroach are — in some ways even more remarkable. Cockroaches are incredibly good at avoiding a swat from a newspaper or the heel of a shoe because they have tiny hairs on their posterior that detect even the most minute changes in air flow around them. This sense (which few other organisms have) allows a cockroach to "surmise the direction of an attack and scurry away to avoid being eaten" (or squished).

By carefully stimulating very small areas of the skin, we can locate areas that are sensitive to temperature. We are convinced that warm and cold temperatures each stimulate specific locations on the skin. Even so, there is no consistent pattern of receptor cells found at these locations, called temperature spots. That is, we have not yet located specific receptor cells for cold or hot. Our experience of hot seems to come from the simultaneous stimulation of both warm and cold spots. A rather ingenious demonstration shows how this works. Cold water is run through one metal tube, and warm water is run through another. The tubes are coiled together. If you grasp the coiled tubes, you would experience heat; the tubes would feel hot even if you knew they weren't.

The Cutaneous (Skin) Senses

The skin contains receptors that respond to touch, pressure, and temperature. The relationships between receptors and the cutaneous sensations are not completely understood. Meissner's corpuscles are sensitive to touch and Pacinian corpuscles to deep pressure. Ruffini endings transmit information about warmth and Krause's bulbs about cold. Information is transmitted from the receptors to nerve fibers that are routed through the spinal cord to the brainstem. From there they are transmitted to an area of cortex in the parietal lobe. Skin senses also undergo various kinds of sensory adaptation. For example, a hot tub can be initially so hot that it is intolerable, but after a while one can sit in it without discomfort.

The Position Senses

Another sensory capacity we often take for granted is our ability to know how and where our bodies are positioned in space. Although we seldom worry about it, we can quickly become aware of how our bodies are positioned in regard to the pull of gravity. We also get sensory information about where various parts of our body are in relation to one another. We can tell if we are moving or standing still. And, unless we are on a rollercoaster or racing across a field, we usually adapt to these sensory messages quickly and pay little attention to them.

Most of the information about where we are in space comes from our sense of vision. If we want to know how we are oriented in space, we simply look around. But we can do the same sort of thing with our eyes closed. We have two systems of position sense over and above what vision can provide. One, the vestibular sense, tells us about balance, about where we are in relation to gravity, and about acceleration or deceleration. The other, the kinesthetic sense, tells us about the movement or position of our muscles and joints.

The receptors for the vestibular sense are located on either side of the head near the inner ears. Five chambers are located there: three semicircular canals and two vestibular sacs. Their orientation is shown. Each of these chambers is filled with fluid. When our head moves in any direction, fluid in the semicircular canals moves, drawn by gravity or the force of our head accelerating in space. The vestibular sacs contain very small solid particles that float in the fluid within the sacs. When we move, these particles are forced against one side of a sac, and they stimulate hair cells that start neural impulses. Overstimulation of the receptor cells in the vestibular sacs or semicircular canals can lead to feelings of dizziness or nausea, reasonably enough called motion sickness.

Pain : A Special Sense

The sense of pain is a curious and troublesome one for psychologists interested in sensory processes. Pain, or the fear of it, can be a strong motivator; we'll do much to avoid it. Pain is surely unpleasant, but it is also very useful. Pain alerts us when a problem occurs somewhere in our bodies and warns us that steps might need to be taken to remove the source of pain. It is the experience of pain that prompts more than 80 percent of all visits to the doctor's office. Feelings of pain are private sensations and are difficult to share or describe.

What is pain? What causes the experience of pain? What are its receptors? We have only partial answers to these questions. Many stimuli cause pain. Intense stimulation of any sense receptor produces pain. Too much light, strong pressures on the skin, excessive temperatures, very loud sounds, and even very "hot" spices cause pain. In the right circumstances, even a light pinprick is painful. Our skin has many receptors for pain, but pain receptors can also be found deep inside our bodies; consider stomachaches, lower back pain, and headaches. Pain is experienced in our brain, and the thalamus seems to play an important role, but pain is the only "sense" for which we cannot find one specific center in the cerebral cortex.

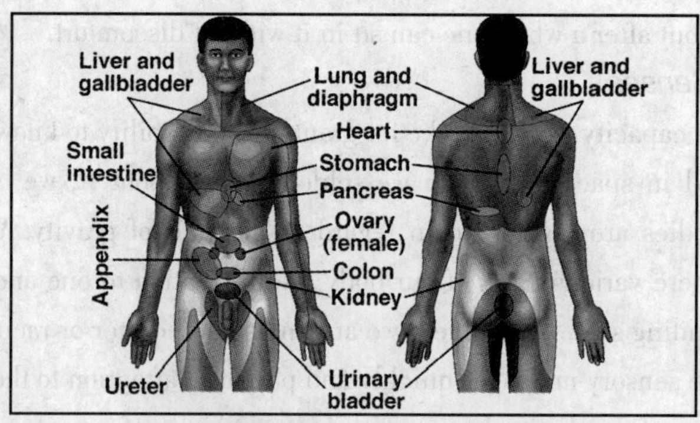

Figure 4.8 Referred Pain Regions

Pain is the most important protective sense. The receptors for pain are widely distributed free nerve endings. They are found in the skin, muscles, and joints and to a lesser extent in most internal organs (including the blood vessels and viscera). See Figure 4.8. Two pathways transmit pain to the CNS. One is for acute, sharp pain, and the other is for slow, chronic pain. Thus, a single strong stimulus produces the immediate sharp pain, followed in a second or so by the slow, diffuse, burning pain that increases in severity with the passage of time.

There are two basic types of pain — nociceptive pain and neuropathic pain.

Nociceptive Pain

Nociceptive pain can be divided into two separate categories.

Somatic Pain

Somatic pain is caused by the activation of pain receptors in either the cutaneous tissues (body surface) or deep tissues (musculoskeletal tissues). When it occurs in the musculoskeletal tissues, it is called deep somatic pain. Deep somatic pain is usually described as dull or aching but localized. Surface somatic pain is usually sharper and may have a burning or pricking quality. Common causes include post-surgical pain or pain related to a laceration.

Visceral Pain

"Viscera" refers to the internal areas of the body that are enclosed within a cavity. Visceral pain is caused by activation of pain receptors resulting from infiltration, compression, extension, or stretching of the chest, abdominal, or pelvic viscera. Visceral pain is not well localized and is usually described as pressure-like, deep squeezing. Examples of visceral pain include pain related to cancer, bone fracture, or bone cancer.

Neuropathic Pain

Neuropathic pain is a neurological disorder resulting from damage to nerves that carry information about pain. Neuropathic pain is reported to feel different from somatic or visceral pain and is often described as "shooting", "electric", "stabbing", or "burning". It may be felt traveling along a nerve path from the spine into the arms and hands or into the buttocks, legs, or feet. Neuropathic pain has very different medication treatment options from other types of pain. For example, opioids (such as morphine) and NSAID's (such as ibuprofen, COX-2 inhibitors) are usually not effective in relieving neuropathic pain. Treatments for neuropathic pain include certain medications, nerve "block" injections, and a variety of interventions generally used for chronic pain. Examples of neuropathic pain conditions include radiculopathies, neuralgias, failed back syndrome, complex regional pain syndrome, arachnoiditis, and painful neuropathies (eg, diabetes or alcohol related).

One theory claims that pain is experienced within the central nervous system rather than in the periphery, and that a gate control mechanism (high in the spinal cord) opens to let pain messages race to the brain or acts to block pain messages by "closing the gate" so that messages never get to the brain for processing. A cognitive-behavioral theory of pain also suggests that central mechanisms are important, noting that pain is influenced by a person's attitudes, expectations, and behaviors.

Even without a full understanding of how pain is sensed, there are techniques that can be used to reduce, or manage, the experience of pain. If pain is really experienced in the brain, what sorts of things can we do to keep pain messages from reaching those brain centers?

Drug therapy is one choice for pain management. Opiates such as morphine, when administered systematical, are believed to inhibit pain messages at the level of the spinal cord, as well as at the specific site of the pain.

Hypnosis and cognitive self-control (trying very hard to convince yourself that the pain you're experiencing is not all that bad and will go away soon) can also be effective in lessening the experience of pain.

That psychological processes can inhibit pain is reinforced by data on placebo effects. A placebo is a substance (perhaps a pill) a person believes will be useful in treating some symptom, such as pain. When a person takes a placebo that he or she believes will alleviate pain, endorphins are released in the brain and effectively keep pain-carrying impulses from reaching the brain. This placebo effect is particularly strong when the health care provider is prestigious, empathic, and shows a positive attitude about the placebo.

Another process that eases the feeling of pain, particularly pain from or near the surface of the skin, is called counterirritation. The idea is to forcefully (but not painfully, of course) stimulate an area of the body near the location of the pain. Dentists have learned that rubbing the patient's gum near the spot of a Novocain injection significantly reduces the pain of the needle.

The ancient Chinese practice of acupuncture is also effective in the treatment of pain. We don't yet know why acupuncture works as well as it does. There are cases where it doesn't work at all, but these usually involve patients who are skeptics, which suggests that at least one of the benefits of acupuncture is its placebo effect. As many as 12 million acupuncture therapies for pain management are performed in the United States each year, although more recent evidence suggests that acupuncture is less effective than pain-killing drugs.

Individual responses to pain are unique and are influenced by many factors, such as prior experience, memory of those experiences, and how one feels about pain. It is clear that gender and cultural differences can be involved in the expression or display of pain. In Japan, for instance, individuals are socialized not to show pain or any intense feeling. In Western culture, men are often socialized not to show pain and to "take it like a man". Among other things, these socialization issues often create difficulties in the diagnosis and treatment of an illness or disease where pain is an informative symptom. Finally, we should also explode the widely-held misconception that newborns cannot feel pain because of immature pain receptors. Research on the newborn's sensitivity to pain clearly shows that newborns do experience pain.

Pain Measurement

There is no way to see pain or objectively measure pain. It does not show up on an X-ray or MRI, and people who have pain may look perfectly normal and unimpaired as you walk past them on the street. This is often a source of frustration to the person with chronic pain who frequently hears "you don't look like you're in pain!" It is also a source of frustration for physicians who are unable to find structural pathology (eg, ruptured disc or torn ligament) to account for a person's pain complaint. Pain is a subjective experience, that is, what one person finds painful may not be painful to another person. Pain patients who visit their physician are often asked to rate their pain on a 0 to 10 scale, with 0 being "no pain" and 10 being "the worst pain imaginable". This is an accurate and simple way to monitor a person's pain. However, you cannot use this to compare across people. For example, my pain rating of a 7 on a 0 to 10 scale may be a 2 for someone else with a higher pain tolerance.

Perception

Stimulus Input: Attention and Set

Perception is the way that sensory information is chosen and transformed so that it has meaning. Once sensory input starts, an individual uses perceptual processes to select among sensory input stimuli and to organize them so that relevant action can occur. (In the computer analogy, the process of perception would represent use of both hardware and software in the central nervous system; many of the perceptual processes are innate — hardware — but some may be modified — software.)

Too many events occur simultaneously in the environment to pay attention to all of them at once, so selective attention is used to focus on those stimuli relevant to current activity. (For example, you might not generally pay much attention to wind direction, but you do if you're flying a kite or hitting a golf ball.)

In terms of perception, a set, a predisposition to respond in a particular fashion, may be one of several types.

When attending to a stimulus, an individual organizes muscular responses, a motor set, to be ready for the particular attention situation. For example, a golfer getting ready to hit a golf ball adopts a particular posture and a practiced way of holding the golf club; similarly, members of basketball teams adopt particular stances, motor sets, as they stand lined up and ready to jump while waiting for the free throw.

A perceptual set is the readiness to interpret a stimulus in a certain way. For example, if you have just run a red traffic light, you might be more inclined to view a flashing light as a police car than as just a bright turn signal. (Note that perceptual sets occur in all of the sensory modalities, not just vision.)

A mental set is a predisposition to think about a situation or a problem in a specific way. For example, a student's poor performance on a math assignment might be because of lack of preparation or because of the mental set "I just can't do well on math problems." Stimulus characteristics that affect set. A variety of stimulus characteristics affect perception and the set that is formed.

Stimulus intensity: if other stimulus factors are comparable, a more intense stimulus attracts more attention than does a more subtle one. For example, a loud siren gets more attention than a faint one.

Stimulus changes: stimulus changes elicit more attention than does sameness or monotony. A flashing light, for example, stands out in a horizon of steady city lights.

Stimulus magnitude: stimulus magnitude is also a factor in attracting attention. For example, a large advertising billboard attracts more attention than a small one.

Stimulus repetition: a repeated stimulus affects attention; the public quickly recognizes a product seen in repeated advertisements.

Organization of Perceptions

Sometimes attention is determined less by the physical characteristics of the stimuli present than by personal characteristics of the perceiver. For example, imagine two students watching a football game on television. Both are presented with identical stimulation from the same TV screen. One asks, "Wow, did you see that tackle?" The other responds, "No, I was watching the cheerleaders." The difference in perception here is hardly attributable to the nature of the stimuli because both students received the same sensory information from the same TV. The difference is due to characteristics of the perceivers, or personal factors, which we categorize as motivation, expectation, or past experience.

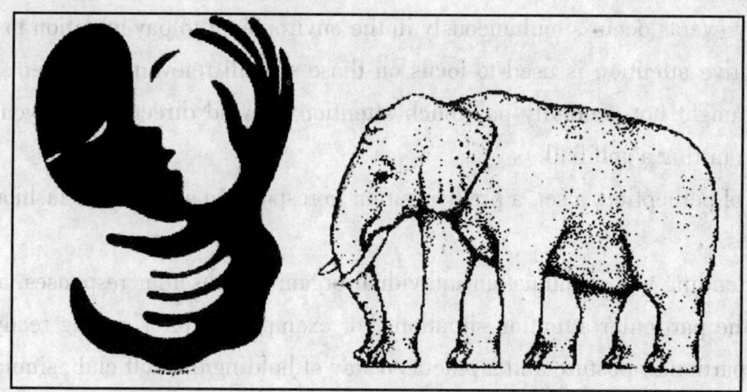

Figure 4.9 Perception

Perception is our sensory experience of the world around us and involves both the recognition of environmental stimuli and actions in response to these stimuli (Figure 4.9). Through the perceptual process, we gain information about properties and elements of the environment that are critical to our survival. Perception not only creates our experience of the world around us, it allows us to act within our environment. Perception includes the five senses: touch, sight, taste smell and taste. It also includes what is known as proprioception, a set of senses involving the ability to detect changes in body positions and movements. It also involves the cognitive processes required to process information, such as recognizing the face of a friend or detecting a familiar scent.

We often perceive what we want to perceive, and we often perceive what we expect to perceive. We may not notice stimuli when they are present simply because we did not "know" they were coming — we didn't expect them. When we are psychologically predisposed to perceive something, we form a mental set.

One of our basic perceptual reactions to the environment is to select certain stimuli from among all those that strike our receptors so they may be processed further. A related perceptual process is to organize and interpret the bits and pieces of experience into meaningful, organized wholes. We do not hear individual sounds of speech; we perceive words, phrases, and sentences. Our visual experience is not one of bits of color and light and dark but of identifiable objects and events. We don't perceive a warm pat on the back as responses from hundreds of individual receptors in our skin.

Perceptual organization was of considerable interest to the Gestalt psychologists. Perhaps you recall that gestalt is a German word that means "configuration" or "whole". You form a gestalt when you see the "big picture". When you perceive the whole as being more than the sum of its parts, you've formed a gestalt.

A basic principle of Gestalt psychology is the figure-ground relationship. Those stimuli you attend to and group together are fix, whereas all the rest are the ground. As you focus your attention on the words on this page, they form figures against the ground (or background, if you'd prefer) provided by the rest of the page. When you hear your instructor's voice during a lecture, it is the figure against the ground of all others grounds in the room. The irate student who barged into the classroom to confront a professor became a figure quite quickly. Do you see the relationship between these classic, Gestalt psychology terms (figure and ground) and the more modern, technical terminology (salient and peripheral details) we introduced at the very beginning of this Topic? What the Gestalt psychologists called a figure, we also can call a salient detail of our sensory world. Those stimuli which make up our perceptual ground are the peripheral details.

The manner in which stimuli are arranged, that is, grouped, (in addition to their individual characteristics) also affects their perception.

Stimulus characteristics that affect organization. Important stimulus characteristics that affect the organization of stimuli and their perception include the following:

Closure

Closure is the completion of an incomplete stimulus. If someone yells at you, "Close the_____," the word door isn't said, but you fill in the blank because of past experience and close the door.

Nearness

Stimuli that are near one another tend to be grouped together; stars near one another are sometimes seen as a pattern or constellation, which is not the case for stars that are far apart.

Similarity

stimuli that are similar to one another are frequently grouped together; people wearing the same band uniforms are seen as similar compared to a group of marching people wearing everyday clothes.

Continuity

the tendency is to view a figure, pattern, or illustration that contains gaps as smooth and continuous rather than as discontinuous. The broken line down the middle of the highway is perceived as a continuous dotted line rather than a long row of blocks.

Contiguity

Contiguity, or nearness in time and space, also influences perception. If certain theme songs and visual stimuli are placed near the beginning or end of television programs, these stimuli are associated with the starting or stopping of the program.

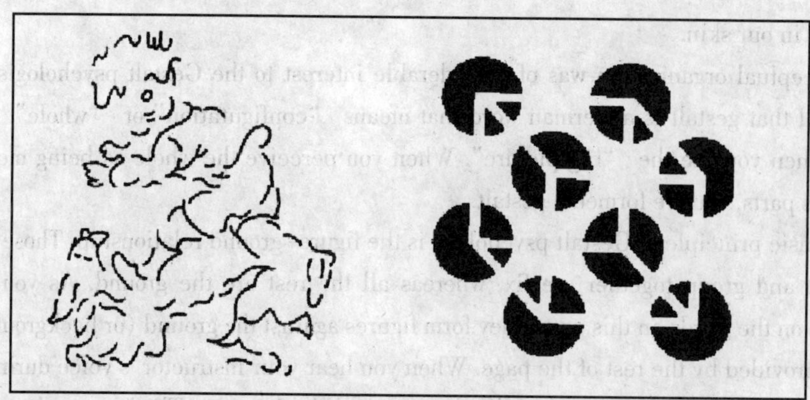

Figure 4.10 Contiguity

The law of continuity holds that points that are connected by straight or curving lines are seen in a way that follows the smoothest path (Figure 4.10). Rather than seeing separate lines and angles, lines are seen as belonging together. Due to our ability to maintain constancy in our perceptions, we see that building as the same height no matter what distance it is. Perceptual constancy refers to our ability to see things differently without having to reinterpret the object's properties. There are typically three constancies discussed, including size, shape, brightness.

Perceptual Constancy

There is a tendency to maintain constancy (of size, color, and shape) in the perception of stimuli even though the stimuli have changed. For example, you recognize that small brownish dog in the distance as your neighbor's large golden retriever, so you aren't surprised by the great increase in size (size constancy) or the appearance of the yellow color (color constancy) when he comes bounding up. And in spite of the changes in the appearance of the dog moving toward you from a distance, you still perceive the shape as that of a dog (shape constancy) no matter the angle from which it is viewed.

The most important stimulus factor in perceptual selection is contrast, the extent to which a stimulus is physically different from the other stimuli around it. One stimulus can contrast with other stimuli in a variety of ways. We are more likely to attend to a stimulus if its intensity is different from the intensities of other stimuli. Generally, the more intense a stimulus, the more likely we are to select it for further processing. Thus, we are more likely to attend to an irate student in a classroom if he is shouting rather than whispering. In other contexts, a bright light is more attention-grabbing than a dim one; an extreme temperature is more likely to be noticed than a moderate one. This isn't always the case, however, as context can make a difference. A shout is more compelling than a whisper, unless everyone is shouting; then it may be the soft, quiet, reasoned tone that gets our attention. If we are faced with a barrage of bright lights, a dim one by contrast may be the one we process more fully.

The same argument holds true for the stimulus characteristic of physical size. In most cases, the bigger the stimulus, the more likely we are to attend to it. There is little point building a small billboard to advertise your motel or restaurant. You want to construct the biggest billboard you can in hopes of attracting attention. Still, faced with many large stimuli, contrast effects often cause us to attend to the one that is smaller. The easiest player to spot on a football field is often the placekicker, who tends to be smaller and not wearing as much protective padding as the other players.

A third dimension for which contrast is relevant is motion. Motion is a powerful factor in determining visual attention. Walking through the woods, you may nearly step on achipmunk before you notice it, as long as it stays still — an adaptive camouflage that chipmunks do well. If it moves to escape, you easily notice it scurrying across the leaves. Again, the contrast created by movement is important.

Although intensity, size, and motion are three characteristics of stimuli that readily come to mind, there are others. Indeed, any way in which two stimuli are different (ie, contrast) can provide a dimension that determines which stimulus we attend to. (Even a small grease spot can easily grab one's attention if it's located in the middle of a solid yellow tie.) Because contrast guides attention, important terms are printed in bold face type throughout this book — so you'll notice them, attend to them, and recognize them as important stimuli.

There is another stimulus characteristic that determines attention, but for which contrast is not relevant; that is repetition. The more often a stimulus is presented, the more likely it will be attended to — with all else being equal. Note that we have to say "all else being equal" or we develop contradictions. If stimuli are repeated too often, we adapt to them as they are no longer novel. Even so, there are many examples that convince us of the value of repetition in getting someone's attention. Instructors who want to make an important point seldom mention it just once, but repeat it. This is why we repeat the definitions of important terms in the text, in the margin, and again in the glossary. The people who schedule commercials on television want you to attend to their messages, and obviously repetition is one of their main techniques.

There are many ways in which stimuli differ. The greater the contrast between any stimulus and the others around it, the greater the likelihood that that stimulus captures our attention. All else being equal, the more often a stimulus is presented, the greater the likelihood that it is perceived and selected for further processing.

Depth and Distance Perception

Perceptual processes function in the three-dimensional organization of stimuli as well as in distance judgments. The processes include use of both monocular and binocular cues.

Perception requires that we select and organize stimulus information. One of the ways in which we organize visual stimuli is to note where they happen to be in the world. We perceive the world as three-dimensional. As long as we pay attention (surely a required perceptual process), we won't fall off cliffs or run into buildings. We know with considerable accuracy just how far we are from objects in our environment. What is remarkable about this ability is that light reflected from objects and events in our environment fall son two-dimensional retinas. The depth and distance in our world is not something we directly sense; it is something we perceive.

The ability to judge depth and distance accurately is an adaptive skill that plays an important role in determining many of our actions. Our ability to make such judgments reflects the fact that we are simultaneously responding to a large number of cues to depth and distance. Some cues are built into our visual systems and are referred to as ocularcues. Physical, or pictorial cues, have to do with our appreciation of the physical environment. We'll also see that our culture plays a role in the perception of depth and distance.

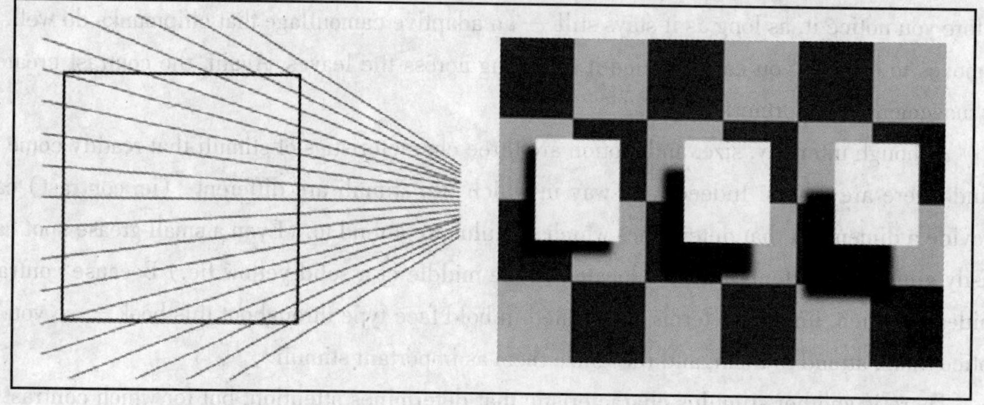

Figure 4.11 Depth and Distance

Depth and distance perception relies on a variety of cues our brain receives through the use of both of our eyes. This can cause problems for those of us who only have the use of one eye. While we are able to perceive certain depths and/or distances using only one eye there are other depths/distances that we will not be able to interpret. If you are someone with the use of only one eye you might experience problems judging the distance of a painting hanging on a nearby wall but have no trouble judging the distance of a building or object several blocks away.

When using our vision to judge depth and distances it is up to us to come up with an acceptable estimate. To establish the distance and/or depth we rely on a variety of cues, some of which require one eye and others require both eyes. These cues make it possible for us to estimate distances using only our vision as a guide.

Other Factors Influencing Perception

Personal Characteristics

Personal characteristics, such as past experience (learning) and motivation, may also affect the way stimuli are perceived. Learning (a musician quickly learns the pattern of tones that make a melody and detects a discordant note) Motivation (while an individual may not initially have a taste for espresso coffee, if the person's group of acquaintances perceives it as an "in" beverage, he or she may then start drinking espresso)

Gestalt Theory

A group of early experimental psychologists known as Gestalt psychologists believed that perceptions are more than the stimuli that create them. By more is meant that a meaningful, whole pattern is created by the stimuli (that is, the total is more than the sum of its parts). These psychologists developed the idea, the principle of Prögnanz, that stimuli can be grouped and seen as a whole. These psychologists believed that the innate, organizing tendencies of the brain would explain organization functions in perception, including many optical illusions, for example, the phi phenomenon and certain figure-ground relationships.

The phi phenomenon occurs when you see two adjacent lights alternately blinking off and on and perceive them as one light moving back and forth. This phi phenomenon illusion is frequently used in signs to suggest movement.

Figure (object)-ground (background) relationships are important in Gestalt theory, which suggests that perceptions are organized to produce a figure-ground effect. One tends to see objects against backgrounds rather than to view each separately. However, when instructed, one may reverse the relationship and see the object as background and vice versa. In the famous figure-ground illustration shown in Figure 4.12, do you see a goblet or the profile of two faces?

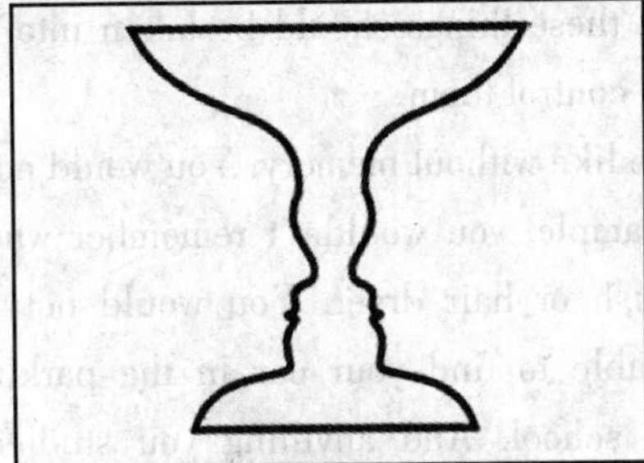

Figure 4.12 A Figure-Ground Illustration

Extrasensory Perception

A phenomenon related to the study of perception and well known in the popular domain is called extrasensory perception (ESP). The belief is that one can have a perceptual experience without any sensory input. Types of reported ESPs include mental telepathy, the ability to read another person's thoughts; forecasting, the ability to predict future incidents accurately (for example, who will win a race or engage in a particular activity); clairvoyance, the awareness of some event that one cannot see (for example, knowing where a body is hidden); psychokinesis, the ability to cause things to move by virtue of thought processes.

Psychologists known as parapsychologists study these phenomena, but the majority of psychologists feel that evidence for the existence of ESP phenomena has not been adequately documented.

Chapter 5 Memory and Intelligence

This chapter focuses on various states of mind, how our memory works, why we forget things, the debate over intelligence and intelligence testing, and the power of the mind to control states of relaxation and hypnosis. Obviously there are a lot of things, both internal and external, that can affect our current state. Emotions, noise, stress, and of course the use of alcohol and drugs all come to mind. All of these things should be taken into consideration when learning about states of mind and how to control them.

Imagine what life would be like without memory. You would not be able to accomplish even the most routine tasks. For example, you wouldn't remember where your bath-room was or where you keep your toothbrush or hair dryer. You would not remember to make yourself breakfast, nor would you be able to find your car in the parking lot. You would have no recollection of how to get to school. And anything you studied for your exam would be nonexistent. In fact, the sentences in your text would make no sense. Without your memory, you would have no idea what a textbook is or why you had it open in front of you. The patterns of print you now — recognize as words would appear as no more than random marks. We care about memory in an academic, study-learn-test sense, but the importance of memory goes well beyond classroom exams. All of those things that define us as individuals, our feelings, beliefs, attitudes, and experiences, are stored in our memories. In this chapter, we'll formulate a working definition of memory. We will consider how information gets into memory and how it is stored there. We will explore the possibility that there are several types of memory and see what these varieties of memory might be. We'll also take a moment to see what scientists can tell us about the physiological changes that occur when new memories are formed.

Human Memory as Information Processing

One way to think about human memory is to consider it as a final step in a series of psychological activities that process information. The processing of information begins when sensory receptors are stimulated above threshold levels. The process of perception then selects and organizes the information provided by the senses. With memory, a record of that information is formed.

Although we often give a single label to what we commonly refer to as memory, it is not a single structure or process. Instead, memory is a set of systems involved in the acquisition, storage, and retrieval of information. Memory comprises systems that can hold information for periods of time ranging from fractions of a second to a lifetime, and have storage capacities that range from the very limited (eg, just a few simple sounds) to the very vast (eg, a complex event, such as a high school graduation ceremony).

Using memory is a cognitive activity that involves three interrelated processes. The first is encoding, a process of putting information into memory, which is a matter of forming cognitive representations of information. Encoding is an active process involving a decision (usually unconscious) as to which details to place into memory. Once die representations are in memory, they must be kept there. This process is called storage. In order to use stored information, it must be gotten out again. This process is called retrieval.

Human memory, like memory in a computer, allows us to store information for later use. In order to do this, however, both the computer and we need to master three processes involved in memory.

The first is called encoding; the process we use to transform information so that it can be stores. For a computer this means transferring data into 1's and 0's. For us, it means transforming the data into a meaningful form such as an association with an existing memory, an image, or a sound.

Next is the actual storage, which simply means holding onto the information. For this to take place, the computer must physically write the 1' and 0's onto the hard drive. It is very similar for us because it means that a physiological change must occur for the memory to be stored.

The final process is called retrieval, which is bringing the memory out of storage and reversing the process of encoding. In other words, return the information to a form similar to what we stored.

The major difference between humans and computers in terms of memory has to do with how the information is stored. For the most part, computers have only two types: permanent storage and permanent deletion. Humans, on the other hand are more complex in that we have three distinct memory storage capabilities (not including permanent deletion). The first is sensory memory, referring to the information we receive through the senses. This memory is very brief lasting only as much as a few seconds.

The Constructive Nature of Memory

By the early 1970s, it was clear that the model had encountered at least two problems. The first of these concerned the learning assumption. Evidence suggested that merely holding an item in STM did not guarantee learning. Much more important was the processing that the item underwent. This is emphasized in the levels - of - processing framework proposed by Craik and Lockhart (1972). They suggested that probability of subsequent recall or recognition was a direct function of the depth to which an item was processed. Hence, if the subject merely noted the visual characteristics of a word, for example whether it was in upper or lower case, little learning would follow. Slightly more would be remembered if the word were also processed acoustically by deciding, for example, whether it rhymed with a specified target word. By far the best recall, however, followed semantic processing, in which the subject made a judgement about the meaning of the word, or perhaps related it to a specified sentence, or to his/her own experience (see Figure 5.1).

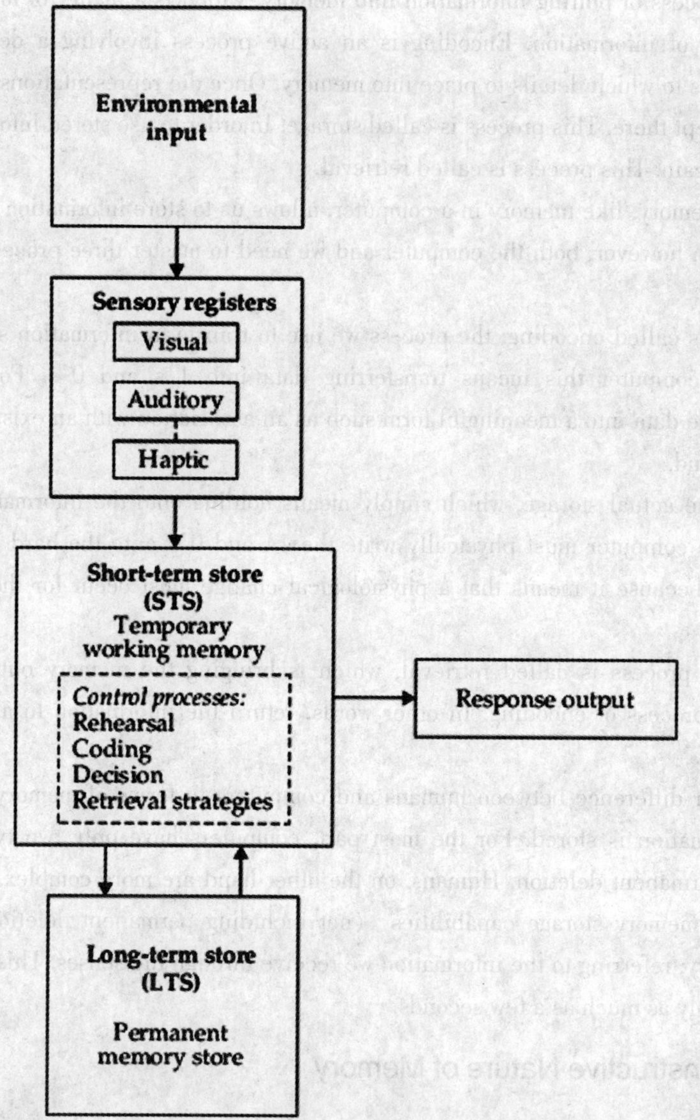

Figure 5.1 Short Term Memory (STM)

Short Term Memory (STM) takes over when the information in our sensory memory is transferred to our consciousness or our awareness (Engle, Cantor, & Carullo, 1993; Laming, 1992). This is the information that is currently active such as reading this page, talking to a friend, or writing a paper. Short term memory can definitely last longer than sensory memory (up to 30 seconds or so), but it still has a very limited capacity. According to research, we can remember approximately 5 to 9 (7 +/- 2) bits of information in our short term memory at any given time.

Participants were read lists of either words or numbers that they had to recall immediately after presentation. Jacobs gradually increased the length of these digits etc until the participant could only accurately recall the information, in the correct order, on 50% of occasions. Recall has to be in the correct order (serial recall).

X N J P T C B D L Y Q H

Jacobs found a difference between capacity for numbers and for letters. On average participants could recall 9 numbers but only 7 letters. He also noticed that recall seemed to increase with age. Eight year olds being able to recall an average of 7 digits whereas by the age of 19 recall had increased to 9 digits. STM has a capacity of between 5 and 9 items of information and as age increases we appear to develop better strategies of recall.

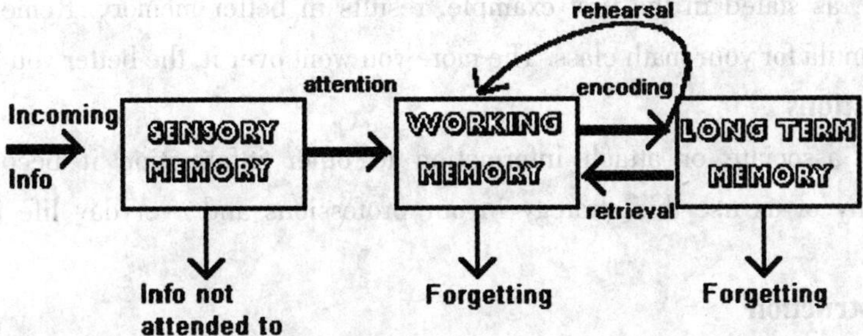

Figure 5.2 Information Processing System of Memory

Obviously rehearsal will help with duration of STM. Try to remember the registration of that speeding car and you will repeat it to yourself over and over.

Amount of information: Murdock 1961 used a version of the Brown - Peterson technique to show that number of chunks affects duration. Participants were given either three letters that spelt a familiar word such as c, a, t or three unrelated three letter words such as sun, pat, lid. The latter deteriorated at the same rate as predicted by B - P so recall after 18 seconds was minimal. However, recall of the three letters was very stubborn to erase and after 18 seconds recall was still at over 90%.

If STM lasts only up to 30 seconds, how do we ever get any work done? Wouldn't we start to lose focus or concentrate about twice every minute? This argument prompted researchers to look at a second phase of STM that is now referred to as Working Memory. Working Memory is the process that takes place when we continually focus on material for longer than STM alone will allow.

What happens when our short term memory is full and another bit of information enters? Displacement means that the new information will push out part of the old information. Suddenly someone says the area code for that phone number and almost instantly you forget the last two digits of the number. We can further sharpen our short term memory skills, however, by mastering chunking and using rehearsal (which allows us to visualize, hear, say, or even see the information repeatedly and through different senses).

Short Term Memory

There are typically six reasons why information is stored in our short term memory.

1. Primary Effect

Information that occurs first is typically remembered better than information occurring later. When given a list of words or numbers, the first word or number is usually remembered due to rehearsing this more than other information.

2. Recently Effect

Often the last bit of information is remembered better because not as much time has past; time which results in forgetting.

3. Distinctiveness

If something stands out from information around it, it is often remembered better. Any distinctive information is easier to remember than that which is similar, usual, or mundane.

4. Frequency Effect

Rehearsal, as stated in the first example, results in better memory. Remember trying to memorize a formula for your math class. The more you went over it, the better you knew it.

5. Associations

When we associate or attach information to other information it becomes easier to remember. Many of us use this strategy in our professions and everyday life in the form of acronyms.

6. Reconstruction

Sometimes we actually fill in the blanks in our memory. In other words, when trying to get a complete picture in our minds, we will make up the missing parts, often without any realization that this is occurring.

Short-term memories can become long-term memory through the process of consolidation, involving rehearsal and meaningful association. Unlike short-term memory (which relies mostly on an acoustic, and to a lesser extent a visual, code for storing information), long-term memory encodes information for storage semantically (ie, based on meaning and association).

Physiologically, the establishment of long-term memory involves a process of physical changes in the structure of neurons (or nerve cells) in the brain, a process known as long-term potentiation, although there is still much that is not completely understood about the process. At its simplest, whenever something is learned, circuits of neurons in the brain, known as neural networks, are created, altered or strengthened. These neural circuits are composed of a number of neurons that communicate with one another through special junctions called synapses. Through a process involving the creation of new proteins within the body of neurons, and the electrochemical transfer of neurotransmitters across synapse gaps to receptors, the communicative strength of certain circuits of neurons in the brain is reinforced. With repeated use, the efficiency of these synapse connections increases, facilitating the passage of nerve impulses along particular neural circuits, which may involve many connections to the visual cortex, the auditory cortex, the associative regions of the cortex, etc.

Several studies have shown that both episodic and semantic long-term memories can be better recalled when the same language is used for both encoding and retrieval.

For example, bilingual Russian immigrants to the United States can recall more autobiographical details of their early life when the questions and cues are presented in Russian than when they are questioned in English.

This process differs both structurally and functionally from the creation of working or short-term memory. Although the short-term memory is supported by transient patterns of neuronal communication in the regions of the frontal, prefrontal and parietal lobes of the brain, long-term memories are maintained by more stable and permanent changes in neural connections widely spread throughout the brain. The hippocampus area of the brain essentially acts as a kind of temporary transit point for long-term memories, and is not itself used to store information. However, it is essential to the consolidation of information from short-term to long-term memory, and is thought to be involved in changing neural connections for a period of three months or more after the initial learning.

Unlike with short-term memory, forgetting occurs in long-term memory when the formerly strengthened synaptic connections among the neurons in a neural network become weakened, or when the activation of a new network is superimposed over an older one, thus causing interference in the older memory.

Over the years, several different types of long-term memory have been distinguished, including explicit and implicit memory, declarative and procedural memory (with a further sub-division of declarative memory into episodic and semantic memory) and retrospective and prospective memory.

Long Term Memory (LTM)

Finally, there is long term memory (LTM), which is most similar to the permanent storage of a computer. Unlike the other two types, LTM is relatively permanent and practically unlimited in terms of its storage capacity. It's been argued that we have enough space in our LTM to memorize every phone number in the U.S. and still function normally in terms of remembering what we do now. Obviously we don't use even a fraction of this storage space.

Long-term memory (LTM) is memory in which associations among items are stored, as part of the theory of a dual-store memory model. The division of long-term and short-term memory has been supported by several double dissociation experiments. According to the theory, long-term memory differs structurally and functionally from working memory or short-term memory, which ostensibly stores items for only around 20 – 30 seconds and can be recalled easily. This differs from the theory of the single-store retrieved context model that has no differentiation between short-term and long-term memory. Long term memory is an important aspect of cognition. LTM can be divided into three processes: encoding, storage, and retrieval. Long-term memory is said to be encoded in the medial temporal lobe. Without it one cannot store new long-term memories.

Some information retained in STM is processed into long-term memory. This information on past experiences is filed away in the recesses of the mind and must be retrieved before it can be used. In contrast to the immediate recall of current experience from STM, retrieval of information from LTM is indirect and sometimes laborious.

Loss of detail as sensory stimuli are interpreted and passed from SIS into STM and then into

LTM is the basis for the phenomenon of selective perception discussed in the previous chapter. It imposes limits on subsequent stages of analysis, inasmuch as the lost data can never be retrieved. People can never take their mind back to what was actually there in sensory information storage or short - term memory. They can only retrieve their interpretation of what they thought was there as stored in LTM.

Long-term Memory Structure

There are no practical limits to the amount of information that may be stored in LTM. The limitations of LTM are the difficulty of processing information into it and retrieving information from it. These subjects are discussed as show in Figure 5.3.

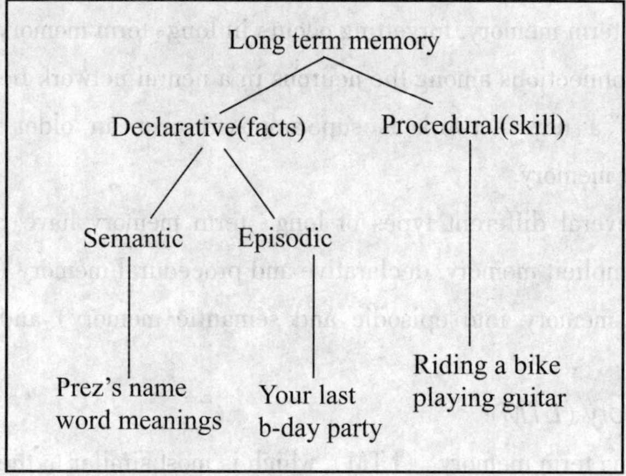

Figure.5.3 Long-term Memory Structure

The three memory processes comprise the storehouse of information or database that we call memory, but the total memory system must include other features as well. Some mental process must determine what information is passed from SIS into STM and from STM into LTM; decide how to search the LTM data base and judge whether further memory search is likely to be productive; assess the relevance of retrieved information; and evaluate potentially contradictory data.

To explain the operation of the total memory system, psychologists posit the existence of an interpretive mechanism that operates on the data base and a monitor or central control mechanism that guides and oversees the operation of the whole system. Little is known of these mechanisms and how they relate to other mental processes.

There are two types of long - term memory: episodic memory and semantic memory. Episodic memory represents our memory of events and experiences in a serial form. It is from this memory that we can reconstruct the actual events that took place at a given point in our lives. Semantic memory, on the other end, is a structured record of facts, concepts and skills that we have acquired. The information in semantic memory is derived from that in our own episodic memory, such that we can learn new facts or concepts from our experiences.

There are several subcategories of LTM. First, memories for facts, life events, and information about our environment are stored in declarative memory. This includes semantic memory, factual knowledge like the meaning of words, concepts, and our ability to do math and episodic memory, memories for events and situations. The second subcategory is often not thought of as memory because it refers to internal, rather than external information. When you brush your teeth, write your name, or scratch your eye, you do this with ease because you previously stored these movements and can recall them with ease. This is referred to as non declarative (or implicit) memory. These are memories we have stored due to extensive practice, conditioning, or habits.

Why We Remember What We Remember

Information that passes from our short term to our long term memory is typically that which has some significance attached to it. Imagine how difficult it would be to forget the day you graduated, or your first kiss. Now think about how easy it is to forget information that has no significance; the color of the car you parked next to at the store or what shirt you wore last Thursday. When we process information, we attach significance to it and information deemed important is transferred to our long term memory.

There are other reasons information is transferred. As we all know, sometimes our brains seem full of insignificant facts. Repetition plays a role in this, as we tend to remember things more the more they are rehearsed. Other times, information is transferred because it is somehow attached to something significant. You may remember that it was a warm day when you bought your first car. The temperature really plays no important role, but is attached to the memory of buying your first car.

What Is Episodic Memory?

Episodic memory is a category of long - term memory that involves the recollection of specific events, situations and experiences. Your first day of school, your first kiss, attending a friend's birthday party and your brother's graduation are all examples of episodic memories. In addition to your overall recall of the event itself, it also involves your memory of the location and time that the event occurred. Closely related to this is what researchers refer to as autobiographical memory, or your memories of your own personal life history. As you can imagine, episodic and autobiographical memories play an important role in your self identity.

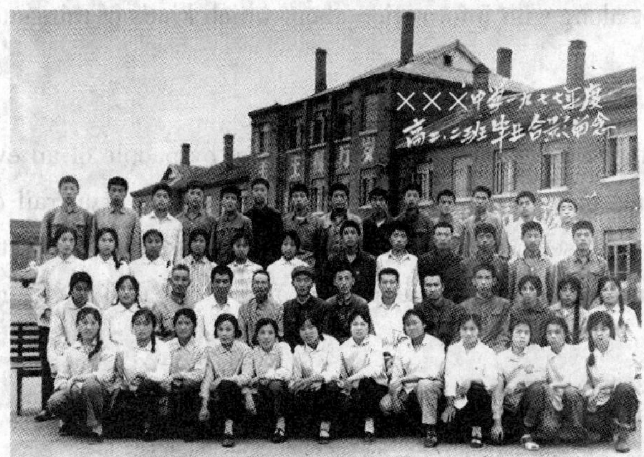

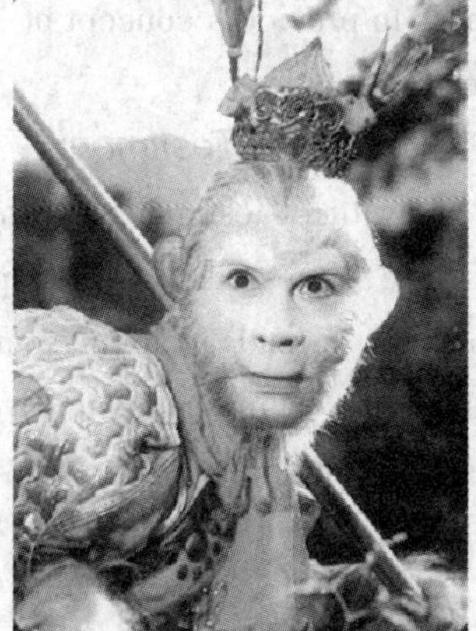

Events that are recorded into episodic memory may trigger episodic learning.

The primary contrast between episodic and semantic memory is that episodic memories are memories which can be explicitly described and stated, while semantic memory is concerned with concepts and ideas. For example, the concept of a table is housed in the semantic memory, but when someone describes his or her kitchen table, this is an episodic memory. Procedural memory can also interact with declarative memory, as for example when someone drives a car, using procedural memory to remember how to drive, semantic memory to define a car, and episodic memory to recall specific driving experiences.

Episodic memories can pertain to general or specific events, such as what it feels like to ride a train, or a specific event which occurred on a train. It can also include facts, such as the names of world leaders, and so-called "flashbulb" memories, which are formed during periods of intense emotion. A classic example of a flashbulb memory from the 20th century is the assassination of President Kennedy, an event which was vividly remembered by people who were alive at the time.

It only takes one exposure to form an episodic memory, which is probably something which evolved early in human evolution, to teach people to avoid making potentially deadly mistakes. For example, someone who almost drowns as a child will often develop a fear of water in response to this single experience. People engage in episodic learning every day, but children often provide very striking examples of episodic learning, since they are exploring a world which is primarily unfamiliar to them, and hence they constantly have new experiences which are filed away in the episodic memory.

This area of the long-term memory is a critical part of identity. People are shaped by the events they participate in and interact with, and loss of episodic memories can cause people to experience confusion or distress, as they lack a context for their identities. Some researchers have suggested that episodic memory sometimes turns into semantic memory over time, with the brain lumping a family of similar experiences together to create a semantic concept. For example, distinct memories of various burns may be bundled together into the semantic memory to provide a concept of "hot", along with information about which kinds of things tend to be hot.

Eyewitness Testimony

Eyewitness testimony is a legal term. It refers to an account given by people of an event they have witnessed. For example they may be required to give a description at a trail of a robbery or a road accident someone has seen. This includes identification of perpetrators, details of the crime scene etc. Eyewitness testimony is an important area of research in cognitive psychology and human memory.

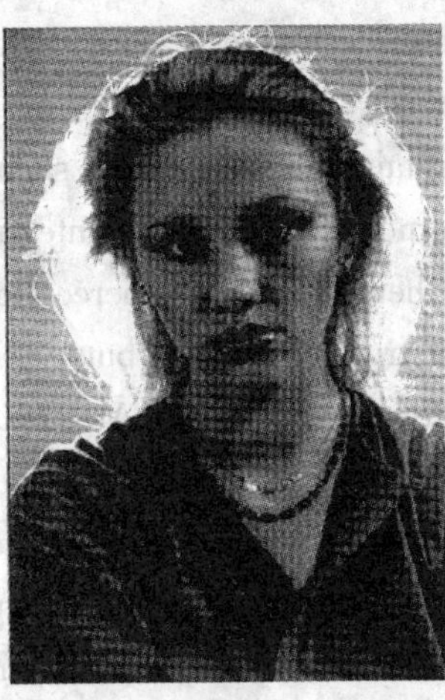

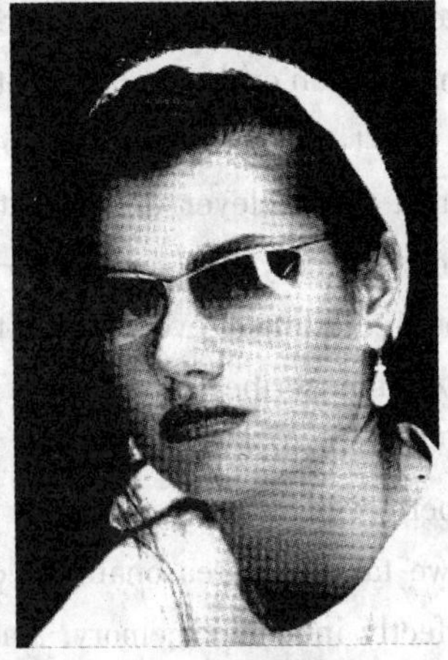

Jurys tend to pay close attention to eyewitness testimony and generally find it a reliable source of information. However, research into this area has found that eyewitness testimony can be affected by many psychological factors.

This recollection is used as evidence to show what happened from an witness' point of view. Memory recall has been considered a credible source in the past, but has recently come under attack as forensics can now support psychologists in their claim that memories and individual perceptions are unreliable; being easily manipulated, altered, and biased. Due to this, many countries and states within the USA are now attempting to make changes in how eyewitness testimony is presented in court. Eyewitness testimony is a specialized focus within forensic psychology.

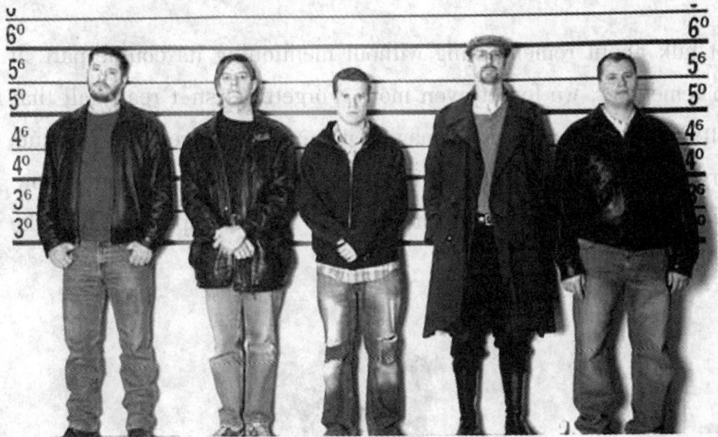

Eyewitness testimony is, at best, evidence of what the witness believes to have occurred. It may or may not tell what actually happened. The familiar problems of perception, of gauging time, speed, height, weight, of accurate identification of persons accused of crime all contribute to making honest testimony something less than completely credible.

The most important foundation for eyewitness testimony is a person's memory — after all, whatever testimony is being reported is coming from what a person remembers. To evaluate the reliability of memory, it is once again instructive to look to the criminal justice system. Police and prosecutors go to great lengths to keep a person's testimony "pure" by not allowing it to be tainted by outside information or the reports of others.

If prosecutors don't make every effort to retain the integrity of such testimony, it will become an easy target for a clever defense attorney. How can the integrity of memory and testimony be undermined? Very easily, in fact — there is a popular perception of memory being something like a tape-recording of events when the truth is anything but.

As Elizabeth Loftus describes in her book *Memory: Surprising New Insights into How We Remember and Why We Forget*:

Memory is imperfect. This is because we often do not see things accurately in the first place. But even if we take in a reasonably accurate picture of some experience, it does not necessarily stay perfectly intact in memory. Another force is at work. The memory traces can actually undergo distortion. With the passage of time, with proper motivation, with the introduction of special kinds of interfering facts, the memory traces seem sometimes to change or become transformed. These distortions can be quite frightening, for they can cause us to have memories of things that never happened. Even in the most intelligent among us is memory thus malleable.

Memory is not so much a static state as it is an ongoing process — and one which never happens in quite the same way twice. This is why we should have a skeptical, critical attitude towards all eyewitness testimony and all reports from memory — even our own and no matter what the subject, however mundane

Forgetting

You can't talk about remembering without mentioning its counterpart. It seems that as much as we do remember, we forget even more. Forgetting isn't really all that bad, and is in actuality, a pretty natural phenomenon. Imagine if you remembered every minute detail of every minute or every hour, of every day during your entire life, no matter how good, bad, or insignificant. Now imagine trying to sift through it all for the important stuff like where you left your keys.

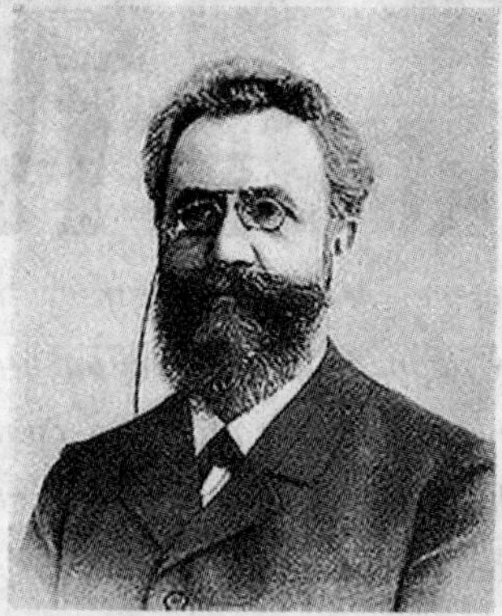

Hermann Ebbinghaus (January 24, 1850 – February 26, 1909) was a German psychologist who pioneered the experimental study of memory, and is known for his discovery of the

forgetting curve and the spacing effect. He was also the first person to describe the learning curve. He was the father of the eminent neo-Kantian philosopher Julius Ebbinghaus.

In 1885, Ebbinghaus published his groundbreaking öber das Gedöchtnis ("*On Memory*", later translated to English as *Memory*. A Contribution to Experimental Psychology) in which he described experiments he conducted on himself to describe the processes of learning and forgetting.

Ebbinghaus made several findings that are still relevant and supported to this day. First, arguably his most famous finding, the forgetting curve. The forgetting curve describes the exponential loss of information that one has learned. The sharpest decline occurs in the first twenty minutes and the decay is significant through the first hour. The curve levels off after about one day.

A typical representation of the forgetting curve. The learning curve described by Ebbinghaus refers to how fast one learns information. The sharpest increase occurs after the first try and then gradually evens out, meaning that less and less new information is retained after each repetition. Like the forgetting curve, the learning curve is exponential. Ebbinghaus had also documented the serial position effect, which describes how the position of an item affects recall. The two main concepts in the serial position effect are recently and primacy. The recency effect describes the increased recall of the most recent information because it is still in the short-term memory. The primacy effect better memory of the first items in a list due to increased rehearsal and commitment to long-term memory.

Another important discovery is that of savings. This refers to the amount of information retained in the subconscious even after this information cannot be consciously accessed. Ebbinghaus would memorize a list of items until perfect recall and then would not access the list until he could no longer recall any of its items. He then would relearn the list, and compare the new learning curve to the learning curve of his previous memorization of the list. The second list was generally memorized faster, and this difference between the two learning curves is what Ebbinghaus called "savings". Ebbinghaus also described the difference between involuntary and voluntary memory, the former occurring "with apparent spontaneity and without any act of the will" and the latter being brought "into consciousness by an exertion of the will".

Prior to Ebbinghaus, most contributions to the study of memory were undertaken by philosophers and centered on observational description and speculation. For example, Immanuel Kant used pure description to discuss recognition and its components and Sir Francis Bacon claimed that the simple observation of the rote recollection of a previously learned list was "no use to the art" of memory. This dichotomy between descriptive and experimental study of memory would resonate later in Ebbinghaus's life, particularly in his public argument with former colleague Wilhelm Dilthey. However, more than a century before Ebbinghaus, Johann Andreas Segner invented the "Segner-wheel" to see the length of after-images by seeing how fast a wheel with a hot coal attached had to move for the red ember circle from the coal to appear complete. Ebbinghaus's effect on memory research was almost immediate. With very few works published on memory in the previous two millennia, Ebbinghaus's works spurred memory research in the United States in the 1890s, with 32 papers published in 1894 alone. This research was coupled with the growing development of mechanized mnemometers, or devices that aided in the recording and study of memory.

The reaction to his work in his day was mostly positive. Noted psychologist William James called the studies "heroic" and said that they were "the single most brilliant investigation in the history of psychology". Edward B. Titchener also mentioned that the studies were the greatest undertaking in the topic of memory since Aristotle.

There are many reasons we forget things and often these reasons overlap. Like in the example above, some information never makes it to LTM. Other times, the information gets there, but is lost before it can attach itself to our LTM. Other reasons include decay, which means that information that is not used for an extended period of time decays or fades away over time. It is possible that we are physiologically preprogrammed to eventually erase data that no longer appears pertinent to us.

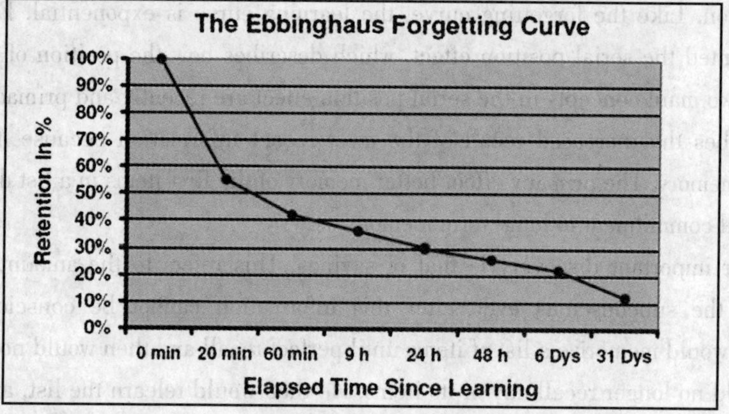

Figure 5.4 The Ebbinghaus Forgetting Curve

This curve asserts, that an average person loses 50% of the memorized data after 20 minutes. After 24 hours 70% are lost. There remains a contingent of 25% of the learned contents which is decreasing constantly, see Figure 5.4.

According to this theory you have to repeat all your knowledge permanently until you reach the point of "over-learning", a point where you don't forget information / skills any more.

Probably you know this situation from car driving. Even after one year of non-driving you are still able to operate your car.

The problem with constant repetition is that we normally don't have the time to recite all of our knowledge permanently. Especially when there are always new information coming that we have to integrate in our memory. If you want to keep pace like this with the information floods of our century, you should have lots of time.

Failing to remember something doesn't mean the information is gone forever though. Sometimes the information is there but for various reasons we can't access it. This could be caused by distractions going on around us or possibly due to an error of association (eg, believing something about the data which is not correct causing you to attempt to retrieve information that is not there). There is also the phenomenon of repression, which means that we purposefully (albeit subconsciously) push a memory out of reach because we do not want to remember the associated feelings. This is often sited in cases where adults "forget" incidences of sexual abuse when they were children. And finally, amnesia, which can be psychological or physiological in origin.

Why do we forget? There are two simple answers to this question. First, the memory has disappeared, it is no longer available. Second, the memory is still stored in the memory system but, for some reason, it cannot be retrieved.

These two answers summarize the main theories of forgetting developed by psychologists. The first answer is more likely to be applied to forgetting in short term memory, the second to forgetting in long term memory. Short term memory (STM) can be explained using the theories of trace decay and displacement. Forgetting from long term memory (LTM) can be explained using the theories of interference and lack of consolidation.

Trace Decay Theory of Forgetting STM

This theory relates to both short term memory and long term memory, and also relates to lack of availability. This theory suggests short term memory can only hold information for between 15 and 30 seconds unless it is rehearsed. After this time the information decays (fades away). This explanation of forgetting in short term memory assumes that memories leave a trace in the brain. A trace is some form of physical and/or chemical change in the nervous system. Trace decay theory states that forgetting occurs as a result of the automatic decay or fading of the memory trace. Trace decay theory focuses on time and the limited duration of short term memory.

No one disputes the fact that memory tends to get worse the longer the delay between learning and recall, but there is disagreement about the explanation for this effect. According to the trace decay theory of forgetting, the events between learning and recall have no affect whatsoever on recall. It is the length of time the information has to be retained that is important. The longer the time, the more the memory trace decays and as a consequence more information is forgotten.

There are a number of methodological problems confronting researchers trying to investigate the trace decay theory. One of the major problems is controlling for the events that occur between learning and recall. Clearly, in any real - life situation, the time between learning something and recalling it will be filled with all kinds of different events. This makes it very difficult to be sure that any forgetting which takes place is the result of decay rather than a consequence of the intervening events.

Intelligence

In this Topic, we focus on the most complex of all cognitive processes: intelligence. We will find that even defining the concept of intelligence is difficult. We'll look at how intelligence is measured, and we'll end the Topic by examining group and individual differences in measured intelligence.

Key Questions to Answer

While reading this Topic, find the answers to the following key questions:

1. How is intelligence defined?
2. How did Spearman define intelligence?
3. How did Sternberg and Gardner define intelligence?
4. What is emotional intelligence?
5. How do Western and non-Western concepts of intelligence differ?
6. What is the definition of a psychological test?
7. What determines the quality of psychological tests?
8. What is the Stanford-Binet intelligence test?
9. What are crystallized and fluid-analytic abilities?
10. What is the intelligence quotient?
11. What are the major features of the Wechsler intelligence scales?
12. What is the difference between a paper-and-pencil intelligence lest?
13. Are there gender differences in IQ?
14. Does intelligence increase, decrease, or remain the same with increasing age?
15. What are fluid and crystallized intelligence?
16. Are there racial differences in IQ scores?
17. What is a stereotype threat and how does it relate to racial differences in IQ?
18. What defines the mentally gifted?
19. How do we define mental retardation?
20. What are the causes of mental retardation?

The assessment of human abilities dates back nearly 4000 years when China used written tests to rate applicants for civil service. Two thousand years later, during the Hans Dynasty, civil service type exams were used in the areas of law, military, agriculture, and geography. In the early 1800s British diplomats observed the Chinese assessments and modified them for use in Britain and eventually the United States for use in civil service placement.

Sir Francis Galton is a key figure in modern intelligence testing. As the first cousin of Charles Darwin, he attempted to apply Darwin's evolutionary theory to the study of human abilities. He postulate that intelligence was quantifiable and normally distributed. In other words, he believed that we could assign a score to intelligence where the majority of people fall in the average range and the percentage of the population decreases the farther from the middle their score gets.

The first workable intelligence test was developed by French psychologist Alfred Binet. He and his partner, Theodore Simon, were commissioned by the French government to improve the teaching methods for developmentally disabled children. They believed that intelligence was the key to effective teaching, and developed a strategy whereby a mental age (MA) was determined and divided by the child's chronological age (CA).

Another theorist, Raymond Cattell, described intelligence as having two distinct factors. The first he called Crystallized Intelligence, representing acquired knowledge, and second, Fluid Intelligence, or our ability to use this knowledge.

Sternberg (1988) argued that there are a number of ways to demonstrate intelligence or adaptive functioning. He proposed a model of intelligence referred to as the theory. According to this model there are three types of intelligence: (1) analytical, or the ability to solve a problem by looking at its components; (2) creative, the ability to use new or ingenious ways to solve problems; and (3) practical, referring to street smarts or common sense. While most IQ tests measure only analytical intelligence, they fail to include practical intelligence which is the most understandable to most of us.

Intelligence is not something we can see or hear, or taste. We can see the results of intelligence sometimes. Many argue that quantifying intelligence correctly is impossible and all that modern IQ tests do is test our knowledge and abilities. While it is true that a person can learn to improve his or her score, this can only occur if correct responses are taught to the person, which is highly unethical. We have also found that our individual IQ score remains quite consistent as we get older. Some argue, however, that modern IQ tests are prejudiced against certain ethnicities and cultures and tend to result in higher scores for others. Where this leaves us, however, is uncertain. As of today, these IQ tests are the best we have in our attempt to quantify the construct known as intelligence.

Just What Is Intelligence

There are probably as many definitions of intelligence as there are experts who study it. Simply put, however, intelligence is the ability to learn about, learn from, understand, and interact with one's environment. This general ability consists of a number of specific abilities, which include these specific abilities:

Adaptability to a new environment or to changes in the current environment;

Capacity for knowledge and the ability to acquire it;

Capacity for reason and abstract thought;

Ability to comprehend relationships;

Ability to evaluate and judge;

Capacity for original and productive thought.

Additional specific abilities might be added to the list, but they would all be abilities allowing a person to learn about, learn from, understand, and interact with the environment. Environment in this definition doesn't mean the environment of the earth, such as the desert, the mountains, etc., although it can mean that kind of environment. It has a wider meaning that includes a person's immediate surroundings, including the people around him or her. Environment in this case can also be something as small as a family, the workplace, or a classroom.

Classic Models of Intelligence

Theoretical models of intelligence are attempts to categorize and organize cognitive or intellectual abilities into groupings that make sense. In a way, they are sophisticated attempts to provide a definition for "intelligence". British psychologist Charles Spearman was one of the pioneers of mental testing and the inventor of many statistical procedures used to analyze test scores. Spearman's characterization of intelligence came from his inspection of scores earned by people on a wide range of psychological tests designed to measure cognitive skills. What impressed Spearman was that no matter what cognitive ability a specific test was designed to measure, some people always seemed to do better than others. People who scored high on some tests tended to score high on all the tests. It seemed as if there was an intellectual power that facilitated performance in general, whereas variations in performance reflected strengths and weaknesses tor specific tasks.

Spearman concluded that intelligence consists of two things: a general intelligence, called a g-factor, and a collection of specific cognitive skills, or s-factors. Spearman believed that "g" was independent of knowledge, of content: it went beyond knowing facts. It involved the ability to understand and apply relationships in all content areas. In this view, everyone has some degree of general intelligence (which Spearman thought was inherited), and everyone has specific skills that are useful in some tasks but not in others. A controversy remains over the extent to which "g" is an all-important, sometimes-important, or never-important factor in intelligence. Still, looking at intelligence in terms of what a variety of tests measure and how such measures are interrelated became a popular way to think about intelligence.

When L. L. Thurstone examined correlations among various tests of cognitive abilities he administered, he found something different from what Spearman had found. Thurstone saw little or no evidence to support the notion of a general g-factor of intellectual ability. Instead, he claimed that abilities fall into seven categories, which he called the seven primary mental abilities (Figure 5.5). Thurstone argued that each factor in his model is independent, and to know one's intelligence requires that you know how one fares on all seven factors.

With the model of J. P. Guilford (1967), matters get more complicated than with either Spearman's or Thurstone's theory. Guilford claimed that intelligence can be analyzed as three intersecting dimensions. Guilford said that any intellectual task can be described in terms of the mental operations used in the task, the content of the material involved, and the product or outcome of the task. Each of these three dimensions has a number of possible values. There are five operations, four contents, and six possible products. The three dimensions of the model, and their values, are found in Figure 5.5.

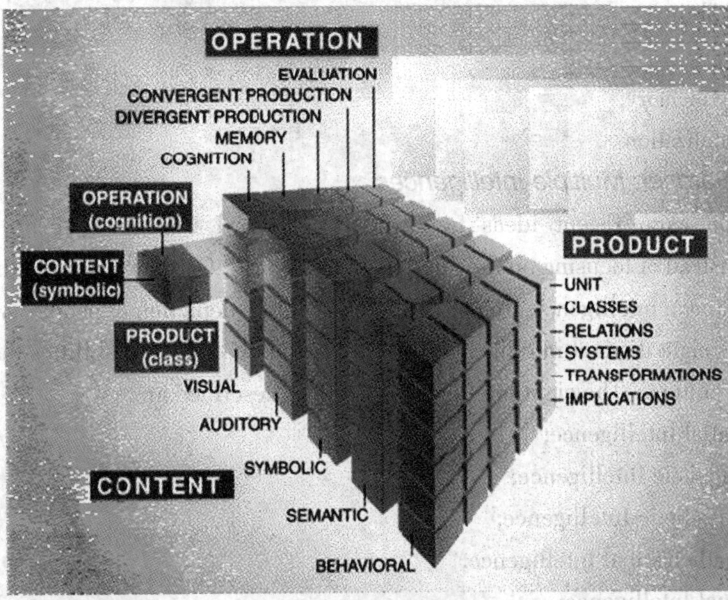

Figure 5.5　Models of Intelligence

If you study Figure 5.5 you will see that there are 120 possible combinations of content. operations, and products in Guilford's model. Just to give yon an idea of how this system works, let's choose one of the "cell" depicted in Figure 5.5 where cognition, figural, and units intersect (the little "block" in the uppermost left comer). What would this intellectual skill be like? Guilford says it's a matter of recognizing (cognitive) diagrams or pictures (figural) of simple, well-defined elements (units). To test this ability, one might be shown an incomplete drawing of a simple object and be asked to identify it as quickly as possible.

The following are some of the major theories of intelligence that have emerged during the last 100 years.

Charles Spearman: General Intelligence

British psychologist Charles Spearman (1863–1945) described a concept he referred to as general intelligence, or the g factor. After using a technique known as factor analysis to examine a number of mental aptitude tests, Spearman concluded that scores on these tests were remarkably similar. People who performed well on one cognitive test tended to perform well on other tests, while those who scored badly on one test tended to score badly on others. He concluded that intelligence is general cognitive ability that could be measured and numerically expressed.

Louis L. Thurstone: Primary Mental Abilities

Psychologist Louis L. Thurstone (1887–1955) offered a differing theory of intelligence. Instead of viewing intelligence as a single, general ability, Thurstone's theory focused on seven different "primary mental abilities". The abilities that he described were:

Verbal comprehension;

Reasoning;

Perceptual speed;

Numerical ability;

Word fluency;

Associative memory;

Spatial visualization.

Howard Gardner: Multiple Intelligences

One of the more recent ideas to emerge is Howard Gardner's theory of multiple intelligences. Instead of focusing on the analysis of test scores, Gardner proposed that numerical expressions of human intelligence are not a full and accurate depiction of people's abilities. His theory describes eight distinct intelligences that are based on skills and abilities that are valued within different cultures. The eight intelligences Gardner described are:

Visual-spatial Intelligence;

Verbal-linguistic Intelligence;

Bodily-kinesthetic Intelligence;

Logical-mathematical Intelligence;

Interpersonal Intelligence;

Musical Intelligence;

Intra personal Intelligence;

Naturalistic Intelligence.

Robert Sternberg :Triarchic Theory of Intelligence

Psychologist Robert Sternberg defined intelligence as "mental activity directed toward purposive adaptation to, selection and shaping of, real-world environments relevant to one's life." While he agreed with Gardner that intelligence is much broader than a single, general ability, he instead suggested some of Gardner's intelligences are better viewed as individual talents. Sternberg proposed what he refers to as "successful intelligence", which is comprised of three different factors:

Analytical intelligence: This component refers to problem-solving abilities.

Creative intelligence: This aspect of intelligence involves the ability to deal with new situations using past experiences and current skills.

Practical intelligence: This element refers to the ability to adapt to a changing environment.

Fluid and Crystallized Intelligence

Raymond Cattell and John Horn suggested that the g-factor should be divided into fluid intelligence and crystallized intelligence.

Fluid intelligence consists of reasoning ability, memory capacity, and speed of information processing. It involves such skills as those requiring spatial and visual imagery and is generally believed to be much less affected by experience and education than is crystallized intelligence.

Crystallized intelligence concerns the application of knowledge to problem solving. It includes abilities such as reasoning and verbal and numerical skills and is generally believed to be affected by experience and formal education.

The concepts of fluid and crystallized intelligence are still used by some psychologists, particularly in the area of aging.

What is Emotional Intelligence?

Emotional intelligence (EI) refers to the ability to perceive, control and evaluate emotions. Some researchers suggest that emotional intelligence can be learned and strengthened, while others claim it is an inborn characteristic.

Since 1990, Peter Salovey and John D. Mayer have been the leading researchers on emotional intelligence. In their influential article "*Emotional Intelligence*", they defined emotional intelligence as, "the subset of social intelligence that involves the ability to monitor one's own and others' feelings and emotions, to discriminate among them and to use this information to guide one's thinking and actions".

The Four Branches of Emotional Intelligence

Salovey and Mayer proposed a model that identified four different factors of emotional intelligence: the perception of emotion, the ability to reason using emotions, the ability to understand emotion and the ability to manage emotions.

1. Perceiving Emotions

The first step in understanding emotions is to accurately perceive them. In many cases, this might involve understanding nonverbal signals such as body language and facial expressions.

2. Reasoning with Emotions

The next step involves using emotions to promote thinking and cognitive activity. Emotions help prioritize what we pay attention and react to; we respond emotionally to things that garner our attention.

3. Understanding Emotions

The emotions that we perceive can carry a wide variety of meanings. If someone is expressing angry emotions, the observer must interpret the cause of their anger and what it might mean. For example, if your boss is acting angry, it might mean that he is dissatisfied with your work; or it could be because he got a speeding ticket on his way to work that morning or that he's been fighting with his wife.

4. Managing Emotions

The ability to manage emotions effectively is a key part of emotional intelligence. Regulating emotions, responding appropriately and responding to the emotions of others are all important aspect of emotional management.

According to Salovey and Mayer, the four branches of their model are, "arranged from more basic psychological processes to higher, more psychologically integrated processes. For example, the lowest level branch concerns the (relatively) simple abilities of perceiving and expressing emotion. In contrast, the highest level branch concerns the conscious, reflective regulation of emotion".

Measuring Emotional Intelligence

"In regard to measuring emotional intelligence — I am a great believer that criterion - report (that is, ability testing) is the only adequate method to employ. Intelligence is an ability, and is directly measured only by having people answer questions and evaluating the correctness of those answers." — John D. Mayer .

Reuven Bar- On's EQ- I

A self - report test designed to measure competencies including awareness, stress tolerance, problem solving, and happiness. According to Bar - On, "Emotional intelligence is an array of noncognitive capabilities, competencies, and skills that influence one's ability to succeed in coping with environmental demands and pressures."

Multifactor Emotional Intelligence Scale (MEIS)

An ability - based test in which test - takers perform tasks designed to assess their ability to perceive, identify, understand, and utilize emotions.

Seligman Attributional Style Questionnaire (SASQ)

Originally designed as a screening test for the life insurance company Metropolitan Life, the SASQ measures optimism and pessimism.

Emotional Competence Inventory (ECI)

Based on an older instrument known as the Self - Assessment Questionnaire, the ECI involves having people who know the individual offer ratings of that person's abilities on a number of different emotional competencies.

Intelligence is not something we can see or hear, or taste. We can see the results of intelligence sometimes. Many argue that quantifying intelligence correctly is impossible and all that modern IQ tests do is test our knowledge and abilities. While it is true that a person can learn to improve his or her score, this can only occur if correct responses are taught to the person, which is highly unethical. We have also found that our individual IQ score remains quite consistent as we get older. Some argue, however, that modern IQ tests are prejudiced against certain ethnicities and cultures and tend to result in higher scores for others. Where this leaves us, however, is uncertain. As of today, these IQ tests are the best we have in our attempt to quantify the construct known as intelligence.

A Psychological Test of Intelligence

Sir Francis Galton, a pioneer in the measurement of individual differences in late nineteenth - century England, was particularly concerned with sensory responses (visual and auditory acuity and reaction times) and their relationship to differences in ability. Several individual tests have been used to test intelligence.

The Binet - Simon intelligence scale, developed by French psychologists Alfred Binet and Theodore Simon, was administered to children to evaluate their performance (mental age) at a given chronological age. The mental age/chronological age measure, called a mental quotient, was used to evaluate a child's learning potential.

Lewis Terman of Stanford University revised the Binet scale in 1916. The revised scale, called the Stanford - Binet intelligence scale, although it retained the concept of mental and chronological ages, introduced the concept of the intelligence quotient (IQ) arrived at by the following widely used formula, which allows comparison between children of different ages.

$$\text{intelligence quotient (IQ)}=\frac{\text{mental age}}{\text{chronological age}}\times 100$$

The 1986 revision of the test, the latest of several, varies the calculation so that the test is useful for adults as well as for children. An individual's score for correct answers is compared to a table of scores of test takers of the same age (with the average score always scaled to 100). Scores between 90 and 110 are labeled as "normal", above 130 as "superior", and below 70 as mentally deficient, or "retarded". The distribution of IQ scores approximates a normal (bell-shaped) curve (Figure 5.6).

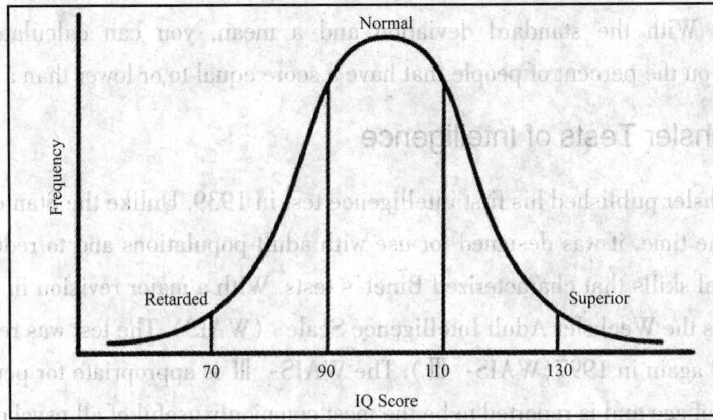

Figure 5.6 The Normal IQ Distribution

David Wechsler developed the Wechsler Adult Intelligence Scale (WAIS) in 1939, revised as the WAIS - R. Wechsler also developed the Wechsler Intelligence Scale for Children (WISC), revised as the WISC - R. The revised forms of these scales are still widely used. They contains two sub - scales, verbal and performance, which provide a verbal IQ and a performance IQ; the subscales are combined for the total IQ. Test score combinations may reveal other strengths and weaknesses to a skilled examiner.

This is a quick explanation of IQ, put up due to popular demand. There are many books on psychology or intelligence that would provide a more rigorous explanation of IQ.

What is intelligence? The definition I like is that intelligence is "the ability to learn or understand or to deal with new or trying situations, also the skilled use of reason". I have heard some people misuse the word smart to mean knowledgeable. That is like confusing velocity with that one can lead to the other does not mean that they are the same thing. IQ tests were created to be able to identify children who might need special education due to their retarded mental development.

(1)Binet's test included varied questions and tasks. The tasks even included unwrapping a piece of candy and comparing the weights of different objects. To relate the mental development of a child to the child's chronological age the IQ was invented. IQ = (MA/CA) * 100. The intelligence quotient was equal to 100 times the Mental Age divided by the Chronological Age. For example, if a certain child started reading, etc., at the age of 3 (CA) and average children start reading, etc., at the age of 6 (MA), the child would get an IQ score of 200. (Such a score is very, very rare). Since people wanted to also use IQs for adults, that formula was not very useful since raw scores start to level off around the age of 16.

(2)Thus the deviation IQ replaced the ratio IQ. It compares people of the same age or age category and assumes that IQ is normally distributed, that the average (mean) is 100 and that the standard deviation is something like 15 (IQ tests sometimes differ in their standard deviations).

What is a standard deviation (SD)? Simply put, the standard deviation is a measure of the spread of the sample from the mean. As a rule of thumb, about 2/3 of a sample is within 1 standard deviation from the mean. About 95% of the sample will be within 2 standard deviations from the mean. With the standard deviation and a mean, you can calculate percentiles. Percentiles tell you the percent of people that have a score equal to or lower than a certain score.

The Wechsler Tests of Intelligence

David Wechsler published his first intelligence test in 1939. Unlike the Stantord-Binet test that existed at the time, it was designed for use with adult populations and to reduce the heavy reliance on verbal skills that characterized Binet's tests. With a major revision in 1955, the test became known as the Wechsler Adult Intelligence Scale (WAIS). The test was revised in 1981 (WAIS-R), and again in 1997(WAIS-Ⅲ). The WAIS-Ⅲ is appropriate for persons between 16 and 74 years of age and is reported to be the most commonly useful of all psychological tests.

A natural extension was the Wechsler Intelligence Scale for Children (WISC), originally published 11 years after the WAIS. With updated nor MS and several new items (among other things, designed to minimize bias against any ethnic group or gender), the WISC-Ⅲ appeared in 1991. It is appropriate for children ages six to it (there is some overlap with the WAIS-Ⅲ). A third test in the series is for younger children, between the ages of four and six. It is called the Wechsler Preschool and Primary Scale of Intelligence, or WPPSI. It was published in 1967, was revised in 19S9 and is now the WPPSI-R. There are some subtle differences among the three Wechsler tests, but each is based on the same logic. Therefore, we will consider only one, the WAIS-Ⅲ in detail.

The WAIS-Ⅲ consists of 14 subtests organized in two categories. Seven subtests define the verbal scale, and seven subtests constitute a performance scale. Each item on each subtest is scored. (Some of the performance items have time limits that affect scoring.) As is now the case with the Stanford-Binet, each subtest score is compared to a score provided by the test's norms. How a person's earned score compares to the scores earned by persons in the norm group (others of the same sex and age who have already taken the test) determines the person's standard score for each Wechsler subtest. Addition to one overall score, the Wechsler tests provide verbal and performance scores, which can tell us something about a person's particular strengths and weaknesses.

There has been controversy for many years about individually administered intelligence tests such as the Wechsler tests and the Stanford - Binet. The extent to which the tests are culturally biased, thus favoring one group of subjects over another, whether they truly measure intelligence and not just academic success, and whether test results can be used for political purposes, perhaps as a basis for racial discrimination, are just some of the concerns that keep surfacing. Although experts allow that the tests may be somewhat biased on racial and socioeconomic grounds, they believe that such tests adequately measure more important elements of intelligence.

High IQ societies ask for certain percentile scores on IQ tests for you to be eligible to join them. Mensa asks for scores at the 98th percentile or higher. For a list of the selection criteria of other societies, click here. There have been various classification systems for IQ.

Terman's classification of IQ was the following

IQ Range	Classification
140 and over	Genius or near genius
120—140	Very superior intelligence
110—120	Superior intelligence
90—110	Normal or average intelligence
80—90	Dullness
70—80	Borderline deficiency
Below 70	Definite feeble-mindedness

Terman wrote the Stanford-Binet test. Later, Wechsler thought that it would be much more legitimate to base his classifications on the Probable Error (PE) so his classification was the following:

Classification	IQ Limits	Percent Included
Very Superior	128 and over	2.2
Superior	120—127	6.7
Bright Normal	111—119	16.1
Average	91—110	50
Dull Normal	80—90	16.1
Borderline	66—79	6.7
Defective	65 and below	2.2

Mental deficiency used to be more finely classified using the following technical terms that later began to be abused by the rest of society as the following:

IQ Range	Classification
70—80	Borderline deficiency
50—69	Moron
20—49	Imbecile
below 20	Idiot

These are now largely obsolete and mental deficiency is now generally called mental retardation. The following is the currently used classification of retardation in the USA:

IQ Range	Classification
50—69	Mild
35—49	Moderate
20—34	Severe
below 20	Profound

Mental Retardation

Mental retardation (MR) is a generalized disorder appearing before adulthood, characterized by significantly impaired cognitive functioning and deficits in two or more adaptive behaviors. It has historically been defined as an Intelligence Quotient score under 70. Once focused almost entirely on cognition, the definition now includes both a component relating to mental functioning and one relating to individuals' functional skills in their environment. As a result, a person with a below - average intelligence quotient may not be considered mentally retarded. Syndromic mental retardation is intellectual deficits associated with other medical and behavioral signs and symptoms. Non - syndromic mental retardation refers to intellectual deficits that appear without other abnormalities.

The terms used for this condition are subject to a process called the euphemism treadmill. This means that whatever term is chosen for this condition, it eventually becomes perceived as an insult. The terms mental retardation and mentally retarded were invented in the middle of the 20th century to replace the previous set of terms, which were deemed to have become offensive. By the end of the 20th century, these terms themselves have come to be widely seen as disparaging and politically incorrect and in need of replacement. The term intellectual disability or intellectually challenged is now preferred by most advocates in most English - speaking countries. The AAIDD have defined intellectual disability to mean the same thing as mental retardation. Currently, the term mental retardation is used by the World Health Organization in the ICD - 10 codes, which has a section titled "Mental Retardation" (codes F70 - F79). In the future, the ICD - 11 is expected to replace the term mental retardation with intellectual disability, and the DSM - V is expected to replace it with intellectual developmental disorder. Because of its specificity and lack of confusion with other conditions, mental retardation is still sometimes used professional medical settings around the world, such as formal scientific research and health insurance paperwork.

Moreover, "educable mentally retarded" is roughly equivalent to mild mental retardation, and "trainable" mentally retarded is roughly equivalent to moderate. The DSM now requires an assessment of a person's adaptive functioning as an additional criterion for labeling someone retarded. IQ is not enough. Maybe the same sort of thing should be done for labeling somebody a genius.

Signs and Symptoms of MR

The signs and symptoms of mental retardation are all behavioral. Most people with mental retardation do not look like they have any type of intellectual disability, especially if the disability is caused by environmental factors such as malnutrition or lead poisoning. The so - called "typical appearance" ascribed to people with mental retardation is only present in a minority of cases, all of which involve syndromic mental retardation.

Children with mental retardation may learn to sit up, to crawl, or to walk later than other children, or they may learn to talk later. Both adults and children with mental retardation may also exhibit some or all of the following characteristics:

Delays in oral language development;

Deficits in memory skills;

Difficulty learning social rules;

Difficulty with problem solving skills;

Delays in the development of adaptive behaviors such as self - help or self - care skills;

Lack of social inhibitors.

Children with mental retardation learn more slowly than a typical child. Children may take longer to learn language, develop social skills, and take care of their personal needs, such as dressing or eating. Learning will take them longer, require more repetition, and skills may need to be adapted to their learning level. Nevertheless, virtually every child is able to learn, develop and become a participating member of the community.

In early childhood, mild mental retardation (IQ 50 - 69, a cognitive ability about half to two - thirds of standard) may not be obvious, and may not be identified until children begin school. Even when poor academic performance is recognized, it may take expert assessment to distinguish mild mental retardation from learning disability or emotional/behavioral disorders. People with mild MR are capable of learning reading and mathematics skills to approximately the level of a typical child aged 9 to 12. They can learn self - care and practical skills, such as cooking or using the local mass transit system. As individuals with mild mental retardation reach adulthood, many learn to live independently and maintain gainful employment.

Moderate mental retardation (IQ 35 - 49) is nearly always apparent within the first years of life. Speech delays are particularly common signs of moderate MR. People with moderate mental retardation need considerable supports in school, at home, and in the community in order to participate fully. While their academic potential is limited, they can learn simple health and safety skills and to participate in simple activities. As adults they may live with their parents, in a supportive group home, or even semi - independently with significant supportive services to help them, for example, manage their finances. As adults, they may work in a sheltered workshop.

A person with severe or profound mental retardation will need more intensive support and supervision his or her entire life. They may learn some activities of daily living. Some will require full - time care by an attendant.

Diagnosis of MR

According to the latest edition of the *Diagnostic and Statistical Manual of Mental Disorders* (DSM - IV), three criteria must be met for a diagnosis of mental retardation: an IQ below 70, significant limitations in two or more areas of adaptive behavior (as measured by an adaptive behavior rating scale, ie, communication, self - help skills, interpersonal skills, and more), and evidence that the limitations became apparent before the age of 18, as the following show .

Class	IQ
Profound mental retardation	Below 20
Severe mental retardation	20—34
Moderate mental retardation	35—49
Mild mental retardation	50—69
Borderline intellectual functioning	70—84

Approximately 85% of the mentally retarded population is in the mildly retarded category. Their IQ score ranges from 50 to 75, and they can often acquire academic skills up to the 6th grade level. They can become fairly self - sufficient and in some cases live independently, with community and social support.

Moderate Mental Retardation

About 10% of the mentally retarded population is considered moderately retarded. Moderately retarded individuals have IQ scores ranging from 35 to 55. They can carry out work and self - care tasks with moderate supervision. They typically acquire communication skills in childhood and are able to live and function successfully within the community in a supervised environment such as a group home.

Severe Mental Retardation

About 3% - 4% of the mentally retarded population is severely retarded. Severely retarded individuals have IQ scores of 20 - 40. They may master very basic self - care skills and some communication skills. Many severely retarded individuals are able to live in a group home.

Profound Mental Retardation

Only 1% - 2% of the mentally retarded population is classified as profoundly retarded. Profoundly retarded individuals have IQ scores under 20 - 25. They may be able to develop basic self - care and communication skills with appropriate support and training. Their retardation is often caused by an accompanying neurological disorder. The profoundly retarded need a high level of structure and supervision.

The American Association on Mental Retardation (AAMR) has developed another widely accepted diagnostic classification system for mental retardation. The AAMR classification system focuses on the capabilities of the retarded individual rather than on the limitations. The categories describe the level of support required. They are: intermittent support, limited support, extensive support, and pervasive support. To some extent, the AAMR classification mirrors the DSM - IV classification. Intermittent support, for example, is support needed only occasionally, perhaps during times of stress or crisis. It is the type of support typically required for most mildly retarded individuals. At the other end of the spectrum, pervasive support, or life - long, daily support for most adaptive areas, would be required for profoundly retarded individuals.

It is formally diagnosed by professional assessment of intelligence and adaptive behavior IQ below 70. The first English - language IQ test, the Terman - Binet, was adapted from an instrument used to measure potential to achieve developed by Binet in France. Terman translated the test and employed it as a means to measure intellectual capacity based on oral language, vocabulary, numerical reasoning, memory, motor speed and analysis skills. The mean score on the currently available IQ tests is 100, with a standard deviation of 15 (WAIS/WISC - IV) or 16 (Stanford - Binet). Sub - average intelligence is generally considered to be present when an individual scores two standard deviations below the test mean. Factors other than cognitive ability (depression, anxiety, etc.) can contribute to low IQ scores; it is important for the evaluator to rule them out prior to concluding that measured IQ is "significantly below average".

The following ranges, based on Standard Scores of intelligence tests, reflect the categories of the American Association of Mental Retardation, the Diagnostic and Statistical Manual of Mental Disorders - IV - TR, and the International Classification of Diseases.

Chapter 6 Motivation, Emotion and Personality

What drives you to want to learn about psychology? Why did you choose your career? Your partner? Where would you live? Are your drives different from other people or do we all share the same goals in life?

This chapter will discuss the various theories related to motivation and emotion. You will learn the different views on motivation, from those deemed instinctual, internal, and those viewed as external. You will also be presented with the theories of emotion, an abstract concept which has yet to have an agreed upon definition.

Motivation

Ever wonder why some people seem to be very successful, highly motivated individuals? Where does the energy, the drive, or the direction come from? Motivation is an area of psychology that has gotten a great deal of attention, especially in the recent years. The reason is that we all want to be successful, we all want direction and drive, and we all want to be seen as motivated.

There are several distinct theories of motivation we will discuss in this section. Some include basic biological forces, while others seem to transcend concrete explanation. These are the five major theories of motivation as the following.

Many people incorrectly view motivation as a personal trait—that is, some people have it, and others don't. But motivation is defined as the force that causes an individual to behave in a specific way. Simply put, a highly motivated person works hard at a job; an unmotivated person does not. Managers often have difficulty motivating employees. But motivation is really an internal process. It's the result of the interaction of a person's needs, his or her ability to make choices about how to meet those needs, and the environment created by management that allows these needs to be met and the choices to be made. Motivation is not something that a manager can "do" to a person.

Theories of Motivation

Darwin explained survival of an organism, and consequently a species, as, in part, resulting from an instinct for survival. Other early attempts to explain motivation (by, for example, William James and William McDougall) also involved instincts, defined by some as unlearned patterns of behavior that aid in the survival of the organism. Explaining behavior in terms of instincts eventually fell out of favor, however, because of the indiscriminate labeling of all motivated behaviors as instincts (till they reached the thousands and included such things as instincts for rivalry, cleanliness, or parental love).

Instinct Theory

Instinct theory is derived from our biological make-up. We've all seen spider's webs and perhaps even witnessed a spider in the tedious job of creating its home and trap. We've all seen birds in their nests, feeding their young or painstakingly placing the twigs in place to form their new home. How do spiders know how to spin webs? How do birds now how to build nests?

The answer is biology. All creatures are born with specific innate knowledge about how to survive. Animals are born with the capacity and often times knowledge of how to survive by spinning webs, building nests, avoiding danger, and reproducing. These innate tendencies are preprogrammed at birth, they are in our genes, and even if the spider never saw a web before, never witnessed its creation, it would still know how to create one.

Humans have the same types of innate tendencies. Babies are born with a unique ability that allows them to survive; they are born with the ability to cry. Without this, how would others know when to feed the baby, know when he needed changing, or when she wanted attention and affection? Crying allows a human infant to survive. We are also born with particular reflexes which promote survival. The most important of these include sucking, swallowing, coughing, blinking. Newborns can perform physical movements to avoid pain; they will turn their head if touched on their cheek and search for a nipple (rooting reflex); and they will grasp an object that touches the palm of their hands.

Drive Reduction Theory

According to Clark Hull (1943, 1952), humans have internal internal biological needs which motivate us to perform a certain way. These needs, or drives, are defined by Hull as internal states of arousal or tension which must be reduced. A prime example would be the internal feelings of hunger or thirst, which motivates us to eat. According to this theory, we are driven to reduce these drives so that we may maintain a sense of internal calmness.

Arousal Theory

Similar to Hull's Drive Reduction Theory, Arousal theory states that we are driven to maintain a certain level of arousal in order to feel comfortable. Arousal refers to a state of emotional, intellectual, and physical activity. It is different from the above theory, however, because it doesn't rely on only a reduction of tension, but a balanced amount. It also does better to explain why people climb mountains, go to school, or watch sad movies.

Psychoanalytic Theory

Remember Sigmund Freud and his five part theory of personality. As part of this theory, he believed that humans have only two basic drives: Eros and Thanatos, or the Life and Death drives. According to Psychoanalytic theory, everything we do, every thought we have, and every emotion we experience has one of two goals: to help us survive or to prevent our destruction. This is similar to instinct theory, however, Freud believed that the vast majority of our knowledge about these drives is buried in the unconscious part of the mind.

Psychoanalytic theory therefore argues that we go to school because it will help assure our survival in terms of improved finances, more money for healthcare, or even an improved ability to find a spouse. We move to better school districts to improve our children's ability to survive and continue our family tree. We demand safety in our cars, toys, and in our homes. We want criminal locked away, and we want to be protected against poisons, terrorists, and any thing else that could lead to our destruction. According to this theory, everything we do, everything we are can be traced back to the two basic drives.

Humanistic Theory

Although discussed last, humanistic theory is perhaps the most well known theory of motivation. According to this theory, humans are driven to achieve their maximum potential and will always do so unless obstacles are placed in their way. These obstacles include hunger, thirst, financial problems, safety issues, or anything else that takes our focus away from maximum psychological growth.

The best way to describe this theory is to utilize the famous pyramid developed by Abraham Maslow (1970) called the Hierarchy of Needs. Maslow believed that humans have specific needs that must be met and that if lower level needs go unmet, we can not possible strive for higher level needs. The Hierarchy of Needs shows that at the lower level, we must focus on basic issues such as food, sleep, and safety. Without food, without sleep, how could we possible focus on the higher level needs such as respect, education, and recognition?

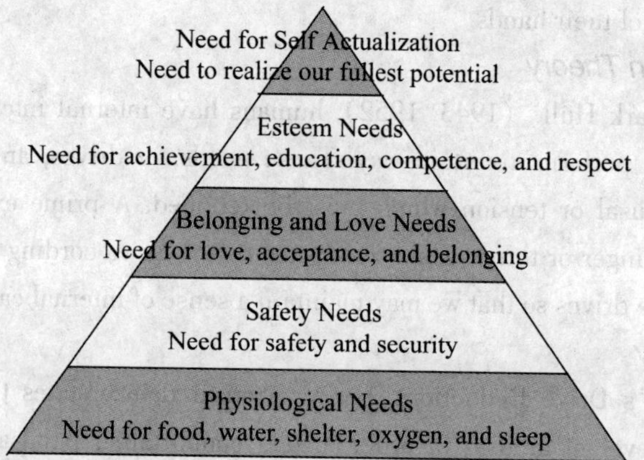

Abraham Maslow (1954) presents a hierarchy of needs model which can be divided into basic (or deficiency) needs (eg, physiological, safety, love, and esteem) and growth needs (cognitive, aesthetics and self-actualization). One must satisfy lower level basic needs before progressing on to meet higher level growth needs. Once these needs have been reasonably satisfied, one may be able to reach the highest level called self-actualization. Every person is capable and has the desire to move up the hierarchy toward a level of self-actualization. Unfortunately, progress is often disrupted by failure to meet lower level needs. Life experiences including divorce and loss of job may cause an individual to fluctuate between levels of he hierarchy. Maslow noted only one in a hundred people become fully self-actualized because our society rewards motivation primarily based on esteem, love and other social needs.

Throughout our lives, we work toward achieving the top of the pyramid, self-actualization, or the realization of all of our potential. As we move up the pyramid, however, things get in the way which slow us down and often knock us backward. Imagine working toward the respect and recognition of your colleagues and suddenly finding yourself out of work and homeless. Suddenly, you are forced backward and can no longer focus your attention on your work due to the need for finding food and shelter for you and your family.

According to Maslow, nobody has ever reached the peak of his pyramid. We all may strive for it and some may even get close, but no one has achieved full self - actualization. Self - actualization means a complete understanding of who you are, a sense of completeness, of being the best person you could possibly be. To have achieved this goal is to stop living, for what is there to strive for if you have learned everything about yourself, if you have experienced all that you can, and if there is no way left for you to grow emotionally, intellectually, or spiritually.

Human's Major Motivation

Hunger Motivation

Hunger is now known to be regulated on a short - term basis by two clusters of cells (called nuclei) in the hypothalamus of the brain, the ventromedial hypothalamic (VMH) and the lateral hypothalamic (LH) nuclei (Figure 6.1).

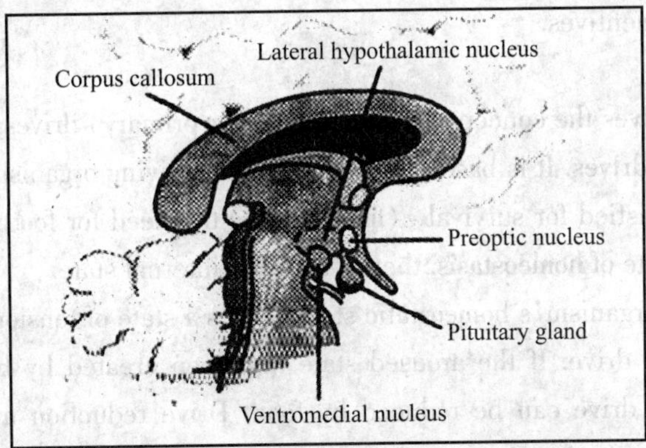

Figure 6.1 The Hypothalamic Nuclei

Lesioning (destruction) produces effects on motivated behavior that are opposite those produced by electrical stimulation of the same nucleus. Damage to a rat's LH causes the rat to stop eating (become aphagic) and eventually starve to death even with an abundance of food. Electrical stimulation of the LH, however, causes it to eat. Conversely, damage to a rat's VMH causes it to overeat (become hyperphagic). (If an adult female rat of a species weighs 350 grams, a hyperphagic rat of the same species can weigh over 1,000 grams.) Electrical stimulation in the same VMH nucleus produces cessation of eating.

Long - term regulation of hunger is less understood, but one theory, the set - point theory, suggests that the body has a weight regulatory system, which establishes a "set - point" that regulates body weight on a long - term basis. This theory could explain, for example, why a hyperphagic rat, even though very overweight, finally stops eating. While the set - point mechanism is not known, one view is that the regulation includes an interaction with the level of body fat. If body fat increases, eating is less frequent and activity increases; the converse is true if body fat decreases.

Other changes can also affect hunger, such as changes in glucose (blood sugar) and hormone levels. For example, the hormone insulin diminishes the blood glucose level, producing hunger and thus increasing eating behavior. In addition, external cues may affect eating behavior, for example, the sight or aroma of food or the sight of other people eating.

Sexual Motivation

Sexual repsonse regulation. Level of sexual motivation, as well as that of thirst and hunger, can be changed by damage to or stimulation of certain areas of the hypothalamus (including the medial preoptic area and the VMH) and other portions of the brain (such as the limbic system). Sexual behavior is also affected by levels of the sexual hormones — primarily, testosterone in males and estrogens in females — produced by the gonads. Sexual hormone production in the gonads is, in turn, controlled by hormones produced in the pituitary gland. Sexual behavior is complex, however, and may be affected by many factors, particularly during development, such as administration of sex hormones or ingestion of drugs that affect production of sex hormones.

Behavioral Perspective of Motivation

The behavioral approach to understanding motivation deals with drives, both learned and unlearned, and with incentives.

Drive Theory

Drive theory involves the concepts of unlearned (or primary) drives, drive reduction, and learned (secondary) drives. It is based on the fact that all living organisms have physiological needs that must be satisfied for survival (for example, the need for food, water, sleep, and so forth) to maintain a state of homeostasis, that is, a steady internal state.

Disruption of an organism's homeostatic state causes a state of tension (arousal) called an unlearned, or primary, drive. If the aroused state has been created by hunger, it is called a hunger drive, and the drive can be reduced by food. Drive reduction moves toward the re-establishment of homeostasis. Drives, then, may be thought of as the consequence of a physiological need, which an organism is impelled to reduce or eliminate. Clark Hull, a learning theorist, developed an equation to show how learning and drive are related.

Drives may also be learned, or secondary. Fear (or anxiety), for example, is often considered a secondary drive that can be learned through either classical or operant conditioning. In Neal Miller's well-known operant conditioning experiment, a rat was placed in a black box and then given a mild electrical shock. Eventually, the rat learned to react to the experience of being put in a black box (with no shock given) with the response of turning a wheel to escape. In this case, the black box is said to have elicited the learned drive of fear. Among other drives considered by some theorists to be learned are the need for affiliation (that is, to belong, to have companionship), the need for security (money), and the need for achievement.

Incentive motivation

Theories of incentive motivation contend that external stimuli can motivate behavior. Humans (and other animals) can learn to value external stimuli (for example, the first prize in a track meet for a human and a pat on the head for a dog) and will work to get them. Incentive motivation is sometimes called "pull" motivation because incentives are said to "pull" in contrast with the "push" associated with drives. Kenneth Spence, well known for his work in incentive motivation, suggested that the incentive value of the reward strengthens the response. (One would run faster for a reward of $100 than for one of $1.)

Emotion

Questions to Answer

1. What are the four components of an emotion?
2. How did Wundt conceptualize emotions?
3. How did Lazarus onceptualize emotions?
4. What are Plutchik's ideas about emotion?
5. What role does emotionality play in motivation?
6. What is the bottom line on how emotions are classified?

In psychology, philosophy, and their many subsets, emotion is the generic term for subjective, conscious experience that is characterized primarily by psychophysiological expressions, biological reactions, and mental states. Emotion is often associated and considered reciprocally influential with mood, temperament, personality, disposition, and motivation, as well as influenced by hormones and neurotransmitters such as dopamine, noradrenaline, serotonin, oxytocin and cortisol. Emotion is often the driving force behind motivation, positive or negative. The physiology of emotion is closely linked to arousal of the nervous system with various states and strengths of arousal relating, apparently, to particular emotions. Although those acting primarily on emotion may seem as if they are not thinking, cognition is an important aspect of emotion, particularly the interpretation of events. For example, the experience of fear usually occurs in response to a threat. The cognition of danger and subsequent arousal of the nervous system (eg, rapid heartbeat and breathing, sweating, muscle tension) is an integral component to the subsequent interpretation and labeling of that arousal as an emotional state. Emotion is also linked to behavioral tendency. Research on emotion has increased significantly over the past two decades with many fields contributing including psychology, neuroscience, medicine, sociology, and even computer science. The numerous theories that attempt to explain the origin, neurobiology, experience, and function of emotions have only fostered more intense research on this topic.

Try to recall the last time you experienced an emotion of sonic significance, perhaps the fear of going to the dentist, the joy of receiving an "A" on a classroom exam, the sadness at the death of a friend, or the anger at being unable to register for a class you wanted to take. You may be able to identify four components to your emotional reaction: (1) You experience a subjective feeling, or affect, which you may label fear, joy, sadness, anger, or the like. (2) You have a cognitive reaction: you recognize, or "know," what happened. (3) You have an internal, physiological reaction, involving glands, hormones, and internal organs, and (4) You engage in an overt behavioral reaction. You tremble as you approach the dentist's office. You run down the hallway, a broad smile on your face, waving your exam over your head. You cry at the news of your friend's death. You shake your fist and veil at the registrar when you find you can't enroll in the class of your choice.

Note that when we add an overt behavioral component to emotions, we can see how emotions and motivation are related. To be motivated is to be aroused to action. Emotional experiences also arouse behaviors. Theorist Richard Lazarus put it this way: Without some version of a motivational principle, emotion makes little sense, inasmuch as what is important or unimportant to us determines what we define as harmful or beneficial, hence emotions.

There has been considerable debate in psychology concerning how best to define emotion. As one researcher puts it. Despite the obvious importance of emotion to human existence, scientists concerned with human nature have not been able to reach a consensus about what emotion is and what place emotion should have in a theory of mind and behavior. For now, however, we need a working definition and we'll say that an emotion is an experience that includes a subjective feeling, a cognitive interpretation, a physiological reaction, and a behavioral expression. With this definition in mind, we turn to the related issue of how to classify emotions.

Emotions give flavor and coloring to our lives. If nothings else, emotions can be classified as pleasant or unpleasant.

Biological/Physiological Factors

Emotion is complex, and the term has no single universally accepted definition. Emotion is, however, closely related to motivation and can sometimes provide motivation (as, for example, a student's fear of failing provides motivation for studying). Psychologists do agree that emotions are reaction patterns that include:

physiological changes;

responses or goal-oriented behaviors;

affective experiences (feelings).

Theorists differ on the order of appearance of the reaction patterns.

The Autonomic Nervous System

The autonomic nervous system (ANS) has two components, the sympathetic nervous system (SNS) and the parasympathetic nervous system (PNS). When activated, the SNS prepares the body for emergency actions; it controls glands of the neuroendocrine system (thyroid, pituitary, and adrenal glands). Activation of the SNS causes the production of epinephrine (adrenaline) from the adrenal glands, increased blood flow to the muscles, increased heart rate, and other readiness reactions. Conversely, the PNS functions when the body is relaxed or at rest and helps the body store energy for future use. PNS effects include increased stomach activity and decreased blood flow to the muscles.

The Role of the Autonomic Nervous System

The autonomic nervous system (ANS) consists of two parts that serve the same organs but have nearly the opposite effect on those organs. The parasytmpathetic division is actively involved in maintaining a relaxed, cairn, and unemotional state. As you strolled down the path into the woods, the parasynipathetic division of your ANS actively directed your digestive processes to do the best they could with the meal you'd just eaten. Blood was diverted from the extremities to the stomach and intestines. Saliva flowed freely. With your stomach full, and with blood diverted to it, you felt somewhat sleepy as your brain responded to the lower levels of blood supply. Your breathing was slow deep, and steady as was your heart rate. Again, all of these activities were under the control of the parasyrnpathetic division of your autonomic nervous system.

Suddenly, there's that bear! Now the sympathetic division of your ANS takes over. Automatically, many physiological changes take place. Changes that are usually quite adaptive.

1. The pupils of your eyes dilate, letting in as much of what light is available, increasing your visual sensitivity.

2. Your heart rate and blood pressure are elevated (energy needs to be mobilized as fast as possible).

3. Blood is diverted away from the digestive tract toward the limbs and brain, and digestion stops; you've got a bear to deal with: dinner can wait until later. Let's get the blood supply out there to the arms and legs where it can do some good.

4. Respiration increases, becoming deeper and more rapid; you'll need all the oxygen you can get.

5. Moisture is brought to the surface of the skin in the form of perspiration: as it evaporates, the body is cooled, thus conserving energy.

6. Blood sugar levels increase, making more energy readily available.

7. Blood will clot more readily than usually for obvious but, it is hoped, unnecessary reasons.

The sympathetic system makes some of these changes directly (for example, stopping salivation and stimulating the cardiac muscle). Others are made indirectly through the release of hormones into the bloodstream, mostly epinephrine and noepinephrine from the adrenal glands. Because part of the physiological aspect of emotion is hormonal, it takes a few seconds for the effect to be experienced. If you were, in fact, confronted by a bear in the woods, you would probably not have the presence of mind to notice, but the reactions of sweaty palms, gasping breaths, and "butterflies in your stomach" take a few seconds to develop.

Is the autonomic and endocrine system reaction the same for every emotion that we experience? There may be slight differences. There appears to be a small difference in the hormones produced during rage and fear reactions. There may be differences in the biological bases of emotions that prepare us for defense or for retreat, fight or flight. Consistent differences in physiological reactions for the various emotional states are at best, very slight indeed. This issue has been controversial in psychology for many years and is likely to remain so.

The reticular activating system (RAS) is a network of neurons that runs through the core of the hind-brain and into the midbrain and forebrain. It has been demonstrated that electrical stimulation of the RAS causes changes in the electrical activity of the cortex (as measured by an electroencephalogram) that are indistinguishable from changes in electrical activity seen when external stimuli (such as loud sounds) are present. The RAS is believed to first arouse the cortex and then to stimulate its wakefulness so that it may more effectively interpret sensory information.

The Limbic System

The limbic system includes the anterior thalamus, the amygdala, the septal area, the hippocampus, the cingulate gyrus, and structures that are parts of the hypothalamus (Figure 6.2). The word limbic means "border" and describes this system because its structures seem to form a rough border along the inner edge of the cerebrum. Studies have associated the limbic system with such emotions as fear and aggression as well with as drives, including those for food and sex.

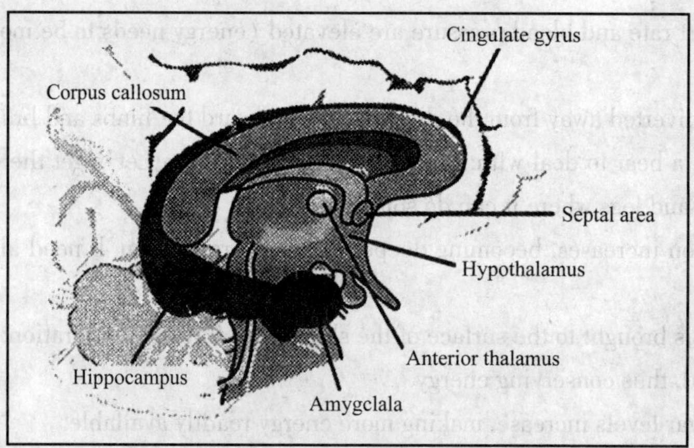

Figure 6.2 The Limbic System

Lie detectors, or polygraphs, rely upon the physiological arousal of the emotions. Concomitant measurements are taken of the heart rate, blood pressure, respiration rate, and galvanic skin response (GSR). (The GSR is a measure of the skin's electrical conductivity, which changes as the sweat glands increase their activity.) Polygraph recordings are used to see if a person is not telling the truth (lying), which usually creates emotional arousal. Because of polygraphs' high error rates, however, their findings are generally not accepted as evidence in the courts.

Cassifying Emotion

Plutchik's Model

Robert Plutchik (1980) offers a three-dimensional model that is a hybrid of both basic-complex categories and dimensional theories. It arranges emotions in concentric circles where inner circles are more basic and outer circles more complex, see Figure 6.3. Notably outer circles are also formed by blending the inner circle emotions. Plutchik's model, as Russell's, emanates from a circumplex representation, where emotional words were plotted based on similarity.

According to Robert Plutchik, there are eight primary human emotions that relate to adaptive behavior. It is believed that these are innate or develop early on due to their survival values. They are made from four pairs of opposites:

1. Anger — blocking goal destruction of object; onset 9-12 months; why?
2. Fear — threat or danger protection; facilitates flight or fight
3. Sadness — loss something valuable seek help/comfort
4. Disgust — gruesome or loathsome object; rejection; push away; poison or sour milk
5. Surprise — unexpected event; turn toward; attend; sharpen our focus
6. Anticipation — new place/event explore & search
7. Trust — acceptance; membership sharing; cooperation; support and reciprocity
8. Joy — gain something valuable; potential mate courting; stimulates paternal nurturing

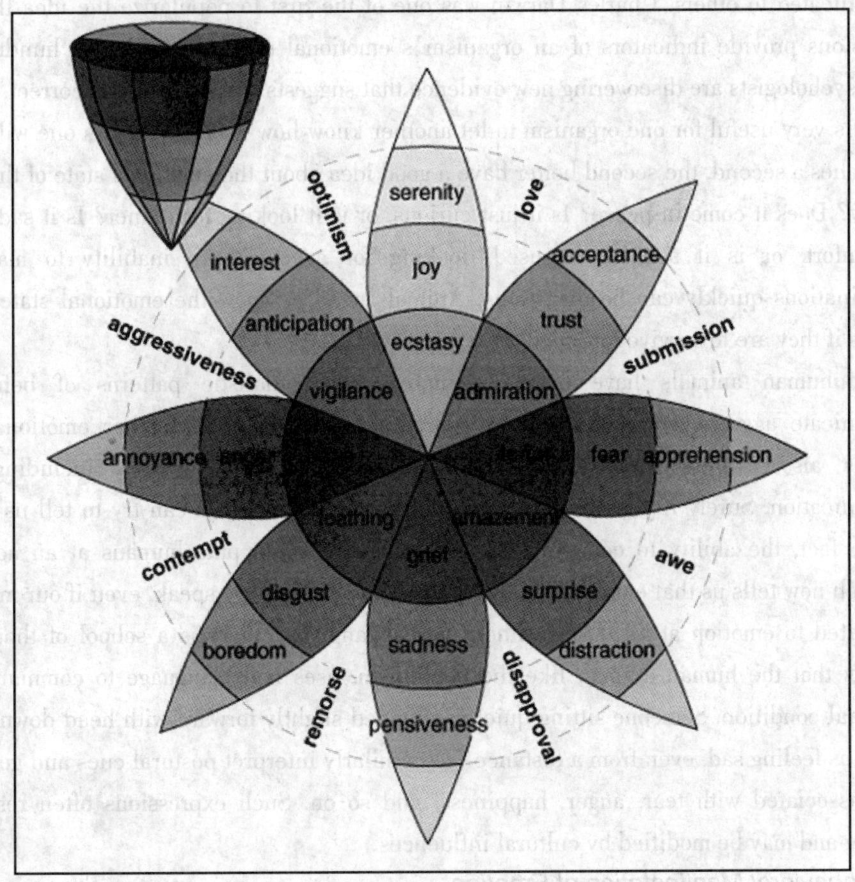

Figure 6.3 Plutchik's Model of Emotion

Parrots' Classification of Emotions

The most nuanced classification of emotions so far is probably Parrots' 2001 theory. Parrot identified over 100 emotions and conceptualized them as a tree structured list:

Primary emotion	Secondary emotion	Tertiary emotions
Love	Affection	Adoration, affection, love, fondness, liking, attaction, caring, tenderness, compassion, sentimentality
	Lust	Arousal, desire, lust, passion, infatuation
	Longing	Longing
Joy	Cheerfulness	Amusement, bliss, cheerfulness, gaiety, glee, jolliness, joviality, joy, delight, enjoyment, gladness, happiness, jubilation, elation, satisfaction, ecstasy, euphona
	Zest	Enthusiasm, zeal, zest, excitement, thrill, exhilaration
	Contentment	Contentment, pleasure
	Pride	Pride, triumph
	Optimism	Eagemess, hope, optimism
	Enthrallment	Enthrallment, rapture
	Relief	Relief
Surprise	Surprise	Amazement, surprise, astonishment

Outward Exoerssion of Emotion

An aspect of emotion that has long intrigued psychologists is how inner emotional states are communicated to others. Charles Darwin was one of the first to popularize the idea that facial expressions provide indicators of an organism's emotional state. More than a hundred years later, psychologists are discovering new evidence that suggests that Darwin was correct.

It is very useful for one organism to let another know how it is feeling. As one wild animal approaches a second, the second better have a good idea about the emotional state of the first. Is it angry? Does it come in peace? Is it just curious, or is it looking for dinner? Is it sad, looking for comfort, or is it sexually aroused, looking for a mate? An inability to make such determinations quickly can be disastrous. Animals need to know the emotional state of other animals if they are to survive for long.

Nonhuman animals have many instinctive and ritualistic patterns of behavior to communicate aggressiveness, interest in courtship, submission, and other emotional states. Humans also express their emotional states in a variety of ways, including verbal communication. Surely if you are happy, sad, angry, or jealous, you can try to tell us how you feel. In fact, the ability to communicate with language often puts humans at an advantage. Research now tells us that emotional states are reflected in how we speak, even if our message is not related to emotion at all. Even without verbal language, there is a school of thought that suggests that the human animal, like the nonhuman, uses body language to communicate its emotional condition. Someone sitting quietly, slumped slightly forward with head down, may be viewed as feeling sad, even from a distance. We similarly interpret postural cues and gestures as being associated with tear, anger, happiness, and so on. Such expressions often result from learning and may be modified by cultural influences.

Behavioral Manifestation of Emotion

Differing facial expressions are not the only way that emotions are expressed. Often, as we know from experience, emotions directly influence behavior. For example, imagine that you are driving home from school one day and you accidentally cut off another motorist. You think nothing of it because it was an accident. The next thing you know you see this other driver in your rearview mirror inches from your rear bumper. He pulls up next to you, and you notice that his face is all red and he is shouting and making obscene gestures at you. Next, to your shock, he tries to run you off the road. You decide to pull over and let this maniac pass you.

In this example, the other motorist was obviously experiencing an emotional episode that was translated into a particular behavior: aggression. Social psychologists define aggression as any behavior that is intended to inflict physical and/or psychological harm on another organism (for example, you) or the symbol of that organism (for example, your car). One of the more popular theories of why aggression occurs in situations like the one just described is the frustration - aggression hypothesis. In its original the frustration - aggression hypothesis stated that "aggression is always a consequence of frustration... the occurrence of aggressive behavior always presupposes the existence of frustration and, contrariwise, ... the existence of frustration leads to some form of aggression." In other words, according to the frustration - aggression hypothesis, when we are frustrated, we behave aggressively.

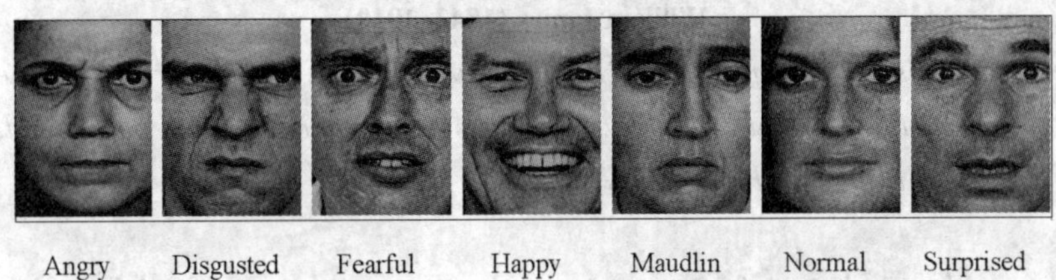

Angry Disgusted Fearful Happy Maudlin Normal Surprised

Means by which we distinguish one emotion from another is a hotly contested issue in emotion research and affective science. This page summarises some of the major theories and the evidence supporting them. The classification of emotions has mainly been researched from two fundamental viewpoints. The first viewpoint is that emotions are discrete and fundamentally different constructs while the second viewpoint asserts that emotions can be characterized on a dimensional basis in groupings.

Theories of Emotion

Darwin believed that body movements and facial expressions (body language, or nonverbal communication) are used by members of a species to communicate meaning. He suggested that although emotional expressions are initially learned behavior, they eventually evolve to become innate in a species because they have survival value. Recognition by one animal that a second animal is afraid rather than angry, for example, allows appropriate survival actions to be undertaken.

James-Lange Theory

In the late 19th century, the most influential theorists were William James (1842–1910) and Carl Lange (1834–1900). James was an American psychologist and philosopher who wrote about educational psychology, psychology of religious experience/mysticism, and the philosophy of pragmatism. Lange was a Danish physician and psychologist. Working independently, they developed the James - Lange theory, a hypothesis on the origin and nature of emotions. The theory states that within human beings, as a response to experiences in the world, the autonomic nervous system creates physiological events such as muscular tension, a rise in heart rate, perspiration, and dryness of the mouth. Emotions, then, are feelings which come about as a result of these physiological changes, rather than being their cause.

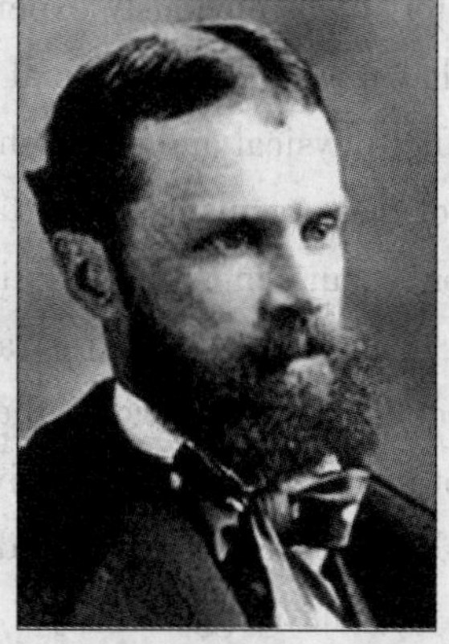

William James (1842–1910)

"When a thing is new, people say: "It is not true." Later, when its truth becomes obvious, they say: "It's not important." Finally, when its importance cannot be denied, they say "Anyway, it's not new."— William James

The James - Lange theory of emotion argues that an event causes physiological arousal first and then we interpret this arousal. Only after our interpretation of the arousal can we experience emotion. If the arousal is not noticed or is not given any thought, then we will not experience any emotion based on this event (Figure 6.4).

EXAMPLE: You are walking down a dark alley late at night. You hear footsteps behind you and you begin to tremble, your heart beats faster, and your breathing deepens. You notice these physiological changes and interpret them as your body's preparation for a fearful situation. You then experience fear.

Cannon- Bard Theory

The Cannon - Bard theory argues that we experience physiological arousal and emotional at the same time, but gives no attention to the role of thoughts or outward behavior(Figure 6.4).

EXAMPLE: You are walking down a dark alley late at night. You hear footsteps behind you and you begin to tremble, your heart beats faster, and your breathing deepens. At the same time as these physiological changes occur you also experience the emotion of fear.

Schachter- Singer Theory

According to this theory, an event causes physiological arousal first. You must then identify a reason for this arousal and then you are able to experience and label the emotion(Figure 6.4).

EXAMPLE: You are walking down a dark alley late at night. You hear footsteps behind you and you begin to tremble, your heart beats faster, and your breathing deepens. Upon noticing this arousal you realize that is comes from the fact that you are walking down a dark alley by yourself. This behavior is dangerous and therefore you feel the emotion of fear.

Lazarus Theory

Lazarus Theory states that a thought must come before any emotion or physiological arousal. In other words, you must first think about your situation before you can experience an emotion(Figure 6.4).

EXAMPLE: You are walking down a dark alley late at night. You hear footsteps behind you and you think it may be a mugger so you begin to tremble, your heart beats faster, and your breathing deepens and at the same time experience fear.

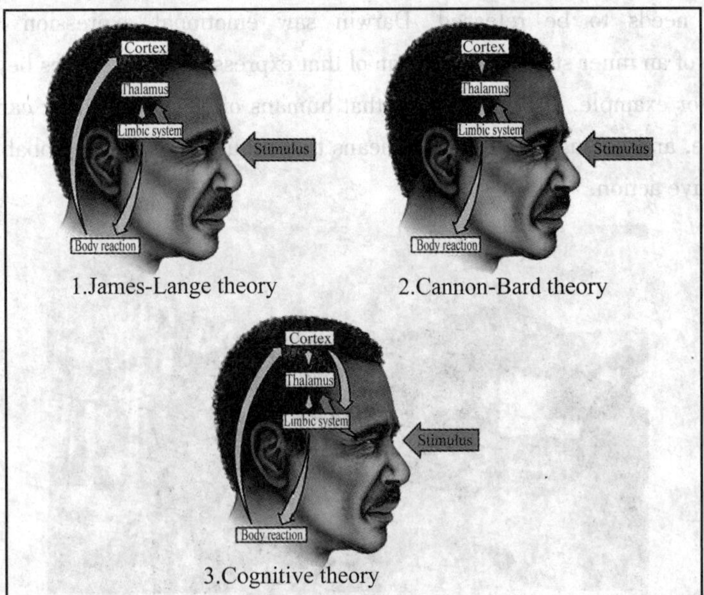

1.James-Lange theory 2.Cannon-Bard theory

3.Cognitive theory

Figure 6.4 Theories of Emotion

Facial Feedback Theory

According to the facial feedback theory, emotion is the experience of changes in our facial muscles. In other words, when we smile, we then experience pleasure, or happiness. When we frown, we then experience sadness. It is the changes in our facial muscles that cue our brains and provide the basis of our emotions. Just as there are an unlimited number of muscle configurations in our face, so to are there a seemingly unlimited number of emotions.

EXAMPLE: You are walking down a dark alley late at night. You hear footsteps behind you and your eyes widen, your teeth clench and your brain interprets these facial changes as the expression of fear. Therefore you experience the emotion of fear.

Emotion in Animals

There is scientific evidence supporting the claim that animals can feel emotions and that human emotions evolved from the same mechanisms. In recent years, research has become available which expands prior understandings of animal language, cognition, tool use, and sexuality.

Darwin's Perspective

Charles Darwin initially planned to include a chapter on emotion in *The Descent of Man* but as his ideas progressed they expanded into a book, *The Expression of Emotion in Man and Animals*. Darwin proposed that emotions are adaptive and serve a communicative and motivational function, and he stated three principles that are useful in understanding emotional expression: First, The Principle of Serviceable Habits takes a Lamarckian stance by suggesting that emotional expressions that are useful will be passed on to the offspring. Second, The Principle of Antithesis suggests that some expressions exist merely because they oppose an expression that is useful. Third, The Principle of the Direct Action of the Excited Nervous System on the Body suggests that emotional expression occurs when nervous energy has passed a threshold and needs to be released. Darwin saw emotional expression as an outward communication of an inner state, and the form of that expression often carries beyond its original adaptive use. For example, Darwin remarks that humans often present their canine teeth when sneering in rage, and he suggests that this means that a human ancestor probably utilized their teeth in aggressive action.

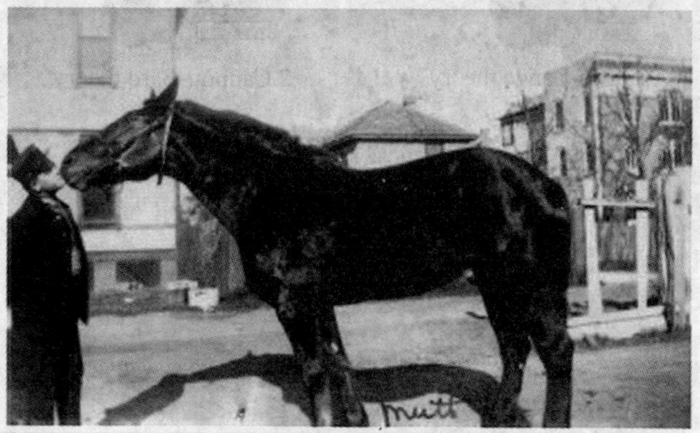

A kiss from a horse

General Evidence

Evidence for emotions in animals has been primarily anecdotal, coming from individuals who interact with pets on a regular basis. However, critics of emotions in animals cite anthropomorphism as motivating factor in the above suggestion. Much of the debates confusion centers around the difficulty in defining emotion and the cognitive requirements necessary to experience emotion in a similar vein to humans. The problem is also furthered by the difficulty in testing for emotion in animals. What is known about human emotion is almost all related or in relation to human communication. Recent attempts in studying emotion in animals have led to new constructions in experimental and information gathering. Mariann Dawkins suggested that emotions could be studied through a functional lens or a mechanistic lens. Functional approaches would rely on understanding what roles emotions play in humans and examining that role in non-human animals. Oatley and Jenkins promote a 3 stage structure to emotion which encompasses a broad range of possibility. The structure, however, may be too broad and could be used to include all the animal kingdom as well as certain plants. The second approach, mechanistic, requires an examination of the mechanisms that drive emotion and search for similarities in non-human animals. The mechanistic approach is utilized extensively by Paul,

Harding and Mend.

Recognizing the difficulty in studying emotion in non - verbal animals, Paul et el demonstrate possible ways to better examine. Observation of the mechanisms that function in human emotion expression, Paul et al suggest that concentration on similar mechanisms in non-human animals can provide clear insights into the animal experience. Paul suggests that cognitive biases vary according to emotional state and suggest this as a possible starting point to examine animal emotion. They propose that researchers may be able to use a controlled stimuli that have accounted appraisal criteria to induce particular emotions in animals and gather which types of basic emotions non - human animals can experience. Dawkins suggests that merely mechanistic or functional research will provide the answer on its own and suggests that a mixture of the two would yield the most significant results.

For Animal Emotion

In recent years, the scientific community has become increasingly supportive of the idea of emotions in animals. Prior to scientific support, evidence for animal emotion was based on anecdotal evidence provided from individuals who had frequent contact with animals. Recent scientific research has provided insight into similarities of physiological changes between human and non-human animals when experiencing emotion. Darwin concluded, through a survey, that humans share universal emotive expressions and suggested that animals likely share in these to some degree. Darwin's results have come under fire by individuals that suggest misinterpretations. Social constructivists disregard the concept that emotions are universal. Others hold an intermediate stance, suggesting that basic emotional expressions and emotion are universal but the intricacies are developed culturally. A study by Elfenbein and Ambady (2002) suggested that individuals within a particular culture are better at reading other cultural members emotions. Most support for animal emotion and it's expression results from the notion that feeling doesn't require significant cognitive processes. Animals would not likely need to employ a significant amount of cognitive processes in order to have emotion, rather, they could be motivated by the processes to act in an adaptive way, as suggested by Darwin.

Against Animal Emotion

Animal emotion is often rejected due to lack of evidence and, those that don't submit to the idea of animal intelligence, often cite that anthropomorphism plays a significant role in individual's perspectives. Those that reject animal's capacity to have emotion mainly do so by citing inconsistencies in studies that have endorsed animal emotion. Having no direct means to communicate emotion, the difficulty of providing an account of emotion in animals relies heavily on work-around experimentation that relies on results from human subjects. Those in opposition to animal emotion suggest that emotions aren't universal, including humans. If emotions aren't universal it suggests that there is not a phylogenic relationship amongst human emotion and animal emotion. The relationship drawn by proponents of animal emotion, then, would be merely a suggestion of mechanistic features that promote adaptivity but lack the complexity of human emotion constructs. Elaborating further on this idea, it's possible that emotions are basic that have been developed from a social construct. Opponents also critique the lack of a precise definition of the term emotion. At times, the term is defined too loosely and includes plants. By not having a sturdy framework, studies in animal emotion cannot verify their results and oftentimes, anthropomorphise animals beyond their actual capacities.

Birds

A few years ago my friend Rod and I were riding our bicycles around Boulder, Colorado, when we witnessed a very interesting encounter among five magpies. Magpies are corvids, a very intelligent family of birds. One magpie had obviously been hit by a car and was laying dead on the side of the road. The four other magpies were standing around him. One approached the corpse, gently pecked at it — just as an elephant noses the carcass of another elephant — and stepped back. Another magpie did the same thing. Next, one of the magpies flew off, brought back some grass, and laid it by the corpse. Another magpie did the same. Then, all four magpies stood vigil for a few seconds and one by one flew off.

Furthermore, in an observational study, Orlaith and Bugnyar sought to explore bystander affiliation (post - conflict affiliation from an uninvolved bystander to the conflict victim) in ravens. Bystander affiliation has been believed to represent an expression of empathy in which the bystander tries to console the victim and alleviate his/her distress. When examining post - conflict behavior in ravens, Orlaith and Bugnyar found that there was strong evidence for bystander affiliation (eg, contact sitting, preening, or beak - to - beak or beak - to - body touching) and also for solicited bystander affiliation, in which there is post - conflict affiliation from the victim to the bystander. Solicited bystander affiliation is thought to reduce the likelihood of renewed aggression against the victims. The researchers concluded that ravens may be sensitive to the emotions of others. However, it is important to note that relationship quality plays an important role in the prevalence and function of these post - conflict interactions. More specifically, bystanders involved in both bystander affiliation and solicited bystander affiliation were likely to share a valuable relationship with the victim. This is similar to findings regarding empathy in humans and non - human primates, in which degree of familiarity between social partners influences the occurrence of empathetic acts.

Dog Communication

Research suggests that canines can experience negative emotions in a similar manner to people, including the equivalent of certain chronic and acute psychological conditions. The classic experiment for this was Martin Seligman's foundational experiments and theory of learned helplessness at the University of Pennsylvania in 1965, as an extension of his interest in depression:

A dog that had earlier been repeatedly conditioned to associate a sound with electric shocks did not try to escape the electric shocks after the warning was presented, even though all the dog would have had to do is jump over a low divider within ten seconds, more than enough time to respond. The dog didn't even try to avoid the "aversive stimulus"; it had previously "learned" that nothing it did mattered. A follow - up experiment involved three dogs affixed in harnesses, including one that received shocks of identical intensity and duration to the others, but the lever which would otherwise have allowed the dog a degree of control was left disconnected and didn't do anything. The first two dogs quickly recovered from the experience, but the third dog suffered chronic symptoms of clinical depression as a result of this perceived helplessness.

A further series of experiments showed that (similar to humans) under conditions of long-term intense psychological stress, around 1/3 of dogs do not develop learned helplessness or long-term depression. Instead these animals somehow managed to find a way to handle the unpleasant situation in spite of their past experience. The corresponding characteristic in humans has been found to correlate highly with an explanatory style and optimistic attitude that views the situation as other than personal, pervasive, or permanent. Since this time, symptoms analogous to clinical depression, neurosis, and other psychological conditions have also been accepted as being within the scope of canine emotion.

In addition, psychology research has shown that human faces are asymmetrical, with the gaze instinctively moving to the right side of a face upon encountering other humans to obtain information about their emotions and state. Research at the University of Lincoln (2008) shows that dogs share this instinct when meeting a human being, and only when meeting a human being (ie, not other animals or other dogs). As such they are the only non-primate species known to do so.

Finally, the existence and nature of personality traits in dogs have been studied (15,329 dogs of 164 different breeds) and five consistent and stable "narrow traits" identified, described as playfulness, curiosity/fearlessness, chase-proneness, sociability and aggressiveness. A further higher order axis for shyness - boldness was also identified.

Felines

The emotions of cats have also been studied scientifically. It has been shown that cats can learn to manipulate their owners through vocalizations that are similar to the cries of human babies. Some cats learn to add a purr to the cry, which makes it less harmonious and more dissonant to humans, and therefore harder to ignore. Individual cats learn to make these cries through operant conditioning; when a particular cry elicits a positive response from a human, the cat is more likely to use that cry in the future.

Growling can be a sign of annoyance or fear, similar to humans. When annoyed or angry, a cat will wriggle and thump its tail much more vigorously than when in a contented state. In bigger cats like Lions, what is and isn't irritating varies from individual. Male may let his cubs play with his mane or tail, or he may hiss and bat them away. Domestic male cats have varying attitudes towards their off springs as well.

Older male siblings tend not to go near new ones, and may even show hostility. The father tom of kittens will tolerate his young for a time, but even he may kill them to drive a female back in heat.

Fish Personality

A 2007 study by the University of Guelph Scientists in Canada suggests that fish may have their own separate personalities. The study examined a group of trout that were visually identical. The study concluded that different fish within the same group exhibited different personality traits. Some fish were more willing to take risks in unknown waters than others when taken from their environment and introduced to a dark tube. Some fish were more social than others, while some preferred being alone. Fish were also shown to have different preferences as far as eating habits.

What then is personality? Few terms have been as difficult to define. Actually, each of the theoretical approaches we will study in this Topic generates its own definition of personality. We'll say that personality' includes the affects, behaviors, and cognitions of people that characterize them in a number of situations overtime. (Here again is our ABC mnemonic.) Personality also includes those dimensions we can use to judge people to be different from one another. With personality theories we are looking for ways that allow us to describe how people remain the same over time and circumstances, and to describe differences that we know exist among people. Note that personality is something a person brings to his or her interactions with the environment. Somehow, personality originates within the individual.

Key Questions to Answer

While reading this Topic, find the answers to the following key questions:

1. What is the definition of personality?
2. What are the main characteristics of Freud's theory of personality?
3. What are the three levels of consciousness proposed by Freud?
4. What role do instincts play in Freud's theory?
5. What are the three structures of personality as Freud saw them?
6. What are defense mechanisms?
7. What were the contributions of Adler Jung, and Homey to the psychoanalytic approach to personality?
8. What are the strengths and weaknesses of the psychoanalytic approach to personality?

What is the Definition of Personality?

Personality includes the affects, behaviors, and cognitions of people that characterize them in a number of situations over time. Personality also includes the dimensions that we can use to judge people to be different from one another. Personality resides within an individual and comprises characteristics that lie or she brings to interactions with the environment.

We begin our discussion of personality with the psychoanalytic approach associated with Sigmund Freud and his students. We begin with Freud because he was the first to present a unified theory of personality.

Freud's theory of personality has been one of the most influential and, at the same time, most controversial in all of science. There are many facets to Freud's theory, but two basic premises characterize the approach: (1) a reliance on innate drives as explanatory concepts for human behavior, and (2) an acceptance of the power of unconscious forces to mold and shape behavior.

Central to Freudian personality theory is the notion that information, feelings, wants, drives, desires, and the like can be found at various levels of awareness or consciousness. Mental events of winch we are actively aware at the moment are conscious or "in consciousness". Aspects of our mental life of which we are not conscious at any moment but that can be easily brought to awareness are stored at preconscious level. When you shift your awareness to think about something you may do this evening, those plans were probably already there, in your preconscious mind.

The Structure of Personality

Freud believed that the mind operates on three interacting levels of awareness: conscious, preconscious, and unconscious. Freud proposed that personality also consists of three separate, though interacting, structures or subsystems: the id, ego, and superego. Each of these structures or subsystems has its own job to do and its own principles to follow.

The id is the totally inborn portion of personality. It resides in the unconscious level of the mind, and it is through the id that basic instincts are expressed. The driving force of the id is libido, or sexual energy; although, it may be more fair to say "sensual" rather than "sexual" so as not to imply that Freud was always talking about adult sexual inter-course. The id operates on the pleasure principle, indicating that the major function of the id is to find satisfaction for basic pleasurable impulses. Although the other divisions of personality develop later, our id remains with us always and is the basic energy source in our lives.

The ego is the part of the personality that develops through one's experience with reality. In many ways, it is our "self", at least the self of which we are consciously aware at any time. It is the rational, reasoning part of our personality. The ego operates on the reality principle. One of the ego's main jobs is to try to find satisfaction for the id, but it does so in ways that are reasonable and rational. The ego may delay gratification of some libidinal impulse or may need to find an acceptable outlet for some need. Freud said that the ego stands for reason and good sense while the id stands for untamed passions.

The last of the three structures to develop is the superego, which we can liken to one's sense of morality or conscience, it reflects our internalization of society's rules. The superego operates on the idealistic principle. One problem we have with our superegos is that they, like our ids, have no contact with reality and, therefore, often place unrealistic demands on the individual. For example, a person's superego may have that person believe that he or she should always be kind and generous and never harbor unpleasant or negative thoughts about someone else, no matter what. The superego demands that we do what it deems right and proper, no matter what the circumstances. Failure to do so may lead to guilt and shame. Again, it falls to the ego to try to maintain a realistic balance between the conscience of the superego and the libido of the id.

Although the dynamic processes underlying personality may appear complicated, the concepts underlying these processes are not as complicated as they sound. Suppose a bank teller discovers an extra $20 in his cash drawer at the end of the day. He certainly could use an extra $20. "Go ahead. Nobody will miss it. The bank can afford a few dollars here and there. Think of the fun you can have with an extra $20," is the basic message from the id. "The odds are that you'll get caught if you take this money. If you are caught, you may lose your job, then you'll have to find another one," reasons the ego. "You shouldn't even think about taking that money. Shame on you! It's not yours, it belongs to someone else and should be returned," the superego protests. Clearly, the interaction of the three components of one's personality isn't always this simple and straightforward but this example illustrates the general idea.

Freud's Theory

Even people who are relatively unfamiliar with psychology as a subject have at least some awareness of psychoanalysis, the school of thought created by Sigmund Freud. While you may have some passing knowledge of key concepts in psychoanalysis like the unconscious, fixations, defense mechanisms and dream symbolism, you might wonder exactly how these ideas fit in together and what influence they really have on contemporary psychologists.

Sigmund Freud originated the psychoanalytic approach based on his experiences in his psychiatric practice and developed a technique called free association, which requires a patient to relax and report everything that comes to mind no matter how trivial or how strange it might seem. Using this technique, he found that patients often revived painful memories reaching back even to early childhood.

Freud believed that the mind is like an iceberg, mostly hidden (Figure 6.5), and that free association would ultimately let a patient retrieve memories from the unconscious, memories not ordinarily available because they are threatening in some way. Conscious awareness (the visible part of the iceberg) floats above the surface. The preconscious (the area only shallowly submerged) contains information which can voluntarily be brought to awareness. The unconscious (the larger, deeply submerged portion of the iceberg) contains thoughts, feelings, and memories of which a person is unaware and many of which have been repressed, or forcibly blocked from consciousness. From his work, Freud developed psychoanalysis, a technique for treating psychological disorders by identifying and resolving problems stored in the unconscious.

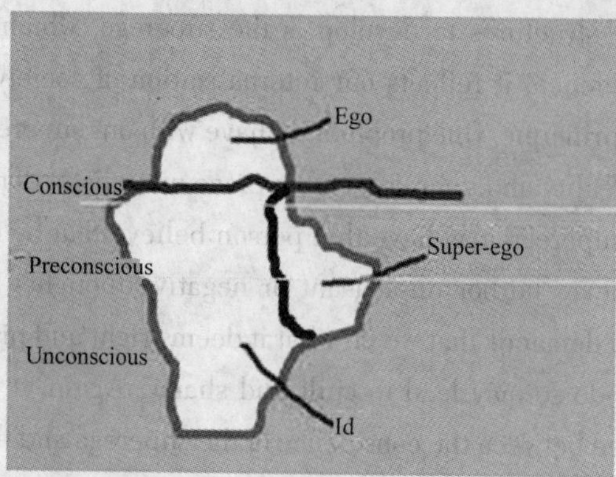

Figure 6.5 Levels of Consciousness

Freudian Personality Theory

Concomitant with his development of psychoanalysis, Freud constructed a theory of personality, which includes the following observations.

Personality has three structures: the id, the ego, and the superego. The id, a reservoir of unconscious psychic energy, operates on the pleasure principle, seeks immediate gratification, and is not restrained by reality. It operates solely at the unconscious level. The ego, which develops in early childhood, operates through the reality principle, which seeks to gratify impulses of the id realistically and to bring long-term pleasure without pain. The ego operates at both the conscious and pre-conscious levels. The superego, a third structure, emerges as children reach 4 or 5 and internalize the morals of parents and society. The superego acts as a voice of conscience and operates mostly at the preconscious level of awareness. People also possess and are driven by a psychological energy called the libido.

Children pass through a series of psychosexual stages during which the id seeks pleasure from body areas, erogenous zones, that change during development. If children have difficulty passing through a particular stage, they are said to have become fixated. Fixation at the phallic stage may create an Oedipus complex for a boy (jealousy of a son toward his father in competing for his mother's attention) or an Electra complex for a girl (who competes with her mother for her father's attention). Children resolve these conflicts by identifying with the parent of the same gender.

During a child's development, the ego strategically uses defense mechanisms to deal with the anxiety produced by conflicting impulses from the id (operating on the pleasure principle) and the superego (using internalized representation of the parents' value system). Defense mechanisms include:

Repression, preventing dangerous or painful thoughts from entering consciousness;

Reaction formation, preventing expression of dangerous impulses by exaggerating opposite behavior;

Projection, attributing one's feelings, shortcomings, or unacceptable impulses to others;

Displacement, directing impulses toward a less threatening or more acceptable person or object;

Regression, retreating to an earlier stage of development;

Sublimation, rechanneling of unacceptable impulses into acceptable activities;

Denial, refusing to perceive reality, acting as if something did not happen;

Compensation, counteracting real or imagined difficulties or weaknesses by emphasizing other traits or excelling in other areas;

Intellectualization, separating emotions from threatening situations by thinking and acting impersonally fantasy, meeting unfulfilled desires by imagination.

Psychopathology can result if an individual does not pass through the stages of psychosexual development and becomes fixated, or fails to pass to the next stage. For example, a person fixated at the oral stage could, among other things, exhibit symptoms of obsessive eating or smoking in adult life. The problem could be identified and treated through psychoanalysis.

The Driving Forces

According to Freud psychoanalytic theory, all psychic energy is generated by the libido. Freud suggested that our mental states were influenced by two competing forces: cathexis and anticathexis. Cathexis was described as an investment of mental energy in a person, an idea or an object. If you are hungry, for example, you might create a mental image of a delicious meal that you have been craving. In other cases, the ego might harness some of the id's energy to seek out activities that are related to the activity in order to disperse some of the excess energy from the id. If you can't actually seek out food to appease your hunger, you might instead browse through a cookbook or browse through your favorite recipe blog.

Anticathexis involves the ego blocking the socially unacceptable needs of the id. Repressing urges and desires is one common form of anticathexis, but it involves a significant investment of energy. Remember, according to Freud's theory, there is only so much libidinal energy available. When a lot of this energy is being devoted to suppressing urges via anticathexis, there is less energy available for other processes. Learn more about how these competing forces work and interact in this overview of cathexis and anticathexis.

Freud also believed that much of human behavior was motivated by two driving instincts: the life instincts and the death instincts. The life instincts are those that relate to a basic need for survival, reproduction and pleasure. They include such things as the need for food, shelter, love and sex. He also suggested that all humans have an unconscious wish for death, which he referred to as the death instincts. Self-destructive behavior, he believed, was one expression of the death drive. However, he believed that these death instincts were largely tempered by the life instincts. Learn more about how these two forces interact and function in this overview of the life and death instincts.

The Basic Structure of Personality

In Freudian theory, the mind is structured into two main parts: the conscious and unconscious mind. The conscious mind includes all the things we are aware of or can easily bring into awareness. The unconscious mind, on the other hand, includes all of the things outside of our awareness — all of the wishes, desires, hopes, urges and memories that lie outside of awareness yet continue to influence behavior. Freud compared the mind to an iceberg. The tip of the iceberg that is actually visible above the water represents just a tiny portion of the mind, while the huge expanse of ice hidden underneath the water represents the much larger unconscious.

In addition to these two main components of the mind, Freudian theory also divides human personality up into three major components: the id, ego and superego. The id is the most primitive part of personality that is the source of all our most basic urges. This part of personality is entirely unconscious and serves as the source of all libidinal energy. The ego is the component of personality that is charged with dealing with reality and helps ensure that the demands of the id are satisfied in ways that are realistic, safe and socially acceptable. The superego is the part of personality that holds all of the internalized morals and standards that we acquire from our parents, family and society at large. You can learn more about each of these three aspects of personality and how they interact in this overview of the id, ego and superego.

The Stages of Development

Freudian theory suggests that as children develop, they progress through a series of psychosexual stages. At each stage, the libido's pleasure - seeking energy is focused on a different part of the body. The successful completion of each stage lead's to a healthy personality as an adult. If, however, a conflict remains unresolved at any particular stage, the individual might remain fixated or stuck at that particular point of development. A fixation can involve an overdependence or obsession with something related to that phase of development. For example, a person with an "oral fixation" is believed to be stuck at the oral stage of development. Signs of an oral fixation might include an excessive reliance on oral behaviors such as smoking, biting fingernails or eating. Discover more about each of the individual stages in this overview of psychosexual development.

Defense Mechanisms

Even if you've never studied Freud's theories before, you have probably heard the term "defense mechanisms" bandied about a few times. When someone seems unwilling to face a painful truth, you might accuse them of being "in denial". When a person tries to look for a logical explanation for unacceptable behavior, you might suggest that they are "rationalizing." These things represent different types of defense mechanisms, or tactics that the ego uses to protect itself from anxiety. Some of the best - known mechanisms of defense include denial, repression and regression, but there are many more. Discover more about the types of defenses and how they work to protect the ego in this overview of the defense mechanisms.

Contemporary Views on Freudian Theory

While Freud's theories have been widely criticized, it is important to remember that his work made important contributions to psychology. His work sparked a major change in how we view mental illness by suggesting that not all psychological problems have physiological causes. His belief that mental problems could be resolved by actually talking about them helped revolutionize psychotherapy.

Since many contemporary psychologists do not give much credence to a lot of Freud's ideas, you might find yourself asking why you should bother learning about Freudian theory at all. First and perhaps most importantly, in order to understand where psychology is at today, it is essential to take a look back at where we've been and how we got here. Freud's work provides an insight into an important movement in psychology that helped transform how we think about mental health and how we approach psychological disorders.

By studying these theories and those that came after, you can gain a better understanding of psychology's rich and fascinating history. Many psychoanalytic terms such as defense mechanism, Freudian slip and anal retentive have become a part of our everyday language. By learning more about his work and theories, you can better understand how these ideas and concepts became woven into the fabric of popular culture.

The Psychoanalytic Approach after Freud

Sigmund Freud was a persuasive communicator. His ideas were challenging, and they attracted many students. Freud founded a psychoanalytic society in Vienna. There was an inner circle of leagues and friends who shared his ideas, but some did not entirely agree with all aspects of his theory. Among other things, they were bothered by the very strong emphasis on biological instincts and libido and what they perceived as a lack of concern for social influences. Some of these analysts proposed theories of their own. They became known as neo - Freudians. Because they had their own ideas, they had to part from Freud: he would not tolerate disagreement with his theory. One had to accept all of Freudian theory, or one had to leave Freud's inner circle.

The theories proposed by the neo - Freudians are complex and comprehensive. Each consists of logically interrelated, assumptions. We realize that it is not possible to do justice to someone's theory of personality in a short paragraph or two. We can, however, sketch the basic idea(s) behind the theories of a few neo-Freudians.

Alfred Adler (1870–1937)

As the psychoanalytic movement was beginning to take shape, Adler was one of Freud's closest friends. However, Adler left Freud's inner circle and, in 1911, founded his own version of a psychoanalytic approach to personality. Two things seemed most to offend Adler: die negativity of Freud's views (for example, the death instinct) and the idea of sexual libido as the prime impulse in life.

Adler argued that we are a product of the social influences on our personality. We are motivated not so much by drives and instincts as we are by goals and incentives. The future and one's hope for what it holds are often more important than one's past. For Adler, the goal in life is the achievement of success or superiority. This goal is fashioned in childhood when, because we are then weak and vulnerable, we develop an inferiority complex, he feeling that we are less able than others to solve life's problems and get along in the world. Although we may seem inferior as children, with the help of social support and our own creativity, we can overcome and succeed. Simply striving for superiority, to be the best, was viewed by Adler as a healthy reaction to early feelings of inferiority, only if it were balanced with a sort of "social interest", or "community feeling", or a genuine desire to be helpful and of service to others.

Carl Jung (1875–1961)

Carl Jung left Freud in 1913. Jung was chosen by Freud to be his successor, but several disagreements developed, mostly about the role of sexuality and the nature of the unconscious, two central themes in psychoanalysis. Jung was more mystical in his approach to personality and, like Adler, was more positive about an individual's ability to control his or her own destiny. He believed the major goal ill life is to unify all of the aspects of our personality, conscious and unconscious, introverted (inwardly directed) and extroverted (outwardly directed). Libido was energy for Jung, but not sexual energy: it was energy for personal growth and development.

Jung accepted the idea of an unconscious mind and expanded on it, claiming that there are two types of unconscious: the personal unconscious, which is very much like Freud's view of the unconscious, and the collective unconscious, which contains very basic ideas that go beyond an individual's own personal experiences. Jung believed that the concepts contained in the collective unconscious are common to all of humanity and are inherited from all past generations. The contents of our collective unconscious include what Jung called archetypes, universal forms and patterns of thought. These are basic "ideas" that transcend generations and all of history. They include certain themes that repeatedly show up in myths: motherhood, opposites, good, evil, masculinity, femininity, and the circle as a symbol representing travel from a beginning back to where one started, or the complete, whole self.

Karen Hornev (1885–1952)

Trained as a psychoanalyst in Germany. Karen Hornev came to the United States in 1934. She held onto a few Freudian concepts but changed most of them significantly. Hornev believed that the idea of levels of consciousness made sense, as did anxiety and repression, but she theorized that the prime impulses that motivate behavior are not biological and inborn or sexual and aggressive. A major concept for Hornev was basic anxiety, which grows out of childhood when the child feels alone and isolated in a hostile environment. If proper parental nurturance is forthcoming, basic anxiety can be overcome. If parents are overly punishing, inconsistent, or indifferent, however, children may develop basic hostitify and may feel very hostile and aggressive toward their parents. However, young children cannot express hostility toward their parents openly, so the hostility gets repressed (into the unconscious), building even more anxiety.

Horney did emphasize early childhood experiences, but from a perspective of social interaction and personal growth. Hornev claimed that there are three distinct ways in which people interact with each other. In some cases, people move away from others, seeking self-sufficiency and independence. The idea here is, "If I am on my own and uninvolved, you won't be able to hurt me." On the other hand, some move toward others, and are compliant and dependent. This style of interaction shields against anxiety in the sense of "If I always do what you want me to do, you won't be upset with me." Horney's third interpersonal style involves moving against others, where the effort is to be in control, to gain power and dominate. "If I am in control, you'll have to do what I want you to." The ideal, of course, is to maintain a balance among these three styles, bill Hornev argued that many people have just one style that predominates their dealings with others.

Hornev also disagreed with Freud's position regarding the biological basis of differences between men and women. Freud's theories have been taken to task several times for their male bias.

Trait Theory of Personality

The trait approach to personality is one of the major theoretical areas in the study of personality. The trait theory suggests that individual personalities are composed broad dispositions. Consider how you would describe the personality of a close friend. Chances are that you would list a number of traits, such as outgoing, kind and even-tempered. A trait can be thought of as a relatively stable characteristic that causes individuals to behave in certain ways.

Unlike many other theories of personality, such as psychoanalytic or humanistic theories, the trait approach to personality is focused on differences between individuals. The combination and interaction of various traits forms a personality that is unique to each individual. Trait theory is focused on identifying and measuring these individual personality characteristics.

Gordon Allport's Trait Theory

In 1936, psychologist Gordon Allport found that one English-language dictionary alone contained more than 4,000 words describing different personality traits. He categorized these traits into three levels:

Cardinal Traits

Traits that dominate an individual's whole life, often to the point that the person becomes known specifically for these traits. People with such personalities often become so known for these traits that their names are often synonymous with these qualities. Consider the origin and meaning of the following descriptive terms: Freudian, Machiavellian, narcissism, Don Juan, Christ-like, etc. Allport suggested that cardinal traits are rare and tend to develop later in life.

Central Traits

These are the general characteristics that form the basic foundations of personality. These central traits, while not as dominating as cardinal traits, are the major characteristics you might use to describe another person. Terms such as intelligent, honest, shy and anxious are considered central traits.

Secondary Traits

These are the traits that are sometimes related to attitudes or preferences and often appear only in certain situations or under specific circumstances. Some examples would be getting anxious when speaking to a group or impatient while waiting in line.

Raymond Cattell's Sixteen Personality Factor Questionnaire

Trait theorist Raymond Cattell reduced the number of main personality traits from Allport's initial list of over 4,000 down to 171,3 mostly by eliminating uncommon traits and combining common characteristics. Next, Cattell rated a large sample of individuals for these 171 different traits. Then, using a statistical technique known as factor analysis, he identified closely related terms and eventually reduced his list to just 16 key personality traits. According to Cattell, these 16 traits are the source of all human personality. He also developed one of the most widely used personality assessments known as the Sixteen Personality Factor Questionnaire (16PF).

Eysenck's Three Dimensions of Personality

British psychologist Hans Eysenck developed a model of personality based upon just three universal trails:

1. Introversion/Extraversion

Introversion involves directing attention on inner experiences, while extraversion relates to focusing attention outward on other people and the environment. So, a person high in introversion might be quiet and reserved, while an individual high in extraversion might be sociable and outgoing.

2. Neuroticism/Emotional Stability

This dimension of Eysenck's trait theory is related to moodiness versus even-temperedness. Neuroticism refers to an individual's tendency to become upset or emotional, while stability refers to the tendency to remain emotionally constant.

3. Psychoticism

Later, after studying individuals suffering from mental illness, Eysenck added a personality dimension he called psychoticism to his trait theory. Individuals who are high on this trait tend to have difficulty dealing with reality and may be antisocial, hostile, non-empathetic and manipulative.

The Five-Factor Theory of Personality

Both Cattell's and Eysenck's theory have been the subject of considerable research, which has led some theorists to believe that Cattell focused on too many traits, while Eysenck focused on too few. As a result, a new trait theory often referred to as the "Big Five" theory emerged. This five-factor model of personality represents five core traits that interact to form human personality. While researchers often disagree about the exact labels for each dimension, the following are described most commonly:

1.Extraversion

2.Agreeableness

3.Conscientiousness

4.Neuroticism

5.Openness

Assessing the Trait Approach to Personality

While most agree that people can be described based upon their personality traits, theorists continue to debate the number of basic traits that make up human personality. While trait theory has objectivity that some personality theories lack (such as Freud's psychoanalytic theory), it also has weaknesses. Some of the most common criticisms of trait theory center on the fact that traits are often poor predictors of behavior. While an individual may score high on assessments of a specific trait, he or she may not always behave that way in every situation. Another problem is that trait theories do not address how or why individual differences in personality develop or emerge.

Evaluating the Psychoanalytic Approach

Given that we have reviewed only a few major ideas from a very complex approach to personality, can we make any value judgments about its contribution? We suspect that you can anticipate our answer. There are critics and supporters of each of the theoretical approaches summarized in this Topic. Each can tell us something about ourselves and about human personality in general.

The psychoanalytic approach, particularly as modified by the neo - Freudians, is the most comprehensive and complex of the theories we'll review. Psychologists have debated the relative merits of Freud's works for decades, and the debate continues. On the positive side, Freud and other psychoanalytically - oriented theorists must be credited for focusing our attention on the importance of the childhood years and for suggesting that some (even biologically determined) impulses may affect our behaviors even though they are beyond our immediate awareness. Although Freud may have overstated the matter, drawing our attention to the impact of sexuality and sexual impulses as influences on personality and human behavior is also a significant contribution. Freud's concept of defense mechanisms has generated considerable research and has found general acceptance, as has the basic notion that the unconscious may influence our pattern at responding to the world.

On the other hand, many psychologists have been critical of several aspects of psychoanalytic theory. We've seen how the neo-Freudians tended to downplay innate biological drives and take a more social approach to personality development than did Freud. One of the major criticisms of the psychoanalytic approach is that so many of its insights appear to be untestable. Freud thought of himself as a scientist, but he tested none of his ideas about human nature experimentally. Some seem beyond testing. Just what ix libidinal energy? How can it be measured? How would we recognize it if we saw it? Concepts such as id, ego, and superego may sound sensible, but how can we prove or (more importantly) disprove their existence? Such a heavy reliance on instincts, especially with sexual and aggressive overtones, as explanatory concepts goes beyond where most psychologists are willing to venture.

Personality Assessment

Personality assessment is conducted through behavioral observations, paper - and - pencil tests, and projective techniques. To be useful, such assessments must be constructed using the established criteria of standardization, reliability, and validity. The information can be used in several areas, including clinical work, vocational counseling, education, and research.

Behavioral Observations

Most people use behavioral observations to form impressions of others. Such observations are also an important part of clinical assessments by clinical psychologists and other professionals.

Interviews, during which subjects' behaviors are observed, may be structured or unstructured. The examiner may ask a standardized set of questions (structured interview) or engage in a conversational interchange with the subject (unstructured interview). During the interview, the examiner forms an opinion about personality characteristics (as is done, for example, also in the nonclinical setting of a job interview).

Paper- and- pencil Tests

The many and various paper - and - pencil tests are used for a variety of purposes. To be useful, such tests must be reliable (that is, they must yield very close scores each time they are administered to a particular individual) and valid (that is, they must measure what they are designed to measure).

The Minnesota Multiphasic Personality Inventory

MMPI is widely used to identify personality problems. The California Personality Inventory (CPI) is also used extensively, generally with people who do not have personality problems. Some tests assess personality as defined by a particular theory. For example, Cattell's 16 PF (personality factor) questionnaire assesses the personality traits defined in Cattell's trait theory.

Projective Techniques

Projective techniques assess personality by presenting ambiguous stimuli and requiring a subject to respond, projecting his or her personality into the responses. The ambiguous inkblots in the well - known Rorschach inkblot test, developed by Hermann Rorschach, are perceived differently by different people, and those perceptions are believed to be related to the subjects' problems.

The Thematic Apperception Test (TAT), developed by Henry Murray, consists of a series of ambiguous pictures, which the subject is requested to describe and tell a story about. The test is used to identify a person's emotions, motives, and problems.

Scoring and interpreting projective tests requires special training, but the tests can be very helpful in identifying personality problems.

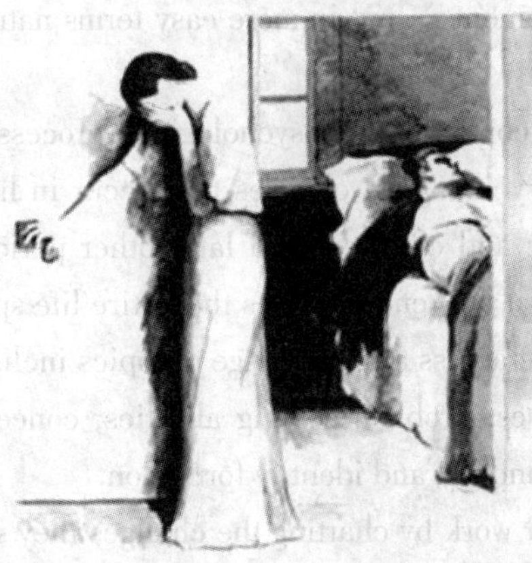

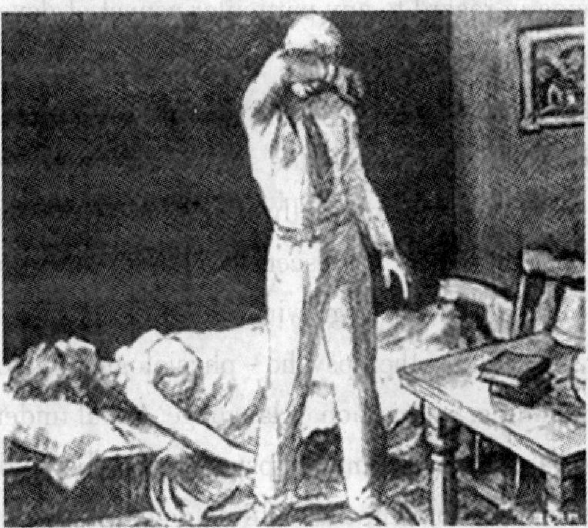

Look at the picture. Your task is to write a complete story about the picture you see above. This should be an imaginative story with a beginning, middle, and an end. Try to portray who the people might be, what they are feeling, thinking, and wishing. Try to tell what led to the situation depicted in the picture and how everything will turn out in the end.

Chapter 7 Child, Adolescent and Adult Development

Developmental Psychology Help Us Understand Ourselves and Others

The study of human development focuses on behavioral and psychological development from conception through later life. Emphasis is on the processes and mechanisms underlying developmental change and stability and the contexts in which development takes place. Psychology is the scientific study of behavior and mental processes. For example, psychology studies the brain, sensation and perception, motivation, intelligence, emotions, memory, psychological disorders, and much more. Developmental Psychology is a subfield of psychology. Its focus is on studying the changes that take place across our life span. Development is defined as changes in our physical structure, thought, and behavior due to genetics or the environment. Development is life long and also can be a very personal thing.

Development incorporates change over time. We all change as we mature. Some of those changes are due to experience and others to our physiology. Developmental psychology is concerned with the patterns and processes of change throughout our lifetimes. A significant question in developmental psychology is the relation between innateness and environmental influence in regard to any particular aspect of development — put in more easy terms nature vs nurture.

Developmental psychology is interested in discovering the psychological processes of development. This is also the study of progressive psychological changes that occur in human beings as they age. Originally concerned with infants and children, and later other periods of great change such as adolescence and early life aging, it now encompasses the entire life span of an individual. This ever growing field examines change across a broad range of topics including: motor skills and other psycho - physiological processes, problem solving abilities, conceptual understanding, acquisition of language, moral understanding, and identify formation.

Although developmental psychologists begin their work by charting the changes they see in the developing human, their ultimate goal is to explain how those changes came about. This is challenging because humans are dynamic, complex beings who are shaped by different people and events. It is often difficult to draw conclusions about exactly which influences and experiences are the most important for particular aspects of cognitive development. Thus, psychologists examine a variety of influences including changes in the brain, the influence of parents, the effect of a child's interaction with siblings and peers, and the role of culture. Typically, in order to accurately characterize aspects of development, psychologists must consider interactions between physiological changes in the brain and the child's or person's social environment. For example, people often use child - directed speech when talking with young children. This type of language accentuates word boundaries and is spoken more slowly compared to adult - directed speech. This aspect of the child's environment may interact with changes in the baby's brain to help the baby comprehend the language spoken around her.

Human development scientific roots date back to fledgling observational and interview studies of children and adolescents in the early part of the twentieth century. In the beginning, description — charting age - related milestones, such as when a child first walked, spoke in sentences, formed a best friendship, and reached puberty — was the principal activity of developmental psychologists. Little attention was accorded to process — the how and why of human change.

Following World War Ⅱ, the field came into its own. Although always a melting pot of interdisciplinary contributions, by the 1960s human development achieved the status of a distinct subdivision within psychology. Empirical work flourished, becoming more sophisticated in methodology and focusing more directly on explanation. Each research was closely tied to a specific domain, or aspect, of human functioning. Together, the grand theories and research brought tension and debate to the field, offering powerfully opposing perspectives on the course and processes of change. A passive child continuously shaped by environmental inputs was pitted against an active, sense - making being undergoing a series of staged shifts rooted in human biology.

Investigators of the mid - century phase had become increasingly sensitive to social and applied issues. Besides traditional topics of enduring interest, such as perception, intelligence, language, personality, and morality, they turned to questions of burning practical concern, such as the impact of poverty, child abuse and neglect, the rising divorce rate, maternal employment and day care, and learning problems in school. In addition to theoretical advances, the field had aligned itself more closely with the goal of improving children's conditions of life.

Developmental Psychology Defined

Developmental psychology is concerned with both physical and psychological changes throughout life — from conception until death. Although theorists differ in their identification of developmental stages and the ages at which they occur, the breakdown is usually similar to that shown in Table 1.

Table 1 Stages in Life

Life Stage	Approximate Age
Prenatal stage	
Conception	Formation of zygote
Germinal	Conception—week 2
Embryo Fetus	Week 2—week 8
Fetus	Week 8—birth
Postnatal stage	
Infancy	Birth—2 years
Toddler	2—3 years
Early childhood	3—6 years
Middle childhood	6—13 years
Adolescence	13—20 years
Young adulthood	20—40 years
Middle adulthood	40—65 years
Late adulthood	65+ years

Nature and Nurture

The relative contributions of nature (genetic and biological inheritance) and nurture (environmental factors) in developmental processes has been and continues to be debated. Psychologists investigate, by using both longitudinal and cross-sectional studies of subjects in each developmental period, how both nature and nurture influence behavior. When put together, the study data provide information about changes over the entire life span.

Identical twins are often studied in nature-nurture investigations (because identical twins develop from one egg, but fraternal twins develop from separate eggs and are genetically no more similar than are any brothers or sisters). Studies have shown that identical twins are more similar in personalities, abilities, and interests than are other siblings, even those identical twins separated at birth and reared apart, a fact that supports the contention that nature (heredity) may be more developmentally important than nurture.

Prenatal Development

The prenatal development period covers the time from conception to birth and is sometimes described in terms of trimesters (first, second, and third) or of three stages (germinal, embryonic, and fetal).

Conception, which occurs when the father's sperm cell penetrates the mother's ovum (egg), marks the beginning of development. The sperm cell/ovum combination creates a zygote, a one-celled organism. All other cells in the body develop from this single cell. Each sperm and each egg cell carry 23 chromosomes, threadlike chains of DNA (deoxyribonucleic acid) that carry genetic information, which unite during fertilization to form 23 pairs of chromosomes. Genes are DNA segments that are functional units in hereditary transmission. After conception, all body cells except gametes (eggs or sperm) contain 23 pairs of chromosomes. The gender of the offspring is determined by the type of sex chromosome in the sperm that fertilizes the ovum; if it is Y bearing, the offspring will be male, and if it is X bearing, the offspring will be female.

The Germinal Stage

The germinal stage extends from conception to two weeks. During this period, the cells in the zygote divide rapidly, and the mass of cells moves slowly along the mother's fallopian tube to the uterus, where it is implanted in the uterine lining. During the implantation process, the placenta is formed. The placenta is a structure that serves as a life-support system for the fetus, allowing oxygen and nutrients to pass into the fetus and waste products to pass out.

The Embryonic Stage

The embryonic stage begins after the cell mass is implanted in the uterus and lasts from two weeks through week eight. Most of the vital organs and body systems form at this time.

The Fetal Stage

The fetal stage is the third stage of prenatal development and covers the period from the end of week eight to birth. Cells continue to divide, body structures become functional, and the fetus becomes capable of movement. When a fetus is from 22 to 26 weeks old, it may survive if birth occurs, but chances for survival increase the closer the term is to 36 weeks.

Prenatal Risks

Risks during the prenatal period include the following.

Development in Infancy and Childhood

Physical Development

In utero, the brain develops rapidly, and an infant is born with essentially all of the nerve cells it will ever have; brain development is particularly rapid during the third trimester. However, after birth, neural connections must form in order for the newborn ultimately to walk, talk, and remember. Mark Rosenweig and David Krech conducted an experiment to demonstrate the importance of enriched environments during development. They compared rats raised alone to those that were allowed to use a playground in the company of other rats. Those in the impoverished (solitary) environment developed a thinner cortex with fewer glial cells, cells that support and nourish the brain's neurons. Other studies have demonstrated that stimulation provided by touch or massage benefits both premature babies and infant rats, a fact that argues for providing an enriched environment for a developing organism.

Infants are born with a surprising number of unlearned (innate) reflexes, that is, unlearned responses to stimuli.

The Moro reflex is an outstretching of the arms and legs in response to a loud noise or sudden change in the environment. The infant's body tenses; arms are extended and then drawn inward as if embracing.

The Babinski reflex is an outward projection of the big toe and fanning of the others when the sole of the foot is touched.

The sucking reflex occurs when an object touches the lips.

The rooting reflex is the turning of an infant's head toward a stimulus such as a breast or hand.

The grasping reflex is the vigorous grasping of an object that touches the palm.

The plantar reflex is the curling under of the toes when the ball of the foot is touched. Physicians sometimes use these reflexes to assess the rate of development. Gradually, learned responses replace the reflex actions as an infant becomes more responsive to the environment.

Although the rate of motor development can vary, the developmental sequence is the same. On average, an infant will learn to roll over at 2.5 months, sit without support at 6 months, and walk alone at 12 months. The growth and body development from infant to child occurs in a cephalocaudal direction; that is, the head and upper trunk develop before the lower trunk and feet.

Sensory and Perceptual Development

Newborn infants can and do respond to a wide ránge of environmental stimuli. All human senses function to some degree at birth; touch is the most highly developed and vision is the least developed sense. At the age of 3 months, however, most infants can recognize a photograph of their mother. An infant's ability to perceive depth has been studied extensively with an apparatus called a visual cliff, a box with a glass platform that extends over a drop of several feet. An adult (mother or experimenter) stands on one side of the glass bridge and calls to the child, who is on the other. Eleanor Gibson and Richard Walk, in a well-known study, found that at about 6 months babies balk at crawling over the edge of the "cliff". Such a response indicates that depth perception is present at this age.

Cognitive Development

The term cognitive development refers to the development of the ability to think and to mentally represent events and to manipulate symbols.

Jean Piaget, a pioneer in the study of children's thinking, was concerned with the way a child organizes information from the environment and adapts to it. He believed that every behavioral act requires two dynamic processes of adaptation: assimilation and accommodation. Assimilation is the process of acquiring new information about the world and fitting it to already acquired information. A child who calls all grown males "daddy", based on the child's perception that they and "daddy" are in some way similar, is practicing assimilation. Accommodation is the process of creating a new concept to handle new information; for example, children come to realize that all toys don't belong to them, that some belong to other children.

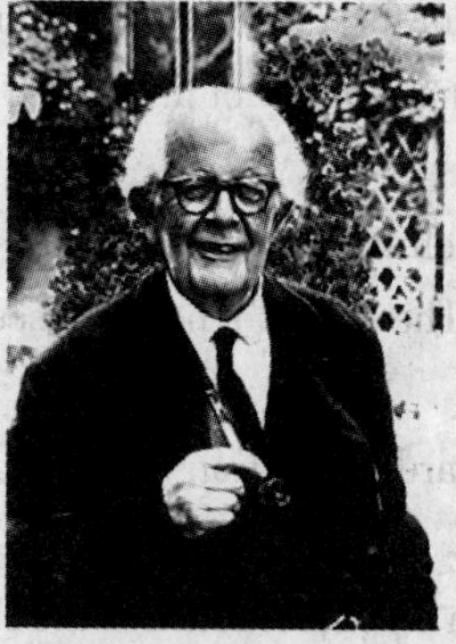

Jean Piaget (1896–1980)

Jean Piaget was a French - speaking Swiss developmental psychologist and philosopher known for his epistemological studies with children. He was the eldest son of Arthur Piaget (Swiss) and Rebecca Jackson (French). His theory of cognitive development and epistemological view are together called "genetic epistemology". Piaget placed great importance on the education of children. As the Director of the International Bureau of Education, he declared in 1934 that only education is capable of saving our societies from possible collapse, whether violent, or gradual. He created the International Center for Genetic Epistemology in Geneva in 1955 and directed it until 1980. He is also the great pioneer of the constructivist theory of knowing.

Piaget, who had a strong biological background, proposed four stages of development: sensorimotor, preoperational, concrete operational, and formal operational. According to Piaget, During the sensorimotor stage (birth to age 2) infants develop their ability to coordinate motor actions with sensory activity. At the start of this stage, children's behavior is dominated by reflexes, but by the end of it, they can use mental images. Also during this stage, children acquire the concept of object permanence, realizing that objects still exist even when the objects are not present.

Much of modern cognitive developmental theory stems from the work of the Swiss psychologist, Jean Piaget. In the 1920s, Piaget observed that children's reasoning and understanding capabilities differed depending on their age. Piaget proposed that all children progress through a series of cognitive stages of development, just as they progress through a series of physical stages of development. According to Piaget, the rate at which children pass through these cognitive stages may vary, but boys and girls eventually pass through all the stagès, in the same order.

Piaget's Sensorimotor Stage

During Piaget's sensorimotor stage (birth to age 2), infants and toddlers learn by doing, looking, hearing, touching, grasping, and sucking. The learning process appears to begin with coordinating movements of the body with incoming sensory data. As infants intentionally attempt to interact with the environment, infants learn that certain actions lead to specific consequences. These experiences are the beginning of the infants' understanding of cause - and - effect relationships.

Piaget divided the sensorimotor stage into six substages. In stage 1 (birth through month 1), infants exclusively use their reflexes, and their cognitive capabilities are limited. In stage 2 (months 1 through 4), infants engage in behaviors that accidentally produce specific effects. Infants then repeat the behavior to obtain the same effect. An example is the infant's learning to suck on a pacifier following a series of trial - and - error attempts to use the new object. In stage 3 (months 4 through 8), infants begin to explore the impact of their behaviors on the environment. In stage 4 (months 8 through 12), infants purposefully carry out goal - directed behaviors.

Object permanence, or the knowledge that out - of - sight objects still exist, may begin to appear at about month 9 as infants search for objects that are hidden from view. In stage 5 (months 12 through 18), toddlers explore cause - and - effect relationships by intentionally manipulating causes to produce novel effects. For example, a toddler may attempt to make her parents smile by waving her hands at them. In stage 6 (months 18 through 24), toddlers begin to exhibit representational (symbolic) thought, demonstrating that they have started to internalize symbols as objects, such as people, places, and things. The child at this stage, for instance, uses words to refer to specific items, such as milk, dog, papa, or mama.

Piaget's model introduces several other important concepts. Piaget termed the infant's innate thinking processes as schemas. In the sensorimotor period, these mental processes coordinate sensory, perceptual, and motor information so that infants eventually develop mental representations. In other words, reflexes provide the basis for schemas, which in turn provide the basis for representational thinking. For example, a child repeatedly touches and sees its rattle and thus learns to identify the rattle by forming an internalized image of it.

According to Piaget, cognitive development occurs from two processes: adaptation and equilibrium.

Adaptation involves children changing their behavior to meet situational demands and consists of two subprocesses: assimilation and accommodation.

Assimilation is the application of previous concepts to new concepts, such as a child who refers to a whale as a fish.

Accommodation is the altering of previous concepts in the face of new information, such as a child who discovers that some creatures living in the ocean are not fish and then correctly refers to a whale as a mammal.

Equilibrium is Piaget's term for the basic process underlying the human ability to adapt, is the search for balance between self and the world. Equilibrium involves the matching of children's adaptive functioning to situational demands, such as when a child realizes that he is one member of a family and not the center of the world. Equilibrium, which helps remove inconsistencies between reality and personal perspectives, keeps children moving along the developmental pathway, allowing them to make increasingly effective adaptations and decisions.

Evaluating Piagetian Theory

The majority of researchers today accept Piaget's primary tenet: New cognitive skills build upon previous cognitive skills. Researchers see infants and toddlers as active learners who purposefully see, touch, and do, and who consequently develop additional cognitive skills. Developmentalists see cognitive development as involving both advancement and limitation. Devlopmentalists also applaud Piaget's role in stimulating professional interest in the cognitive world of children.

Piaget's research and theories are not unchallenged, however. Some of the more prominent critics of Piaget include Robbie Case, Pierr Dasen, Kurt Fischer, and Elizabeth Spelke. These critics and others maintain that the stages of development described by Piaget are not so distinct and clearly defined as Piaget originally indicated. These detractors also note that all children do not necessarily pass through Piaget's stages in precisely the same way or order. Piaget was aware of this phenomenon, which he termed decalage, but he never adequately explained decalage in light of the rest of his model.

Critics also suggest that toddlers and preschoolers are not as egocentric or as easily deceived as Piaget believed. Preschoolers may empathize with others, or put themselves into another person's shoes, and young children may make inferences and use logic. Preschoolers also develop cognitive abilities in relation to particular social and cultural contexts. These abilities may develop differently within enriched or deprived cultural environments. In other words, children who grow up in middle and upper-class families may have more opportunities to develop cognitive skills than those who grow up in lower-class families.

Children appear to employ and more deeply understand symbols at an earlier age than was previously thought. In as early as the first 3 months, infants display a basic understanding of how the world works. For example, infants pay closer attention to objects that seem to defy physical laws, such as balls that appear to roll through walls or rattles that appear to hang in mid-air as opposed to stationary objects.

Memory

Central to early cognitive development is memory development. Memory is the ability to encode, retain, and recall information over time. Researchers generally refer to sensory (less than 1 second), short-term (less than 30 seconds), and long-term (indefinite) memory stores. Children are not able to habituate or learn if they are unable to encode objects, people, and places and eventually recall them from long-term memory.

Researchers are unclear about the exact nature of infantile memory, however. The unclear facts about infantile memory include how long such memories last, as well as how easily memories are retrieved from long-term stores. Evidence suggests that babies begin forming long-term memories during the first 6 months. Infants may recognize and remember primary caretakers, as well as familiar surroundings. Early memory experiences help infants and toddlers to understand basic concepts and categories, all of which are central to more completely understanding the world around them.

Language

Language skills begin to emerge during the first 2 years. Psycholinguists, specialists in the study of language, indicate that language is an outgrowth of children's ability to use symbols. Physical development determines the timing of language development. As the brains develop, preschoolers acquire the capacity for representational thinking, which lays the foundation for language. In this way, cognitive development also determines the timing of language development. Observational learning (imitation) and operant conditioning (reinforcement) play important roles in the early acquisition of language. Children are reinforced to speak meaningfully and reasonably by imitating the language of their caregivers; in turn caregivers are prompted to respond meaningfully and reasonably to the children.

Psycholinguists are especially interested in three elements of language: content (what is meant), form (what is actually said), and use (how and to whom it is said). Psycholinguists claim that all members of the human race use these three elements in some combination to communicate with each other. Noam Chomsky suggested that the learning of a language is rooted in an inborn capacity to comprehend and structure language, which he defined as the language acquisition device.

Language acquisition is one of the most important aspects of a child's development.

Moral Development

Lawrence Kohlberg proposed that moral development occurs in three levels, with two stages at each level.

The Preconventional Level:

At stage 1, punishment orientation, judgments are guided by the prospect of punishment.

At stage 2, pleasure-seeking orientation, activities are undertaken primarily to satisfy one's own needs; needs of others are important only as they relate to one's own needs.

The Conventional Level:

At stage 3, good girl/good boy orientation, behavior is engaged in that brings approval or pleases others in a child's immediate group.

At stage 4, authority orientation, behavior is influenced by respect for authority, performing one's duty, and doing what is right.

The Postconventional Level:

At stage 5, contract and legal orientation, behavior is based on support of rules and regulations because society's right to exact such support is accepted.

At stage 6, ethical and moral principles orientation, behavior is directed by self-chosen ethical and moral principles.

Kohlberg found that the first two stages are reached by most children, that stages 3 and 4 are reached by older children and most adults, but that the stage 6 is reached by only 20% of the population.

Carol Gilligan examined certain differences between the moral development of males and that of females. In younger children, she found that girls are more concerned with a morality based on caring and boys with a morality based on justice. Gilligan proposed that this gender difference is in part due to children's relationship with their mother.

Social Development

Social development begins at birth as a child forms an attachment (a strong emotional bond) with the primary caregiver (s), usually the mother. Harry Harlow studied attachment deprivation with baby monkeys raised in isolation. Although their physical needs were met and they were given surrogate mothers made of cloth, these monkeys suffered severe behavior pathologies. They recovered if the isolation was limited to three months, but longer periods produced abnormal adults. Ethically, this type of study could not be conducted with humans, but parallels have been found with children reared in cold, isolated, emotionally deprived environments. Emotional attachments to caregivers are thought to be essential for social development.

Konrad Lorenz studied imprinting, a rapid and relatively permanent type of learning that occurs for a limited time (called a critical period) early in life, particularly in birds. Baby ducks learn to follow their mother if they see her moving during the first 30 - hour period after their birth. If, however, they don't see their mother, they can imprint on and follow a human or even a moving object instead. Imprinting demonstrates that attachments by the young to a parent can occur early and can have lifelong consequences.

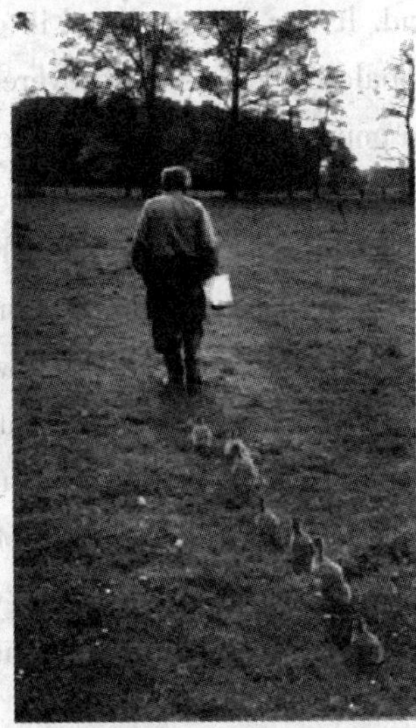

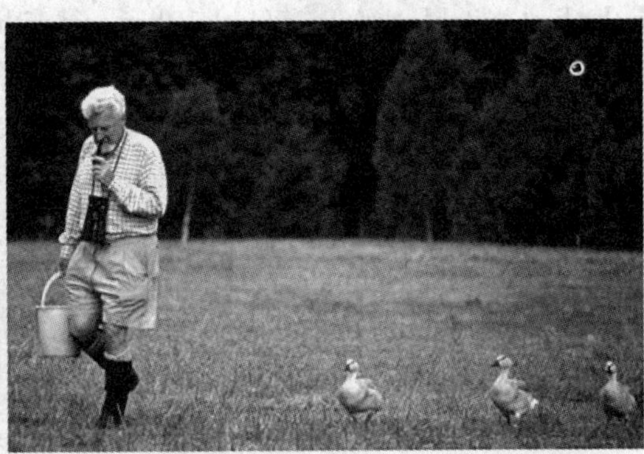

Konrad Lorenz is best known among biologists for his pioneering work on imprinting in young animals. During a critical period early in their lives, many young animals learn the identity of their mother and father. Once learned, this identity is firmly fixed and may be used later in life in identifying mates, forming flocks, and in other social interactions. Lorenz found that by substituting himself for the mother during this critical period, he could induce young geese to imprint on him. Famous photographs of Lorenz show him being followed by geese imprinted in this way.

A prolific writer, Lorenz synthesized much early ethological thought about communication, learning, and social interactions. In addition to his work on imprinting, he set the stage for understanding the instinctive basis of animal behavior, and for the role of learning within the framework set by instinct. Lorenz attempted to draw on his experiences with animals to analyze human behavior and culture. On Aggression, his analysis of the role of aggression in shaping human and animal societies, generated substantial controversy because of its argument, in part, that behavioral tendencies are instinctive and unmodifiable by experience. This met fierce political resistance from American psychologists, who were strongly aligned on the nurture side of the nature - nurture argument. More recent work, such as that by American psychologist Robert Plomin, demonstrates a very credible role for genetics (nature) in shaping human personalities.

Imprinting is the term used in psychology and ethology to describe any kind of phase-sensitive learning (learning occurring at a particular age or a particular life stage) that is rapid and apparently independent of the consequences of behavior. It was first used to describe situations in which an animal or person learns the characteristics of some stimulus, which is therefore said to be "imprinted" onto the subject.

The best-known form of imprinting is filial imprinting, in which a young animal acquires several of its behavioral characteristics from its parent. It is most obvious in nidifugous birds, which imprint on their parents and then follow them around. It was first reported in domestic chickens, by the 19th-century amateur biologist Douglas Spalding. It was rediscovered by the early ethologist Oskar Heinroth, and studied extensively and popularized by his disciple Konrad Lorenz working with grey lag geese. Lorenz demonstrated how incubator-hatched geese would imprint on the first suitable moving stimulus they saw within what he called a "critical period" between 13–16 hours shortly after hatching. For example, the goslings would imprint on Lorenz himself (to be more specific, on his wading boots), and he is often depicted being followed by a gaggle of geese who had imprinted on him. Lorenz also found that the geese could imprint on inanimate objects. In one experiment, they followed a box placed on a model train in circles around the track. Filial imprinting is not restricted to non-human animals that are able to follow their parents, however. In child development, the term is used to refer to the process by which a baby learns who its mother and father are. The process is recognised as beginning in the womb, when the unborn baby starts to recognize its parents' voices.

The filial imprinting of birds was a primary technique used to create the movie Winged Migration, which contains a great deal of footage of migratory birds in flight. The birds imprinted on handlers, who wore yellow jackets and honked horns constantly. The birds were then trained to fly along with a variety of aircraft, primarily ultra lights.

The Italian hang-glider pilot Angelod Arrigo extended this technique. Arrigo noted that the flight of a non-motorised hang-glider is very similar to the flight patterns of migratory birds: Both use updrafts of hot air (thermal currents) to gain altitude that then permits soaring flight over distance. He used this fact to enable the reintroduction into the wild of threatened species of raptors.

Birds that are hatched in captivity have no mentor birds to teach them their traditional migratory routes. Arrigo had one solution to this problem. The chicks hatched under the wing of his glider, and imprinted on him. Then, he taught the fledglings to fly and to hunt. The young birds followed him not only on the ground (as with Lorenz) but also in the air as he took the path of various migratory routes. He flew across the Sahara and over the Mediterranean Sea to Sicily with eagles, from Siberia to Iran (5,500 km) with a flock of Siberian cranes, and over Mount Everest with Nepalese eagles. In 2006, he worked with a condor in South America.

In a similar project, orphaned Canada Geese were trained to their normal migration route by the Canadian ultra light enthusiast Bill Lishman, as shown in the fact-based movie drama *Fly Away Home*.

Chicks of domestic chickens prefer to be near large groups of objects that they have imprinted on. This behavior was used to determine that very young chicks of a few days old have rudimentary counting skills. In a series of experiments, they were made to imprint on plastic balls and could figure out which of two groups of balls hidden behind screens had the most balls.

The term gender stereotyping refers to patterns of behavior expected of people according to their gender. The development of gender-related differences is complex. Gender stereotyping occurs not only because of parental differences in rearing children of each gender but also because of socialization experiences. Eleanor Maccoby has observed that children with widely different personalities play together simply because they are of the same gender.

Personality Development

Developmental psychologists also study personality development in children.

Developing Gender Identity

The theories of Piaget, Kohlberg, and Erikson deal with how (and when) children develop concepts or cognitions about themselves and the world in which they live. In this section we'll focus on the concept of gender one's maleness or femaleness, as opposed to one's sex, which is a biological term. Gender has been defined as "the socially ascribed characteristics of females and males, their roles and appropriate behaviors" (Amaro, 1995) and "the meanings that societies and individuals ascribe to female and male categories" (Eagly, 1995).

One of the first proclamations made upon the birth of a baby is "It's a girl!" or "It's a boy!" Parents wrap little girls in pink, boys in blue, and dress an infant or small child in clothes that clearly label the child as a boy or a girl.

One question we might ask is what differences do we find between boys and girls in childhood? Let's discuss the general answer first and then go into specifics. Differences between male and female infants and children are few and subtle. They are more likely to be in the eye of the beholder than in the behaviors of children.

As infants, boys develop a bit more slowly than girls, have a little more muscle tissue than girls, and are somewhat more active, but even these differences are slight (Eaton & Enns, 1986). During the first year of life there are virtually no differences in temperament or "difficulty" between boys and girls (Thomas & Chess, 1977). Adults often believe that there ought to be differences between the sexes (Paludi & Gullo, 1986) and choose toys, clothing, and playmates based on what they believe is acceptable (Schau et al, 1980). However, when averaged over many studies, there are few areas in which parents consistently treat their sons and daughters differently (Lytton & Romney, 1991).

The only area in which North American parents show significant differentiation is the encouragement of different sex-typed activities for girls and boys. For example, in one study (Snow et al., 1983), fathers were more likely to give dolls to one-year-old girls than to boys. However, even at this age, children themselves already have their own toy preferences; when offered dolls, boys are less likely to play with them. In the first few years of elementary school, girls have a different view of areas of their own competence and activities of value than boys do. Girls tend to value (and see themselves as competent ill) reading and instrumental music, for example, whereas boys value math and sports activities (Eccles et al, 1993.)

Children's peer groups provide significant experiences for both girls and boys (Macoby, 1988). By the age of three or four, girls and boys gravitate toward playmates of the same sex, a pattern that is shown cross-culturally. Boys tend to dominate in mixed-sex interactions (Jacklin & Maccoby, 1978). Boys develop the tendency to use direct commands to influence others, whereas girls tend to use polite suggestions, which are effective with other girls but not with boys (Serbin et al, 1984). Girls develop more intensive friendships than boys and are more distressed when those friend-ships end. Maccoby (1990) has suggested that the interactive styles that develop in same sex groups in childhood lay the foundation for differences in social relationships of adult men and women, with more supportive, intimate relationships among women and more direct, hierarchical relationships among men.

Here's a different but related question: At what age do boys and girls begin to see each other as "different"? When do children develop gender identity, the basic sense or self-awareness of maleness or femaleness? Even five-month-old infants are able to distinguish gender in faces shown to them in pictures. Most of us develop a sense of gender identity by the time we are two or three years old. By the age of four, most children demonstrate gender stereotypes, showing that they believe that certain occupations, activities, or toys go better with males and some go better with females. By the time they are ready to start school, most children have a notion of associating various personality traits with men and women. This pattern has been found in several cultures. Once gender identity is established, it remains quite invulnerable to change.

Cognitive psychologists believe that once children can discriminate between the sexes, they develop schemas for gender-related information. You'll recall that a schema is an organized system of general information, stored in memory that guides the processing of new information. For example, children remember toys better if they are gender consistent than if they are gender inconsistent. That is, male children remember male-oriented toys better than female-oriented toys and female children remember female-oriented toys better than male-oriented toys. This effect extends to when children are asked to remember situations depicting gender-consistent versus gender-inconsistent information. In one experiment, male and female children were asked to recall a series of pictures depicting men and women in either traditional or nontraditional roles. The results showed that male children remembered more pictures showing a male in a traditional male role (eg, firefighter) than a male in a nontraditional role (eg, schoolteacher). Female children better remembered a female in a traditional role than in a nontraditional role (Liben & Signorella, 1993). According to Liben and Signorella, this gender difference is most likely due to distorting or forgetting material in memory that is inconsistent with one's gender schemes. These memory distortions help perpetuate a child's gender schema because information that does not fit with the schema is changed so that it fits with the schema.

Developing Social Attachments

To a large degree, we adapt and thrive in this world to the extent that we can profit from interpersonal relationships. The roots of social development can be found in early infancy in the formation of attachment. Attachment is a strong emotional relationship between a child and in other or primary caregiver (Bowlby, 2004). Attachment has survival value, "increasing the chances of an infant being protected by those to whom he or she keeps proximity" (Ainsworth, 1989). A well-fanned attachment provides a child with freedom to explore the environment, curiosity, adaptive problem solving, and competence when interacting with peers.

Forming an attachment between infant and mother, for example, involves regular interaction and active give-and-take between the two. Strong attachments are most likely to be formed if the parent is optimally sensitive and responsive to the needs of the child. Sensitivity refers to the parent's ability to correctly read the signals coining from an infant (for example, correctly identifying when the infant is hungry by the nature of the infant's crying pattern). Responsiveness refers to how the parent responds to the child's signals, for example picking up the infant when he or she cries, changing the diaper as soon as it is soiled, feeding on a regular basis, and so on. Interestingly, there is an optimal level of sensitivity and responsiveness that relates to positive, secure attachments. Too much or too little can result in negative, insecure attachment (Belsky, Rovine & Taylor, 1984).

Simply spending time with an infant is seldom enough to produce successful attachment. Attachment is promoted by spontaneous bugging, smiling, eye contact, and vocalizing (Lamb et al, 1982). It is fostered by qualities such as warmth and gentleness. When the process is successful, we say that the child is "securely attached". Forming an attachment is a two-way street. Attachment will be most secure when the baby reciprocates by smiling, cooing, and clinging to mother when attended to (Ainsworth, 1979; Pedersoii et al, 1990). About 65% of American children become securely attached by the age of one year — a percentage close to that found in seven other countries (van Ijzendoom & Kroonenberg, 1988).

Are there long-term benefits of becoming securely attached? Yes. Secure attachment is related to: (1) sociability (less fear of strangers, better relationships with peers, more popularity, and more friends); (2) higher self-esteem; (3) better relationships with sib-lings; (4) fewer tantrums or less aggressive behaviors; (5) less concern by teachers over controlling behaviors in the classroom; (6) more empathy and concern for the feelings of others; (7) fewer behavioral problems at later ages, and (8) better attention spans (from Bee, 1992). Securely attached children also show greater persistence at problem solving and are less likely to seek help from adults when injured or disappointed.

We need to make it clear that infants can and do form attachments with persons other than their mothers. Father-child attachments are quite common and are beneficial for the long-term development of the child. One researcher found that she could predict the extent to which a child showed signs of attachment to its father simply by knowing how often Dad changed the baby's diaper (Ross et al, 1975). There is no evidence that fathers are less sensitive to the needs of their children than are mothers (Parke, 1981); although, they may be a little more physical and a little less verbal in their interactions (Parke & Tinsley, 1987).

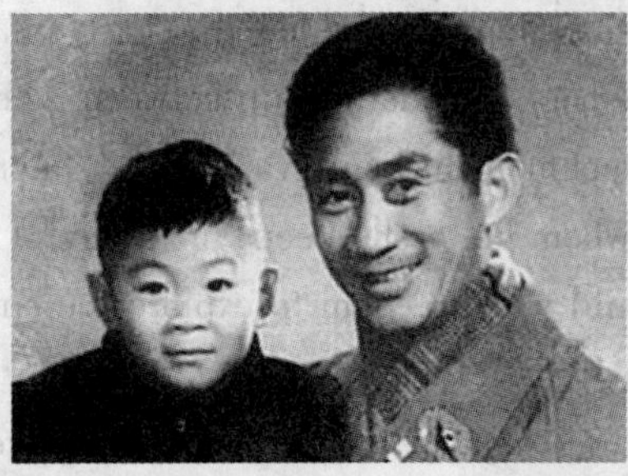
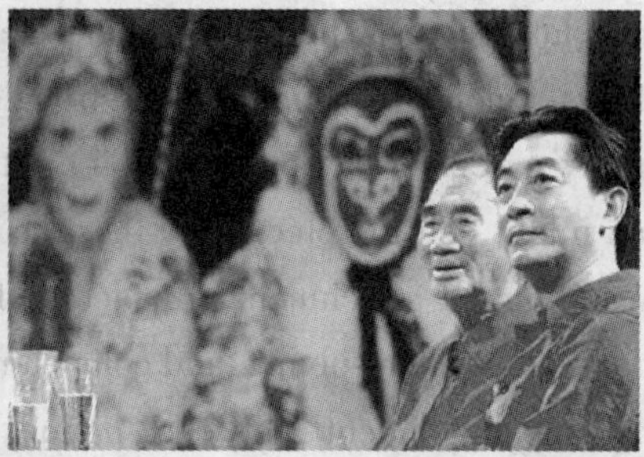

Early experiences with caregivers gradually give rise to a system of thoughts, memories, beliefs, expectations, emotions and behaviors about the self and others. Attachment is an emotional bond to another person. Psychologist John Bowlby was the first attachment theorist, describing attachment as a "lasting psychological connectedness between human beings" (Bowlby, 1969, p. 194). Bowlby believed that the earliest bonds formed by children with their caregivers have a tremendous impact that continues throughout life. According to Bowlby, attachment also serves to keep the infant close to the mother, thus improving the child's chances of survival.

The central theme of attachment theory is that mothers who are available and responsive to their infant's needs establish a sense of security in their children. The infant knows that the caregiver is dependable, which creates a secure base for the child to then explore the world.

Whether an adult is secure or insecure in his or her adult relationships may be a partial reflection of his or her experiences with his or her primary caregivers. Bowlby believed that the mental representations or working models (ie, expectations, beliefs, "rules" or "scripts" for behaving and thinking) that a child holds regarding relationships are a function of his or her caregiving experiences. For example, a secure child tends to believe that others will be there for him or her because previous experiences have led him or her to this conclusion. Once a child has developed such expectations, he or she will tend to seek out relational experiences that are consistent with those expectations and perceive others in a way that is colored by those beliefs. According to Bowlby, this kind of process should promote continuity in attachment patterns over the life course, although it is possible that a person's attachment pattern will change if his or her relational experiences are inconsistent with his or her expectations. In short, if we assume that adult relationships are attachment relationships, it is possible that children who are secure as children will grow up to be secure in their romantic relationships. Or, relatedly, that people who are secure as adults in their relationships with their parents will be more likely to forge secure relationships with new partners.

Attachment Pattern of Behavior Patterns before the Age of 18 Months

Attachment-pattern	Child	Caregiver
Secure	Uses caregiver as a secure base for exploration. Protests caregiver's departure and seeks proximity and is comforted on return, returning to exploration. May be comforted by the stranger but shows clear preference for the caregiver.	Responds appropriately, promptly and consistently to needs. Caregiver has successfully formed a secure parental attachment bond to the child.
Avoidant	Little affective sharing in play. Little or no distress on departure, little or no visible response to return, ignoring or turning away with no effort to maintain contact if picked up. Treats the stranger similarly to the caregiver. The child feels that there is no attachment; therefore, the child is rebellious and has a lower self-image and self-esteem.	Little or no response to distressed child. Discourages crying and encourages independence.
Ambivalent/ Resistant	Unable to use caregiver as a secure base, seeking proximity before separation occurs. Distressed on separation with ambivalence, anger, reluctance to warm to caregiver and return to play on return. Preoccupied with caregiver's availability, seeking contact but resisting angrily when it is achieved. Not easily calmed by stranger. In this relationship, the child always feels anxious because the caregiver's availability is never consistent.	Inconsistent between appropriate and neglectful responses. Generally will only respond after increased attachment behavior from the infant.
Disorganized	Stereotypies on return such as freezing or rocking. Lack of coherent attachment strategy shown by contradictory, disoriented behaviours such as approaching but with the back turned.	Frightened or frightening behaviour, intrusiveness, withdrawal, negativity, role confusion, affective communication errors and maltreatment. Very often associated with many forms of abuse towards the child.

We need to consider attachment formation for those children who spend time, sometimes a lot of time, in day care facilities. In the United States, more than half the mothers of children younger than three are employed, and the care of those children is at least, in part, taken over by others. There is evidence that children who are placed in high quality day care benefit cognitively and socially (Shaffer, 1999). How do these children fare with respect to attachment? It depends to a large extent on the quality of the care the children are given no matter where they get it. Children who receive warm, supportive, attentive care, adequate stimulation, and opportunities for exploration demonstrate secure attachment (Howes, 1990). The impact of day care depends on the likelihood that the child would have received good, warm, supportive, loving care at home. Additionally, the quality of day care and quality of maternal care combine to affect attachment security. Children who experience both low quality day care and insensitive/unresponsive parenting show the poorest attachment security.

The benefits or harm of nonparental child care may also depend on the age of the child. There is little dispute about the conclusion that children who enter day care at 18 months, two years, or later show no consistent loss of security of attachment to their parents. The debate centers on children less than one year old, and there is some evidence that secure attachment is less likely among those children who are cared for at home during their first year. Two other studies suggest that early infant day care has little effect on a child's later social and emotional development. In one study conducted in France, there was no difference in the amount of aggression and other behavior problems between three to four-year-old children who had attended day care during the first three years of life and those who had not. Early day care has also been found not to affect mother-infant interactions or cognitive outcomes for the child. Thus, it appears that there is no consistent relationship between early infant day care and later social and emotional development.

It may tentatively be concluded that forming secure attachments is important for the later development of the child. There are long-term benefits (ranging from improved emotional stability to improved problem-solving skills) to be derived from the development of strong attachments formed early in childhood. Further, attachments formed with the father or other caregivers seem as useful for long-term development as do attachments to the mother.

There is now an increasing amount of research that suggests that adult romantic relationships function in ways that are similar to infant-caregiver relationships, with some noteworthy exceptions, of course. Naturalistic research on adults separating from their partners at an airport demonstrated that behaviors indicative of attachment-related protest and caregiving were evident, and that the regulation of these behaviors was associated with attachment style (Fraley & Shaver, 1998). For example, while separating couples generally showed more attachment behavior than nonseparating couples, highly avoidant adults showed much less attachment behavior than less avoidant adults. In the sections below I discuss some of the parallels that have been discovered between the way that infant-caregiver relationships and adult romantic relationships function.

There is now an increasing amount of research that suggests that adult romantic relationships function in ways that are similar to infant-caregiver relationships, with some noteworthy exceptions, of course. Naturalistic research on adults separating from their partners at an airport demonstrated that behaviors indicative of attachment-related protest and caregiving were evident, and that the regulation of these behaviors was associated with attachment style (Fraley & Shaver, 1998). For example, while separating couples generally showed more attachment behavior than nonseparating couples, highly avoidant adults showed much less attachment behavior than less avoidant adults. In the sections below I discuss some of the parallels that have been discovered between the way that infant-caregiver relationships and adult romantic relationships function.

Partner Selection

Cross - cultural studies suggest that the secure pattern of attachment in infancy is universally considered the most desirable pattern by mothers (see van IJzendoorn & Sagi, 1999). For obvious reasons there is no similar study asking infants if they would prefer a security-inducing attachment figure. Adults seeking long-term relationships identify responsive caregiving qualities, such as attentiveness, warmth, and sensitivity, as most "attractive" in potential dating partners (Zeifman & Hazan, 1997). Despite the attractiveness of secure qualities, however, not all adults are paired with secure partners. Some evidence suggests that people end up in relationships with partners who confirm their existing beliefs about attachment relationships (Frazier et al., 1997).

Secure Base and Safe Haven Behavior

In infancy, secure infants tend to be the most well adjusted, in the sense that they are relatively resilient, they get along with their peers, and are well liked. Similar kinds of patterns have emerged in research on adult attachment. Overall, secure adults tend to be more satisfied in their relationships than insecure adults. Their relationships are characterized by greater longevity, trust, commitment, and interdependence (eg, Feeney, Noller & Callan, 1994), and they are more likely to use romantic partners as a secure base from which to explore the world (eg, Fraley & Davis, 1997). A large proportion of research on adult attachment has been devoted to uncovering the behavioral and psychological mechanisms that promote security and secure base behavior in adults. There have been two major discoveries thus far. First and in accordance with attachment theory, secure adults are more likely than insecure adults to seek support from their partners when distressed. Furthermore, they are more likely to provide support to their distressed partners (eg, Simpson et al., 1992). Second, the attributions that insecure individuals make concerning their partner's behavior during and following relational conflicts exacerbate, rather than alleviate, their insecurities (eg, Simpson et al., 1996).

Avoidant Attachment and Defense Mechanisms

According to attachment theory, children differ in the kinds of strategies they use to regulate attachment - related anxiety. Following a separation and reunion, for example, some insecure children approach their parents, but with ambivalence and resistance, whereas others withdraw from their parents, apparently minimizing attachment - related feelings and behavior. One of the big questions in the study of infant attachment is whether children who withdraw from their parents — avoidant children — are truly less distressed or whether their defensive behavior is a cover - up for their true feelings of vulnerability. Research that has measured the attentional capacity of children, heart rate, or stress hormone levels suggests that avoidant children are distressed by the separation despite the fact that they come across in a cool, defensive manner.

Recent research on adult attachment has revealed some interesting complexities concerning the relationships between avoidance and defense. Although some avoidant adults, often called fearfully - avoidant adults, are poorly adjusted despite their defensive nature, others, often called dismissing-avoidant adults, are able to use defensive strategies in an adaptive way. For example, in an experimental task in which adults were instructed to discuss losing their partner, Fraley and Shaver (1997) found that dismissing individuals (ie, individuals who are high on the dimension of attachment-related avoidance but low on the dimension of attachment-related anxiety) were just as physiologically distressed (as assessed by skin conductance measures) as other individuals. When instructed to suppress their thoughts and feelings, however, dismissing individuals were able to do so effectively. That is, they could deactivate their physiological arousal to some degree and minimize the attention they paid to attachment-related thoughts. Fearfully-avoidant individuals were not as successful in suppressing their emotions.

Development in Middle Childhood

Ages 7 through 11 comprise middle childhood. Some authorities divide middle childhood into early-middle (ages 7-9) and late-middle (ages 10-11) periods. Like infants, toddlers, and preschoolers, these older children grow both physically and cognitively, although their growth is slower than it was during early childhood.

Physical development in middle childhood is characterized by considerable variations in growth patterns. These variations may be due to gender, ethnic origin, genetics, hormones, nutrition, environment, or disease. While children of this age group follow the same basic developmental patterns, they do not necessarily mature at the same rate. Most girls experience a preadolescent growth spurt around age 9 or 10, while most boys experience the same growth spurt around age 11 or 12. Children who do not receive adequate nutrition or medical attention may be at risk for stunted or delayed growth development. For example, children who live in countries where malnutrition is not a problem tend to be taller than children who live in countries where malnutrition is a problem.

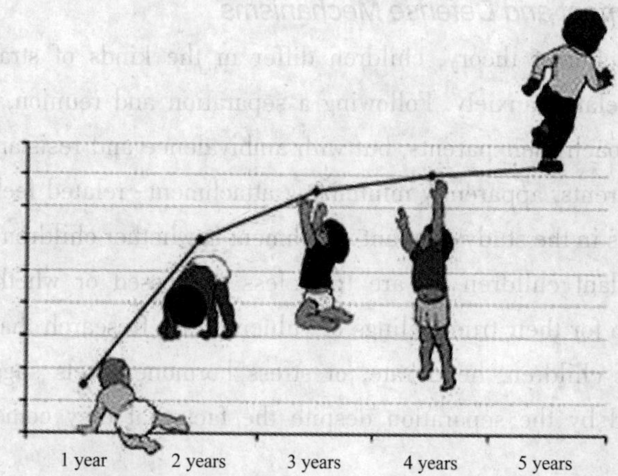

Physical changes, brain and nervous system development, gross and fine motor skills, and health issues are important aspects of physical development during middle childhood as in previous developmental stages.

Physical Changes

By the beginning of middle childhood, children typically have acquired a leaner, more athletic appearance. Girls and boys still have similar body shapes and proportions until both sexes reach puberty, the process whereby children sexually mature into teenagers and adults. After puberty, secondary sexual characteristics — breasts and curves in females, deeper voice and broad shoulders in males — make distinguishing females from males much easier.

Girls and boys grow about 2 to 3 inches and gain about 7 pounds per year until puberty. Skeletal bones and muscles broaden and lengthen, which may cause children (and adolescents) to experience growing pains. Skeletal growth in middle childhood is also associated with losing the deciduous teeth, or baby teeth.

Throughout most of middle childhood, girls are smaller than boys and have less muscle mass. As girls enter puberty, however, they may be considerably larger than boys of the same age, who enter puberty a few years later. Once boys begin sexually maturing, their heights and weights eventually surpass the heights and weights of girls of the same age.

Brain and Nervous System Development

Brain and nervous system developments continue during middle childhood. More complex behavioral and cognitive abilities become possible as the central nervous system matures.

Early in middle childhood, a growth spurt occurs in the brain so that by age 8 or 9, the organ is nearly adult - size. Brain development during middle childhood is characterized by growth of specific structures, especially the frontal lobes. These lobes, located in the front of the brain just under the skull, are responsible for planning, reasoning, social judgment, and ethical decision making, among other functions. Damage to this part of brain results in erratic emotional outbursts, inability to plan, and poor judgment. The most anterior (front) portion of the frontal lobes is the prefontal cortex, which appears to be responsible for personality.

As the size of the frontal lobes increases, children are able to engage in increasingly difficult cognitive tasks, such as performing a series of tasks in a reasonable order. An example is assembling a mechanical toy: unpacking the pieces, connecting the parts, making the model move by adding a power source, a series of tasks that must be completed in the correct order to achieve certain results.

Lateralization of the two hemispheres of the brain, also continues during middle childhood, as does maturation of the corpus callosum (the bands of neural fibers connecting the two cerebral hemispheres), and other areas of the nervous system. Interestingly, children achieve concrete operations around age 7 when the brain and nervous systems have developed a certain amount of neural connections. When these neural connections have developed, a child's ability to perceive and think about the world advances from an egocentric, magical viewpoint to a more concrete and systematic way of thinking.

Motor Skills

Motor skills are behavioral abilities or capacities. Gross motor skills involve the use of large bodily movements, and fine motor skills involve the use of small bodily movements. Both gross and fine motor skills continue to refine during middle childhood.

Children love to run, jump, leap, throw, catch, climb, and balance. Children play baseball, ride bikes, roller skate, take karate lessons, take ballet lessons, and participate in gymnastics. As school - age children grow physically, they become faster, stronger, and better coordinated. Consequently, during middle childhood, children become more adept at gross motor activities.

Children enjoy using their hands in detailed ways, too. From early in preschool, children learn and practice fine motor skills. Preschool children cut, paste, mold, shape, draw, paint, create, and write. These children also learn such skills as tying shoelaces, untying knots, and flossing their teeth. Some fortunate children are able to take music lessons for piano, violin, flute, or other instruments. Learning to play an instrument helps children to further develop their fine motor skills. In short, along with the physical growth of children comes the development of fine motor skills, including the sense of competence and confidence to use these skills.

Health

Middle childhood tends to be a very healthy period of life in Western societies. The typical minor illnesses of early childhood — colds, coughs, and stomachaches — are likely to lessen in frequency in middle childhood. This improved resistance to common illnesses is probably due to a combination of increased immunity from previous exposures and improved hygiene and nutritional practices. Minor illnesses occur, but most illnesses do not require medical attention. Minor illnesses may help children learn psychological coping skills and strategies for dealing with physical discomforts.

Major illnesses for school - age children are the same as major illnesses for younger children: influenza, pneumonia, cancer, human immunodeficiency virus (HIV), and acquired immunodeficiency syndrome (AIDS). But obesity, or being 20 percent or more above one's ideal weight, is a special health problem that occurs during the school years. About 25% of school - age children in the United States today are obese, and the majority of these children go on to become obese adults. Obesity in adulthood is related to heart problems, high blood pressure, and diabetes. Although obese children are not at the same medical risks as obese adults, these children should master effective eating and exercise habits as early as possible to decrease the risk of later obesity - and health - related problems.

The majority of disabilities and deaths in middle childhood are the result of injuries from accidents. In the United States, nearly 22 million children are hurt in accidents each year. For children, the most common deadly accidents result from being struck by moving vehicles. Accidents may occur at, near, and away from home; therefore, adequate adult supervision is always important. Injuries occurring at school are usually the result of playground - and sports - related accidents. Consequently, children should always wear protective headgear and other safety gear when playing sports and riding bikes. Other causes of death in middle childhood include cancer, congenital defects, homicide, and deadly infections.

Cognitive Development in Middle Childhood

School - age children think systematically about multiple topics more easily than preschoolers. Older children have keener metacognition, a sense of their own inner world. These children become increasingly skilled at problem solving.

Piaget referred to the cognitive development occurring between ages 7 and 11 as the concrete operations stage. Piaget used the term operations to refer to reversible abilities that the child has not yet developed. By reversible, Piaget referred to mental or physical actions that can occur in more than one way, or in differing directions. While in the concrete operations stage, older children cannot think both logically and abstractly. School - age children are limited to thinking concretely — in tangible, definite, exact, and uni - directional terms, based on real and concrete experiences rather than on abstractions. Older children do not use magical thinking and are not as easily misled as younger children. Unlike preschoolers, school - age children know better than to ask their parents to take them flying in the air just like the birds do.

Piaget noted that children's thinking processes change significantly during the concrete operations stage. School - age children can engage in classification, or the ability to group according to features, and serial ordering, or the ability to group according to logical progression. Older children come to understand cause - and - effect relationships and become adept at mathematics and science. Comprehending the concept of stable identity, that one's self remains consistent even when circumstances change, is another concept grasped by older children. For example, older children understand the stable identity concept of a father maintaining a male identity regardless of what he wears or how old he becomes.

In Piaget's view, children at the beginning of the concrete operations stage demonstrate conservation, or the ability to see how physical properties remain constant as appearance and form change. Unlike preschoolers, school - age children understand that the same amount of clay molded into different shapes remains the same amount. A concrete operational child will tell you that five golf balls are the same number as five marbles, but the golf balls are larger and take up more space than the marbles.

Piaget believed that preoperational cognitive abilities are limited by egocentrism, the inability to understand the point of view of others. But egocentrism is not found in children in the concrete operations stage. By the school years, children have usually learned that other people have their own views, feelings, and desires.

Piaget's model of cognitive development has come under increasing attacks in recent years. Modern developmentalists have frequently referred to experimental research that contradicts certain aspects of Piaget's theories. For example, cognitive theorists like Robert Siegler have explained the phenomenon of conservation as a slow, progressive change in the rules that children use to solve problems, rather than a sudden change in cognitive capacities and schemas. Other researchers have shown that younger and older children develop by progressing through a continuum of capacities rather than a series of discrete stages. In addition, these researchers believe that children understand far more than Piaget theorized. With training, for instance, younger children may perform many of the same tasks as older children. Researchers have also found that children are not as egocentric, suggestible, magical, or concrete as Piaget held, and that their cognitive development is largely determined by biological and cultural influences.

Memory

School - age children are better at the skill of remembering than are younger children. Experiencing more of the world, older children have more to draw upon when encoding and recalling information. In school, older children also learn how to use mnemonic devices, or memory strategies. Creating humorous lyrics, devising acronyms, chunking facts (breaking long lists of items into groups of three's and four's), and rehearsing facts (repeating them many times) help children memorize increasingly complicated amounts and types of information.

Youngsters may remember more when participating in cooperative learning, in which adult-supervised education relies on peers interacting, sharing, planning, and supporting each other. Develop - mentalists disagree on the relative value of cooperative learning versus didactic learning, in which a teacher lectures to students.

School - age children also begin to evince metamemory, or the ability to comprehend the nature of memory and predict how well one will remember something. Metamemory helps children sense how much study time is needed for next week's math test.

Childhood Intelligence

Psychologists and other authorities are keenly interested in childhood intelligence. Intelligence is an inferred cognitive capacity that relates to a person's knowledge, adaptation, and ability to reason and act purposefully. Around the beginning of the twentieth century, Alfred Binet and Theophile Simon measured perception, memory, and vocabulary in children. These researchers divided a child's mental age, or level of intellectual attainment, by his or her chronological age, or actual age, to yield the child's intelligence quotient (IQ). Years later, the average IQ for a child was set at 100. Today, the two most famous IQ tests for children are the Stanford - Binet Intelligence Scale and the Wechsler Intelligence Scale for Children (WISC), both of which have been updated numerous times.

Some psychologists indicate that the multifaceted nature of intelligence necessitates a distinction between basic intelligence (academic IQ) and applied intelligence (practical IQ). For instance, Howard Gardner proposed that children exhibit multiple intelligences, including musical ability, complex movement, and empathy. Similarly, Robert Sternberg proposed the triarchic theory of intelligence, which states that intelligence consists of three factors: information - processing skills, context, and experience. These three factors determine whether cognition or behavior is intelligent.

An individual's intelligence, at least as measured by IQ tests, remains fairly constant throughout life. Yet considerable differences in IQ scores exist across a range of individuals. These individual differences are probably the result of some combination of genetics, home and educational environment, motivation, nutrition and health, socioeconomic status, and culture.

Critics repeatedly question the value of measuring intelligence, especially when the most commonly used testing instruments are inherently culture - specific. Critics point out that minorities score lower on IQ tests that are devised and standardized using white, middle - class subjects. These same minorities score higher on IQ tests devised and standardized using subjects from their own cultural background. Proponents of IQ tests suggest that it is possible to develop culture - fair (fair for all members in a culture) and culture - free (without cultural content) IQ tests, such as Raven's Progressive Matrices Test. This IQ test gauges the subject's ability to solve problems that are presented in unfamiliar designs. Proponents also claim that IQ scores effectively predict future academic performance — what these tests were originally designed to measure.

A great deal of uproar occurred in the 1970s in response to schools placing minorities into special education classes based on their IQ scores. These scores were obtained from culturally biased IQ tests. Today, IQ tests cannot be used as academic achievement or placement tests.

Physical Development in Adolescence

Adolescence is the transition period from childhood to adulthood, a period that brings sometimes tumultuous physical, social, and emotional changes. Adolescence begins with the onset of puberty and extends to adulthood, usually spanning the years between 12 and 20. Puberty is the period during which the reproductive system matures, a process characterized by a marked increase in sex hormones.

Adolescence — the transition period between childhood and adulthood — encompasses ages 12 to 19. It is a time of tremendous change and discovery. During these years, physical, emotional, and intellectual growth occurs at a dizzying speed, challenging the teenager to adjust to a new body, social identity, and expanding world view.

Perhaps no aspect of adolescence is as noticeable as the physical changes that teenagers experience. Within the span of a few years, a dependent child becomes an independent and contributing adult member of society. The start of adolescence also marks the beginning of Freud's final stage of psychosexual development, the genital stage, which pertains to both adolescence and adulthood.

Puberty is the time of rapid physical development, signaling the end of childhood and the beginning of sexual maturity. Although puberty may begin at different times for different people, by its completion girls and boys without any developmental problems will be structurally and hormonally prepared for sexual reproduction. The speed at which adolescents sexually mature varies; the beginning of puberty in both genders falls within a range of 6 to 7 years. In any grouping of 14 - year - olds, for example, one is likely to see teenagers in assorted stages of development — some appearing as older children and others as fully mature adolescents. Eventually, though, everyone catches up.

Hormones are responsible for the development of both primary sex characteristics (structures directly responsible for reproduction) and secondary sex characteristics (structures indirectly responsible for reproduction). Examples of primary sex characteristics are the penis in boys and the uterus in females. An example of secondary sex characteristics is the growth of pubic hair in both genders. During childhood, males and females produce roughly equal amounts of male (androgen) and female (estrogen) hormones. At the onset of puberty, the pituitary gland stimulates hormonal changes throughout the body, including in the adrenal, endocrine, and sexual glands. The timing of puberty seems to result from a combination of genetic, environmental, and health factors.

An early sign of maturation is the adolescent growth spurt, or a noticeable increase in height and weight. The female growth spurt usually begins between ages 10 and 14, and ends by age 16. The male growth spurt usually begins between ages 10 and 16, and ends by age 18.

Girls generally begin puberty a few years earlier than boys, somewhere around ages 11 to 12. Increasing levels of estrogen trigger the onset of puberty in girls. They grow taller; their hips widen; their breasts become rounder and larger; hair grows on the legs, under the arms, and around the genitals; the labia thicken; the clitoris elongates; and the uterus enlarges. Around the age of 12 or 13, most girls today begin menstruating, or having menstrual periods and flow. The onset of menstruation is termed menarche. At this time, females can become pregnant.

Health Issues: Age 12–19

Adolescent health problems are often correlated with low socioeconomic status, poor diet, inadequate health care, risk-taking activities, personality issues, and a sedentary lifestyle. Yet the teenage years are typically healthy, although major health problems can emerge. Three possible major health problems include eating disorders, depression, and substance abuse.

Eating Disorders

Eating disorders involve a preoccupation with food. The most common of these among teenagers is obesity, which is defined as a skin-fold measurement in the 85th percentile for one's height. Obesity carries with it the potential for social stigma, psychological distress, and chronic health problems. Approximately 15% to 20% of adolescents are obese.

A preoccupation with not becoming obese can lead to anorexia nervosa, or self-starvation. The typical anorexic is a model teenager who is obsessed with food — buying, cooking, and preparing it — but who eats very little herself. She is probably a perfectionist and has a distorted self-perception of her body, believing herself to be too fat. The anorexic is generally 20% under her ideal weight. As many as 1 percent of adolescent girls are anorexic, and 2 to 8 percent of them eventually die from starvation.

Related to anorexia is bulimia nervosa, a disorder that follows a pattern of binge-purge eating. After eating an enormous amount of food, bulimics vomit, take laxatives, or exercise vigorously to burn off recently consumed calories. Bulimics, like anorexics, are obsessed with food, weight, and body shape. Unlike anorexics, they maintain a relatively normal body weight. Both anorexia and bulimia are far more common among females than males. They also cross all levels of society. The exact causes of these eating disorders are unknown.

Depression

As many as 40 percent of adolescents have periods of depression, a type of mood disorder characterized by feelings of low self-esteem and worthlessness, loss of interest in life activities, and changes in eating and sleeping patterns. Adolescent depression is often due to hormonal changes, life challenges, and/or concerns about appearance. More teenage females than males suffer from depression.

A real and tragic consequence of teenage depression is suicide. As many as 13 percent of adolescents report having attempted suicide at least once. Risk factors include feelings of hopelessness, suicidal preoccupation, a previous suicide attempt, having a specific plan to carry out the suicide, having access to firearms or sleeping pills, and stressful life events. As with adults, more teenage females attempt suicide, but more teenage males actually die from their attempts. Females use less violent methods (such as taking pills) than males, who tend to use more extreme and irreversible methods (such as shooting themselves).

Substance abuse is a major health threat. Legal and illegal substances available to adolescents include tobacco, caffeine, alcohol, glue, paint vapors, and pills. In one survey, 30% of the adolescents reported using illicit drugs, such as amphetamine and cocaine. The spread of AIDS infections by use of dirty needles increases the seriousness of this health threat.

Cognitive Development: Age 12–19

Most adolescents reach Piaget's stage of formal operations (ages 12 and older), in which they develop new tools for manipulating information. Previously, as children, they could only think concretely, but in the formal operations stage they can think abstractly and deductively. Adolescents in this stage can also consider future possibilities, search for answers, deal flexibly with problems, test hypotheses, and draw conclusions about events they have not experienced firsthand.

Cognitive maturity occurs as the brain matures and the social network expands, which offers more opportunities for experimenting with life. Because this worldly experience plays a large role in attaining formal operations, not all adolescents enter this stage of cognitive development. Studies indicate, however, that abstract and critical reasoning skills are teachable. For example, everyday reasoning improves between the first and last years of college, which suggests the value of education in cognitive maturation.

Intellectual Development in Adolescence

According to Robert Sternberg's triarchic theory, intelligence is comprised of three aspects: componential (the critical aspect), experiential (the insightful aspect), and contextual (the practical aspect). Most intelligence tests only measure componential intelligence, although all three are needed to predict a person's eventual success in life. Ultimately, adolescents must learn to use these three types of intelligence.

Componential intelligence is the ability to use internal information-processing strategies when identifying and thinking about solving a problem, including evaluating results. Individuals who are strong in componential intelligence do well on standardized mental tests. Also involved in componential intelligence is metacognition, which is the awareness of one's own cognitive processes — an ability some experts claim is vital to solving problems.

Experiential intelligence is the ability to transfer learning effectively to new skills. In other words, it is the ability to compare old and new information, and to put facts together in original ways. Individuals who are strong in experiential intelligence cope well with novelty and quickly learn to make new tasks automatic.

Contextual intelligence is the ability to apply intelligence practically, including taking into account social, cultural, and historical contexts. Individuals who are strong in contextual intelligence easily adapt to their environments, can change to other environments, and are willing to fix their environments when necessary. An important part of contextual intelligence is tacit knowledge, or savvy, which is not directly taught. Tacit knowledge is the ability to work the system to one's advantage. Examples are knowing how to cut through institutional red tape and maneuvering through educational systems with the least amount of hassle. People with tacit knowledge are often thought of as street-smart.

Moral Development and Judgment

Another facet of cognitive development is moral development and judgment, or the ability to reason about right and wrong. Lawrence Kohlberg proposed a theory of moral development with three levels consisting of six stages. The first level, preconventional morality, has to do with moral reasoning and behavior based on rules and fear of punishment (Stage 1) and nonempathetic self-interest (Stage 2). The second level, conventional morality, refers to conformity and helping others (Stage 3) and obeying the law and keeping order (Stage 4). The third level, postconventional morality, is associated with accepting the relative and changeable nature of rules and laws (Stage 5) and conscience-directed concern with human rights (Stage 6).

Moral development depends, in part, on the appearance of empathy, shame, and guilt. Internalization of morality begins with empathy, the ability to relate to others' pain and joy. Children in their first year begin to show signs of basic empathy in that they become distressed when those around them do likewise. Internalization of morality also involves shame (feelings of not living up to others' standards) and guilt (feelings of not living up to personal standards). Shame develops around age 2, and guilt develops between ages 3 and 4. As children mature cognitively, they evidence an increasing ability to weigh consequences in light of self-interest and the interest of those around them. Teenagers typically demonstrate conventional morality as they approach their 20s, although some may take longer to gain the experience they need to make the transition.

Research tends to support much of Kohlberg's model; however, the theory has been criticized on several counts. According to some experts, the model favors educated individuals who are verbally sophisticated. People may also regress in their moral reasoning or behave differently than their moral reasoning may predict. Culture, family factors, and gender affect the attainment of the higher levels of moral judgment; hence, Kohlberg's model has been criticized as limited in terms of certain cultures, family styles, and distinction between differences in male and female moral development.

Personality Development

Two widely cited approaches to personality development are those of Sigmund Freud and Erik Erikson.

Sigmund Freud's Stages of Psychosexual Development

Sigmund Freud developed a treatment theory called psychoanalysis, which is based upon a theory of psychosexual stages of development (Table 2).

Table 2 Freudian Psychosexual Stages of Development

Stage	Age	Erogenous Zone/Activities
Oral	0 to 18 months	Mouth/sucking, biting, chewing
Anal	18 to 36 months	Anus/bowel and bladder control
Phallic	3 to 6 years	Genitals/masturbation
Latency	6 years to puberty	Repression of sexual feelings
Genital	puberty	Maturation of sexual orientation

Erik Erikson's Stages of Development

Erik Erikson proposed a theory of development that continues throughout the life span. His theory states that there are universal life stages and that a specific psychosocial dilemma occurs at each phase of development. These problems (crises) must be resolved before an individual can move to the next developmental stage (Table 3). Erikson's theory has been credited for accounting for continuity and changes in personality development. It has also been criticized for vagueness and has not stimulated a great deal of empirical research.

Table 3 Erik Erikson's Stages of Development

Age	Psychological Stage	Period
Birth to 1 year	Trust vs. Mistrust Learning that the provider of comfort is reliable, consistent, and predictable	Oral-sensory
2 to 3 years	Autonomy vs. Shame and Doubt Learning to exercise independence and freedom of choice along with self-control	Muscular-anal
3 to 5 years	Initiative vs. Guilt Planning and executing a task for the sake of actively doing it	Locomotor-genital
6 to 11 years	Industry vs. Inferiority Developing as a worker and producer	Latency
Adolescence	Identity vs. Role Confusion Evolving a sense of self that is reliable and consistent, both for oneself and for others	Puberty
Young adulthood	Intimacy vs. Isolation Preparing for a commitment to affiliation with others and developing the ethical strength to abide by such commitments	Young adulthood
Middle age	Generativity vs. Stagnation Finding a way to support in the establishment and guidance of the next generation	Adulthood
Old age	Integrity vs. Despair Integrating the earlier stages into an acceptance of oneself and a sense of fulfillment rather than looking back in regret at what might have been	Maturity

The Search for Identity in Adolescence

Adolescence is the period of transition between childhood and adulthood. Developmentalists have traditionally viewed adolescence as a time of psychosocial storm and stress, of bearing the burdens of wanting to be an adult long before becoming one. Developmentalists today are more likely to view adolescence as a positive time of opportunities and growth, as most adolescents make it through this transition without serious problems or rifts with parents.

Freud termed the period of psychosexual development beginning with puberty as the genital stage. During this stage, sexual development reaches adult maturity, resulting in a healthy ability to love and work if the individual has successfully progressed through previous stages. Because early pioneers in development were interested only in childhood, Freud explained that the genital stage encompasses all of adulthood, and he described no special difference between adolescent and adult years.

In contrast, Erikson noted that the chief conflict facing adolescents at this stage is one of identity versus identity confusion. Hence, the psychosocial task for adolescents is to develop individuality. To form an identity, adolescents must define a personal role in society and integrate the various dimensions of their personality into a sensible whole. They must wrestle with such issues as selecting a career, college, religious system, and political party.

Researchers Carol Gilligan and Deborah Tannen have found differences in the ways in which males and females achieve identity. Gilligan has noted that females seek intimate relationships, while males pursue independence and achievement. Deborah Tannen has explained these differences as being due, at least in part, to the dissimilar ways in which males and females are socialized.

The hormonal changes of puberty affect the emotions of adolescents. Along with emotional and sexual fluctuations comes the need for adolescents to question authority and societal values, as well as test limits within existing relationships. This is readily apparent within the family system, where adolescents' need for independence from the parents and siblings can cause a great deal of conflict and tension at home.

Societal mores and expectations during adolescence now restrain the curiosity so characteristic of young children, even though peer pressure to try new things and behave in certain ways is also very powerful. Added to this tug-of-war are teenagers' increasing desires for personal responsibility and independence from their parents, along with an ever-growing, irresistible interest in sexuality.

Sexual Identity, Orientation in Adolescence

A part of discovering one's total identity is the firming of sexual orientation, or sexual, emotional, romantic, and affectionate attraction to members of the same sex, the other sex, or both. A person who is attracted to members of the other sex is heterosexual. A person who is attracted to members of the same sex is homosexual. Many use the term gay to refer to a male homosexual, and lesbian to refer to a female homosexual. A person who is attracted to members of both sexes is bisexual.

In the 1940s and 1950s, Alfred Kinsey and his associates discovered that sexual orientation exists along a continuum. Prior to Kinsey's research into the sexual habits of United States residents, experts generally believed that most individuals were either heterosexual or homosexual. Kinsey speculated that the categories of sexual orientation were not so distinct. In his surveys, many Americans reported having had at least minimal attraction to members of the same gender, although most had never acted out on this attraction. In short, Kinsey and colleagues brought to the attention of medical science the notion of heterosexuality, homosexuality, and bisexuality all being separate but related sexual orientations. The etiology of heterosexuality, homosexuality, and bisexuality continues to elude researchers. Today's theories of sexual orientation fall into biological, psychological, social, and interactional categories.

Biological Theories

Attempts to identify the specific physiological causes of homosexuality have been inconclusive. Traditional physiological theories include too little testosterone in males, too much testosterone in females, prenatal hormonal imbalances, prenatal biological errors due to maternal stress, differences in brain structures, and genetic differences and influences.

Psychological and Social Theories

Early childhood seems to be the critical period in which sexual orientation forms, suggesting that learning plays a part in causing homosexuality. Freudians have traditionally held that homosexuality is rooted in early childhood developmental conflicts, particularly the Oedipal conflict. Freudians believe homosexuality develops in response to troubled family relationships, an overly affectionate and dominant mother and a passive father, and/or the loss of one or both parents. However, these theories cannot explain why homosexuality occurs in individuals not coming from these types of families. More recently, researchers have proposed that social-learning factors may be account for homosexuality. The sexual preference may develop when a child engages in early cross-gender behaviors (behaviors stereotypical of the other sex) or when a teenager's sexual drive emerges during a period of primarily same-gender friendships.

Interactional Theories

Proponents of the interactional theory of homosexuality allege that sexual orientation develops from a complex interaction of biological, psychological, and social factors. John Money explains that prenatal hormones first act on the embryo's and fetus's brain, which creates a physiological predisposition toward a particular sexual orientation. During early childhood, social-learning factors influence the child, either facilitating or inhibiting the predisposition.

Sexuality: Age 12–19

Adolescents struggle to find appropriate sexual outlets for articulating their desires. They participate in the same sexual activities as do adults, while usually in the absence of a committed and long-term relationship. Sexually active teenagers may think they are in love and date one person exclusively for extended periods, but they lack the level of maturity necessary to maintain intimate and loving relationships. Adolescent promiscuity may be indicative of emotional problems, including low self-esteem, dependence, immaturity, insecurity, or deep-seated hostility.

Teenagers find a variety of means to express themselves sexually. Most young people relieve sexual tension through masturbation, which by this age is an erotically motivated behavior. About 90 percent of males and 60 percent of females report having masturbated at least once by age 17. A second sexual expression for teenagers is mutual petting, or sexual activities other than intercourse. Petting is either heavy (below the waist) or light (above the waist). A third sexual outlet for adolescents is intercourse. The mechanics of sex are the same whether the participants are teenagers or adults. However, although the passion of sex may be present, the commitment and intimacy of a mature relationship are usually missing from the teenage experience.

According to U.S. statistics, which may vary, the average age for a first sexual intercourse is between 16 and 17. Complicating matters is the fact that sexually active adolescents either use contraception on an irregular basis, or they do not use it all. They also do not consistently take precautions against sexually transmitted diseases, even in this day of HIV and AIDS.

Five percent of adolescents experiment with homosexual activity with same-age partners, according to one national survey. These data probably do not represent the number of teenagers who are truly homosexual, because many adolescent homoerotic experiences are nothing more than sexual experimentation.

Homosexual teenagers may be hesitant to reveal their perceived preferences, or come out of the closet, because of society's and their peers' negative attitudes about homosexuality. These teenagers may avoid homosexual experiences or, if they have them, worry about their significance. Homosexual teenagers may also avoid disclosure for fear of being victimized by heterosexual teenagers. Homophobia involves negative remarks, social ostracizing, and threats; it can also involve gay bashing, or violently attacking homosexuals. People probably gay bash because of peer pressure and discomfort with their own sexual identity.

Problems resulting from adolescent sex, perhaps the greatest potential problem, faced by sexually active teenagers is an unplanned pregnancy. With so many teenagers refusing to use contraception consistently, teenage pregnancy has reached an unimaginable level in the United States. Each year, about 500,000 babies are born to adolescent mothers, who typically face many serious problems. Medically, pregnancy and childbirth during adolescence are risky to both child and mother. An adolescent girl's body is not fully developed, and she may not have access to adequate medical care or understand the importance of proper nutrition. Thus, she is at higher risk of having a miscarriage or a premature, low birth-weight baby. The young mother also may die during childbirth.

Financially, many adolescent mothers are single and live in poverty. If they drop out of high school, they have limited earning power. With less money and more expenses, they are forced to accept welfare to support their children and themselves.

Teenage mothers who are married face similar problems. About 50 percent of teenage mothers are married, and according to statistics they struggle financially just as much as unwed teenage mothers. Not surprisingly, teenage marriages are plagued by poverty, again because of limited education and earning power. They are also highly susceptible to divorce because of their emotional and financial instability, some of which is due to immaturity and marrying for the wrong reasons.

Juvenile Delinquency

Peer pressure during adolescence is strong, sometimes so much so that teenagers engage in antisocial acts. Juvenile delinquency is the breaking of the law by minors. Two categories of delinquency are: (1) Minors who commit crimes punishable by law (such as robbery). (2) Minors who commit offenses ordinarily not considered criminal for adults (such as truancy). Adolescents, especially males, are responsible for nearly half of crimes committed, especially against property.

The likelihood of a teenager becoming a juvenile delinquent is determined more by lack of parental supervision and discipline than socioeconomic status. Adolescent rebellion may grow out of tension between adolescents' desire for immediate gratification and parents' insistence on delayed gratification. Parents who are unwilling or unavailable to socialize younger children may be setting them up for problems later in adolescence.

While some offenders are sent to juvenile reform facilities, others are given lesser punishments, such as probation or community service. Still others are court-mandated to seek mental health therapy. Fortunately, most juvenile delinquents eventually grow up to be law-abiding and contributing citizens.

Development in Late Adulthood

Late adulthood (old age) is generally considered to begin at about age 65. Erik Erikson suggests that at this time it is important to find meaning and satisfaction in life rather than to become bitter and disillusioned, that is, to resolve the conflict of integrity vs. despair. It has been estimated that by the year 2030, Americans over 65 will make up 20% of the population. Despite the problems associated with longevity, studies of people in their 70s have shown that growing old is not necessarily synonymous with substantial mental or physical deterioration. Many older people are happy and engaged in a variety of activities. Gerontology, an interdisciplinary field that studies the process of aging and the aging population, involves psychology, biology, sociology, and other fields.

Independence

Psychosocial development in adulthood consists of changes in lifestyles and relationships. According to Erikson, the primary task of early adulthood is to establish identity and intimacy (sharing one's total self with someone else) after wrestling with the intimacy versus isolation psychosocial crisis, which poses commitment to others opposite the possibility of self-absorption. Much psychosocial development occurring during this period is in conjunction with significant life changes, such as leaving home, finding a long-term romantic relationship, beginning a career, and starting a family.

An important aspect of establishing intimacy with a partner is first being able to separate from the family of origin, or family of procreation. Most young adults have familial attachments from which they are separating. This process normally begins during Daniel Levinson's early adult transition (ages 17–22), when many young adults first leave home to attend college or to take a job in another city.

By age 22, young adults have attained at least some level of attitudinal, emotional, and physical independence. They are ready for Levinson's entering the adult world (ages 22–28) stage of early adulthood, during which relationships take center stage. Moreover, dating and marriage are natural extensions of the eventual separating from the family of origin — a key process in becoming an adult. Early bonding and separation experiences, then, set the stage for later independence from the family and the ability to form healthy attachments.

Relationships

Love, intimacy, and adult relationships go hand-in-hand. Robert Sternberg proposed that love consists of three components: passion, decision/commitment, and intimacy. Passion concerns the intense feelings of physiological arousal and excitement (including sexual arousal) present in a relationship, while decision/commitment concerns the decision to love the partner and maintain the relationship. Intimacy relates to the sense of warmth and closeness in a loving relationship, including the desire to help the partner, self-disclose, and keep him or her in one's life. People express intimacy in the following three ways:

Physical intimacy, or mutual affection and sexual activity;

Psychological intimacy, or the sharing of feelings and thoughts;

Social intimacy, or having the same friends and enjoying the same types of recreation.

The many varieties of love described by Sternberg consist of varying degrees of passion, commitment, and intimacy. For example, infatuation, or puppy love so characteristic of adolescence, involves passion, but not intimacy or commitment. In addition to love and intimacy, a deeper level of sexuality is realized during young adulthood within the context of one or more long- or short-term relationships. While the maturity level of the participants affects adolescent sexuality, adult sexuality is fully expressive. Following are discussions of some of the most common types of adult relationships.

Singlehood

Today, many people are choosing singlehood, or remaining single, over marriage or other long-term committed relationships. Many singles clearly lead satisfying and rewarding lives, whatever their reasons for not marrying. Many claim that singlehood gives them freedom from interpersonal obligations, as well as personal control over their living space. As of the late 1990s, 26 percent of men and 19 percent of women in the United States were single adults. Most singles date; many are sexually active. Typical sexual activities for singles are the same as those for other adults. Some singles are celibate, abstaining from sexual relationships.

Cohabitation and Marriage

The two most common long-term relationships of adulthood are cohabitation and marriage. Cohabitors are unmarried people who live and have sex together. Of the more than 3 million Americans who cohabitate, most are between the ages of 25 and 45. Many individuals claim they cohabitate as a test for marital compatibility, but no solid evidence supports the idea that cohabitation increases later marital satisfaction. In contrast, some research suggests a relationship between premarital cohabitation and increased divorce rates. Other individuals claim that they cohabitate as an alternative to marriage, not as a trial marriage.

The long-term relationship most preferred by Americans is marriage. Over 90 percent of Americans will marry at least once, with the average age for first-time marriage being 24 for females and 26 for males.

Marriage can be advantageous. Married people tend to be healthier and happier than their never-married, divorced, and widowed counterparts. On average, married males also live longer than single males. Marriages seem to be happiest in the early years, although marital satisfaction increases again in the later years once parental responsibilities have ended and finances have stabilized. Marriage can also be disadvantageous. Numerous problems and conflicts arise in long-term relationships. Unrealistic expectations about marriage, as well as differences over sex, finances, household responsibilities, and parenting are only a few potential problem areas. Severe problems may lead one or both spouses to engage in extramarital affairs.

Extramarital Relationships

Nonconsensual extramarital sexual activity (not agreed upon in advance by both partners) is a violation of commitment and trust between spouses. People express various reasons for engaging in extramarital activities; in any case, such affairs can irreparably damage a marriage. Marriages in which one or both partners are unfaithful typically end in divorce. Some couples may choose to stay together for monetary reasons or until the children are grown.

Divorce

When significant problems in a marital relationship arise, some couples decide to divorce, or to legally terminate their marriage. About 50 percent of all marriages in the United States end in divorce, with the average duration of these marriages being about 7 years.

Both the process and aftermath of divorce are very stressful on both partners. Divorce can lead to increased risk of experiencing financial hardship, developing medical conditions (ulcers, for example) and mental problems (such as anxiety or depression), having a serious accident, attempting suicide, or dying prematurely. The couple's children and the extended families also suffer during a divorce, especially when disagreements occur over custody of the children. Most divorcees and their children and families eventually cope, and about 75 percent of divorcees remarry.

Friends

Friends play an important role in the lives of young adults. Most human relationships, including casual acquaintances, are nonloving in that they do not involve true passion, commitment, or intimacy. According to Sternberg, friendships are loving relationships characterized by intimacy, but not by passion or commitment. In other words, closeness and warmth are present without feelings of passionate arousal and permanence. Friends normally come from similar backgrounds, share the same interests, and enjoy each other's company.

While many young adults experience the time constraints of going to school, working, and starting a family, they usually manage to maintain at least some friendships, though perhaps with difficulty. That is, as life responsibilities increase, time for socializing with others may diminish.

Physical Development: Age 45–65

Although no longer at the peak level of their young adult years, middle-aged adults still report good health and physical functioning, However, as a result of the passage of time, middle adults undergo various physical changes. Decades of exposure and use take their toll on the body as wrinkles develop, organs no longer function as efficiently as they once did, and lung and heart capacities decrease. Other changes include decreases in strength, coordination, reaction time, sensation (sight, hearing, taste, smell, touch), and fine motor skills. Also common among middle adults are the conditions of presbyopia (farsightedness or difficulty reading) and presbycusis (difficulty hearing high-pitched sounds). Still, none of these changes is usually so dramatic that the middle adult cannot compensate by wearing glasses to read, taking greater care when engaging in complex motor tasks, driving more carefully, or slowing down at the gym. Of course, people age at different rates, so some 40 year olds may feel middle-aged long before their 50-year-old counterparts. Most people, however, describe feeling that they have reached midlife by their mid-50s.

The biopsychosocial changes that accompany midlife — specifically, menopause (the cessation of menstruation) in women and the male climacteric (male menopause) in men — appear to be major turning points in terms of the decline that eventually typifies older adulthood. None of the biological declines of middle and late adulthood needs to be an obstacle to enjoying all aspects of life, including sex. For example, too often society has erroneously determined that menopause inevitably means the end of female sexuality. However, while menopause gives rise to uncomfortable symptoms, such as hot flashes, headaches, irritability, dizziness, and swelling in parts of the body, post-menopausal women frequently report improved sexual enjoyment and desire, perhaps because they no longer worry about menstruation and pregnancy. For these same reasons, women who have undergone a hysterectomy, or surgical removal of the uterus, frequently report improved sexual response.

Men also experience biological changes as they age, although none is as distinct and pronounced as female menopause. Testosterone production lessens, which creates physical symptoms, such as weakness, poor appetite, and inability to focus on specific tasks for extended periods. However, this reduction in testosterone does not fully explain the psychological symptoms of anxiety and depression that may accompany middle adulthood, indicating that the male climacteric probably has more to do with emotional rather than physical events. During middle age, men are faced with the realization that they are no longer 20 years old and that they are not going to accomplish all they wanted to in life. They may also feel less sexually attractive and appealing, as they discover that seemingly overnight they have gained extra weight around the waist, are balding, and are feeling less energetic than they used to.

Because of society's emphasis on youthfulness and physical appearances, middle - aged men and women may sometimes suffer from diminished self - esteem. Women, for instance, experience the American double standard of aging: Men who are graying are perceived as distinguished, mature, and sexy, while women who are graying are viewed as being over the hill or past their prime. This double standard, coupled with actual physical changes and decline, does little to help middle adults avoid a midlife crisis.

Intellectual Development: Age 45–65

Cross - sectional studies of IQ show young adults performing better than middle or older adults, while longitudinal studies of IQ tend to show the same people increasing in intelligence at least until their 50s. The results of the cross - sectional studies may be due more to cohort influences: the effects of practice, increased comfort taking such tests, and the tendency for those who remain in the studies to perform better than those who drop out.

Young adults score higher on tests of fluid intelligence, which is the ability to think abstractly and deal with novel situations, while middle adults improve over time on tests of crystallized intelligence, which involves using learned information collected throughout a life span. In summary, the results of traditional IQ tests imply that intelligence continues at approximately the same level at least into middle adulthood, and probably beyond.

Thinking patterns

Middle - age adult thinking differs significantly from that of adolescents and young adults. Adults are typically more focused in specific directions, having gained insight and understanding from life events that adolescents and young adults have not yet experienced. No longer viewing the world from an absolute and fixed perspective, middle adults have learned how to make compromises, question the establishment, and work through disputes. Younger people, on the hand, may still look for definitive answers.

Many middle - age adults have attained Piaget's stage of formal operations, which is characterized by the ability to think abstractly, reason logically, and solve theoretical problems. Many of the situations facing adults today require something more than formal operations. That is, the uncertain areas of life may pose problems too ambiguous and inconsistent for such straightforward thinking styles. Instead, middle adults may develop and employ postformal thinking, which is characterized by the objective use of practical common sense to deal with unclear problems. An example of postformal thinking is the middle adult who knows from experience how to maneuver through rules and regulations and play the system at the office. Another example is the middle adult who accepts the reality of contradictions in his or her religion, as opposed to the adolescent who expects a concrete truth in an infallible set of religious doctrines and rules. Postformal thinking begins late in adolescence and culminates in the practical wisdom so often associated with older adulthood.

Adult learners

Does intellectual development stop at age 22? Not at all. In fact, in recent years, colleges and universities have reported an increased enrollment of adult learners — students age 25 or older. Of course, labeling this age group as adult learners is not to imply that the typical college student is not also an adult. Academic institutions typically identify those outside the 18–21 range as adults, because most have been working and rearing families for some time before deciding to enter or reenter college. Compared with younger students, adult learners may also have special needs: anxiety or low self - confidence about taking classes with younger adults, feelings of academic isolation and alienation, fears of not fitting in, or difficulties juggling academic, work, and domestic schedules.

Adults most often choose to go to college for work - related purposes. Many employers require workers to attain certain levels of education in order to qualify for promotions. Other workers go to college to learn new skills in preparation for another career. Additionally, certain organizations, such as state licensing boards, may require professionals to have a certain number of continuing education hours each year to maintain their licenses. Finally, adults may also return to college simply for personal enrichment.

Many adults today choose distance education as their primary learning method. Numerous educational institutions offer accredited courses, certificates, and undergraduate and graduate degrees by correspondence or via alternative learning formats, such as intensive study classes conducted one weekend per month, telecourses provided over the television, or virtual classrooms set up on the Internet. Some of the programs have minimal residency requirements (time actually spent on campus); others do not, which benefits adults in rural areas who use these alternative methods to access studies that were previously unavailable to them. Adult students who successfully complete external programs tend to be highly self-motivated and goal-oriented.

Retirement

Retirement at age 65 is the conventional choice for many people, although some work until much later. People have been found to be happier in retirement if they are not forced to retire before they are ready and if they have enough income to maintain an adequate living standard. Chronic health problems such as arthritis, rheumatism, and hypertension increasingly interfere with the quality of life of most individuals as they age.

Widowhood

Women tend to marry men older than they are and, on average, live 5 to 7 years longer than men. One study found ten times as many widows as widowers. Widowhood is particularly stressful if the death of the spouse occurs early in life; close support of friends, particularly other widows, can be very helpful.

Theories of Aging

Erik Erikson, who took a special interest in this final stage of life, concluded that the primary psychosocial task of late adulthood (65 and beyond) is to maintain ego integrity (holding on to one's sense of wholeness), while avoiding despair (fearing there is too little time to begin a new life course). Those who succeed at this final task also develop wisdom, which includes accepting without major regrets the life that one has lived, as well as the inescapability of death. However, even older adults who achieve a high degree of integrity may feel some despair at this stage as they contemplate their past. No one makes it through life without wondering if another path may have been happier and more productive.

Two major theories explain the psychosocial aspects of aging in older adults. Disengagement theory views aging as a process of mutual withdrawal in which older adults voluntarily slow down by retiring, as expected by society. Proponents of disengagement theory hold that mutual social withdrawal benefits both individuals and society. Activity theory, on the other hand, sees a positive correlation between keeping active and aging well. Proponents of activity theory hold that mutual social withdrawal runs counter to traditional American ideals of activity, energy, and industry. To date, research has not shown either of these models to be superior to the other. In other words, growing old means different things for different people. Individuals who led active lives as young and middle adults will probably remain active as older adults, while those who were less active may become more disengaged as they age.

As older adults approach the end of their life span, they are more apt to conduct a life review. The elderly may reminisce for hours on end, take trips to favorite childhood places, or muse over photo albums and scrapbooks. Throughout the process, they look back to try to find the meaning and purpose that characterized their lives. In their quest to find life's meaning, older adults often have a vital need to share their reminisces with others who care, especially family.

Thanatology: Study of Death and Dying

At the end of the human life span, people face the issues of dying and death (the permanent cessation of all life functions). North American society in recent years has witnessed an increased interest in the thanatology, or the study of death and dying. Thanatologists examine all aspects of death, including biological (the cessation of physiological processes), psychological (cognitive, emotional, and behavioral responses), and social (historical, cultural, and legal issues).

Death and dying has been studied extensively by Elisabeth Kübler-Ross, who suggested that terminally ill patients display the following five basic reactions.

Denial, an attempt to deny the reality and to isolate oneself from the event, is frequently the first reaction.

Anger frequently follows, as the person envies the living and asks, "Why should I be the one to die?"

Bargaining may occur; the person pleads to God or others for more time. As the end nears, recognition that death is inevitable and that separation from family will occur leads to feelings of exhaustion, futility, and deep depression.

Acceptance often follows if death is not sudden, and the person finds peace with the inevitable. People who are dying are sometimes placed in a hospice, a hospital for the terminally ill that attempts to maintain a good quality of life for the patient and the family during the final days. In a predictable pattern after a loved one's death, initial shock is followed by grief, followed by apathy and depression, which may continue for weeks. Support groups and counseling can help in successfully working through this process.

Life Meaning and Death

Human beings think about the impact and inevitability of death throughout much of their lives. Most children understand by the ages of 5 to 7 that death is the irreversible ending of all life functions, and that it happens to all living beings. Adolescents fully comprehend the meaning of death, but they often believe that they are somehow immortal. As a result, they may engage in risky behavior, such as driving recklessly or smoking, with little thought of dangerous consequences.

Although most young and middle adults have gained a more realistic view of death through the death of some family members or friends, anxiety about death may be more likely to peak in middle adulthood. As people continue aging, they gradually learn to accept the eventual deaths of loved ones, as well as their own deaths. By later adulthood, most people come to accept — perhaps with some tranquility if they feel they have lived meaningfully — the inevitability of their own demise, which prompts them to live day by day and make the most of whatever time remains. If they do not feel they have lived meaningfully, older adults may react to impending death with feelings of bitterness or even passivity.

The concept of searching for meaning in life through death is one of the foundations of existential psychology. Existential psychologists like Rollo May believe that individuals must accept the inevitability of their own deaths and the deaths of loved ones; otherwise, they cannot fully embrace or find true meaning in life. This theory tracks with research that indicates that the more purpose and meaning that individuals see in their lives, the less they fear death. In contrast, the denial of death leads to existential anxiety, which can be a source of emotional troubles in daily life.

The Stages of Dying and Death

Perhaps the best - known pioneer in thanatology is Elisabeth Kubler - Ross, who after interviewing 200 terminally ill people proposed five stages of coming to terms with death. Upon learning of their own impending death, dying people's first reaction is often denial, in which they refuse to acknowledge the inevitable, perhaps believing a mistake has been made. They may seek other medical opinions and diagnoses or pretend that the situation will simply go away on its own. Gradually, as they realize that they are going to die, the terminally ill experience anger at having their lives end prematurely. They may become envious and resentful of those who will continue on, especially if they feel that their own life plans and dreams will go unfulfilled. Individuals who are dying will then attempt to bargain, often with God or another religious figure, and will promise to change or make amends or atone for their wrongdoings. When bargaining fails, they experience depression and hopelessness. During this stage, the terminally ill may mourn the loss of health that has already occurred, as well as the impending losses of family and plans. Finally, those dying learn to accept the inevitable, paving the way for a smoother transition both for themselves and loved ones.

Kubler - Ross pointed out that although the above five stages are typical, they are not absolute. Not all people progress predictably through all the stages, nor do people experience the stages in one particular order. Additionally, these stages do not necessarily represent the healthiest pattern for all individuals under all circumstances. Kubler- Ross and others also have noted that people whose loved ones are dying may progress through the same five stages as the dying person.

An individual who is not facing an immediate death has more time to adjust to the idea. In fact, dying can be a time of increased personal growth. The life review, or process of reminiscing, can help people examine the significance of their lives and prepare for death by making changes and finishing uncompleted tasks. Many dying individuals report that they are finally able to sort out who and what is the most important to them and are able to enjoy to the fullest what time remains. Many also report that dying is a time of religious awakening and transcendence.

Following the death of a loved one, survivors normally experience bereavement, or a change in status, as in the case of a spouse becoming a widow or widower. The behavioral response of the bereaved person is termed mourning; the emotional response is termed grief. People vary in their patterns of mourning and grief, both within and across cultures. People may also experience anticipatory grief, or feelings of loss and guilt, while the dying person is still alive.

Grieving typically begins with shock or disbelief, and is quickly followed by intense and frequent memories of the dead person. When those who are grieving finally attain resolution, or acceptance of the person's passing, they resume everyday activities and are able to move on with their lives.

People grieve in considerably different ways. Some adults are very vocal in their expressions of grief, while others prefer to be alone to quietly gather their thoughts and reflect on the loss of the loved one. Of course, cultural groups around the world handle grief according to their own customs. Egyptian mourners, for example, may cry loudly in public as a sign of grief, while Japanese mourners may talk quietly to the deceased person while kneeling in front of a home altar.

Dealing with Dying and Death

A variety of options are available for individuals seeking to cope with dying and death. Grief therapy counseling, and support groups can help individuals deal with their grief and bereavement. Hospice, which can occur at home or in a hospital or other institution, can provide care for dying persons and their families. Hospices are designed for terminally ill patients to live out their remaining days as independently, fully, and affordably as possible. Death education can also help by providing people with information on dying, legal issues, and various practical matters. Classes on death and dying are available at colleges, hospitals, and community centers. Many people take comfort in bibliotherapy, or reading books about dying, perhaps explaining the popularity of the life - after - life books. These testimonials detail the alleged journeys of people who were clinically dead into the afterlife before they were resuscitated.

Section Ⅱ

As a scientific discipline, mental disorders has enormous breadth. This relevant and essential section will give readers a practical insights in the field of contemporary mental disorders. It comprises diagnosis and treatment, as in the research in mood and personality disorders, eating and sexual dysfunction, gender identity disorders and childhood mental disorders, as in the insights and support therapeutically given when a clinician treats a patient. The Section II has 10 chapters, it present the classification of mental disorders, common symptoms, psychological assessment. The special areas of mental disorders like psychology care for dying patient and legal aspects are covered in the last section, equips the clinical readers with a sure and knowledgeable grasp of the many facets of mental disorders and psychiatry.

Chapter 1 Dementia, Delirium and Amnestic Disorders

Prior editions of this book discussed delirium, dementia and amnestic disorders in a broader chapter entitled *Organic Mental Disorders* (following the convention in the *Diagnostic and Statistical Manual of Mental Disorders* [DSM]). This category encompassed psychological and behavioral disorders whose abnormalities resulted from known biological causes and pathophysiological mechanisms. In contrast to these organic disorders, psychiatric illnesses such as schizophrenia or bipolar disorder were categorized as "functional disorders" with no identifiable organic etiology. This organic/functional dichotomy became increasingly problematic as evidence grew for central nervous system dysfunction in the major "functional" menial disorders. In addition, this dichotomy left clinicians with no satisfactory alternative term for conditions that were not "organic mental disorders". Finally, the organic versus nonorganic distinction encouraged the continued stigmatization of mentally ill individuals by suggesting that "functional" disorders such as schizophrenia were not true medical disorders.

In the *Diagnostic and Statistical Manual of Mental Disorders*, 4th edition (DSM - Ⅳ), the section on organic mental disorder is completely reorganized, and the term "organic" is eliminated. The disorders of delirium, dementia, and amnesia are classified as cognitive disorders and will be presented in this chapter. Other diagnoses previously classified within the *Organic Mental Disorder* section of DSM - Ⅲ - R are now called secondary if caused by a specific medical disorder (eg, mood disorder resulting from hypothyroidisin or personality change resulting from stroke) or substance induced if substance intoxication or withdrawal is judged to be etiologically related to the disturbance (eg, cocaine psychotic disorder with delusions). The secondary disorders are now classified phenomenologically with related disorders. For example, secondary mood disorders are in the *Mood Disorder* section of DSM - Ⅳ and are discussed in Section Ⅱ Chapter 2 of this book. The substance - induced disorders are all classified together in DSM - Ⅳ under the title *Substance - Related Disorders*. If a patient presents with depression, for example, the clinician can readily use DSM - Ⅳ criteria to assess whether the depression (1) is secondary to an underlying condition such as hypothyroidisin, (2) is caused by withdrawal from a substance such as cocaine or by intoxication with a substance such as a barbiturate, or (3) is a primary psychiatric condition.

Symptoms and Signs of Cognitive Disorders

A. Common Symptoms and Signs

In evaluating a patient with a psychological or behavioral disturbance, certain signs and symptoms suggest that the disorder is a cognitive disorder, as described in this chapter. These signs and symptoms include the following:

1. Fluctuating performance on serial mental status examinations.
2. Memory impairment.
3. Disorientation.
4. Cognitive impairment, eg, dyscalculia, or reduced fund of information.
5. Visual hallucinations or illusions.
6. Tactile hallucinations or illusions.
7. Motor restlessness.
8. Impaired judgment and poor impulse control.
9. Autonomic symptoms (tachycardia, fever, sweating, hypertension).
10. Sudden onset without any previous personal or family psychiatric history, at any age, but particularly in a patient over 40.
11. Lack of expected response to traditional treatment.
12. Prior physical illness or current physical symptoms.
13. History of recent drug or medication intake.

Although any of these symptoms and signs may be present in any psychiatric disorder, when they are elicited, it is important first to consider cognitive disorders or secondary or substance-induced disorders in the differential diagnosis.

B. Etiology

A single psychiatric syndrome may have many organic causes, and a single cause can result in different syndromes. For example, nenrosyphilis can cause dementia, delirium, secondary psychotic disorder, secondary mood disorder, or secondary personality change. Even in the same patient, a given cause may lead first to one syndrome and then to another. For example, nenrosyphilis may first present as a secondary mood disorder or a secondary personality change, but then may progress to dementia. Similarly, infection with the human immunodeficiency virus (HIV) may cause a variety to disorders, including delirium, dementia, secondary psychotic disorder, and secondary mood disorder.

C. Factors Affecting Symptoms and Signs

Even if a specific, identifiable cause is present. The course of illness for a given individual depends on physical, psychological, and social factors.

1. Physical factors affecting symptoms and signs include the following:

a. The degree, of insult sustained by the central nervous system (CNS). For example, brain tumor is manifested differently depending on the size and location of the tumor and whether intracranial pressure is increased. Pernicious anemia is manifested differently depending on the serum level of vitamin B_{12}.

b. The rate at which whole-brain involvement occurs. For example, the sequelae of a brain tumor depend on whether the tumor grows slowly or rapidly. In the case of heavy metal poisoning, effect depend on whether intoxication is gradual or acute.

c. The physical condition of the patient. For example, an elderly patient with several concurrent medical diagnoses is more prone to developing a substance-induced delirium when prescribed a CNS-active medication than is a younger, healthier patient.

2. Psychological factors affecting symptoms and signs include the following:

a. The patient's personality and psychological defense mechanisms. For example, in response to the same specific brain insult, a patient with a paranoid personality may become more paranoid, and a patient with an obsessive personality may become more obsessive.

b. The patient's intelligence and education. For example, the signs of dementia are often quite subtle in a well-educated patient with above average intelligence who can still do very well on a cognitive examination.

c. The patient's level of premorbid psychological adjustment. For example, a patient who was relatively well adjusted before dementia may be better able to tolerate a mild deficit than a patient with preexisting psychological difficulties.

d. The patient's level of current psychological stress and conflict. For example, a patient who has recently lost a spouse or has been forced to retire may have more difficulty tolerating even mild deficits in cognitive functioning than patient without current stress.

3. Social factors affecting symptoms and signs include the following:

a. The degree of social isolation versus support. For example, a patient with dementia of the Alzheimer's type may function well while living with a healthy spouse, but may then deteriorate if the spouse becomes ill and needs hospitalization.

b. The degree of familiarity patients have with their environment. For example, patient is with dementia often function poorly and become easily confused in an unfamiliar hospital environment (a phenomenon known as "sundowning" because it lends to worsen at night), although they may be able to take care of themselves fairly well in their own home.

c. The level of sensory input. Either insufficient or excessive sensory input (eg, being in a darkened room in a nursing home without a calendar or at attempting to rest in an Intensive Care Unit surrounded by lights, noise, and constant activity) may cause increased confusion in inpatient with delirium and/or dementia.

Dementia

Dementia is a syndrome manifested by several cognitive deceits that include memory impairment involving at least one of the following: aphasia, agnosia, apraxia, or a disturbance in executive functioning (the ability to plan, sequence, abstract and organize) than interferes with social, occupational, or interpersonal skills. Table 1, table 2, table 3 and table 4 list the DSM-Ⅳ criteria for dementias.

The patient with dementia is forgetful, has difficulty learning new information, and will often try to minimize or deny deficits. Typically, recent memory is worse than remote memory. A patient may be unable to recall names of three objects after 5 minutes, but may have excellent recall of events that occurred in childhood. The most commonly used brief test for cognitive function is the Folstein Mini-Mental Status Examination (MMSE) (Table 5).

Table 1 Diagnostic criteria for dementia (all types)

The development of multiple cognitive deficits manifested by both of the following:
1. Memory impairment (inability to learn new information and to recall previously learned information)
2. At least one of the fallowing cognitive disturbances:
a. Aphasia (language disturbance)
b. Apraxia (inability to carry out motor activities despite intact motor function)
c. Agnosia (failure to recognize or identify objects despite intact sensory function)
d. Disturbance in executive functioning (eg, planning organizing, sequencing, abstracting)

Table 2 DSM-Ⅳ diagnostic criteria for dementia of the Alzheimer's type

A. See Table 1
B. The course is characterized by gradual onset and continuing cognitive decline
C. The cognitive deficits cause significant impairment in social or occupational functioning and represent a significant decline from a previous level of functioning
D. The cognitive deficits in A are not caused by any of the following:
1. Central nervous system conditions that cause progressive deficits in memory and cognition (eg, cerebrovascular disease, Parkinson's disease, Huntinglon's disease, subdural hematoma, normal - pressure hydrocephalus)
2. Systemic conditions that are known to cause dementia (eg, hypothyroidism, vitamin B_{12} or folic acid deficiency, niacin deficiency, hypercalcemia, neurosyphilis, HIV infection)
3. Substance-induced conditions
E. The deficits do not occur exclusively during the course of delirium
F. Not better accounted for by another Axis I disorder (eg, major depressive disorder, schizophrenia)

In addition to defects in memory, language skills and constructional abilities are also frequently impaired. Patients may have difficult repeating a phrase or naming objects pointed to by the examiner. Constructional ability may be tested by having the patient draw intersecting pentagons or a clock face with the hands set at a certain time.

Patients with dementia also develop difficulty with abstract thinking. For instance, they may be unable to state how a chair and a desk are similar. Interpretations of proverbs are usually concrete.

It is not unusual, as the dementia progresses, for patients to develop accentuation of their piemorbid character trails; for example, a normally suspicious patient may develop frank paranoia. With frontal lobe disease patients may lose normal social inhibitions and consequently may demonstrate inappropriate sexual behaviors.

Table 3 DSM-Ⅳ diagnostic criteria for vascular dementia.

A. See Table 1
B. Focal neurological signs and symptoms (eg, exaggeration of deep tendon reflexes, extensor plantar response, psedobulbar palsy, gait abnormalities, weakness of an extremity) or laboratory evidence indicative of cerebrovascuiar disease (eg, multiple infarctions involving cortex and underlying white matter) that are judged to be etiologically related to the disturbance
C. The cognitive deficits cause significant impairment in social or occupational functioning and represent a significant decline from a previous level of functioning
D. The deficits do not occur exclusively during the course of delirium

Patients with dementia will often have abnormalities either than cognitive ones. Their grooming and hygiene may be impaired. Their affect may be labile or shallow. Mood may be depressed, particularly early in the course of the illness when patients are more aware of their cognitive deficits. The thought process is often remarkable for perserveration. Delusional thinking or hallucinations may develop, with paranoid delusions being particularly common. Confabulation may occur. Insight and judgment become progressively more impaired.

The DSM-Ⅳ allows clinicians to characterize the nature of an individual's dementia, such as Alzheimer's type or vascular type. Different codes exist for an uncomplicated dementia and for dementias with delirium, delusions, hallucinations, affective disturbances, behavioral disturbances, or communication disturbances. The diagnosis is made on the basis of the predominant features of the patient's presentation.

Dementia of the Alzheimer's type is further characterized by age of onset; a patient is diagnosed with early onset if symptoms develop at age 65 or younger or with late onset if symptoms develop after 65 years of age.

Table 4 DSM-Ⅳ diagnostic criteria for dementia other than Alzheimer's or vascular

A. See Table 1
B. The cognitive deficits cause significant impairment in social or occupational functioning and represent a significant decline from a previous level of functioning
C. The deficits do not occur exclusively during the course of delirium
D. There is evidence from the history, physical examination, or laboratory findings of a medical condition for dementia from other general medical conditions) or substance use (for substance-induced persisting dementia) judged to be etiologically related to the disturbance, or (for dementia of multiple etiologies) there is evidence of multiple etiologies (eg, head trauma plus chronic alcohol use, dementia of the Alzheimer's type with the subsequent development of vascular dementia)

Epidemiology

Dementia is found predominantly in elderly persons, although certain etiological factors may cause dementia at any age. The diagnosis of dementia may be made at any time after the IQ is fairly stable (usually by age four). Chronic neurological disorders are the cause of such early dementias.

Dementia of the Alzheimer's type is by far the most common form of dementia, accounting for approximately 40% - 65% of all cases. Prevalence is 1% at 65 years of age, and doubles every 5 years. Alzheimer's dementia (AD) affects as many as four million citizens of the United States. This number is likely to double over the next 30 years. The annual economic toll of AD in the United States in terms of health care expenses and lost wages of both patients and their caregivers is estimated at 80-100 billion dollars.

Of the remaining types of dementia, the second most common type is vascular dementia (10% - 40%) followed by mixed Alzheimer's - vascular dementia and less common forms of dementia.

Table 5 Instructions administration of Mini-Mental Status Examination (MMSE)

A. Orientation Ask for the date. Then ask specifically for parts omitted, eg, "Can you also tell me what season it is?" One point for each correct. Ask in turn "Can you tell me the name of this hospital? (town, county, etc)". One point for each correct. B. Registration Ask the patient if you may test his memory. Then say the names of 3 unrelated objects, clearly and slowly, about one second to each. After you have said 3, ask him to repeat them. This first repetition determines his score (0-3) but keep saying them until he can repeat all 3, up to 6 trials. If he does not eventually learn all 3, recall can not be meaningfully tested. C. Attention and calculation Ask the patient to begin with 100 and count backwards by 7. Stop after 5 subtractions (93, 86, 79, 72, 65). Score the total number of correct answers. If the patient cannot or will not perform this task, ask him to spell the word "world" backwards. The score is the number of letters in correct order, eg dlow = 5, dlow = 3. D. Language Naming: Show the patient a wrist watch and ask him what it is. Repeat for pencil. Score 0-2. Repetition: Ask the patient to repeat the sentence after you. Allow only one trial. Score 0 or 1. 3-Stage command: Give the patient a piece of plain blank paper and repeat the command. Score 1 point for each part correctly executed. Reading: On a blank piece of paper print the sentence "Close your eyes" in letters large enough for the patient to see clearly. Ask him to read it and do what it says. Score 1 point only if he actually closes his eyes. Writing: Give the patient a blank piece of paper and ask him to write a sentence for you. Do not dictate a sentence, it is to be written spontaneously. It must contain a subject and verb and be sensible. Correct grammar and punctuation are not necessary. Copying: On a clean piece of paper, draw intersecting pentagons, each side about 1 inch, and ask him to copy it exactly as it is. All 10 angles must be present and 2 must intersect to score 1 point. Tremor and rotation are ignored. Estimate the patient's level of sensorium along a continuum, from alert on the left to coma on the right.

Etiology and Pathogenesis

The pathogenesis of dementia depends largely, on the etiology. Approximately 5-15 of all dementias are reversible, and if their cause is identified and treated the prognosis is good. On the other hand, neurodegenerative dementias such as AD are progressive and incurable and ultimately end in death.

A. Dementia of the Alzheimer's Type

AD is a neurodegenerative disease of the brain with an average duration of 8 - 10 years between onset and death, and a variable course of progression that ranges from 4 to 20 years. AD has an insidious onset, most commonly after the age of 60 years, although in rare instances as early as 40 years of age, followed by progressive deterioration.

AD is divided into three stages based on functional and cognitive capacity. Although variable, the MMSE can be used to track the course of cognitive impairment. Typically, early AD MMSE is equal to or greater than 18, moderate AD MMSE is between 12 and 18, and severe AD MMSE is less than 12. On average the MMSE score declines by 3 points per year.

In terms of functional capacity, with early AD, judgment is typically intact as are activities of daily living (ADL). With moderate AD, judgment is severely impaired and patients generally require assistance with ADLs and some form of supervised care. With severe AD, judgment is essentially lost and patients are completely dependent on others for ADL and self - care. They may not be oriented to family members or to self, may become bed bound, and may consequently develop decubiti, infection, or other illness, which ultimately may lead to death.

Short - term memory loss is usually the earliest manifestation of AD. This is typically associated with mild aphasia and impaired visuospatial ability, which evolve into fluent aphasia and constructional apraxia. Other cognitive functions such as calculations, reasoning, judgment, and executive functioning also become impaired. Typically behavioral aggression, psychomotor agitation, frank psychosis, and affective or personality changes, although not an early consequence of AD, may ensue as the illness progresses.

The major neuropathological features of AD are neuritic plaques, amyloid deposition in plaques, and neurofibrillary tangles spread diffusely through the cerebral cortex and hippocampus. These features remain the pathognomic findings for diagnosis, which can be made histologically only definitively at autopsy. Hence the clinical diagnosis of AD is based on clinical presentation and on exclusion of other causes of dementia.

In AD degeneration in the cortical neurons and the associated reduction in the number of cortical synapses have been correlated with the severity of dementia. The most common distribution is in the hippocampus, a structure deep in the brain involved with encoding memory, and in the temporal and parietal lobes. In general, the greater the involvement of the frontal lobe, the more likely the development of mood and behavioral symptoms.

As noted, the two key abnormal findings in the brain of individuals with AD are amyloid plaques and neurofibrillary tangles. Plaques are dense deposits of an amyloid protein (called p-amyloid) and other associated proteins and nonnerve cells (glial cells and microglia) that gradually build up outside and around neurons, forming insoluble deposits that interrupt synaptic transmission, resulting in neuronal cell death. β- amyloid is a protein fragment snipped from a larger protein, called the amyloid precursor protein (APP), during metabolism. APPs are normally associated with nerve cell membranes (transmembrane). For reasons that are not clear, β-amyloid may develop when APP is abnormally cleaved by proteases. The abnormally large β-amyloid peptide (40-42 amino acids) rapidly forms insoluble "sticky" aggregates that are key to the development of plaques and consequent cell death. Theories regarding the toxicity of β-amyloid to neuronal cells include formation of free radicals, local inflammatory response, depletion of intracellular choline, and disruption of potassium channels.

Neurofibrillary tangles are abnormal collections of intracellular phosphorylated proteins. The primary component of tangles is one form of the protein, tau, which is involved in microtubule stability in normal neurons. Abnormal tau proteins of AD result in microtubule disintegration and the consequent development of neurofibrillary tangles, which consist primarily of paired helical abnormal tau proteins.

Although AD is a generalized neurodegenerative disorder, the cholinergic (acetylcholine) pathways are the neurotransmitter system most aggressively affected early in the disease. Ninety percent of cholinergic neurons arise from the nucleus basalis of Meynert in the basal forebrain, with projections to frontal, parietal, temporal, and subcortical structures. This is consistent with short-term memory loss as the presenting symptom of AD, as the temporal lobe projections to the hippocampus are part of the core circuit that encodes new memories. There are also decreased levels of choline acetyltransferase (CAT), the enzyme involved in the synthesis of acetyicholine, and decreased concentrations of acetylcholine in the cerebrospinal fluid. The depletion of acetylcholine concentrations has been correlated with memory and cognitive impairment in AD and restoration of cholinergic function is a primary goal in current pharmacological treament strategies.

In addition to its effects on the cholinergic system, AD also results in the loss of noradrenergic neurons in the locus ceruleus and of serotoneigic neurons in the dorsal raphe nuclei. In addition, researchers have found decreased levels of γ-aminonutyric acid (GABA), substance P, somatostatin. and corticotropin-releasing factor.

The two most significant risk factors for AD are advanced age and positive family history. As noted previously, the prevalence of AD doubles every 5 years after the age of 65. The prevalence of dementia is 25-30 in the 85- to 90-year-old population. The prevalence trend in the very old (greater than 90) is unclear due to the limitations of study size and data in this population.

Genetic familial risk factors can be seen in the effect of positive family history in sporadic cases (90 of AD) as well as in the 10 of AD that appears to be familial. Having one affected sibling or parent doubles the risk of AD, having two affected parents or one parent and one sibling increases the risk three-to fourfold.

Mutations on chromosomes 1, 14, and 21 are associated with some forms of early familial AD (FAD). The defective gene on chromosome 1 has been named present 2, which is involved in the development of β-amyloid plaques. The presenilin 2 gene has been linked to the abnormally high prevalence of AD among families descended from a group of Germans (called

Volga Germans). Only a very small traction of early - onset FAD is caused by this presenilin 2 gene mutation. The detective gene on chromosome 14 has been named presenilin, which is more commonly implicated in the development of β - amyloid plaques. The defective gene on chromosome 21 results in the abnormal processing of APP, resulting in the accumulation of neuritic plaques. Further more, patients with Down syndrome (trisomy 21) who survive die fifth decade of life show the neuropathological brain changes of AD and may suffer significant cognitive decline.

Together, presenilins 1 and 2 and mutations in the APP gene account for nearly 50 of early-onset FAD. The gene(s) for the remaining 50 has yet to be identified.

Another important risk factor in late - onset familial and sporadic AD may be the inheritance of the E4 allele of apolipoprotein E (Apo E), a cholsterol carrier protein whose gene is located on chromosome 19. Every person has two Apo E genes, one inherited from each parent. Of the three common alleles of Apo E, E2 may be protective against AD. E3 appears neutral, and E4 appears linked to an increased risk for developing AD, both in laic - onset familial AD and in sporadic AD. The greatest risk is in individuals with two copies of Apo E E4, with studies suggesting up to 90 developing AD by age 85. How Apo E E4 increases a person's susceptibility to AD is not known.

Currently genetic testing is not part of routine clinical practice. Since 90 of AD is sporadic, Apo E testing would have no negative or positive predictive value, assuming individuals live to age 85.

Age and positive family history are the only clear risk factors for AD. Head injury, gender, education, diet, occupational exposures, and thyroid disease have shown to be possible risk factors in AD. However, these other risk factors have not been found to be very significant consistently and appear to be sensitive to sampling methodology. Recent studies have made clear that there is a long preclinical phase of AD, with disease expression occurring when a critical threshold of neuronal compromise is reached. This would suggest that many vectors of neuronal injury, particularly cerebrovascular disease, would enhance and hasten the expression of AD.

The etiology of AD is likely multifactorial in which genetic and environmental factors combine with aging to overcome the ability of neurons to maintain homeostasis. This impaired neuronal metabolism results in damaged mitochondria, damaged cyloskeleton, increased release of excitotoxic neurotransmitler glutamate, activation of local inflammatory mechanisms, aberrant phosphorylation of membrane proteins, and, ultimately, premature dysfunction and neuronal cell death.

B. Vascular Dementia

Vascular dementia accounts for approximately 15 of all dementias. Typically, patients have risk factors such as hypertension, cardiac disease, diabetes, and strokes. Vascular dementia was classically characterized by an abrupt onset and stepwise deterioration of dementia, as opposed to the insidious onset and gradual progression seen more commonly in AD. However, it is possible for vascular dementia to resemble AD in its onset and course. The pattern of cognitive impairment is often patchy, depending on the location of vascular com - promise and there are often focal upper motor neuron signs (eg, reflex or tone asymmetry).

There are two forms of vascular dementia. Classical multiinfarct dementia involves multiple completed strokes in cortical and possibly subcortical areas. The other form is associated with the small vessel disease and microangiopathy of chronic vascuar risk factors (eg, hypertension, diabetes mellitus, smoking, hypercholesteremia), and was classically described as Binswanger's disease. The classic presentation of this type of primarily slibcortical vascular dementia is diminished attention and concentration and prolonged response latency. Due to the extensive subcortical - fronlal connections, frontal lobe behavioral syndromes (eg, apathy, disinhibition) can be frequently seen. The decrement in verbal fluency and the ablation of short - term memory are less prominent than in AD. Behavioral manifestations are variable depending on the vascular region involved. Brain imaging studies usually show multiple vascular lesions of cortical and subcortical regions. Functional imaging scans with positron emission tomography (PET) or single - photon emission computed tomography (SPECT) will usually show a patchy reduction in cerebral blood flow.

Although hypertension, cerebrovascuiar disease, diabetes, and AD are all common diseases of aging, the prevalence of mixed (AD and vascular) dementia has been underreported, due to unrealistic efforts to define dementia distinctly as either of the Alzheimer or vascular type. Previous studies suggesting higher prevalences of vascular dementia probably included mixed disease. AD, vascular dementia, and mixed AD/vascular dementia comprise 80 - 90 of clinical dementia.

C. Alcohol - Related Dementia

Chronic alcohol use has been considered an etiology of dementia. This has been subject to debate as a neuropathological entity, has been hard to identify, and there has been no clear dose relationship between alcohol use and cognitive functioning. However, the heavy neuiological comorbidity due to nuintiona compromise, increased cerebrovascular disease, head injuries. Wernicke's encephalopathy and Korsakoff's syndrome may be the etiology for alcohol - related dementia, or at least heavy risk factors for developing dementia.

D. Dementia due to Parkinson's Disease

Parkinson's disease (PD) induced dementia accounts tor 5%–10% of all dementias. Parkinson's disease is a slowly progressive neurologic condition associated with dopainine deficiency and characterized by the triad of resting tremor, bradykinesia, and rigidity. Its onset is usually in middle to late life. Approximately 40%–50% of patients with PD develop dementia. The dementia of PD is insidious in onset and develops late in the disease course. Subcortical patterns cf cognitive deficits (eg, diminished attention and concentration, slowing of response, and apathy) are common. Histopathologically, there is neuronal loss and gliosis primarily in the lateral substantia nigra.

E. Dementia due to Lewy Body Disease

Lewy body disease (LBD) typically has a more rapid onset with a fluctuating course. Visual hallucinations, parkinsonian symptoms, and susceptibility to delirium are common carly in the course. Patients with LBD are remarkably sensitive to extrapyramidal side effects of antipsychotic medications. The pathognomonic histopathologic feature of LBD is the presence of Lewv inclusion bodies in the cerebral cortex.

F. Frontal Lobe Dementias

Pick's disease and other forms of frontotemporal dementias are noteworthy for the early presentation of impaired executive functioning and personality and behavioral changes, including disinhibition, affective blunting, and deterioration of social skills. Memory deficits become more apparent as the disease progresses. In Pick's disease, there is profound atrophy of the frontal and/or temporal lobes, with characteristic Pick inclusion bodies found on autopsy. It typically presents between the ages of 50 and 60 year, though if, may begin later. There is also a non-Pick body form of frontotemporal dementia.

G. Other Progressive Dementing Disorders

Other progressive neurodegenerative diseases cause irreversible dementias. Creutzteldt-Jakob disease is a rapidly progressive spongiform encephalopathy associated with a slow virus or prion. Individuals with Creutzfeldt-Jakob disease frequently demonstrate a heightened startle response. Huntington's disease is an antosornal dominant neurodegeneracive disorder that affects the basal ganalia and other subcortical structures. Onset is usaully before age 50, is associated with a clear autosomal dominant transmission family history, and presents with involuntary movements and behavioral changes, with dementia being a later complication. Progressive suprannclear palsy is another dementia presenting with more rapid course and extrapyramidal symptoms. A distinguishing feature may be the prominence of vertical voluntary gaze paresis while retaining involuntary vertical gaze reflexes.

H. Dementia due to Other Causes

Many other medical conditions can present as a dementia and are important to consider in the differential diagnosis because they are potentially reversible. These reversible dementias account for approximately 10 of dementias. Reversible causes of dementia, include endocrine disturbances (eg, hypothyrodism. hypoglycemia), nutritional deficiencies (eg, thiamine. niacin, or vitamin B_{12} deficiency), structural abnormalities heniatoma, normal - pressure hydrocephalus), infectious conditions (eg, neurosyphilis, HIV), renal and hepatic disorders, the toxic effect of long standing substance abuse (eg, ethanol abuse), and iatrogenic, phannocological toxicity due to undiagnosed CNS side effects, toxicity. or polypharmacy interactions.

The extent of the reversibility is contingent on the nature of the disorder and the timeliness of diagnosis and treatment. For instance, dementia secondary to HIV, although not fully reversible, may be improved by antiviral medications. On the other hand, dementia secondary to normal - pressure hydrocephalus, which may presents dementia, ataxia, and urinary incontinence, may be fully or partially reversed it the diagnosis is made and treatment (shunt placement) is initiated promptly.

Differential Diagnosis

Distinguishing dementia from other cognitive disorders and from both primary and secondary - psychiatric disorders is critical. Common clinical dilemmas in geriairic care are distinguishing dementia from depression, delirium, or the cognitive changes of normal aging. Chronically mentally ill patients may also be incorrectly diagnosed with dementia. There is also debate whether chronic schizophrenia can be a primary etiology of dementia. A chronic schizophrenic patient with profound social regression and severe negative symptoms may be difficult to distinguish from a patient with dementia.

A. Major Depression and Related Affective Disorders

Depression in older individuals frequently presents with atypical features such as prdominant cognitive deficits. Some older individuals with depression may even deny feeling sad. The cognitive dulling associated with depression in older people has been described as pseudodementia or the dementia syndrome of depression. The cognitive impairment in these patients is temporary and improves as the depression resolves. Table 6 contrasts the clinical features of cognitive consequences of depression (pseudodementia) and dementia. Clinical features that suggest an underlying depressive disorder include a more sudden onset of cognitive decline. This may or may not be preceded by depressive symptoms. These individuals may have a prior history of affective disorders, may present with neurovegetative signs such as appetite, sleep, and energy disturbance, and may have various somatic complaints. In addition, depressed patients tend to exaggerate their cognitive deficits and display poor effort on cognitive examination, frequently answering with the words "I don't know." In contrast, patients with dementia frequently minimize, rationalize, and attempt to conceal and compensate for their deficits. Depressed patients often show inconsistent deficits of both recent and remote memory, whereas patients with early dementia tend to have a more intact remote memory, with severe short-term deficits. Depressed patients' memory deficits are more responsive to prompting and encouragement than patients with AD. In content, the responses of depressed patients are characterized more by "near misses" and poor effort than the gross errors of truly demented patients.

Even with these clues to differentiating between cognitive changes due to depression and dementia, it may be difficult to make the distinction. In addition, patients with dementia may become secondarily depressed. In a patient in whom the distinction is quite unclear, a reasonable approach would be to treat a suspected depression and then see if the patient continues to show signs of dementia well after the depressive episode has resolved.

B. Delirium

Although cognitive impairment exists in both delirium and dementia, the clinical course of each is quite distinct. Delirium has a widely fluctuating clinical course with an acute onset, whereas dementia typically has a more insidious progressive course with less acute onset. Critical in the distinction is assessing the level of consciousness and measuring cognitive capacity serially. It should be stressed that for patients with dementia (as well as any neurologically vulnerable patient) the risk of developing a superimposed delirium is great.

C. Normal Aging

In normal aging memory losses are slight and do not interfere with activities of daily living. The speed of mental processing may slow with aging, but aging is not synonymous with dementia. Cognitive changes associated with normal aging include prolonged latency of response, slower set shift, decreased attention and concentration, slower acquisition and processing, and less efficient memory. However, with normal aging, language, acquired skills, judgment, personality, and social or occupational functioning remain intact.

Table 6 Differentiation of pseudodementia and dementia.

The Dementia Syndrome of	Depression
Sudden onset	Gradual onset
Vegetative signs common	Vegetative signs less common
Patients expose cognitive deficits	Patients conceal cognitive deficits
Patients often respond "I don't know"	Patients attempt to answer questions
Variability in cognitive performance	Consistently poor cognitive performance
Inconsistent effort	Consistent effort
Recent and remote memory may be r equally poor	Recent memory worse than remote memory
Sundowning uncommon	Sundowning uncommon

D. Schizophrenia

Both schizophrenia and dementia cause a deterioration from a previous level of functioning, impaired abstract thinking, and poor judgment. However, although schizophrenia can be of late onset, it typically manifests during adolescence or young adulthood. In addition, patients with schizophrenia have prominent thought disorganization or psychotic symptoms that may fluctuate over time, with cognitive capacity frequently changing with exacerbation of level of illness.

E. Factitious Illness

In factitious disorders, patients present with psychological symptoms in a conscious attempt to mimic psychiatric illness. In these individuals, symptoms are worse when the patient is aware of being observed, and the symptoms are not consistent with what is observed in true dementia. For example, a patient simulating memory impairment will often show equal difficulty with both recent and remote memory, whereas in true dementia recent memory is usually more impaired than remote memory. Also, in true dementia a patient will often be oriented to his or her name but not to time or place, patients with factitious illness often state they do not know their own name, a finding seen only in the very late stages of true dementia.

Diagnosis

In diagnosing a dementia the clinician must first aggressively rule out any potential reversible causes of the disorder. Ideally, a complete history should be obtained from someone who knows the patient well, as well as from the patient. Attention should be paid to medications, drug and alcohol use, onset and course of impairment, as well as psychosocial and medical antecedents. A physical examination should be performed with full neurological evaluation. A comprehensive mental status examination should be performed, as should a standardized cognitive measure such as the MMSE.

The following laboratory tests should be obtained as part of the dementia workup: complete blood count, complete chemistry profile, urinalysis, thyroid function tests, for late and vitamin B_{12} levels, and syphilis serology. These may include toxicology screen, sedimentation rate, HIV and Lyme disease serology, heavy metal screen, antinuclear antibody, neuropsychological testing, chest X - ray, lumbar puncture, and neuroimaging. A chest X - ray may assist in determining the presence of pneumonia, congestive heart failure, and chronic obstructive pulmonary disease. Cerebiospinal fluid (CSF) is not routinely evaluated. A lumbar puncture may be performed for cases with unusual presentation (early onset, rapid progression), suspicion of neuroosyphilis, neuroborreliosis, or metastatic carcinoma. Recently developed CSF diagnostic markers for Alzheimer's disease include decreased amyloid precursor protein or tau-related markers (eg, Alzheimer 50 antigen). However, the sensitivity and specificity of these tests do not supersede the diagnostic accuracy of a good clinical history and examination. Neuroimaging is not routinely obtained as part of a dementia workup but is often useful. Structure neuroimaging such as computed tomography (CT) or magnetic resonance imaging (MRI) can demonstrate atrophy, white matter ischemic changes, infarcts, space occupying lesions, and normal - pressure hydrocephalus. Quantitative studies of hippocampal atrophy may have some predictive diagnostic value in dementia. Functional imaging such as SPECT or PET provide information on metabolic function by measuring cerebral blood flow or cell uptake of glucose. In Alzheimer's dementia parietotemporal deficits are typically seen earlier than frontal deficits. Panetolemporal hypoinetabolism and right - left asymmetry are the most consistent findings in functional imaging of Aizheimer's disease. Vascular dementias, on the other hand, show asymmetric cortical and subcortical focal deficits often with a patchy distribution.

The early signs of dementia are very subtle and vague, and may not be immediately obvious. Early symptoms also vary a great deal. Usually, though, people first seem to notice that there is a problem with memory, particularly in remembering recent events. Other common symptoms include:

Confusion;

Personality change;

Apathy and withdrawal;

Loss of ability to do everyday tasks.

Sometimes people fail to recognise that these symptoms indicate that something is wrong. They may mistakenly assume that such behavior is a normal part of the ageing process. Or symptoms may develop gradually and go unnoticed for a long time. Sometimes, people may refuse to act even when they know something is wrong.

Ten Warning Signs

Go through the following list and note the symptoms that are present. If there are several ticks, a doctor should be consulted for a complete examination of the person with the symptoms.

1.Recent memory loss that affects day to day functions

It is normal to forget meetings, colleagues' names or a friend's telephone number occasionally, but then remember them later. A person with dementia may forget things more often, and not remember them at all.

2. Difficulty performing familiar tasks

Busy people can be so distracted from time to time that they may leave the carrots on the stove and only remember to serve them when the meal has finished. A person with dementia might prepare a meal and not only forget to serve it, but also forget they made it.

3. Problems with language

Everyone has trouble finding the right word sometimes, but a person with dementia may forget simple words or substitute inappropriate words, making sentences difficult to understand.

4. Disorientation to time and place

It is normal to forget the day of the week or your destination for a moment. But people with dementia can become lost on their own street, not knowing where they are, how they got there or how to get back home.

5. Poor or decreased judgement

Dementia affects a person's memory and concentration, and this in turn affects their judgement. Many activities, such as driving, require good judgement and when this ability is affected, the person will be a risk, not only to themselves, but also to others on the road.

6. Problems with abstract thinking

Balancing a cheque book may be difficult for many of us. Someone with dementia could forget completely what the numbers are and what needs to be done with them.

7. Misplacing things

Anyone can temporarily misplace a wallet or keys. A person with dementia may repeatedly put things in inappropriate places.

8. Changes in mood or behavior

Everyone becomes sad or moody from time to time. Someone with dementia can have rapid mood swings, for no apparent reason. They can become confused, suspicious or withdrawn.

9. Changes in personality

People's personalities can change a little with age. But a person with dementia can become suspicious or fearful, or apathetic and uncommunicative. They may also become disinhibited, over familiar or more outgoing than previously.

10. Loss of initiative

It is normal to tire of housework, business activities or social obligations. The person with dementia may lose interest in previously enjoyed activities, or become very passive and require cues prompting them to become involved.

Remember that many conditions have symptoms similar to dementia, so it is important not to assume that someone has dementia just because some of the above symptoms are present.

Strokes, depression, alcoholism, infections, hormone disorders, nutritional deficiencies and brain tumours can all cause dementia-like symptoms. Many of these conditions can be treated.

Consulting a Cognitive Dementia and Memory Service (CDAMS) clinic or doctor to obtain a diagnosis is critical at an early stage. A complete medical and psychological assessment may identify a treatable condition and ensure that it is treated correctly, or it may confirm the presence of dementia. Such an assessment might include the following:

A detailed medical history, provided, if possible, by the person with the symptoms and a close relative or friend. This helps to establish whether there is a slow or sudden onset of symptoms and their progression. A thorough physical and neurological examination, including tests of the senses and movements to rule out other causes of dementia and to identify medical illnesses which may worsen the confusion associated with dementia.

Treatment

A multitiered approach to management of dementia includes psychosocial support to the patient and caregivers and psychopharmacological support to the patient for cognitive, behavioral dysfunction and psychotic or affective symptoms. The main goals of treatment are to optimize function, slow the progression of the dementia, and improve the quality of life. By maximizing functional capacity and improving cognition, mood, and behavior, institutionalization may be prevented or delayed.

Treatment of dementia may help slow or minimize the development of symptoms.

Cholinesterase Inhibitors

These drugs, donepezil (Aricept), rivastigmine (Exelon) and galantamine hydrobromide (Razadyne), are Alzheimer's drugs that work by boosting levels of a chemical messenger involved in memory and judgment. Side effects can include nausea, vomiting and diarrhea. Although primarily used as Alzheimer's drugs, they're also used to treat vascular, Parkinson's and Lewy body dementias.

Memantine (Namenda)

This drug for Alzheimer's disease works by regulating the activity of glutamate, another chemical messenger involved in all brain function, including learning and memory. Its most common side effect is dizziness. Some research has shown that combining memantine with a cholinesterase inhibitor may have even better results. Although primarily used to treat Alzheimer's disease, it may help improve symptoms in other dementias.

Other Medications

Although no standard treatment for dementia exists, some symptoms can be treated. Additional treatments aim to reduce the risk factors for further brain damage.Treatment of the underlying causes of dementia can also slow or sometimes stop its progress. To prevent a stroke, for example, your doctor may prescribe medications to control high blood pressure, high cholesterol, heart disease and diabetes. Doctors may also prescribe medication to treat conditions such as blood clots, anxiety and insomnia for people with vascular dementia.

In addition, some specific symptoms and behavioral problems can be treated with sedatives, antidepressants and other medications, but some of these drugs may worsen other symptoms.

Creutzfeldt - Jakob disease has no known treatments. Care is focused on making sure the person is comfortable.

Delirium

Delirium is a serious disturbance in a person's mental abilities that results in a decreased awareness of one's environment and confused thinking. The onset of delirium is usually sudden, often within hours or a few days. Delirium can often be traced to one or more contributing factors, such as a severe or chronic medical illness, medication, infection, surgery, or drug or alcohol abuse. The symptoms of delirium and dementia can be similary, and input from a family member or caregiver may be important for a doctor to make an accurate diagnosis.

It is a transient, potentially reversible dysfunction in cerebral metabolism, etiologically related to metabolic derangements, that has an acute or subacute onset and is typically manifested by alterations of levels of consciousness and change in cognition. It is the most common psychiatric syndrome found in a general medical hospital, particularly among older patients.

Numerous physiological insults are potential putative agents for inducing the delirium syndrome. Whether the syndrome develops depends on the vulnerability of the patient's brain and the intensity of the putative agent. Hence, individuals with dementia may develop a delirium when confronted with what otherwise might be a minor insult, such as a urinary tract infection, or the addition of a medication with anticholinergic side effects.

The delirium syndrome may manifest itself in numerous ways, but key to the presentation is a change in the level of consciousness, from a hyperactive state (ie, increased arousal and psychomotor activity), a hypoactive state (ie, decreased arousal and psychomotor activity), or a mixed form with fluctuations between states.

The Diagnostic and Statistical Manual of Mental Disorders (DSM) is the key reference regarding the criteria for the diagnosis of delirium. Since its inception in 1952, different editions have contained different criteria (see Table 7). The diagnostic features of delirium in the current DSM (DSM-Ⅳ) are as follows:

1. Disturbance of consciousness (ie, reduced clarity of awareness of the environment), with reduced ability to focus, sustain, or shift attention.

2. Change in cognition (such as memory deficit, disorientation, language disturbance) or the development of a perceptual disturbance that is not better accounted for by a preexisting or evolving dementia.

3. The disturbance that develops over a short period of time (usually hours to days) and tends to fluctuate during the course of the day.

4. Evidence from the history, physical examination, or laboratory findings of a general medical condition, substance intoxication or withdrawal and/or medication side effect judged to

be etiologically related to the disturbance.

Epidemiology

There are few definitive data on the epidemiology of delirium. Past research has been confounded in part by variability of diagnostic criteria.

Current data indicate that delirium occurs in 10 - 20 of patients on acute medical/surgical wards. Some authors report that the incidence of delirium in elderly patients presenting to the emergency room is as high as 80. Delirium is infrequent in the young and middle - aged and, when present, is often associated with alcohol or illicit drug use. The incidence of delirium increases progressively with each decade past the age of 40.

Certain groups are most at risk for developing delirium: (1) elderly patients; (2) patients with preexisting brain damage (eg, dementia, strokes); (3) patients on polyphamiacy or withdrawing from addictive substances; and (4) medically compromised patients (eg, individuals with AIDS, burn patients).

Table 7 DSM - Ⅳ diagnostic criteria for delirium

A. Disturbance of consciousness (ie, reduced clarity of awareness of the environment) with reduced ability to focus, sustain, or shift attention
B. Change in cognition (such as memory deficit, disorientation, language disturbance) or development of a perceptual disturbance that is not better accounted for by a pre - existing, established, or evolving dementia
C. The disturbance develops over a short period of time (usually hours to days) and lends to fluctuate during the course of the day

Delirium occurs in between 10% - 20% of inpatients and is more common in post - operative patients, especially orthopedic and ICU patients. Of those without delirium upon admission, from 5% - 30% go on to develop it during the hospital stay. Delirium is associated with the following:

More severe illness;

Higher mortality and morbidity;

Longer hospital stays;

More severe functional decline during and after hospital stays;

A significantly higher risk of institutionalization.

The prognosis of patients who have had delirium is significantly poorer than that of other patients hospitalized with the same diagnoses. Age does not seem to be a separate risk factor in most studies. However, dementia increases the risk of delirium substantially, and other risk factors for delirium include the following:

Dehydration or renal dysfunction;

Infections;

Hypoxia;

Hypoperfusion;

Metabolic disorders.

Medications which increase the risk of delirium include the following:

Narcotics (especially meperidine);

Sedative-hypnotics;

H2-blockers;

Drugs for Parkinson's disease;

Anticholinergic agents;

Digoxin.

Delirium occurs very frequently in postoperative patients, especially those with hip fractures (>50% in some studies). Risk factors for developing delirium post-operatively include the following:

Dementia;

Perioperative hypotension;

Perioperative hypoxia;

Use of meperidine, benzodiazepines, or anticholinergic drugs.

Symptoms

The signs and symptoms of delirium appear over a short period of time, from a few hours to a few days. They often fluctuate throughout the day, so a person may have periods of no symptoms. Primary signs and symptoms include those below. Reduced awareness of the environment , this may result in:

An inability to stay focused on a topic or to change topics	Poor memory, particularly of recent events	Behavior changes
Wandering attention	Disorientation, or not knowing where one is, who one is or what time of day it is	Seeing things that don't exist (hallucinations)
Getting stuck on an idea rather than responding to questions or conversation	Difficulty speaking or recalling words	Restlessness, agitation, irritability or combative behavior
Being easily distracted by unimportant things	Rambling or nonsense speech	Disturbed sleep habits
Being withdrawn, with little or no activity or little response to the environment	Difficulty understanding speech	Extreme emotions, such as fear, anxiety, anger or depression
Poor thinking skills (cognitive impairment)	Difficulty reading or writing	

Other medical conditions can result in symptoms associated with delirium. Dementia and delirium may be particularly difficult to distinguish, and a person may have both. In fact, frequently delirium occurs in people with dementia.

Tests and Diagnosis

A doctor will diagnose delirium based on the answers to questions about a person's medical history, tests to assess mental status and the identification of possible contributing factors. An examination may include the following:

Mental Status Assessment

A doctor starts by assessing awareness, attention and thinking. This can be done informally through conversation, or more formally with tests or screening checklists that assess mental state, confusion, perception and memory.

Physical and Neurological Exams

The doctor will perform a physical exam, checking for signs of dehydration, infection, alcohol withdrawal and other problems. The physical exam can also help detect underlying disease. Delirium may be the first or only sign of a serious condition, such as respiratory failure or heart failure. A neurological exam — checking vision, balance, coordination and reflexes can help determine if a stroke or another neurological disease is causing the delirium.

Other Possible Tests

If the cause or trigger of delirium can't be determined from the medical history or exam, the doctor may order blood, urine and other diagnostic tests. Brain-imaging tests may be used when a diagnosis can't be made with other available information.

Treatment

The first goal of treatment for delirium is to address any underlying causes or triggers by stopping use of a particular medication, for example, or treating an infection. Treatment then focuses on creating the best environment for healing the body and calming the brain. Supportive care aims to prevent complications by protecting the airway, providing fluids and nutrition, assisting with movement, treating pain, addressing incontinence and keeping people with delirium oriented to their surroundings. A number of simple, nondrug approaches may be of some help:

Clocks and calendars to help a person stay oriented;

A calm, comfortable environment that includes familiar objects from home;

Regular verbal reminders of current location and what's happening;

Involvement of family members;

Avoidance of change in surroundings and caregivers;

Uninterrupted periods of sleep at night, with low levels of noise and minimal light;

Open blinds during the day to promote daytime alertness and a regular sleep-wake cycle;

Avoidance of physical restraints and bladder tubes;

Adequate nutrition and fluid;

Use of adequate light, music, massage and relaxation techniques to ease agitation;

Opportunities to get out of bed, walk and perform self-care activities;

Provision of eyeglasses, hearing aids and other adaptive equipment as needed.

Talk with the doctor about avoiding or minimizing the use of drugs that may trigger delirium. However, certain drug treatment may calm a person who misinterprets the environment in a way that leads to severe paranoia, fear or hallucinations, and when severe agitation or confusion:

Prevents the performance of a necessary medical exam or treatment;

Endangers the person or threatens the safety of others;

Doesn't lessen with nondrug treatments.

Amnestic Disorders

Victor et al (1971) defines the amnestic syndrome as an abnormal mental state in which memory and learning are affected out of all proportion to other cognitive functions in an otherwise alert and responsive patient. Amnestic disorders have been broadly classified into transient amnesias and persistent memory disorders. Transient amnesias include transient global amnesia, transient epileptic amnesia, posttraumatic amnesia and alcoholic blackouts, while persistent memory disorders include Korsakoff syndrome and amnestic syndromes that follow herpes encephalitis, severe hypoxia, vascular disorders or head injury (Kopelman, 2000).

The disorders are a group of disorders that involve loss of memories previously established, loss of the ability to create new memories, or loss of the ability to learn new information. As defined by the mental health professional's handbook, the *Diagnostic and Statistical Manual of Mental Disorders*, fourth edition, text revision, the amnestic disorders result from two basic causes: general medical conditions that produce memory disturbances; and exposure to a chemical (drug of abuse, medication, or environmental toxin). An amnestic disorder whose cause cannot be definitely established may be given the diagnosis of amnestic disorder not otherwise specified. The amnestic disorders are characterized by problems with memory function. There is a range of symptoms associated with the amnestic disorders, as well as differences in the severity of symptoms. Some people experience difficulty recalling events that happened or facts that they learned before the onset of the amnestic disorder. This type of amnesia is called retrograde amnesia. Other people experience the inability to learn new facts or retain new memories, which is called anterograde amnesia. People with amnestic disorders do not usually forget all of their personal history and their identity, although memory loss of this degree of severity occurs in rare instances in patients with dissociative disorders.

In general, amnestic disorders are caused by structural or chemical damage to parts of the brain. Problems remembering previously learned information vary widely according to the location and the severity of brain damage. The ability to learn and remember new information, however, is always affected in an amnestic disorder. Amnestic disorder due to a general medical condition can be caused by head trauma, tumors, stroke, or cerebrovascular disease (disease affecting the blood vessels in the brain). Substance - induced amnestic disorder can be caused by alcoholism, long - term heavy drug use, or exposure to such toxins as lead, mercury, carbon monoxide, and certain insecticides. In cases of amnestic disorder caused by alcoholism, it is thought that the root of the disorder is a vitamin deficiency that is commonly associated with alcoholism, known as Korsakoff's syndrome. The causes of transient global amnesia, or TGA, are unclear.

Etiology

Amnestic disorders are caused by general medical conditions or substance use. Common general medical conditions include head trauma, hypoxia, herpes simplex encephalitis, and posterior cerebral artery infarction. Amnestic disorders often are associated with damage of the mammillary bodies, fornix, and hippocampus. Bilateral damage to these structures produces the most severe deficits. Amnestic disorders due to substance - related causes may be due to substance abuse, prescribed or over - the - counter medications, or accidental exposure to toxins. Alcohol abuse is a leading cause of substance - related amnestic disorder. Persistent alcohol use may lead to thiamine deficiency and induce Wernicke - Korsakoff's syndrome.

Demographics

Individuals affected by a general medical condition or alcoholism are at risk for amnestic disorders. The overall incidence of the amnestic disorders is difficult to estimate. Amnestic disorders related to head injuries may affect people in any age group. Alcohol - induced amnestic disorder is most common in people over the age of 40 with histories of prolonged heavy alcohol use. Amnestic disorders resulting from the abuse of drugs other than alcohol are most common in people between the ages of 20 and 40. Transient global amnesia usually appears in people over 50. Only 3% of people who experience transient global amnesia have symptoms that recur within a year.

Symptoms

In addition to problems with information recall and the formation of new memories, people with amnestic disorders are often disoriented with respect to time and space, which means that they are unable to tell an examiner where they are or what day of the week it is. Most patients with amnestic disorders lack insight into their loss of memory, which means that they will deny that there is anything wrong with their memory in spite of evidence to the contrary. Others will admit that they have a memory problem but have no apparent emotional reaction to their condition. Some persons with amnestic disorders undergo a personality change; they may appear apathetic or bland, as if the distinctive features of their personality have been washed out of them.

Some people experiencing amnestic disorders confabulate, which means that they fill in memory gaps with false information that they believe to be true. Confabulation should not be confused with intentional lying. It is much more common in patients with temporary amnestic disorders than it is in people with long - term amnestic disorders. Transient global amnesia (TGA) is characterized by episodes during which the patient is unable to create new memories or learn new information, and sometimes is unable to recall past memories. The episodes occur suddenly and are generally short. Patients with TGA often appear confused or bewildered. Common symptoms associated with Amnestic Disorders include:

Loss of memory;

Disorientation with time and space;

Lack of insight to their loss of memory;

Difficulty learning or recalling information;

In some cases, awareness of their loss of memory but unable to understand why.

Diagnosis

Amnestic disorders may be self-reported, if the patient has retained insight into his or her memory problems. More often, however, the disorder is diagnosed because a friend, relative, employer, or acquaintance of the patient has become concerned about the memory loss or recognizes that the patient is confabulating, and takes the patient to a doctor for evaluation. Patients who are disoriented, or whose amnesia is associated with head trauma or substance abuse, may be taken to a hospital emergency room.

The doctor will first examine the patient for signs or symptoms of traumatic injury, substance abuse, or a general medical condition. He or she may order imaging studies to identify specific areas of brain injury, or laboratory tests of blood and urine samples to determine exposure to environmental toxins or recent consumption of alcohol or drugs of abuse. If general medical conditions and substance abuse are ruled out, the doctor may administer a brief test of the patient's cognitive status, such as the mini-mental state examination or MMSE. The MMSE is often used to evaluate a patient for dementia, which is characterized by several disturbances in cognitive functioning (speech problems, problems in recognizing a person's face, etc.) that are not present in amnestic disorders. The doctor may also test the patient's ability to repeat a string of numbers (the so-called digit span test) in order to rule out delirium. Patients with an amnestic disorder can usually pay attention well enough to repeat a sequence of numbers where as patients with delirium have difficulty focusing or shifting their attention. In some cases the patient may also be examined by a neurologist (a doctor who specializes in disorders of the central nervous system)

If there is no evidence of a medical condition or substance use that would explain the patient's memory problems, the doctor may test the patient's memory several times in order to rule out malingering or a factitious disorder. Patients who are faking the symptoms of an amnestic disorder will usually give inconsistent answers to memory tests if they are tested more than once.

DSM-Ⅳ-TR specifies three general categories of amnestic disorders. These are: amnestic disorder due to a general medical condition, substance-induced persisting amnestic disorder, and amnestic disorder not otherwise specified. The basic criterion for diagnosing an amnestic disorder is the development of problems remembering information or events that the patient previously knew, or inability to learn new information or remember new events. In addition, the memory disturbance must be sufficiently severe to affect the patient's social and occupational functioning, and to represent a noticeable decline from the patient's previous level of functioning. DSM-Ⅳ-TR also specifies that the memory problems cannot occur only during delirium, dementia, substance use or withdrawal.

Treatments

Psychosis may pose a greater challenge than cognitive decline for patients with dementia and their caregivers. The nature and frequency of psychotic symptoms varies over the course of illness, but in most patients, these symptoms occur more often in the later stages of disease.

Management of psychosis requires a comprehensive nonpharmacologic and pharmacologic approach, including an accurate assessment of symptoms, awareness of the environment in which they occur, and identification of precipitants and how they affect patients and their caregivers. Nonpharmacologic interventions include counseling the caregiver about the nonintentional nature of the psychotic features and offering coping strategies. Approaches for the patient involve behavior modification; appropriate use of sensory intervention; environmental safety; and maintenance of routines such as providing meals, exercise, and sleep on a consistent basis. Pharmacologic treatments should be governed by a "start low, go slow" philosophy; a monosequential approach is recommended, in which a single agent is titrated until the targeted behavior is reduced, side effects become intolerable, or the maximal dosage is achieved. Atypical antipsychotics have the greatest effectiveness and are best tolerated. Second - line medications include typical antipsychotics for short - term therapy; and, less often, anticonvulsants, acetylcholinesterase inhibitors, antidepressants, and anxiolytics. Goals of treatment should include symptom reduction and preservation of quality of life.

Virtually all patients with dementia will develop changes in behavior and personality as the disease progresses. The nature and frequency of symptoms vary over the course of the illness, and psychotic features tend to present later, particularly when the patient becomes more dependent. Psychotic manifestations and other behavior problems may be more troubling and challenging than cognitive losses; these features result in an increased burden for caregivers, earlier institutionalization, and an acceleration in cognitive decline.

Psychotic features of dementia include hallucinations (usually visual), delusions, and delusional misidentifications. Hallucinations are false sensory perceptions that are not simply distortions or misinterpretations. They usually are not frightening and therefore may not require treatment. Delusions are unshakable beliefs that are out of context with a person's social and cultural background. Delusional misidentification may result from a combined decline in visual function and cognition. For example, patients may suspect that their family members are impostors (ie, Capgras' syndrome), believe that strangers are living in their home, or fail to recognize their own reflection in a mirror.

In studies of patients with Alzheimer's disease, psychotic features were present in 15 to 75 percent of patients. Delusional misidentifications are thought to occur in at least 30 percent of patients with dementia.

Nonpsychotic behaviors associated with dementia include agitation, wandering, and aggression. Agitation represents a cluster of physical manifestations that suggest emotional distress or motor restlessness. Patients with agitation should be evaluated for an underlying precipitating cause, such as hunger, thirst, drug use (including alcohol and caffeine), or an undetected infection. Patients who display physical or verbal aggression, which often is associated with delusional misidentification, may require a combination of pharmacologic and non-pharmacologic treatments.

There are no treatments that have been proved effective in most cases of amnestic disorder, as of 2002. Many patients recover slowly over time, and sometimes recover memories that were formed before the onset of the amnestic disorder. Patients generally recover from transient global amnesia without treatment. In people judged to have the signs that often lead to alcohol induced persisting amnestic disorder, treatment with thiamin may stop the disorder from developing.

Nonpharmacologic Management

Nonpharmacologic interventions are important adjuncts to psychopharmacologic agents and have been proven effective in patients with dementia. These interventions may be used in most patients with dementia-related behavior disorders.

Before introducing an intervention, the behavior problem or symptom must be identified and quantified in terms of frequency and severity. Identification and elimination of precipitating causes are essential. Goals of care should be negotiated with caregivers; the targeted behavior often cannot be eliminated completely, but it may be reduced to tolerable or acceptable levels.

Approaches for the Caregiver

Caregivers of patients with dementia should be educated about the disease process and the disease manifestations being exhibited. Attendance at support group meetings, personal discussion with the physician, and resources such as the 36-Hour Day 7 and the Alzheimer's Association may be helpful. In most situations, coping strategies include remaining calm and using touch, music, toys, and familiar personal items. Helping the caregiver understand the lack of intentionality of the behaviors is essential.

Behavior Approaches

Approaches that were helpful in the past should be tried initially. It is better to distract patients who are angry or aggressive than to try to reason with them. Asking closed-ended questions (eg, "Would you like cereal for breakfast?") instead of open-ended questions (eg, "What would you like for breakfast?") may be less confusing and stressful for the patient. Validation therapy focuses on responding to the emotion rather than the content of what the patient says. The use of reminiscence therapy to recount pleasurable experiences and the use of therapeutic activities such as dance, art, music, and exercise have proven to be useful. Reality orientation is not recommended except in the very early stages of the disease. When nonthreatening hallucinations or delusions are reported, reassurance to the caregiver may be the only treatment needed.

Environment Modification

Patients with physically nonaggressive behavior, such as pacing and wandering, may respond to the creation of a safe environment where they can walk without risk. Items such as guns and knives should be removed. Making the environment safe is a work in progress; further modifications will be necessary as the disease progresses. For patients in the later stages of the disease, a safe environment may be attained only in specialized settings such as Alzheimer's units or long-term care facilities.

Developing and Maintaining Routines

Patients with dementia benefit from consistency. Serving meals at the same time each day reduces stress and lessens the likelihood of troublesome behaviors.

Sensory Intervention

Touch may be beneficial in many older adults who are delusional. Music therapy and pet therapy, which create a homelike environment in nursing homes, seem to lessen behaviors associated with psychosis and enhance patients' quality of life.

Pharmacologic Treatment

The axioms "first do no harm" and "start low, go slow" form the cornerstone of psychopharmacologic treatment for patients with dementia. Sequential monotherapy for a targeted behavior is recommended until improvement is achieved, side effects become intolerable, or the maximal dosage is reached. A recent systematic review of studies of single-agent pharmacotherapy found that the reduction in symptoms is modest, but that small improvements may benefit the patient and caregiver. The goal of pharmacologic treatment should be reduction, not eradication, of the most troublesome behaviors. Control of symptoms in most patients will require clear identification of target behaviors (ie, those that are most troublesome or that interfere with care), careful dosage titration, and consideration of alternate or additional agents if the behavior is inadequately controlled.

Periodic reassessment of behaviors and reprioritization of goals should be part of an ongoing management plan. Behaviors may be assessed with a caregiver interview that uses the brief version of the Behavioral Pathology in Alzheimer's Disease scale (BEHAVEAD) or the Neuropsychiatric Inventory (NPI-Q). Although the BEHAVEAD is useful in specialty clinics, it may be cumbersome in a busy primary care practice. Family physicians should ask pertinent questions to identify problem behaviors, assess the reduction or increase in behaviors, detect changes in function, and identify the most common adverse effects of therapy. The expected effects and side effects of medication, especially the emergence of extrapyramidal dysfunction and falls, should be discussed with caregivers during every office visit. Providing caregivers with an opportunity to discuss problems by telephone may be helpful.

Several classes of drugs may be beneficial in the management of psychotic symptoms in patients with dementia. Atypical antipsychotics are the first-line agents for pharmacotherapy of psychotic symptoms. Anticonvulsants and acetylcholinesterase inhibitors may be considered in patients who have an inadequate response to the initial agent. Benzodiazepines may be useful for episodes of acute agitation. Systematic reviews, of these results have been published, as has a review of studies of patients in long-term care.

Atypical Antipsychotics

Atypical antipsychotics are the most thoroughly studied class of medications for patients with dementia and are the most common drugs used in clinical practice. They are better tolerated than typical neuroleptic agents, with less risk of causing extrapyramidal syndrome (EPS). In the absence of contraindications such as serious extrapyramidal dysfunction (eg, EPS, parkinsonism), an atypical neuroleptic agent should be initiated at the lowest effective dosage and titrated weekly. Tremor, rigidity, dystonia, and dyskinesia are identified in a significant number of patients at baseline and may be exacerbated by the use of atypical antipsychotics, particularly when these agents are taken at higher dosages. Physicians must use caution when increasing dosages and observe the patient closely for the emergence of EPS. Based on the results of clinical trials, there appears to be a narrow window of tolerated effective dosages. All of these agents may be administered once daily, usually at night to take advantage of their sedative effects. Two randomized controlled trials found that risperidone (Risperdal) is effective in the management of psychotic disorders of dementia. However, a retrospective analysis of 17 placebo - controlled studies of the use of atypical antipsychotic agents to treat behavior disorders in patients with dementia found an increased mortality rate. Most deaths were from cerebrovascular events or infections. This prompted the U.S. Food and Drug Administration to issue a safety alert for all agents in this class. Quetiapine (Seroquel) is the least likely drug in this class to increase symptoms in patients with Parkinson's disease or EPS. Intramuscular administration of olanzapine (Zyprexa) has been tested in acutely agitated patients, with favorable responses compared with patients who received placebo and lorazepam (Ativan). Once symptoms are acceptably controlled, the use of medications on an "as - needed" basis should be discouraged. Improvement in aberrant behavior often occurs more quickly and at lower dosages of these agents than reduction of psychotic symptoms. Although the response to medication may be modest, it has the potential for significant improvement in quality of life for patients and their caregivers.

Typical Antipsychotics

Although the use of haloperidol (Haldol) is discouraged in long - term care facilities, it is widely used in the management of delirium and acute agitation in other settings. Haloperidol has been used with acceptable side effects in the management of behavior disorders of dementia. If used, it should be prescribed at low dosages and for short periods (typically days), after which the patient should be switched to another agent such as an atypical antipsychotic.

A meta - analysis of older trials of antipsychotic treatment for agitation in older patients with dementia suggests no clear differences in clinical response. However, side effects (primarily prolonged rigidity) limit the use of haloperidol. It is one of the few drugs not implicated in the risk of falls in older adults, but this effect may be a result of marked impairment in patient mobility or its use in patients who are unresponsive to other agents

Anticonvulsants

Anticonvulsant agents typically are used when psychotic behaviors result in aggressive behavior. Increasing evidence supports the use of divalproex (Depakote) or carbamazepine (Tegretol). These drugs are recommended as second - line agents in patients with inadequate response to antipsychotic agents. Multiple small, relatively short - term trials have proven anticonvulsants to be effective and well - tolerated. In practice, however, side effects, drug interaction, and a narrow therapeutic window may limit the use of carbamazepine. Data suggest that patients taking divalproex have continued symptomatic improvement on a stable dosage over time, although this effect may reflect the natural history of behavior disorders. Sedation is a common side effect of these agents and may limit their use. Most of the data on gabapentin (Neurontin) has been anecdotal.

Acetylcholinesterase Inhibitors

Acetylcholinesterase inhibitors such as donepezil (Aricept), galantamine (Razadyne: formerly Reminyl), and rivastigmine (Exelon) have been associated with a reduction in problem behaviors in patients with dementia. However, these drugs should not be considered first - line agents in the treatment of psychosis but rather adjunctive treatment. Data on primary endpoints of cognitive function in patients taking acetylcholinesterase inhibitors consistently show a delay in time to institutionalization, which may reflect improved behavior, a delay in onset of behavior symptoms, or retention of function. Although the responses are modest, even small gains or stabilization of symptoms may lower the burden for patients and their caregivers.

Antidepressant

The distinction between depression with psychotic features and psychotic symptoms of dementia may be problematic, especially in patients with a history of depression or prominent negative symptoms. Small series results suggest that the use of selective serotonin reuptake inhibitors and trazodone (Desyrel) may be effective and could be considered in selected patients.

Anxiolytics

Benzodiazepines should not be considered first - line therapy for management of chronic behavior disorders of dementia, even in patients with prominent anxiety. However, community surveys show that these drugs are commonly used in these patients. No published studies support the routine use of benzodiazepines for the management of psychotic symptoms of dementia. Chronic benzodiazepine use may worsen the behavior abnormality because of the amnestic and disinhibitory effects of these drugs. In clinical practice, benzodiazepine use should be limited to management of acute symptoms that are unresponsive to redirection or other agents. A short - acting benzodiazepine with prompt sedative effects may be useful to empower the caregiver or nursing facility during an episode of acute agitation that fails to respond to reassurance or removal of the precipitant. Short - acting benzodiazepines should be discontinued after the symptoms are controlled with other agents. Benzodiazepines with short half - lives, no active metabolites, and little potential for drug interaction are recommended.

In patients with intractable symptoms, hospitalization in a geriatric psychiatry unit, if available, may be necessary. Patients with Lewy body disease, who often present with hallucinations, may be particularly resistant to neuroleptics and may worsen when treated with these agents. Behavior problems are dynamic and variable and may resolve spontaneously. A reduction in dosage or elimination of agents is appropriate when target symptoms are improved. In long - term care settings, stepwise reduction in medication is more easily monitored and often will be requested by the consulting pharmacist. Although the patient's behavior may vary over time, no data support the notion that tapering medications will lead to the emergence of uncontrollable symptoms.

More research is needed on the pharmacologic management of behavior problems and psychosis associated with dementia. Community-based clinical trials with a stepwise, multiple-agent design will provide a stronger basis for recommendations and a better understanding of the impact of pharmacologic interventions in these patients.

Prognosis

Amnestic disorders caused by alcoholism do not generally improve significantly over time, although in a small number of cases the patient's condition improves completely. In many cases the symptoms are severe, and in some cases warrant long-term care for the patient to make sure his or her daily needs are met. Other substance induced amnestic disorders have a variable rate of recovery, although in many cases full recovery does eventually occur. Transient global amnesia usually resolves fully.

Amnestic disorders resulting from trauma are not generally considered preventable. Avoiding exposure to environmental toxins, refraining from abuse of alcohol or other substances, and maintaining a balanced diet may help to prevent some forms of amnestic disorders.

Chapter 2 Anxiety and Mood Disorder

Anxiety and fear are ubiquitous emotions. The terms anxiety and tear have specific scientific meanings, but common usage has made them interchangeable. For example, a phobia is a kind of anxiety that is also defined in the *Diagnostic and Slallsiicaf Manual of Menial Disorder*, 4th edition (DSM - Ⅳ) as a "persistent or irrational fear." Fear is defined as an emotional and physiological response to a recognized external threat (eg, a runaway car or an impending crash in an airplane). Anxiety is an unpleasant emotional state, the sources of which are less readily identified. It is frequently accompanied by physiological symptoms that may lead to fatigue or even exhaustion. Because fear of recognized threats causes similar unpleasant mental and physical changes, patients use the term fear and anxiety interchangeably. Thus, there is little need to differentiate anxiety from fear. However, distinguishing among different anxiety disorders is important, since accurate diagnosis is more likely to result in effective treatment and a better prognosis.

The intensity of anxiety has many gradations ranging from minor qualms to noticeable trembling and even complete panic, the most extreme form of anxiey.

The course of anxiety also varies, with peak severity being reached within a few seconds or more gradually over minutes, hours, or days. Duration also varies from a few seconds to hours or even days or months, although episodes of panic usually abate within 10 minutes and seldom last more than 30 minutes.

Anxiety Disorders

Anxiety and depression share common symptoms and can result from similar circumstances, and there is evidence that treatments for each condition can benefit patients with the other. But in theory, at least, the two are distinguishable and anxiety is not generally seen as an aspect of depression. On the other hand, discriminating between them may focus attention on the trees rather than the forest; Brown et al noted "Of further concern is the possibility that our classification systems have become overly precise to the point that they are now erroneously distinguishing symptoms and disorders that actually reflect inconsequential variations of broader, underlying syndromes."

There is a dialectical conflict in perspectives on the links between anxiety and depression: a unitary theory sees them as expressions of the same pathology; the opposing perspective sees them as fundamentally different, while the compromise is to view them as having common roots but different expressions for a variety of reasons. Probably they are linked, but anxiety suggests arousal and an attempt to cope with the situation; depression suggests lack of arousal and withdrawal. An anxious person might say "That terrible event is not my fault but it may happen again, and I may not be able to cope with it but I've got to be ready to try." A depressed person might say "That terrible event may happen again and I won't be able to cope with it, and it's probably my fault anyway so there's really nothing I can do."

A 1991 paper by Clark and Watson formed a watershed in formulating the conceptual distinction between anxiety and depression. Based on an analysis of patterns of association between measures of anxiety and depression, they proposed a tripartite hierarchical model that holds that anxiety and depression have common, and unique, features. Common to both conditions is general affective distress or negative affect, plus symptoms such as sleep disturbances, irritability, and loss of appetite. Beyond these nonspecific symptoms, depression is uniquely characterized by anhedonia and low levels of positive affect. These refer to a loss of pleasure and interest in life, a lack of enthusiasm, sluggishness, apathy, social withdrawal and disinterest. Thus, negative affect is nonspecific, while positive affect (or, in this case, its absence) is specific to depression. Anxiety, meanwhile, is uniquely characterized by physiological hyperarousal, exhibited in racing heart, seating, shakiness, trembling, shortness of breath and feelings of panic. The nonspecific distress factor reflects a "temperamental sensitivity to negative stimuli" that is related to neuroticism and predicts the development of either depression or anxiety disorders. Clark, Watson and Mineka reviewed evidence for this idea, and noted that people who score highly on trait neuroticism appear more likely to develop depression, concluding that neuroticism forms a vulnerability factor to depression.

Although conceptual distinctions are drawn between anxiety and depression, the two share many common symptoms and may result from similar circumstances; there may also be bidirectional causal links between them, so that they occur together quite commonly. For example, the limitations in everyday function brought on by anxiety may lead to pessimism and general despondency; conversely, the lack of energy and the poor self-esteem of depression may undermine the sense of self-efficacy and thereby lead to anxiety.

Anxiety is a common emotion and as such is often a normal response to the vicissitudes of life. In its mild forms, anxiety may be adaptive. A little anxiety, forexample, helps a student prepare for examinations. In its extreme forms, however, anxiety is incapacitating or terrifying. High anxiety may cause the same student to lose concentration, memory, or even his or her voice.

Physicians observe anxiety most commonly in patients experiencing an acute external stress. Although short - term treatment with antianxiety or sedative drugs, such as benzodiazepines, has a place in the management of such patients, physicians often can offer more help by their presence, reassurances, and attitude. Anxiety states often resolve spontaneously with time, although clinicians should be aware that acute stress can lead to chronic anxiety or posttraumatic stress disorder.

The word anxiety has more precise diagnostic meaning in psychiatry. It refers to both paroxysmal and persistent psychological feelings (dread, irritability, ruminations) and physiologic changes (dyspnea, sweating, insomnia, trembling) which endure over time and impair normal functioning. These are often chronic disorders in which symptoms persist in the absence of obvious contemporaneous external stresses or in which the degree of symptoms seems out of proportion to the degree of external stress. Anxiety disorders were formerly lumped together under the term "anxiety neurosis". It is now recognized that a number of relatively distinct clinical syndromes exist under the general rubric of anxiety disorders, as reflected in the diagnostic criteria in the third edition of the *Diagnostic and Statistical Manual* (DSM - Ⅲ).

At least three - fourths of patients with primary depression complain of feeling anxious, worried, or fearful. Extreme anxiety may occur in agitated depression in the form of anguished facial expressions: tip biting, picking at fingers, nails, or clothing, hand - wringing, constant pacing, and inability to sit quietly. Conversely, primary anxiety can be depressing in its own right. If anxiety persists, particularly if it interferes with functioning, secondary depression is the rule rather than the exception. Some patients have both primary anxiety and primary depressive disorders. Although most patients with anxiety or depression fall clearly into the respective DSM - Ⅳ categories, differential diagnosis of anxiety and depression can be challenging and require several interviews, further evaluation, and trials of treatment.

Theories of Anxiety

It is important to recognize a distinction between psychological and medical models of anxiety. The medical approach is categorical; to receive a diagnosis of anxiety, a patient must meet specified criteria, as laid out, for example, in the DSM - Ⅳ. The categorical approach is practical and provides a basis for deciding whether or not to treat a patient. The underlying assumption is that there is a qualitative distinction between those who are well and those who are sick; although sickness can vary in severity, cases either do not lie on the same continuum as non-cases, or at least form a distinctive cluster at one end of a continuum.

This conception is widely challenged, however. Psychologists take a dimensional approach that treats anxiety as a continuum of severity (or, in some models, a set of continua) with no intrinsic threshold. The arguments for a dimensional conception point out that there does not seem to be a bimodal distribution of scores representing well and sick groups; there also seems to be a continuum of impairments due to anxiety, with no threshold beyond which rising anxiety scores would indicate an anxiety disorder. Similarly, a dimensional model has been proposed in mental status testing, where there is a diagnostic dilemma of how to classify people who do not meet the criteria for dementia, but who are also not normal. Most of the anxiety scales we review provide intensity or severity scores that reflect an underlying dimensional model of anxiety.

Anxiety has long been recognized but only relatively recently studied systematically. Fear was apparently portrayed in ancient Egyptian hieroglyphics, and the Roman orator Cicero distinguished between a character predisposition to anxiety (anxietas) and emotional responses to situations (angor). Nineteen hundred years later, Darwin analyzed the role of fear as an adaptive response involving common signs such as heart palpitations, dilation of the pupils and increased perspiration. Freud subsequently distinguished between objective and neurotic anxiety, based on whether the source of anxiety was external or internal. The feelings of apprehension, irritability and physiological arousal are the same in both conditions. Objective anxiety, synonymous with fear, is an internal reaction to a real external threat, while Freud characterized internal or neurotic anxiety as a reaction to the person's own repressed sexual or aggressive impulses that threaten to enter consciousness. For Freud, neurotic anxiety arises especially in response to unacceptable impulses such as Oedipal conflicts or sexual feelings that may have been punished in childhood and are accordingly repressed. If a person's repression of their impulses should partially break down, placing them in danger of re-experiencing repressed psychological trauma, they may experience a free-floating anxiety that appears to have no specific object save a fear of punishment if the inner impulses are expressed openly. Neurotic anxiety may be inferred when anxiety reactions appear disproportionate to the level of threat. Freud also described moral anxiety, in which the conflict lies between the person's impulses or unconscious desires and external prohibitions as perceived through the person's conscience. Thus, a high school student who is attracted to a teacher will feel anxious about meeting the teacher in the corridor.

A limitation of Freud's theory is that it did not adequately distinguish among the resulting feelings of stress, guilt, anxiety or depression, which tended to be grouped under the general label of "neurotic" symptoms. Freud's perspective was also strictly clinical and he opposed formal measurement; this orientation seemed to delay the development of anxiety scales for roughly 30 years.

The 1950s saw the development of an experimental tradition in studying anxiety. Laboratory studies assessed the links between personal drive, anxiety and the complexity of an experimental task, and feelings of fear and frustration. In 1953, Taylor presented her Manifest Anxiety Scale which built on Freud's theme of neurotic anxiety. The scale was widely used in experimental research; common findings were that people with higher drive, or "manifest anxiety", showed superior performance in simple response tasks, but less adequate performance in complex tasks that included many possible types of error. Anxiety came to be viewed more comprehensively as a process that involves stressful threats, personality characteristics and defences, and behavioral reactions.

During the 1960s, this reference to personality led to Spielberger's empirical demonstration of a distinction between anxiety as a reaction, versus an underlying tendency to respond to threats. Cattell and others had applied newly developed multivariate analysis techniques to measures of anxiety, also showing two distinct facets of anxiety that were not included in Taylor's measure. Traits refer to enduring and general dispositions to react to situations in a consistent manner; trait anxiety involves a tendency to experience anxious symptoms in non-threatening situations; it implies vulnerability to stress. State anxiety is a discrete response to a specific threatening situation: Freud's objective anxiety. State anxiety involves transitory unpleasant feelings of apprehension, tension, nervousness or worry, often accompanied by activation of the autonomic nervous system. It presumably forms a natural defence and adaptation mechanism in the face of threat. People with high trait anxiety are assumed to be more prone to experiencing state anxiety, perhaps to excess. Freud had anticipated this in his recognition of the variations in response to objective threats among normal and neurotic persons.

Etiological theories of anxiety are diverse, but may be grouped into biological theories which emphasize the relevance of hormone levels, neurochemical patterns and genetics, versus cognitive - behavioral theories which argue that such biological changes may result from psychological reactions. A synthesis between these perspectives has also been proposed. Behavioral theorists tend to emphasize the relevance of parenting styles and early learning experiences that may foster a fear response and a sense of powerlessness. Cognitive theorists point out the relevance of beliefs and perceptions for the maintenance of anxiety reactions. Clark, for example, showed that panic attacks may be triggered by a misinterpretation of normal physical sensations as presaging a threat; a vicious circle involves a reaction of heightened anxiety which produces more physical sensations leading to more catastrophic interpretations, spiralling into a panic attack. Biological theorists have tended to focus on the role of particular neurotransmitter systems in particular anxiety disorders; the noradrenergic system may be linked to panic disorder, while the serotonergic system appears relevant in obsessive - compulsive disorders and dopamine may be relevant in social phobia.

Panic Disorder

In many cases, panic attacks strike out of the blue, without any warning. Often, there is no clear reason for the attack. They may even occur when you're relaxed or asleep. A panic attack may be a one - time occurrence, but many people experience repeat episodes. Recurrent panic attacks are often triggered by a specific situation, such as crossing a bridge or speaking in public, especially if that situation has caused a panic attack before. Usually, the panic - inducing situation is one in which you feel endangered and unable to escape. You may experience one or more panic attacks, yet be otherwise perfectly happy and healthy. Or your panic attacks may occur as part of another disorder, such as panic disorder, social phobia, or depression. Regardless of the cause, panic attacks are treatable. There are many effective treatments and coping strategies you can use to deal with the symptoms.

Symptoms and Signs

A typical panic attack often begins abruptly and without warning while a patient is involved in a relatively nonthreatening and nonstressful activity, like entering a store, driving a car, or sitting at a desk working. The patient becomes flushed, lightheaded, and sweaty and is overwhelmed by feelings of terror, apprehension, and impending doom. Dyspnea may occur with a subjective sense of choking or smothering, and palpitations or chest pain are often so severe that patients believe they are having a heart attack or are dying. The symptoms of panic attacks usually peak in less than 10 minutes and resolve in 20 to 30 minutes. Most patients experiencing their first panic attack obtain help, sometimes going to a doctor's office or emergency room, but the fear has usually subsided by this time. Fatigue or exhaustion frequently follows a panic attack, and the patient may sleep.

The cardinal feature of panic disorder is the sudden, unexpected, and often overwhelming feeling of terror and apprehension accompanied by somatic symptoms in multiple organ systems such as dyspnea, palpitations, and faintness. The symptoms and signs of panic disorder are similar to those occurring during intense physical exertion or in a life-threatening situation.

Many people experience panic attacks without further episodes or complications. There is little reason to worry if you've had just one or two panic attacks. However, some people who've experienced panic attacks go on to develop panic disorder. Panic disorder is characterized by repeated panic attacks, combined with major changes in behavior or persistent anxiety over having further attacks. You may be suffering from panic disorder if you:

Experience frequent, unexpected panic attacks that aren't tied to a specific situation;

Worry a lot about having another panic attack;

Are behaving differently because of the panic attacks, such as avoiding places where you've previously panicked.

While a single panic attack may only last a few minutes, the effects of the experience can leave a lasting imprint. If you have panic disorder, the recurrent panic attacks take an emotional toll. The memory of the intense fear and terror that you felt during the attacks can negatively impact your self-confidence and cause serious disruption to your everyday life. Eventually, this leads to the following panic disorder symptoms:

Anticipatory Anxiety

Instead of feeling relaxed and like yourself in between panic attacks, you feel anxious and tense. This anxiety stems from a fear of having future panic attacks. This "fear of fear" is present most of the time, and can be extremely disabling.

Phobic Avoidance

You begin to avoid certain situations or environments. This avoidance may be based on the belief that the situation you're avoiding caused a previous panic attack. Or you may avoid places where escape would be difficult or help would be unavailable if you had a panic attack. Taken to its extreme, phobic avoidance becomes agoraphobia.

Is It a Heart Attack or a Panic Attack?

Most of the symptoms of a panic attack are physical, and many times these symptoms are so severe that people think they're having a heart attack. In fact, many people suffering from panic attacks make repeated trips to the doctor or the emergency room in an attempt to get treatment for what they believe is a life-threatening medical problem. While it's important to rule out possible medical causes of symptoms such as chest pain, heart palpitations, or difficulty breathing, it's often panic that is overlooked as a potential cause not the other way around.

Differential Diagnosis

Many patients with panic disorder complain of chest pain, cardiac extrasystoles, and palpitations. The diagnostic challenge is to differentiate anxiety with cardiovascular symptoms from the organic diseases it mimics. Because there may be an increased prevalence of mitral valve prolapse in patients with panic disorder this condition should be investigated; however, in the vast majority of patients wtih panic disorder, no significant cardiac pathology is ever found.

Other diagnostic possibilities include both hyperthyroidism and hypothyroidism, a catecholamine-secreting pheochromocytoma, complex partial seizures, and hypoglycemia. Drug ingestions (amphetamine, cocaine, caffeine, sympathomimetic nasal decongestants) and drug withdrawal (alcohol, barbiturates, opiates, minor tranquilizers) may produce symptoms that simulate panic attacks.

Etiology and Pathophysiology

Panic disorder often coexists with mood disorders, with mood symptoms potentially following the onset of panic attacks. Lifetime prevalence rates of major depression may be as much as 50%-60%.

Other medical conditions that apparently share significant comorbidity with panic disorder include chronic obstructive pulmonary disorder, irritable bowel syndrome, migraine headache, obsessive-compulsive disorder, restless leg syndrome, fatigue, specific phobias, social phobia, and agoraphobia. Comorbidities also include cardiovascular disorders (eg, mitral valve prolapse, hypertension, cardiomyopathy, stroke), with panic patients being nearly twice as likely to develop coronary artery disease. Patients with panic disorder who have coronary disease can experience myocardial ischemia during their panic episodes. Panic disorder is also associated with a higher risk of sudden death.

However, panic disorder is also present in 30% of patients with chest pain and normal findings on angiography.

Panic disorder is found in 5% - 40% of persons with asthnia, 15% of patients with headache, 20% of patients with epilepsy, and 10% of patients in primary care settings.

In addition, individuals with panic disorder tend to have lower oxygen consumption and exercise tolerance than does the general population. Individuals with panic disorder have a suicide rate many times higher than the population. The rate of substance abuse (especially stimulants, cocaine, and hallucinogens) in persons with panic disorder is 7%-28%, a risk 4-14 times greater than that of the population. In addition, panic disorder is found in 8% - 15% of individuals in alcohol treatment programs. Pregnant mothers with panic disorder during pregnancy are more likely to have preterm labor and infants of smaller birth - weight for gestational age. Data on prevalence in different racial groups are inconsistent. Symptom manifestations may differ, with African Americans more often presenting with somatic symptoms and more likely seeking help in medical rather than psychiatric settings. One-month prevalence estimates for women are 0.7%, versus 0.3% for men (ie, women are more likely to be affected than men by a 2- to 3-fold factor). Panic is more common in women who have never been pregnant and during the postpartum period, but it is less common during pregnancy.

Although panic can occur in people at any age, it usually develops between the ages of 18 and 45 years. The average age of onset, as with most anxiety disorders, is in the third decade of life. Patients with late - onset panic disorder have a tendency toward less mental health use, lower comorbidity and hypochondriasis, and better coping behavior.

Treatment

Cognitive Behavioral Therapy

Cognitive behavioral therapy is generally viewed as the most effective form of treatment for panic attacks, panic disorder, and agoraphobia. Cognitive behavioral therapy focuses on the thinking patterns and behaviors that are sustaining or triggering the panic attacks. It helps you look at your fears in a more realistic light.

For example, if you had a panic attack while driving, what is the worst thing that would really happen? While you might have to pull over to the side of the road, you are not likely to crash your car or have a heart attack. Once you learn that nothing truly disastrous is going to happen, the experience of panic becomes less terrifying.

Exposure Therapy for Panic Attacks and Panic Disorder

In exposure therapy for panic disorder, you are exposed to the physical sensations of panic in a safe and controlled environment, giving you the opportunity to learn healthier ways of coping. You may be asked to hyperventilate, shake your head from side to side, or hold your breath. These different exercises cause sensations similar to the symptoms of panic. With each exposure, you become less afraid of these internal bodily sensations and feel a greater sense of control over your panic.

If you have agoraphobia, exposure to the situations you fear and avoid is also included in treatment. As in exposure therapy for specific phobias, you face the feared situation until the panic begins to go away. Through this experience, you learn that the situation isn't harmful and that you have control over your emotions.

Medication can be used to temporarily control or reduce some of the symptoms of panic disorder. However, it doesn't treat or resolve the problem. Medication can be useful in severe cases, but it should not be the only treatment pursued. Medication is most effective when combined with other treatments, such as therapy and lifestyle changes, that address the underlying causes of panic disorder. The medications used for panic attacks and panic disorder include:

Antidepressants. It takes several weeks before they begin to work, so you have to take them continuously, not just during a panic attack.

Benzodiazepines. These are antianxiety drugs that act very quickly (usually within 30 minutes to an hour). Taking them during a panic attack provides rapid relief of symptoms. However, benzodiazepines are highly addictive and have serious withdrawal symptoms, so they should be used with caution.

When it comes to panic attacks, professional treatment and therapy can make a big difference. But there are many things you can do to help yourself, too:

Learn about panic. Simply knowing more about panic can go a long way towards relieving your distress. So read up on anxiety, panic disorder, and the fight - or - flight response experienced during a panic attack. You'll learn that the sensations and feelings you have when your panic are normal and that you aren't going crazy. Smoking and caffeine can provoke panic attacks in people who are susceptible. As a result, it's wise to avoid cigarettes, coffee, and other caffeinated beverages. Also be careful with medications that contain stimulants, such as diet pills and non-drowsy cold medications.

Learn how to control your breathing. Hyperventilation brings on many sensations (such as lightheadedness and tightness of the chest) that occur during a panic attack. Deep breathing, on the other hand, can relieve the symptoms of panic. By learning to control your breathing, you develop a coping skill that you can use to calm yourself down when you begin to feel anxious. If you know how to control your breathing, you are also less likely to create the very sensations that you are afraid of.

Practice relaxation techniques. When practiced regularly, activities such as yoga, meditation, and progressive muscle relaxation strengthen the body's relaxation response — the opposite of the stress response involved in anxiety and panic. And not only do these relaxation practices promote relaxation, but they also increase feelings of joy and equanimity. So make time for them in your daily routine.

Agoraphobia

Agoraphobia is a fear of being caught in a situation from which a graceful and speedy escape to safety would be difficult or embarrassing if the patient felt discomfort (often in the form of panic). Situations likely to induce fear and avoidance include attendance at auditoriums, eating out (especially at formal sitdown restaurants), shopping in supermarkets, standing in lines, using public transportation, and driving under conditions in which opportunities to pull over, stop or get off the highway quickly may be restlicted. Being accompanied by a trusted family member or friend permits many agoraphobic individuals to increase the number of possibly uncomfortable situations they can endure and lo extend the range ol their excursions.

Symptoms and Signs

The term agoraphobia has been widely misunderstood. Its literal definition suggests a fear of "open spaces". However, this is an incomplete and misleading view. Agoraphobics are not necessarily afraid of open spaces. Rather, they are afraid of having panicky feelings, wherever, these fearful feelings may occur. For many, they happen at home, in houses of worship, or in crowded supermarkets, places that are certainly not "open". In fact, agoraphobia is a condition which develops when a person begins to avoid spaces or situations associated with anxiety. Typical "phobic situations" might include driving, shopping, crowded places, traveling, standing in line, being alone, meetings and social gatherings.

Agoraphobia is a type of phobia. A phobia is the excessive fear of a specific object, circumstance or situation. Agoraphobia is excessive worry about having a panic attack in a public place. Commonly feared places and situations are elevators, sporting events, bridges, public transportation, shopping malls, airplanes, crowds or lines of people. The difference between typical agoraphobia symptoms and symptoms similar to a panic attack are showed as following.

Typical agoraphobia symptoms	Signs and symptoms similar to a panic attack
Fear of being alone in any situation	Light headedness
Fear of being in crowded places	Trouble breathing
Fear of losing control in a public place	Dizziness
Fear of being in places where it may be hard to leave, such as an elevator or train	Excessive sweating
Inability to leave your house for long periods (housebound)	Rapid heart rate
Sense of helplessness	Flushing
Overdependence on others	Nausea
A sense that your body is unreal	Upset stomach or diarrhea
	Chest pain
	Feeling a loss of control
	Trouble swallowing

Etiology and Pathogenssis

As of 2002, the causes of agoraphobia are complex and not completely understood. It has been known for some years that anxiety disorders tend to run in families. Recent research has confirmed earlier hypotheses that there is a genetic component to agoraphobia, and that it can be separated from susceptibility to PD. In 2001 a team of Yale geneticists reported the discovery of a genetic locus on human chomosome 3 that governs a person's risk of developing agoraphobia. PD was found to be associated with two loci: one on human chromosome 1 and the other on chromosome 11q. The researchers concluded that agoraphobia and PD are common; they are both inheritable anxiety disorders that share some, but not all, of their genetic loci for susceptibility.

A number of researchers have pointed to inborn temperament as a broad vulnerability factor in the development of anxiety and mood disorders. In other words, a person's natural disposition or temperament may become a factor in developing a number of mood or anxiety disorders. Some people seem more sensitive throughout their lives to events, but upbringing and life history are also important factors in determining who will develop these disorders. Children who manifest what is known as "behavioral inhibition" in early infancy are at increased risk for developing more than one anxiety disorder in adult life — particularly if the inhibition remains over time. (Behavioral inhibition refers to a group of behaviors that are displayed when the child is confronted with a new situation or unfamiliar people.) These behaviors include moving around, crying, and general irritability, followed by withdrawing, seeking comfort from a familiar person, and stopping what one is doing when one notices the new person or situation. Children of depressed or anxious parents are more likely to develop behavioral inhibition.

Another factor in the development of PD and agoraphobia appears to be a history of respiratory disease. Some researchers have hypothesized that repeated episodes of respiratory disease would predispose a child to PD by making breathing difficult and lowering the threshold for feeling suffocated. It is also possible that respiratory diseases could generate fearful beliefs in the child's mind that would lead him or her to exaggerate the significance of respiratory symptoms.

About 42% of patients diagnosed with agoraphobia report histories of real or feared separation from their parents or other caretakers in childhood. This statistic has been interpreted to mean that agoraphobia in adults is the aftermath of unresolved childhood separation anxiety. The fact that many patients diagnosed with agoraphobia report that their first episode occurred after the death of a loved one, and the observation that other agoraphobics feel safe in going out as long as someone is with them, have been taken as supportive evidence of the separation anxiety hypothesis.

There are also theories about human learning that explain agoraphobia. It is thought that a person's initial experience of panic - like symptoms in a specific situation, for example, being alone in a subway station may lead the person to associate physical symptoms of panic with all subway stations. Avoiding all subway stations would then reduce the level of the person's discomfort. Unfortunately, the avoidance strengthens the phobia because the person is unlikely to have the opportunity to test whether subway stations actually cause uncomfortable physical sensations. One treatment modality, exposure therapy, is based on the premise that phobias can be "unlearned" by reversing the pattern of avoidance.

Gender role socialization has been suggested as an explanation for the fact that the majority of patients with agoraphobia are women. One form of this hypothesis maintains that some parents still teach girls to be fearful and timid about venturing out in public. Another version relates agoraphobia to the mother - daughter relationship, maintaining that mothers tend to give daughters mixed messages about becoming separate individuals. As a result, girls grow up with a more fragile sense of self, and may stay within the physical boundaries of their home because they lack a firm sense of their internal psychological boundaries.

The differential diagnosis of agoraphobia is described differently in DSM - Ⅳ - TR and in ICD - 10, the European diagnostic manual. The U.S. diagnostic manual specifies that agoraphobia must be defined in relation to PD, and that the diagnoses of specific phobias and social phobias are the next to consider. The DSM - Ⅳ - TR also specifies that the patient's symptoms must not be related to substance abuse; and if they are related to a general medical condition, they must have excessive symptoms usually associated with that condition. For example, a person with Crohn's disease has realistic concerns about an attack of diarrhea in a public place and should not be diagnosed with agoraphobia unless the fear of losing bowel control is clearly exaggerated. The DSM Ⅳ - TR does not require a person to experience agoraphobia within a set number of circumstances in order to meet the diagnostic criteria.

In contrast, the European diagnostic manual primarily distinguishes between agoraphobia and delusional or obsessive disorders, and depressive episodes. In addition, ICD - 10 specifies that the patient's anxiety must be restricted to or occur primarily within two out of four specific situations: crowds; public places; traveling alone; or traveling away from home. The primary area of agreement between the American and European diagnostic manuals is that both specify avoidance of the feared situation as a diagnostic criterion.

Diagnosis of agoraphobia is usually made by a physician after careful exclusion of other mental disorders and physical conditions or diseases that might be related to the patient's fears. Head injury, pneumonia, and withdrawal from certain medications can produce some of the symptoms of a panic attack. In addition, the physician may ask about caffeine intake as a possible dietary factor. As of 2002, there are no laboratory tests or diagnostic imaging studies that can be used to diagnose agoraphobia.

Furthermore, there are no widely used diagnostic interviews or screening instruments specifically for agoraphobia. One self-report questionnaire, however, is under development by Dutch researchers who recently reported on its validity. The test is called the Agoraphobic Self-Statements Questionnaire, or ASQ, and is intended to evaluate thinking processes in patients with agoraphobia, as distinct from their emotional responses.

Treatment

Treatment of agoraphobia usually consists of medication plus cognitive-behavioral therapy (CBT). The physician may also recommend an alternative form of treatment for the anxiety symptoms associated with agoraphobia. Some patients may be advised to cut down on or give up coffee or tea, as the caffeine in these beverages can be contribute to their panic symptoms.

Medications that have been used with patients diagnosed with agoraphobia include the benzodiazepine tranquilizers, the MAO inhibitors (MAOIs), tricyclic antidepressants (TCAs), and the selective serotonin uptake inhibitors, or SSRIs. In the past few years, the SSRIs have come to be regarded as the first-choice medication treatment because they have fewer side effects. The benzodiazepines have the disadvantage of increasing the symptoms of agoraphobia when they are withdrawn, as well as interfering with CBT. (Benzodiazepines can decrease mental sharpness, making it difficult for patients taking these medications to focus in therapy sessions.) The MAO inhibitors require patients to follow certain dietary guidelines. For example, they must exclude aged cheeses, red wine, and certain types of beans. TCAs may produce such side effects as blurred vision, constipation, dry mouth, and drowsiness.

CBT is regarded as the most effective psychotherapeutic treatment for agoraphobia. The specific CBT approach that seems to work best with agoraphobia is exposure therapy. Exposure therapy is based on undoing the association that the patient originally formed between the panic symptoms and the feared situation. By being repeatedly exposed to the feared location or situation, the patient gradually learns that he or she is not in danger, and the anxiety symptoms fade away. The therapist typically explains the procedure of exposure therapy to the patient and reassures him or her that the exposure can be stopped at any time that his or her limits of toleration have been reached. The patient is then exposed in the course of a number of treatment sessions to the feared situation, usually for a slightly longer period each time. A typical course of exposure therapy takes about 12 weeks. On the other hand, one group of German researchers reported good results in treating patients with agoraphobia with individual high-density exposure therapy. The patients were exposed to their respective feared situations for an entire day for two–three weeks. One year later, the patients had maintained their improvement.

Exposure treatment for agoraphobia may be combined with cognitive restructuring. This form of cognitive behavioral therapy teaches patients to observe the thoughts that they have in the feared situation, such as, "I'll die if I have to go into that railroad station," and replace these thoughts with positive statements. In this example, the patient with agoraphobia might say to himself or herself, "I'll be just fine when I go in there to buy my ticket."

Although insight - oriented therapies have generally been considered relatively ineffective in treating agoraphobia, a recent trial of brief psychodynamic psychotherapy in patients with PD with agoraphobia indicates that this form of treatment may also be beneficial. Of the 21 patients who participated in the 24 - session course of treatment (twice weekly for 12 weeks), 16 experienced remission of their agoraphobia. There were no relapses at six - month follow - up. Patients diagnosed with agoraphobia have reported that alternative therapies, such as hypnotherapy and music therapy, were helpful in relieving symptoms of anxiety and panic. Ayurvedic medicine, yoga, religious practice, and guided imagery meditation have also been helpful.

Prognosis

The prognosis for untreated agoraphobia is considered poor by most European as well as most American physicians. The DSM - Ⅳ - TR remarks that little is known about the course of agoraphobia without PD, but that anecdotal evidence indicates that it may persist for years with patients becoming increasingly impaired. The ICD - 10 refers to agoraphobia as "the most incapacitating of the phobic disorders", to the point that some patients become completely housebound. With proper treatment, however, 90% of patients diagnosed with agoraphobia can recover and resume a normal life.

Posttraumatic Stress Disorder

Posttraumatic stress disorder, often abbreviated as PTSD, is a complex disorder in which the affected person's memory, emotional responses, intellectual processes, and nervous system have all been disrupted by one or more traumatic experiences. It is sometimes summarized as "a normal reaction to abnormal events." The DSM - Ⅳ - TR classifies PSTD as an anxiety disorder.

PTSD has a unique position as the only psychiatric diagnosis (along with acute stress disorder) that depends on a factor outside the individual, namely, a traumatic stressor. A patient cannot be given a diagnosis of PTSD unless he or she has been exposed to an event that is considered traumatic. These events include such obvious traumas as rape, military combat, torture, genocide, natural disasters, and transportation or workplace disasters. In addition, it is now recognized that repeated traumas or such traumas of long duration as child abuse, domestic violence, stalking, cult membership, and hostage situations may also produce the symptoms of PTSD in survivors.

A person suffering from PTSD experiences flashbacks, nightmares, or daydreams in which the traumatic event is experienced again. The person may also experience abnormally intense startle responses, insomnia, and may have difficulty concentrating. Trauma survivors with PTSD have been effectively treated with group therapy or individual psychological therapy, and other therapies have helped individuals, as well. Some affected individuals have found support groups or peer counseling groups helpful. Treatment may require several years, and in some cases, PTSD may affect a person for the rest of his or her life.

Etiology

Whether or not PTSD develops appears to depend upon the nature of the trauma, the characteristics of the individual, and the context in which these events take place. The trauma can be anticipated or not, acute or chronic, constant or repetitive, due to natural events (eg, an earthquake) or malevolence (eg, rape, child abuse, torture). PTSD can develop in individuals who were apparently healthy, successful, and well-adjusted prior to the traumatic experiences. Among the factors which influence the development of PTSD are (1) the extent to which the individual's life-space is affected; (2) the duration of the impact; (3) the extent to which the individual perceives human malevolence behind the traumatic event (eg, a fire attributed to arson will probably be more traumatic than one attributed to lightning); and (4) social isolation.

When PTSD was first suggested as a diagnostic category for DSM-Ⅲ in 1980, it was controversial precisely because of the central role of outside stressors as causes of the disorder. Psychiatry has generally emphasized the internal weaknesses or deficiencies of individuals as the source of mental disorders; prior to the 1970s, war veterans, rape victims, and other trauma survivors were often blamed for their symptoms and regarded as cowards, moral weaklings, or masochists. The high rate of psychiatric casualties among Vietnam veterans, however, led to studies conducted by the Veterans Administration. These studies helped to establish PTSD as a legitimate diagnostic entity with a complex set of causes.

Present neurobiological research indicates that traumatic events cause lasting changes in the human nervous system, including abnormal secretions of stress hormones. In addition, in PTSD patients, researchers have found changes in the amygdala and the hippocampus, the parts of the brain that form links between fear and memory. Experiments with ketamine, a drug that inactivates one of the neurotransmitter chemicals in the central nervous system, suggest that trauma works in a similar way to damage associative pathways in the brain. Positron emission tomography (PET) scans of PTSD patients suggest that trauma affects the parts of the brain that govern speech and language.

Studies of specific populations of PTSD patients (combat veterans, survivors of rape or genocide, former political hostages or prisoners, etc.) have shed light on the social and cultural causes of PTSD. In general, societies that are highly authoritarian, glorify violence, or sexualize violence have high rates of PTSD even among civilians.

Persons whose work exposes them to traumatic events or who treat trauma survivors may develop secondary PTSD (also known as compassion fatigue or burnout). These occupations include specialists in emergency medicine, police officers, firefighters, search-and-rescue personnel, psychotherapists, disaster investigators, etc. The degree of risk for PTSD is related to three factors: the amount and intensity of exposure to the suffering of trauma victims; the worker's degree of empathy and sensitivity; and unresolved issues from the worker's personal history.

Although the most important causal factor in PTSD is the traumatic event itself, individuals differ in the intensity of their cognitive and emotional responses to trauma; some persons appear to be more vulnerable than others. In some cases, this greater vulnerability is related to temperament or natural disposition, with shy or introverted people being at greater risk. In other cases, the person's vulnerability results from chronic illness, a physical disability, or previous traumatization — particularly abuse in childhood. As of 2001, researchers have not found any correlation between race and biological vulnerability to PTSD.

Epidemiology

It is difficult to gauge the extent of PTSD following a traumatic event because the studies that have been done have often followed subjects for only a short period of time, and the nature of the events is often so situation-specific. About 15 percent or more of the civilian population may experience mental distress severe enough to require treatment following a major natural disaster. For example, in a study that followed survivors of a shipboard tire for 31 to 51 years, one-third were found to be unable to return to sea because of psychological symptoms. Following extreme prolonged harsh conditions such as combat, prisoner-of-war camps, or Nazi death camps, a higher incidence of both acute and delayed FTSD is likely. Some evidence, based on follow-up of World War Ⅱ veterans 20 years after the war, indicates an increasing incidence of new patients seeking psychiatric care for war-associated symptoms. The vicissitudes of normal aging may unmask a latent traumatic stress disorder.

Symptoms

DSM-Ⅳ-TR specifies six diagnostic criteria for PTSD:

Traumatic Stressor

The patient has been exposed to a catastrophic event involving actual or threatened death or injury, or a threat to the physical integrity of the self or others. During exposure to the trauma, the person's emotional response was marked by intense fear, feelings of helplessness, or horror. In general, stressors caused intentionally by human beings (genocide, rape, torture, abuse, etc.) are experienced as more traumatic than accidents, natural disasters, or "acts of God".

Intrusive Symptoms

The patient experiences flashbacks, traumatic daydreams, or nightmares, in which he or she relives the trauma as if it were recurring in the present. Intrusive symptoms result from an abnormal process of memory formation. Traumatic memories have two distinctive characteristics: (1) they can be triggered by stimuli that remind the patient of the traumatic event; (2) they have a "frozen" or wordless quality, consisting of images and sensations rather than verbal descriptions.

Avoidant Symptoms

The patient attempts to reduce the possibility of exposure to anything that might trigger memories of the trauma, and to minimize his or her reactions to such memories. This cluster of symptoms includes feeling disconnected from other people, psychic numbing, and avoidance of places, persons, or things associated with the trauma. Patients with PTSD are at increased risk of substance abuse as a form of self-medication to numb painful memories.

Hyperarousal

Hyperarousal is a condition in which the patient's nervous system is always on "red alert" for the return of danger. This symptom cluster includes hypervigilance, insomnia, difficulty concentrating, general irritability, and an extreme startle response. Some clinicians think that this abnormally intense startle response may be the most characteristic symptom of PTSD.

Duration of Symptoms

The symptoms must persist for at least one month.

Significance

The patient suffers from significant social, interpersonal, or work-related problems as a result of the PTSD symptoms. A common social symptom of PTSD is a feeling of disconnection from other people (including loved ones), from the larger society, and from spiritual or other significant sources of meaning.

Differential Diagnosis

In adjustment disorder, symptoms such as reexperiencing the trauma are absent. Other considerations include major depressive disorder, generalized anxiety disorder, phobic disorder, organic mental disorders, and other conditions such as "compensation neurosis" and "postconcussion syndrome."

In the case of a known trauma of recent occurrence, most often a civilian disaster or war — the diagnosis of PTSD is relatively straightforward, based on the criteria listed above.

DSM-Ⅳ introduced a new diagnostic category, acute stress disorder, to differentiate between time-limited and longer-term stress reactions. In acute stress disorder, the hyperarousal and intrusive symptoms last between two days and four weeks. If the symptoms last beyond four weeks, and all of the above criteria are met, the diagnosis is changed to PTSD.

The diagnosis of PTSD is more difficult in cases of delayed reaction to trauma. Some individuals do not develop symptoms of PTSD until months or even years after the traumatic event. DSM-Ⅳ-TR specifies an interval of at least six months between the event and the development of symptoms for a diagnosis of PTSD with delayed onset. Delayed symptoms are often triggered by a situation that resembles the original trauma, as when a person raped in childhood experiences workplace sexual harassment.

DSM-Ⅲ and its successors included the category of adjustment disorder to differentiate abnormal reactions to such painful but relatively common life events ("ordinary stressors") as divorce, job loss, or bereavement from symptoms resulting from overwhelming trauma. The differential diagnosis (the process of determining that the diagnosis is one disorder although it may resemble another) is complicated, however, by the fact that "ordinary stressors" sometimes reawaken unresolved childhood trauma, producing the delayed-reaction variant of PTSD.

Most patients with PTSD (as many as 80%) have been diagnosed with one of the anxiety (30%-60%), dissociative, mood (26%-85%), or somatoform disorders as well as with PTSD. Between 40%-60% of persons with delayed-reaction PTSD are diagnosed with a personality disorder, most often borderline personality disorder. Another common dual diagnosis is PTSD/ substance abuse disorder. Between 60%–80% of patients who develop PTSD turn to alcohol or narcotics in order to avoid or numb painful memories. According to the NVVRS, the estimated lifetime prevalence of alcohol abuse among male Vietnam veterans is 39.2%, and the estimated lifetime prevalence of drug abuse is 5.7%. Dual diagnoses complicate treatment because the therapist must decide whether to treat the disorders in sequence or concurrently. PTSD patients diagnosed with personality disorders are regarded as the most difficult to treat.

As of 2002, there are no physical tests to establish a diagnosis of PTSD. The diagnosis is usually made on the basis of the patient's history and results from one or more short-answer interviews or symptom inventories. The instruments most often used to evaluate patients for PTSD include the Anxiety Disorders Interview Scale (ADIS), the Beck Depression Inventory, the Clinician-Administered PTSD Scale (CAPS), the Disorders of Extreme Stress Inventory (DESI), the Dissociative Experiences Scale (DES), the Hamilton Anxiety Scale, and the Impact of Event Scale (IES).

Prophylaxis

Military experience suggests that PTSD can be prevented partially if soldiers are taught that a degree of fear and anxiety are normal concomitants of battle rather than signs of cowardice or mental illness. Furthermore, the development of chronic PTSD can often be prevented if the soldier with acute PTSD is seen close to the battle front under the principles of immediate treatment, expectancy of return to normal duties, and brevity of treatment contact.

Treatment

In general, there have been few well-controlled clinical trials of treatment options for PTSD, particularly for severely affected patients.

Critical incident stress debriefing (CISD) is a treatment offered to patients within 48 hours following a civilian disaster or war zone trauma. It is intended to weaken the acute symptoms of the trauma and to forestall the development of full-blown PTSD. CISD usually consists of four phases:

Description of the traumatic event;

Sharing of survivors' emotional reactions to the event;

Open discussion of symptoms caused by the event;

Reassurance that the symptoms are normal responses to trauma, followed by discussion of coping strategies.

Critical incident stress management is a system of interventions designed to help emergency/disaster response workers, public safety personnel, and therapists deal with stress reactions before they develop secondary PTSD.

Other mainstream treatment methods used with patients who have already developed PTSD include:

Cognitive-behavioral Therapy

There are two treatment approaches to PTSD included under this heading: exposure therapy, which seeks to desensitize the patient to reminders of the trauma; and anxiety management training, which teaches the patient strategies for reducing anxiety. These strategies may include relaxation training, biofeedback, social skills training, distraction techniques, or cognitive restructuring.

Psychodynamic Psychotherapy

This method helps the patient recover a sense of self and learn new coping strategies and ways to deal with intense emotions related to the trauma. Typically, it consists of three phases: (1) establishing a sense of safety for the patient; (2) exploring the trauma itself in depth; (3) helping the patient reestablish connections with family, friends, the wider society, and other sources of meaning.

Discussion or Peer-counseling Groups

These groups are usually formed for survivors of specific traumas, such as combat, rape/incest, and natural disasters. They help patients to recognize that other survivors of the shared experience have had the same emotions and reacted to the trauma in similar ways. They appear to be especially beneficial for patients with guilt issues about their behavior during the trauma (such as submitting to rape to save one's life, or surviving the event when others did not).

Family Therapy

This form of treatment is recommended for PTSD patients whose family life has been affected by the PTSD symptoms.

In general, medications are used most often in patients with severe PTSD to treat the intrusive symptoms of the disorder as well as feelings of anxiety and depression. These drugs are usually given as one part of a treatment plan that includes psychotherapy or group therapy. As of 2002, there is no single medication that appears to be a "magic bullet" for PTSD. The selective serotonin reuptake inhibitors (SSRIs) appear to help the core symptoms when given in higher doses for five to eight weeks, while the tricyclic antidepressants (TCAs) or the monoamine oxidase inhibitors (MAOIs) are most useful in treating anxiety and depression. Some alternative therapies for PTSD include:

Spiritual/religious counseling. Because traumatic experiences often affect patients' spiritual views and beliefs, counseling with a trusted religious or spiritual advisor may be part of a treatment plan. A growing number of pastoral counselors in the major Christian and Jewish bodies have advanced credentials in trauma therapy.

Yoga and various forms of bodywork are often recommended as ways of releasing physical tension or muscle soreness caused by anxiety or hypervigilance.

Martial arts training can be helpful in restoring the patient's sense of personal effectiveness and safety. Some martial arts programs, such as Model Mugging, are designed especially for survivors of rape and other violent crimes.

Art therapy, journaling, dance therapy, and creative writing groups offer safe outlets for the strong emotions that follow traumatic experiences.

Since the mid - 1980s, several controversial methods of treatment for PTSD have been introduced. Some have been developed by mainstream medical researchers while others are derived from various forms of alternative medicine. They include:

Eye Movement Desensitization and Reprocessing

This is a technique in which the patient reimagines the trauma while focusing visually on movements of the therapist's finger. It is claimed that the movements of the patient's eyes reprogram the brain and allow emotional healing.

Tapas Acupressure Technique (TAT)

TAT was derived from traditional Chinese medicine (TCM), and its practitioners maintain that a large number of acupuncture meridians enter the brain at certain points on the face, especially around the eyes. Pressure on these points is thought to release traumatic stress.

Thought Field Therapy

This therapy combines the acupuncture meridians of TCM with analysis of the patient's voice over the telephone. The therapist then provides an individualized treatment for the patient.

Traumatic Incident Reduction

This is a technique in which the patient treats the trauma like a videotape and "runs through" it repeatedly with the therapist until all negative emotions have been discharged.

Emotional Freedom Techniques (EFT)

EFT is similar to TAT in that it uses the body's acupuncture meridians, but it emphasizes the body's entire "energy field" rather than just the face.

Counting Technique

Developed by a physician, this treatment consists of a preparation phase, a counting phase in which the therapist counts from 1 to 100 while the patient reimagines the trauma, and a review phase. Like Traumatic Incident Reduction, it is intended to reduce the patient's hyperarousal.

Obsessive - compulsive Disorder

Obsessive - compulsive disorder (OCD) is currently classified as an anxiety disorder marked by the recurrence of intrusive or disturbing thoughts, impulses, images or ideas (obsessions) accompanied by repeated attempts to suppress these thoughts through the performance of certain irrational and ritualistic behaviors or mental acts (compulsions). The obsessions and compulsions take up large amounts of the patient's time (an hour or longer every day) and usually cause significant emotional distress for the patient and difficulties in his or her relationships with others.

Some researchers have questioned whether OCD really belongs with the other anxiety disorders. They think that it should be grouped with the spectrum of such obsessive - compulsive disorders as Tourette's syndrome, which are known to have biological causes. OCD should not be confused with obsessive - compulsive personality disorder even though the two disorders have similar names. Obsessive - compulsive personality disorder is not characterized by the presence of obsessions and compulsions; rather, it is a lifelong pattern of insistence on control, orderliness, and perfection that begins no later than the early adult years. It is possible, however, for a person to have both disorders.

The major characteristics are recurrent obsessions (persistent intrusive thoughts) and compulsions (intrusive behaviors) which the patient experiences as involuntary, senseless, or repugnant. Common obsessions include thoughts of violence (eg, killing a loved one), obsessive slowness, fears of germs or contamination, and doubt (eg, a priest who worries excessively that he had not said his prayers properly). Examples of compulsions include repeated checking to be assured that something was done properly, hand washing, extreme neatness, and counting rituals, as in numbering steps while walking. Obsessions and compulsions do not invariably coexist in the same individual. The relationship of the obsessive - compulsive disorder to obsessive or compulsive characterologic traits remains controversial.

Etiology and Pathophysiology

The etiology of the obsessive - compulsive state is uncertain, but it can be viewed from psychodynamic, psychosocial, and biologic perspectives. Obsessions and compulsions often seem to symbolize unconscious wishes, impulses, and fears and to reflect dynamic adaptations to unwanted aggressive or sexual urges. Biologic factors are suggested by reports of an increased incidence of obsessive compulsive disorder in monozygotic twins and first - degree relatives of probands, of biologic markers associated with the disorder, and of favorable response to certain tricyclic antidepressants and monoamine oxidase inhibitors.

In the early part of the century, Sigmund Freud theorized that OCD symptoms were caused by punitive, rigid toilet - training practices that led to internalized conflicts. Other theorists thought that OCD was influenced by such wider cultural attitudes as insistence on cleanliness and neatness, as well as by the attitudes and parenting style of the patient's parents. Cross - cultural studies of OCD indicate that, while the incidence of OCD seems to be about the same in most countries around the world, the symptoms are often shaped by the patient's culture of origin. For example, a patient from a Western country may have a contamination obsession that is focused on germs, whereas a patient from India may fear contamination by touching a person from a lower social caste.

Studies of families with OCD members indicate that the particular expression of OCD symptoms may be affected by the responses of other people. Families with a high tolerance for the symptoms are more likely to have members with more extreme or elaborate symptoms. Problems often occur when the OCD member's obsessions and rituals begin to control the entire family.

There is considerable evidence that OCD has a biological component. Some researchers have noted that OCD is more common in patients who have suffered head trauma or have been diagnosed with Tourette's syndrome. Recent studies using positron emission tomography (PET) scanning indicate that OCD patients have patterns of brain activity that differ from those of people without mental illness or with some other mental illness. Other studies using magnetic resonance imaging (MRI) found that patients diagnosed with OCD had significantly less white matter in their brains than did normal control subjects. This finding suggests that there is a widely distributed brain abnormality in OCD. Some researchers have reported abnormalities in the metabolism of serotonin, an important neurotransmitter, in patients diagnosed with OCD. Serotonin affects the efficiency of communication between the front part of the brain (the cortex) and structures that lie deeper in the brain known as the basal ganglia. Dysfunction in the serotonergic system occurs in certain other mental illnesses, including major depression. OCD appears to have a number of features in common with the so-called obsessive-compulsive spectrum disorders, which include Tourette's syndrome, Sydenham's chorea, eating disorders, trichotillomania and delusional disorders.

There appear to be genetic factors involved in OCD. The families of persons who are diagnosed with the disorder have a greater risk of OCD and tic disorders than does the general population. Childhood-onset OCD appears to run in families more than adult-onset OCD, and is more likely to be associated with tic disorders. Twin studies indicate that monozygotic, or identical twins, are more likely to share the disorder than dizygotic, or fraternal twins. The concordance (match) rate between identical twins is not 100%, however, which suggests that the occurrence of OCD is affected by environmental as well as genetic factors. In addition, it is the general nature of OCD that seems to run in families rather than the specific symptoms; thus, one family member who is affected by the disorder may have a compulsion about washing and cleaning while another is a compulsive counter.

Large epidemiological studies have found a connection between streptococcal infections in childhood and the abrupt onset or worsening of OCD symptoms. The observation that there are two age-related peaks in the onset of the disorder increases the possibility that there is a common causal factor. Patients with childhood-onset OCD often have had one of two diseases caused by a group of bacteria called Group A beta-hemolytic streptococci ("strep" throat and Sydenham's chorea) prior to the onset of the OCD symptoms. The disorders are sometimes referred to as pediatric autoimmune neuropsychiatric disorders associated with streptococcal infections, or PANDAS. It is thought that antibodies in the child's blood cross-react with structures in the basal ganglia, producing or worsening the symptoms of OCD or tic disorders.

Symptoms

The symptoms of OCD should not be confused with the ability to focus on detail or to check one's work that is sometimes labeled "compulsive" in everyday life. This type of attentiveness is an important factor in academic achievement and in doing well in fields that require close attention to detail, such as accounting or engineering. By contrast, the symptoms of OCD are serious enough to interfere with the person's day-to-day functioning. Historical examples of OCD include a medieval Englishman named William of Oseney, who spent twelve hours per day reading religious books in order to be at peace with God; and Freud's Rat Man, a patient who had repeated dreams of cursing Freud and covering him with dung. While the Rat Man was ashamed of these impulses and had no explanation for them, he could not control them.

More recent accounts of OCD symptoms include those of a young man who compulsively touched every electrical outlet as he passed, washed his hands several times an hour, and returned home repeatedly to check that the doors and windows were locked. Another account describes a firefighter who was worried that he had throat cancer. He spent three hours a day examining his throat in the mirror, feeling his lymph nodes, and asking his wife if his throat appeared normal. Brief descriptions of the more common obsessions and compulsions follow.

Contamination

People with contamination obsessions are usually preoccupied with a fear of dirt or germs. They may avoid leaving home or allowing visitors to come inside in order to prevent contact with dirt or germs. Some people with contamination obsessions may wear gloves, coats, or even masks if they are forced to leave their house for some reason. Obsessions with contamination may also include abnormal fears of such environmental toxins as lead, asbestos, or radon.

Washing compulsions are commonly associated with contamination obsessions. For example, a person concerned about contamination from the outside may shower and launder all clothing immediately upon coming home. The compulsion may be triggered by direct contact with the feared object, but in many cases, even being in its general vicinity may stir up intense anxiety and a strong need to engage in a washing compulsion. One man who was afraid of contamination could not even take a short walk down the street without experiencing a compulsion to disinfect the soles of his shoes, launder all his clothing, and wash his hands until they were raw after he returned to his apartment.

Washing compulsions may not always be caused by a fear of germs. That is, a need for perfection or for symmetry may also lead to unnecessary washing. In such cases, the individual may be concerned about being "perfectly" clean, or feel that he cannot leave the shower until his left foot has been washed exactly as many times as his right foot. Other people with washing compulsions may be unable to tolerate feeling sweaty or otherwise not clean.

Obsessional Doubting

Obsessional doubting refers to the fear of having failed to perform some task adequately, and that dire consequences will follow as a result. Although the person may try to suppress the worrisome thoughts or images, he or she usually experiences a rising anxiety which then leads to a compulsion to check the task. For example, someone may worry about forgetting to lock the door or turn off the gas burner on the stove and spend hours checking these things before leaving home. In one instance, a man was unable to throw away old grocery bags because he feared he might have left something valuable inside one of them. Immediately after looking into an empty bag, he would again have the thought, "What if I missed something in there?" In many cases, no amount of checking is sufficient to dispel the maddening sense of doubt.

Need for Symmetry

Persons suffering from an obsession about symmetry often report feeling acutely uncomfortable unless they perform certain tasks in a symmetrical or balanced manner. Thus, crossing one's legs to the right must be followed by crossing legs to the left; scratching one side of the head must be followed by scratching the other; tapping the wall with a knuckle on the right hand must be followed by tapping with one on the left, etc. Sometimes the person may have a thought or idea associated with the compulsion, such as a fear that a loved one will be harmed if the action is not balanced, but often there is no clearly defined fear, only a strong sense of uneasiness.

Aggressive and Sexual Obsessions

Aggressive and sexual obsessions are often particularly horrifying to those who experience them. For some people, obsessive fears of committing a terrible act in the future compete with fears that they may already have done something awful in the past. Compulsions to constantly check and confess cause such individuals to admit to evildoing they had no part in, a phenomenon familiar to law enforcement following highly publicized crimes. These obsessions often involve violent or graphic imagery that is upsetting and disgusting to the person, such as rape, physical assault, or even murder. One case study concerned a young woman who constantly checked the news to reassure herself that she had not murdered anyone that day; she felt deeply upset by unsolved murder cases. A middle-aged man repeatedly confessed to having molested a woman at work, despite no evidence of such an action ever occurring in his workplace.

Obsessions and compulsions in children are often focused on germs and fears of contamination. Other common obsessions include fears of harm coming to self or others; fears of causing harm to another person; obsessions about symmetry; and excessive moralization or religiosity. Childhood compulsions frequently include washing, repeating, checking, touching, counting, ordering and arranging. Younger children are less likely to have full-blown anxiety-producing obsessions, but they often report a sense of relief or strong satisfaction (a "just right" feeling) from completing certain ritualized behaviors. Since children are particularly skillful in disguising their OCD symptoms from adults, they may effectively hide their disorder from parents and teachers for years.

Unusual behaviors in children that may be signs of OCD include:

Avoidance of scissors or other sharp objects. A child may be obsessed with fears of hurting herself or others.

Chronic lateness or dawdling. The child may be per forming checking rituals (repeatedly making sure all her school supplies are in her bookbag, for example).

Daydreaming or preoccupation. The child may be counting or performing balancing rituals mentally.

Spending long periods of time in the bathroom. The child may have a handwashing compulsion.

Schoolwork handed in late or papers with holes erased in them. The child may be repeatedly checking and correcting her work.

For both children and adults, the symptoms of OCD wax and wane in severity; and the specific content of obsessions and compulsions may change over time. The disorder, however, very seldom goes away by itself without treatment. People with OCD in all age groups typically find that their symptoms worsen during major life changes or following highly stressful events.

As noted above, OCD is a relatively common mental disorder, with about 2.3% of the population of the United States being diagnosed with the condition at some point in their lives. As of 2000, the annual social and economic costs of OCD in the United States are estimated at $9 billion. Although the disorder may begin at any age, the typical age of onset is late adolescence to young adulthood, with slightly more women than men being diagnosed with OCD. Interestingly, childhood OCD is more common in males, and the sex ratio does not favor females until adulthood. People with OCD appear to be less likely to marry than persons diagnosed with other types of mental disorders.

Epidemiology

The lifetime prevalence of obsessive compulsive disorder, based upon interviews of the general population 18 years and older, varies between 1.9 and 3.0 percent. The prevalence tends to be slightly higher in females than males but does not vary significantly by race, education, or urbanization of area of residence.

These disorders usually begin in adolescence or young adulthood, with about 65% of cases beginning before age 25. They are rarely seen in children. Long term prognosis appears to be variable. Some patients (perhaps 10%) show a chronic, unremitting course; some show periods of complete remission, the majority show an episodic course with periods of incomplete remission.

Differential Diagnosis

OCD is a disorder that may not be diagnosed for years. People who suffer from its symptoms are often deeply ashamed, and go to great lengths to hide their ritualistic behaviors. The disorder may be diagnosed when family members get tired of the impact of the patient's behaviors on their lives, and force the patient to consult a doctor. In other cases, the disorder may be self-reported. The patient may have come to resent the amount of time wasted by the compulsions; or he or she may have taken a screening questionnaire such as the brief screener available on the NIMH website (listed in the Resources section below).

The diagnosis of OCD may be complicated because of the number of other conditions that resemble it. For example, major depression may be associated with self-perceptions of being guilty, bad, or worthless that are excessive and unreasonable. Similarly, eating disorders often include bizarre thoughts about size and weight, ritualized eating habits, or the hoarding of food. Delusional disorders may entail unusual beliefs or behaviors, as do such other mental disorders as trichotillomania, hypochondriasis, the paraphilias, and substance use disorders. Thus, accurate diagnosis of OCD depends on the careful analysis of many variables to determine whether the apparent obsessions and compulsions might be better accounted for by some other disorder, or to the direct effects of a substance or a medical condition.

In addition, OCD may coexist with other mental disorders, most commonly depression. It has been estimated that about 34% of patients diagnosed with OCD are depressed at the time of diagnosis, and that 65% will develop depression at some point in their lives.

Colored positron emission tomography scans (PET scans) of a human brain, showing active areas in obsessive-compulsive disorder. In this patient, some parts of the brain show increased activity as the symptoms strengthen (areas shown in the top row), while other brain areas show decreased activity as symptoms strengthen (bottom row).

Repetitive self - destructive behaviors, such as gambling, drinking, drug abuse, and overeating, should not be diagnosed as "obsessive - compulsive" disorder since the individual normally derives pleasure from the activity. Stereotyped behavior is also common in schizophrenia, Tourette's syndrome, and depression.

Treatment

Controlled studies have shown that both behaviorally oriented psychotherapy and psychopharmacology can be helpful in these disorders. Compulsions and rituals probably respond more than do obsessions and ruminations to behavior therapy. The tricyclic antidepressant drugs and monoamine oxidase inhibitors are relatively effective but require chronic administration. In severe unresponsive cases of obsessional - compulsive disorder cingulotomy or modified frontal leukotomy is reported to be helpful.

As of 2002, a combination of behavioral therapy and medications appears to be the most effective treatment for OCD. The goal of treatment is to reduce the frequency and severity of the obsessions and compulsions so that the patient can work more efficiently and have more time for social activities. Few OCD patients become completely symptom - free, but most benefit considerably from treatment.

Behavioral treatments using the technique of exposure and response prevention are particularly effective in treating OCD. In this form of therapy, the patient and therapist draw up a list, or hierarchy, of the patient's obsessive and compulsive symptoms. The symptoms are arranged in order from least to most upsetting. The patient is then systematically exposed to the anxiety - producing thoughts or behaviors, beginning with the least upsetting. The patient is asked to endure the feared event or image without engaging in the compulsion normally used to lower anxiety. For example, a person with a contamination obsession might be asked to touch a series of increasingly dirty objects without washing their hands. In this way, the patient learns to tolerate the feared object, reducing both worrisome obsessions and anxiety - reducing compulsions. About 75%–80% of patients respond well to exposure and response prevention, with very significant reductions in symptoms.

Other types of psychotherapy have met with mixed results. Psychodynamic psychotherapy is helpful to some patients who are concerned about the relationships between their upbringing and the specific features of their OCD symptoms. Cognitive - behavioral psychotherapy may be valuable in helping the patient to become more comfortable with the prospect of exposure and prevention treatments, as well as helping to identify the role that the patient's particular symptoms may play in his or her own life and what effects family members may have on the maintenance and continuation of OCD symptoms. Cognitive - behavioral psychotherapy is not intended to replace exposure and response prevention, but may be a helpful addition to it.

The most useful medications for the treatment of OCD are the selective serotonin reuptake inhibitors (SSRIs), which affect the body's reabsorption of serotonin, a chemical in the brain that helps to transmit nerve impulses across the very small gaps between nerve cells. These drugs, specifically clomipramine (Anafranil), fluoxetine (Prozac), fluvoxamine (Luvox), sertraline (Zoloft), and paroxetine (Paxil) have been found to relieve OCD symptoms in over half of the patients studied. It is not always possible for the doctor to predict which of the SSRIs will work best for a specific patient. Lack of response to one SSRI does not mean that other drugs within the same family will not work. Treatment of OCD often proceeds slowly, with various medications being tried before the most effective one is found. While studies report that about half of those treated with SSRIs show definite improvement, relapse rates may be as high as 90% when medications are discontinued.

Some treatments that have been used for OCD include electroconvulsive therapy (ECT) and, as a technique of last resort, psychosurgery for truly intractable OCD. Some patients have benefited from ECT; however, the National Institute of Mental Health (NIMH) recommends reserving ECT for OCD patients who have not responded to psychotherapy or medication.

Prognosis

While most patients with OCD benefit from a combination of medications and psychotherapy, the disorder is usually a lifelong condition. In addition, the presence of personality disorders or additional mental disorders is associated with less favorable results from treatment. The total elimination of OCD symptoms is very rare, even with extended treatment.

The onset of OCD in childhood is the single strongest predictor of a poor prognosis. Treatment in children is also complicated by the fact that children may find the response and exposure techniques very stressful. It is also hard for children to understand the potential value of such treatments; however, creative therapists have learned to use anxiety reduction strategies, education, and behavioral rewards to help their young patients with the treatment tasks. Concern about the long-term use of medications in children with OCD has further encouraged the use of cognitive-behavioral techniques whenever possible.

Mood Disorders

The British physician Aubrey Lewis once noted that the history of the diagnosis and treatment of melancholia could serve as a history of psychiatry itself. That observation seems particularly relevant today, since advances in the diagnosis and treatment of mood disorders have led to a dramatic increase in their perceived prevalence and to more rigorous criteria for placement in competing nosological categories.

The distinguishing characteristic of these disorders is a primary pervasive disturbance in mood. In this context, the term "mood" denotes an emotional state that may affect all aspects of the individual's life. The syndromes are characterized by palliologically elevated or depressed mood and should be regarded as existing on a continuum with normal mood. A diagnosis is appropriate when the mood disturbance is "primary" and central to the illness and not secondary to some other physical or psychological state. In the latter instance, the diagnosis would be incomplete without a reference to the precip itating cause. Although historically a precipitating stressful event was thought to be a critical element in the differential diagnosis of mood disorders, current opinion is that data of this sort lack diagnostic specificity and prognostic validity. Even so, when a mood disturbance following a siressful life event is a mild one that does not meet the criteria for any of the disorders discussed in this chapter, a diagnosis of adjustment disorder with depressed mood is warranted.

In this chapter, the class of mood disorders is divided into disorders in which there is a full major mood syndrome, disorders in which there is only a partial but persistent mood syndrome, and disorders that cannot be classified in either of these two ways. Major mood disorders are further classified according to whether the patient has a history of a manic episode. A past or present history of a manic episode justifies a diagnosis of bipolar I disorder, which may be further subdivided on the basis of the presenting or most recent mood state (manic, depressed, or mixed). Some investigators have suggested that the spectrum of bipolar illness contains distinct subtypes characterized by the prominence of either mania or depression. If there is no history of a manic episode, and if the criteria of severity are met, a diagnosis of major depressive disorder is warranted. Major depression is further subclassitied according to whether it is a first episode or a recurrence. Additional clinical features such as the presence of psychotic ideation or vegetative signs should also be specifically recorded. Although not authorized by the *Diagnostic and Statistical Manual of Mental Disorders*, 4th edition (DSM - Ⅳ), the term "unipolar" is sometimes used to describe this group of disorders.

Other specific mood disorders include cyclothymic disorder and dysthymic disorder. The term cyclothymic disorder encompasses individuals whose symptoms resemble those of bipolar disorder but are neither severe enough nor of sufficient duration to meet the criteria for diagnosis of bipolar or major depressive disorder. The term dysthymic disorder partially encompasses the group of individuals historically classified as suffering from depressive neurosis. These individuals have chronic depression that is not of sufficient severity or duration to meet the criteria for major depressive episode.

The terms bipolar disorder NOS ("nol otherwise specified") and depressive disorder NOS are reserved for individuals who do not precisely meet any of the criteria just described. One example would be patients with a history of mood change occurring regularly during the preinenstrual period.

Bipolar Disorder

Symptoms and Signs

One essential criterion for a diagnosis of bipolar I disorder is a past or present history of a manic episode. Manic episodes are characterized by a predominantly elevated, expansive, or irritable mood that presents as a prominent or persistent part of the illness. Manic patients classically have abundant resources of energy and engage in multiple activities and ventures. At baseline and between episodes, the bipolar manic patient may indeed function at a high level of productivity, particularly in areas requiring creative talent. In the initial stages of an episode and sometimes in attenuated episodes the ventures may appear.

One of the primary early symptoms of a manic episode is a decreased need for sleep, so that in many cases the individual may not sleep for 3 or 4 days at a time. A "hunger" for social interchange may be manifested by frequent and inappropriate phone calls to distant acquaintances, particularly during late - night periods when social stimulation is minimal. Hypergraphia (excessive writing) and a fascination with music and playing musical instruments are frequently noted. Manic palients may also have a tendency to wear bright colors and unusual combinations of eccentric attire or may exhibit an attitude of carelessness about clothes or makeup. Public disrobing is also common.

Manic speed is characteristically rapid and discursive. Manic patients are difficult to interrupt and have difficulty not interrupimg others who are speaking. The speech itself may involve rhyming, punning, and bizarre associations, but there are no pathognomonic elements. Manic patients are readily distractible and respond to both internal and external stimuli in a selfreferential manner. Manic episodes that are more severe or that are observed later in the natural history of the disorder may be characterized by paranoia and irritability rather than euphoria and grandiosity. Anxiety and feelings of suspicion can cause the verbal output of such individuals to be markedly decreased, leading to erroneous diagnostic conclusions. Significant social aggression is rare, although acute mania and hyponiania are coininon diagnoses in individuals with a history of psychiatric trealnient who coiiurnt violent crimes. In some cases, severe depression may occur concomitantly with the manic state ("mixed state") or in abnipt alternation with the manic Mate. Suicidal risk is significantly elevated over the base rate for bipolar disorders in such individuals. True delusions and auditory halluicinations may be present, giving rise to difficult problems of differential diagnosis. The content of the delusions or hallucinations is often consistent with the predominant mood (mood- congruent).

In severe cases, mania can present as a state of catatonia. In such cases, the individual appears "will - fully" unresponsive, often assuming a fixed posture and appearing mute except for occasional shouts or guttural sounds. Less severe stales mav be characterized by primitive delusions, fecal smearing, and extremes of tearfulness and emotional lability.

According to DSM - Ⅳ - TR, patients with bipolar I disorder have had at least one episode of mania (criteria for a manic episode are presented in Table 1). Some patients have had previous depressive episodes (Table 2), and most patients will have subsequent episodes that can be either manic or depressive. Hypomanic and mixed episodes (Table 3 and Table 4, respectively) can occur, as well as significant subthreshold mood lability between episodes. Patients meeting criteria for bipolar II disorder have a history of major depressive episodes and hypomanic episodes only. Patients may also exhibit significant evidence of mood lability, hypomania, and depressive symptoms but fail to meet duration criteria for bipolar II disorder, thereby leading to a diagnosis of bipolar disorder not otherwise specified. Finally, cyclothymic disorder may be diagnosed in those patients who have never experienced a manic, mixed, or major depressive episode but who experience numerous periods of depressive symptoms and numerous periods of hypomanic symptoms for at least 2 years (1 year in children), with no symptom - free period greater than 2 months. Summary of Manic and Depressive Symptom Criteria in DSM - Ⅳ - TR Mood Disorders in Table 5.

Table 1 Diagnostic Criteria for a Manic Episode

A. A distinct period of abnormally and persistently elevated, expansive, or irritable mood, lasting at least 1 week (or any duration if hospitalization is necessary).
B. During the period of mood disturbance, three (or more) of the following symptoms have persisted (four if the mood is only irritable) and have been present to a significant degree:
(1) Inflated self-esteem or grandiosity
(2) Decreased need for sleep (eg, feels rested after only 3 hours of sleep)
(3) More talkative than usual or pressure to keep talking
(4) Flight of ideas or subjective experience that thoughts are racing
(5) Distractibility (ie, attention too easily drawn to unimportant or irrelevant external stimuli)
(6) Increase in goal-directed activity (either socially, at work or school, or sexually) or psychomotor agitation
(7) Excessive involvement in pleasurable activities that have a high potential for painful consequences (eg, engaging in unrestrained buying sprees, sexual indiscretions, or foolish business investments)
C. The symptoms do not meet criteria for a mixed episode.
D. The mood disturbance (1) is sufficiently severe to cause marked impairment in occupational functioning, usual social activities, or relationships with others, (2) necessitates hospitalization to prevent harm to self or others, or (3) has psychotic features.
E. The symptoms are not due to the direct physiological effects of a substance (eg, a drug of abuse, a medication, or other treatment) or a general medical condition (eg, hyperthyroidism).

Table 2 Diagnostic Criteria for a Major Depressive Episode

A. Five (or more) of the following symptoms have been present nearly every day during the same 2-week period and represent a change from previous functioning; at least one of the symptoms is either depressed mood or loss of interest or pleasure:
(1) Depressed mood at most of the day as indicated by either subjective report (eg, feels sad or empty) or observation made by others (eg, appears tearful)
(2) Markedly diminished interest or pleasure in all, or almost all, activities most of the day (as indicated by either subjective account or observation made by others)
(3) Significant weight loss when not dieting, weight gain (eg, a change of more than 5% of body weight in a month), or a decrease or increase in appetite
(4) Insomnia or hypersomnia
(5) Psychomotor agitation or retardation (observable by others, not merely subjective feelings of restlessness or being slowed down)
(6) Fatigue or loss of energy
(7) Feelings of worthlessness or excessive or inappropriate guilt (which may be delusional)
(8) Diminished ability to think or concentrate or indecisiveness (either by subjective account or as observed by others)
(9) Recurrent thoughts of death (not just fear of dying), recurrent suicidal ideation without a specific plan, or previous suicide attempt or a specific plan for committing suicide
B. The symptoms do not meet criteria for a mixed episode.
C. The symptoms cause clinically significant distress or impairment in social, occupational, or other important areas of functioning.
D. The symptoms are not due to the direct physiological effects of a substance (eg, a drug of abuse, a medication) or a general medical condition (eg, hypothyroidism).
E. The symptoms are not better accounted for by bereavement (ie, after the loss of a loved one) and have persisted for longer than 2 months or are characterized by marked functional impairment, morbid preoccupation with worthlessness, suicidal ideation, psychotic symptoms, or psychomotor retardation.

Table 3 Diagnostic Criteria for a Hypomanic Episode

A. A distinct period of persistently elevated, expansive, or irritable mood, lasting at least 4 days, that is clearly different from the usual nondepressed mood.

B. During the period of mood disturbance, three (or more) of the following symptoms have persisted (four if the mood is only irritable) and have been present to a significant degree:

(1) Inflated self-esteem or grandiosity

(2) Decreased need for sleep (eg, feels rested after only 3 hours of sleep)

(3) More talkative than usual or pressure to keep talking

(4) Flight of ideas or subjective experience that thoughts are racing

(5) Distractibility (ie, attention too easily drawn to unimportant or irrelevant external stimuli)

(6) Increase in goal-directed activity (either socially, at work or school, or sexually) or psychomotor agitation

(7) Excessive involvement in pleasurable activities that have a high potential for painful consequences (eg, engaging in unrestrained buying sprees, sexual indiscretions, or foolish business investments)

C. The episode is associated with an unequivocal change in functioning that is uncharacteristic of the person when not symptomatic.

D. The disturbance in mood and the change in functioning are observable by others.

E. The episode (1) is not severe enough to cause marked impairment in social or occupational functioning, (2) does not necessitate hospitalization, and (3) does not have psychotic features.

F. The symptoms are not due to the direct physiological effects of a substance (eg, a drug of abuse, a medication, or other treatment) or a general medical condition (eg, hyperthyroidism).

Table 4 Diagnostic Criteria for a Mixed Episode

A. The criteria are met both for a manic episode and for a major depressive episode (except for duration) nearly every day during at least a 1-week period.

B. The mood disturbance (1) is sufficiently severe to cause marked impairment in occupational functioning, usual social activities, or relationships with others, (2) necessitates hospitalization to prevent harm to self or others, or (3) has psychotic features.

C. The symptoms are not due to the direct physiological effects of a substance (eg, a drug of abuse, a medication, or other treatment) or a general medical condition (eg, hyperthyroidism).

Table 5 Summary of Manic and Depressive Symptom Criteria in DSM-Ⅳ-TR Mood Disorders

Disorder	Manic Symptom Criteria	Depressive Symptom Criteria
Major depressive disorder	No history of mania or hypomania	History of major depressive episodes (single or recurrent)
Dysthymic disorder	No history of mania or hypomania	Depressed mood, more days than not, for at least 2 years (but not meeting criteria for a major depressive episode)
Bipolar I disorder	History of manic or mixed episodes	Major depressive episodes typical but not required for diagnosis
Bipolar II disorder	One or more episodes of hypomania; no manic or mixed episodes	History of major depressive episodes
Cyclothymic disorder	For at least 2 years, the presence of numerous periods with hypomanic symptoms	Numerous periods with depressive symptoms that do not meet criteria for a major depressive episode
Bipolar disorder not otherwise specified	Manic symptoms present, but criteria not met for bipolar I, bipolar II, or cyclothymic disorder	Not required for diagnosis

In addition to providing definitions of bipolar disorder, DSM-Ⅳ-TR also includes specifiers describing the course of recurrent episodes, such as seasonal pattern, longitudinal course (with or without full interepisode recovery), and rapid cycling.

Some investigators have advocated moving from a categorical to a more dimensional perspective in characterizing bipolar disorder. In particular, this perspective includes the concept of a bipolar spectrum that would encompass a range of presentations not currently considered bipolar. For example, a patient with antidepressant - induced hypomanic symptoms would be considered to have a form of bipolar disorder under the spectrum conceptualization.

Natural History

Bipolar disorder is generally an episodic, lifelong illness with a variable course. The first episode of bipolar disorder may be manic, hypomanic, mixed, or depressive. Men are more likely than women to be initially manic, but both are more likely to have a first episode of depression. Patients with untreated bipolar disorder may have more than 10 total episodes of mania and depression during their lifetime, with the duration of episodes and interepisode periods stabilizing after the fourth or fifth episode. Often, 4 years or more may elapse between the first and second episodes, but the intervals between subsequent episodes usually narrow. However, it must be emphasized that variability is the hallmark of this illness. Thus, when taking a history, a number of longitudinal issues must be considered, including the number of prior episodes, the average length and severity of episodes, average interepisode duration, and the interval since the last episode of mania or depression.

Frequently, a patient will experience several episodes of depression before a manic episode occurs. Consequently, bipolar disorder should always be considered in the differential diagnosis of depression. Patients very often do not report prior episodes of mania and hypomania and instead seek treatment for complaints of depression, delaying correct diagnosis. For a patient who is not educated about bipolar disorder, symptoms of dysphoric hypomania may not be recognized or reported. Therefore, the psychiatrist needs to ask explicitly about prior manic or hypomanic episodes, since knowledge of their presence can influence treatment decisions. The psychiatrist should also ask about a family history of mood disorders, including mania and hypomania. Consultation with family members and significant others may be extremely useful in establishing family history and identifying prior affective episodes.

In addition to substance abuse and risk - taking behavior, other cross - sectional features that can have an impact on diagnosis and treatment planning include the presence of psychotic symptoms or cognitive impairment and the risk of suicide or violence to persons or property.

Suicide rates are high among bipolar disorder patients. Completed suicide occurs in an estimated 10% - 15% of individuals with bipolar I disorder. Suicide is more likely to occur during a depressive or a mixed episode. Pharmacotherapy may substantially reduce the risk of suicide. For example, in an 11 - year follow - up study of 103 patients with bipolar disorder who were receiving lithium, death rates were well below those expected for this group on the basis of age and sex.

Bipolar disorder causes substantial psychosocial morbidity, frequently affecting patients' relationships with spouses or partners, children, and other family members as well as their occupation and other aspects of their lives. Even during periods of euthymia, patients may experience impairments in psychosocial functioning or residual symptoms of depression or mania/hypomania. It is estimated that as many as 60% of people diagnosed with bipolar I disorder experience chronic interpersonal or occupational difficulties and subclinical symptoms between acute episodes. Divorce rates are substantially higher in patients with bipolar disorder, approaching two to three times the rate of comparison subjects. The occupational status of patients with bipolar disorder is twice as likely to deteriorate as that of comparison subjects. Patients' ability to care for themselves, degree of disability or distress, childbearing status or plans, availability of supports such as family or friends, and resources such as housing and finances also bear on treatment plans.

Epidemiology

Bipolar I disorder affects approximately 0.8% of the adult population, with estimates from community samples ranging between 0.4% and 1.6%. These rates are consistent across diverse cultures and ethnic groups. Bipolar Ⅱ disorder affects approximately 0.5% of the population. While bipolar Ⅱ disorder is apparently more common in women, bipolar I disorder affects men and women fairly equally. These estimates of prevalence are considered conservative. Reasons for this underestimate may include differences in diagnostic definitions and inclusion of persons who fall within the bipolar spectrum but who do not meet DSM-Ⅳ-TR criteria for bipolar I or bipolar Ⅱ disorder.

The Epidemiologic Catchment Area study reported a mean age at onset of 21 years for bipolar disorder. When studies examining age at onset are stratified into 5-year intervals, the peak age at onset of first symptoms falls between ages 15 and 19, followed closely by ages 20-24. There is often a 5- to 10-year interval, however, between age at onset of illness and age at first treatment or first hospitalization. Onset of mania before age 15 has been less well studied. Bipolar disorder may be difficult to diagnose in this age group because of its atypical presentation with ADHD. Thus, the true age at onset of bipolar disorder is still unclear and may be younger than reported for the full syndrome, since there is uncertainty about the symptom presentation in children. Research that follows cohorts of offspring of patients with bipolar disorder may help to clarify early signs in children.

Onset of mania after age 60 is less likely to be associated with a family history of bipolar disorder and is more likely to be associated with identifiable general medical factors, including stroke or other central nervous system lesion.

Evidence from epidemiological and twin studies strongly suggests that bipolar disorder is a heritable illness. First-degree relatives of patients with bipolar disorder have significantly higher rates of mood disorder than do relatives of nonpsychiatrically ill comparison groups. However, the mode of inheritance remains unknown. In clinical practice, a family history of mood disorder, especially of bipolar disorder, provides strong corroborative evidence of the potential for a primary mood disorder in a patient with otherwise predominantly psychotic features.

Likewise, the magnitude of the role played by environmental stressors, particularly early in the course of the illness, remains uncertain. However, there is growing evidence that environmental and lifestyle features can have an impact on severity and course of illness. Stressful life events, changes in sleep - wake schedule, and current alcohol or substance abuse may affect the course of illness and lengthen the time to recovery.

Treatment

Bipolar disorder requires lifelong treatment, even during periods when you feel better. Treatment is usually guided by a psychiatrist skilled in treating the condition. You may have a treatment team that also includes psychologists, social workers and psychiatric nurses. The primary treatments for bipolar disorder include medications; individual, group or family psychological counseling (psychotherapy); or education and support groups.

Hospitalization

Your doctor may have you hospitalized if you are behaving dangerously, you feel suicidal or you become detached from reality (psychotic).

Initial Treatment

Often, you'll need to begin taking medications to balance your moods right away. Once your symptoms are under control, you'll work with your doctor to find the best long - term treatment.

Continued Ttreatment

Maintenance treatment is used to manage bipolar disorder on a long - term basis. People who skip maintenance treatment are at high risk of a relapse of symptoms or having minor mood changes turn into full - blown mania or depression.

Substance Abuse Treatment

If you have problems with alcohol or drugs, you'll also need substance abuse treatment. Otherwise, it can be very difficult to manage bipolar disorder.

Medications

A number of medications are used to treat bipolar disorder. If one doesn't work well for you, there are a number of others to try. Your doctor may suggest combining medications for maximum effect. Medications for bipolar disorder include those that prevent the extreme highs and lows that can occur with bipolar disorder (mood stabilizers) and medications that help with depression or anxiety. Medications for bipolar disorder include:

Lithium

Lithium (Lithobid, others) is effective at stabilizing mood and preventing the ex treme highs and lows of certain categories of bipolar disorder and has been used for many years. Periodic blood tests are required, since lithium can cause thyroid and kidney problems. Common side effects include restlessness, dry mouth and digestive issues.

Anticonvulsants

These mood - stabilizing medications include valproic acid (Depakene, Stavzor), divalproex (Depakote) and lamotrigine (Lamictal). The medication asenapine (Saphris) may be helpful in treating mixed episodes. Depending on the medication you take, side effects can vary. Common side effects include weight gain, dizziness and drowsiness. Rarely, certain anticonvulsants cause more serious problems, such as skin rashes, blood disorders or liver problems.

Antipsychotics

Certain antipsychotic medications, such as aripiprazole (Abilify), olanzapine (Zyprexa), risperidone (Risperdal) and quetiapine (Seroquel), may help people who don't benefit from anticonvulsants. The only antipsychotic that's specifically approved by the U.S. Food and Drug Administration (FDA) for treating bipolar disorder is quetiapine. However, doctors can still prescribe other medications for bipolar disorder. This is known as off - label use. Side effects depend on the medication, but can include weight gain, sleepiness, tremors, blurred vision and rapid heartbeat. Weight gain in children is a significant concern. Antipsychotic use may also affect memory and attention and cause involuntary facial or body movements.

Antidepressants

Depending on your symptoms, your doctor may recommend you take an antidepressant. In some people with bipolar disorder, antidepressants can trigger manic episodes, but may be OK if taken along with a mood stabilizer. The most common antidepressant side effects include reduced sexual desire and problems reaching orgasm. Older antidepressants, which include tricyclics and MAO inhibitors, can cause a number of potentially dangerous side effects and require careful monitoring.

Symbyax

This medication combines the antidepressant fluoxetine and the antipsychotic olanzapine. It works as a depression treatment and a mood stabilizer. Symbyax is approved by the FDA specifically for the treatment of bipolar disorder. Side effects can include weight gain, drowsiness and increased appetite. This medication may also cause sexual problems similar to those caused by antidepressants.

Benzodiazepines

These anti - anxiety medications may help with anxiety and improve sleep. Examples include clonazepam (Klonopin), lorazepam (Ativan), diazepam (Valium), chlordiazepoxide (Librium) and alprazolam (Niravam, Xanax). Benzodiazepines are generally used for relieving anxiety only on a short - term basis. Side effects can include drowsiness, reduced muscle coordination, and problems with balance and memory.

Finding the right medication

Finding the right medication or medications for you will likely take some trial and error. This requires patience, as some medications need weeks to months to take full effect. Generally only one medication is changed at a time so your doctor can identify which medications work to relieve your symptoms with the least bothersome side effects. This can take months or longer, and medications may need to be adjusted as your symptoms change. Side effects improve as you find the right medications and doses that work for you, and your body adjusts to the medications.

Medications and pregnancy

A number of medications for bipolar disorder can be associated with birth defects. Use effective birth control (contraception) to prevent pregnancy. Discuss birth control options with your doctor, as birth control medications may lose effectiveness when taken along with certain bipolar disorder medications.

If you plan to become pregnant, meet with your doctor to discuss your treatment options. Discuss breast - feeding with your doctor, as some bipolar medications can pass through breast milk to your infant.

Psychotherapy

Psychotherapy is another vital part of bipolar disorder treatment. Several types of therapy may be helpful. These include:

Cognitive behavioral therapy

This is a common form of individual therapy for bipolar disorder. The focus of cognitive behavioral therapy is identifying unhealthy, negative beliefs and behaviors and replacing them with healthy, positive ones. It can help identify what triggers your bipolar episodes. You also learn effective strategies to manage stress and to cope with upsetting situations.

Psychoeducation

Counseling to help you learn about bipolar disorder (psychoeducation) can help you and your loved ones understand bipolar disorder. Knowing what's going on can help you get the best support and treatment, and help you and your loved ones recognize warning signs of mood swings.

Family therapy

Family therapy involves seeing a psychologist or other mental health provider along with your family members. Family therapy can help identify and reduce stress within your family. It can help your family learn how to communicate better, solve problems and resolve conflicts.

Group therapy

Group therapy provides a forum to communicate with and learn from others in a similar situation. It may also help build better relationship skills.

Other therapies

Other therapies that have been studied with some evidence of success include early identification and therapy for worsening symptoms (prodrome detection) and therapy to identify and resolve problems with your daily routine and interpersonal relationships (interpersonal and social rhythm therapy). Ask your doctor if any of these options may be appropriate for you.

Transcranial magnetic stimulation

This treatment applies rapid pulses of a magnetic field to the head. It's not clear exactly how this helps, but it appears to have an antidepressant effect. However, not everyone is helped by this therapy, and it's not yet clear who is a good candidate for this type of treatment. More research is needed. The most serious potential side effect is a seizure.

Electroconvulsive Therapy (ECT)

Electroconvulsive therapy can be effective for people who have episodes of severe depression or feel suicidal or people who haven't seen improvements in their symptoms despite other treatment. With ECT, electrical currents are passed through your brain. Researchers don't fully understand how ECT works. But it's thought that the electric shock causes changes in brain chemistry that leads to improvements in your mood. ECT may be an option if you have mania or severe depression when you're pregnant and cannot take your regular medications. ECT can cause temporary memory loss and confusion.

Hospitalization

In some cases, people with bipolar disorder benefit from hospitalization. Getting psychiatric treatment at a hospital can help keep you calm and safe and stabilize your mood, whether you're having a manic episode or a deep depression. Partial hospitalization or day treatment programs also are options to consider. These programs provide the support and counseling you need while you get symptoms under control.

Treatment in Children and Adolescents

Children and adolescents with bipolar disorder are prescribed the same types of medications as those used in adults. However, there's little research on the safety and effectiveness of bipolar medications in children, so treatment decisions are based on adult research. Treatments are generally decided on a case - by - case basis, depending on exact symptoms, medication side effects and other factors. As with adults, ECT may be an option for adolescents with severe bipolar I symptoms or for whom medications don't work. Most children diagnosed with bipolar disorder require counseling as part of initial treatment and to keep symptoms from returning. Psychotherapy, along with working with teachers and school counselors can help children develop coping skills, address learning difficulties and resolve social problems. It can also help strengthen family bonds and communication. Psychotherapy may also be necessary to resolve substance abuse problems, common in older children with bipolar disorder.

Cyclothymic Disorder

Cyclothymia (si - klo - THIGH - me - uh), also called cyclothymic disorder, is a mood disorder. Cyclothymia causes emotional ups and downs, but they're not as extreme as in bipolar disorder type I or II. With cyclothymia, you experience periods when your mood noticeably shifts up and down from your baseline. You may feel on top of the world for a time, followed by a low period when you feel somewhat blue. Between these cyclothymic highs and lows, you may feel stable and fine. Compared with bipolar disorder I or Ⅱ, the highs and lows of cyclothymia are less extreme. Still, it's critical to seek help managing these symptoms because they increase your risk of bipolar disorder I or Ⅱ. Treatment options for cyclothymia include talk therapy (psychotherapy), medications and close, ongoing follow-up with your doctor.

Symptoms and Signs

Cyclothymia symptoms alternate between emotional highs and lows. The highs of cyclothymia are characterized by symptoms of an elevated mood (hypomanic symptoms), which resemble those of mania but are less severe. The lows consist of mild or moderate depressive symptoms.

Cyclothymia symptoms are similar to those of bipolar disorder Ⅰ or Ⅱ, but they're less severe. When you have cyclothymia, you can typically function in your daily life, though not always well. The unpredictable nature of your mood shifts may significantly disrupt your life because you never know how you're going to feel.

Hypomanic Phase of Cyclothymia

The highs (hypomania) of cyclothymia meet the same diagnostic definition of hypomania for type Ⅱ bipolar disorder. Signs and symptoms may include:

An exaggerated feeling of happiness or well-being (euphoria);

Extreme optimism;

Inflated self-esteem;

Poor judgment;

Rapid speech;

Racing thoughts;

Aggressive or hostile behavior;

Being inconsiderate of others;

Agitation;

Excessive physical activity;

Risky behavior;

Spending sprees;

Increased drive to perform or achieve goals;

Increased sexual drive;

Decreased need for sleep;

Tendency to be easily distracted;

Inability to concentrate.

Depressive Phase of Cyclothymia

Depressive episodes of cyclothymia may include a combination of these signs and symptoms:

Sadness;

Hopelessness;

Suicidal thoughts or behavior;

Anxiety;

Guilt;

Sleep problems;

Appetite problems;

Fatigue;

Loss of interest in activities once considered enjoyable;

Decreased sex drive;

Problems concentrating;

Irritability;

Chronic pain without a known cause.

For the first two years after symptoms begin, the highs and lows of cyclothymia are less extreme. After that time, your highs and lows may become more pronounced. You may have depressive episodes that meet the criteria for full-blown major depressive episodes. Or you could experience full manic episodes.

Differential Diagnosis

Doctor or other health care provider must determine if you have cyclothymia, bipolar disorder I or Ⅱ, depression or another condition that may be causing your symptoms. To help pinpoint a diagnosis for your symptoms, you'll likely have several exams and tests, which generally include:

General Medical Exam

During this exam, your doctor measures your blood pressure and listens to your heart and lungs, among other things — or reviews results of recent physical exams — to determine if there could be any medical reasons for your symptoms.

Lab Tests

These may include a complete blood count as well as thyroid tests and other blood tests. You may also have a urinalysis or tests for drug and alcohol use.

Psychological Evaluation

A doctor or mental health provider will talk to you about your thoughts, feelings and behavior patterns. You may also fill out psychological self-assessments and questionnaires. You may be asked about substance or alcohol abuse. And with your permission, family members or close friends may be asked to provide information about your symptoms and possible episodes of mania or depression.

To be diagnosed with cyclothymia, you must meet the criteria spelled out in the *Diagnostic and Statistical Manual of Mental Disorders* (DSM). This manual is published by the American Psychiatric Association and is used by mental health providers to diagnose mental conditions and by insurance companies to reimburse for treatment. Diagnostic criteria for cyclothymia include those below.

You've had numerous periods of elevated mood (hypomania) and many periods of depressive symptoms for at least two years.

Your periods of stable moods usually last less than two months.

Your symptoms significantly affect you socially, at work, at school or in other important functions.

You don't have manic episodes, major depression or schizoaffective disorder — a combination of schizophrenia symptoms, such as hallucinations or delusions, and mood disorder symptoms, such as mania or depression.

Your symptoms aren't caused by substance abuse or a medical condition.

Treatment

Cyclothymia requires lifelong treatment, even during periods when you feel better — usually guided by a mental health provider skilled in treating the condition. To treat cyclothymia, your doctor or mental health provider aims to: Decrease your risk of bipolar disorder I or Ⅱ, since cyclothymia carries a high risk of developing into more severe bipolar disorder; reduce the frequency and severity of your symptoms, allowing you to live a more balanced and enjoyable life; prevent a relapse of symptoms, through continued treatment during periods of remission (maintenance treatment); treat alcohol or other substance abuse problems, since they can worsen cyclothymia symptoms. The main treatments for cyclothymia are medications and psychotherapy.

Medications may help control cyclothymia symptoms and prevent episodes of hypomania and depression. Medications used to treat cyclothymia include:

Mood Stabilizers

Mood stabilizers help regulate and stabilize mood so that you don't swing between depression and hypomania. Lithium (Lithobid) has been widely used as a mood stabilizer. Anti-seizure medications, also known as anticonvulsants, are also used to prevent mood swings. Examples include valproic acid (Depakene), divalproex sodium (Depakote), carbamazepine (Tegretol, Equetro, others) and lamotrigine (Lamictal). Your doctor may recommend that you take mood stabilizers for the rest of your life to prevent and treat hypomanic episodes. Certain antipsychotic medications — such as olanzapine (Zyprexa), quetiapine (Seroquel) and risperidone (Risperdal) — may help people who don't benefit from the mood-stabilizing effects of anti-seizure medications.

Antianxiety Medications

Antianxiety medications, such as benzodiazepines, may help improve sleep.

Antidepressants

Use of antidepressants for cyclothymia is typically not recommended, unless they're combined with a mood stabilizer or antipsychotic. As with bipolar disorder I or II, taking antidepressants alone can trigger potentially dangerous manic episodes. Before taking antidepressants, carefully weigh the pros and cons with your doctor. If one medication doesn't work well for you, there are many others to consider. Keep trying until you find one that works well for you. Your doctor may advise combining certain medications for maximum effect. It can take several weeks after first starting a medication to notice an improvement in your cyclothymia symptoms. All medications have side effects and possible health risks. Talk to your doctor about the benefits and risks. Medications such as mood stabilizers may harm a developing fetus or nursing infant. Women with cyclothymic disorder who want to become pregnant or do become pregnant must fully explore with their health care providers the benefits and risks of medications.

Psychotherapy

Psychotherapy, also called counseling or talk therapy, can help you understand what cyclothymia is and how it's treated. Types of therapy that may help cyclothymia include:

Cognitive behavioral therapy

Cognitive behavioral therapy helps you identify unhealthy, negative beliefs and behaviors and replace them with healthy, positive ones. In addition, you can explore what triggers your hypomanic or depressive episodes and learn how to manage stress and cope with upsetting situations.

Family therapy

Family therapy helps you and your family members learn how to communicate, solve problems and resolve conflicts with each other. Family therapy helps identify stressors within the family that may contribute to unhealthy behavior patterns. Your family may also gain a better understanding of your condition and why you think and behave the way you do.

Group therapy

Group therapy provides a forum to communicate with and learn from others in a similar situation. It may also help build better relationship skills.

Interpersonal social rhythm therapy

This type of therapy helps you manage your daily routines (including your sleep schedule), improve your relationships and develop better communication skills so that interpersonal problems don't disrupt your routines.

Major Depression

Depression is a medical illness that causes a persistent feeling of sadness and loss of interest. Depression can cause physical symptoms, too. Also called major depression, major depressive disorder and clinical depression, it affects how you feel, think and behave. Depression can lead to a variety of emotional and physical problems. You may have trouble doing normal day-to-day activities, and depression may make you feel as if life isn't worth living. More than just about of the blues, depression isn't a weakness, nor is it something that you can simply "snap out" of. Depression is a chronic illness that usually requires long-term treatment, like diabetes or high blood pressure. But don't get discouraged. Most people with depression feel better with medication, psychological counseling or other treatment.

Symptoms and Signs

A constant sense of hopelessness and despair is a sign you may have major depression, also known as clinical depression. With major depression, it may be difficult to work, study, sleep, eat, and enjoy friends and activities. Some people have clinical depression only once in their life, while others have it several times in a lifetime. Major depression seems to occur from one generation to the next in some families, but may affect people with no family history of the illness. Most people feel sad or low at some point in their lives. But clinical depression is marked by a depressed mood most of the day, particularly in the morning, and a loss of interest in normal activities and relationships — symptoms that are present every day for at least 2 weeks.

Depression Symptoms Include:

Feelings of sadness or unhappiness;

Irritability or frustration, even over small matters;

Loss of interest or pleasure in normal activities;

Reduced sex drive;

Insomnia or excessive sleeping;

Changes in appetite, depression often causes decreased appetite and weight loss, but in some people it causes increased cravings for food and weight gain;

Agitation or restlessness, for example, pacing, hand-wringing or an inability to sit still;

Irritability or angry outbursts;

Slowed thinking, speaking or body movements;

Indecisiveness, distractibility and decreased concentration;

Fatigue, tiredness and loss of energy — even small tasks may seem to require a lot of effort;

Feelings of worthlessness or guilt, fixating on past failures or blaming yourself when things aren't going right;

Trouble thinking, concentrating, making decisions and remembering things;

Frequent thoughts of death, dying or suicide;

Crying spells for no apparent reason;

Unexplained physical problems, such as back pain or headaches.

For some people, depression symptoms are so severe that it's obvious something isn't right. Other people feel generally miserable or unhappy without really knowing why. Depression affects each person in different ways, so symptoms caused by depression vary from person to person. Inherited traits, age, gender and cultural background all play a role in how depression may affect you.

Depression Symptoms in Children and Teens

Common symptoms of depression can be a little different in children and teens than they are in adults. In younger children, symptoms of depression may include sadness, irritability, hopelessness and worry.

Symptoms in adolescents and teens may include anxiety, anger and avoidance of social interaction.

Changes in thinking and sleep are common signs of depression in adolescents and adults but are not as common in younger children.

In children and teens, depression often occurs along with behavior problems and other mental health conditions, such as anxiety or attention-deficit/hyperactivity disorder (ADHD). Schoolwork may suffer in children who are depressed. Depression symptoms in older adults, is not a normal part of growing older, and most seniors feel satisfied with their lives. However, depression can and does occur in older adults. Unfortunately, it often goes undiagnosed and untreated. Many adults with depression feel reluctant to seek help when they're feeling down.

In older adults, depression may go undiagnosed because symptoms, for example, fatigue, loss of appetite, sleep problems or loss of interest in sex, may seem to be caused by other illnesses.

Older adults with depression may have less obvious symptoms. They may feel dissatisfied with life in general, bored, helpless or worthless. They may always want to stay at home, rather than going out to socialize or doing new things. Suicidal thinking or feelings in older adults is a sign of serious depression that should never be taken lightly, especially in men. Of all people with depression, older adult men are at the highest risk of suicide.

Differential Diagnosis

Because depression is common and often goes undiagnosed, some doctors and health care providers may ask questions about your mood and thoughts during routine medical visits. They may even ask you to fill out a brief questionnaire to help check for depression symptoms. When doctors suspect someone has depression, they generally ask a number of questions and may do medical and psychological tests. These can help rule out other problems that could be causing your symptoms, pinpoint a diagnosis and also check for any related complications. These exams and tests generally include:

Physical Exam

This may include measuring your height and weight; checking your vital signs, such as heart rate, blood pressure and temperature; listening to your heart and lungs; and examining your abdomen.

Laboratory Tests

For example, your doctor may do a blood test called a complete blood count (CBC) or test your thyroid to make sure it's functioning properly.

Psychological Evaluation

To check for signs of depression, your doctor or mental health provider will talk to you about your thoughts, feelings and behavior patterns. He or she will ask about your symptoms, and whether you've had similar episodes in the past. You'll also discuss any thoughts you may have of suicide or self-harm. Your doctor may have you fill out a written questionnaire to help answer these questions.

Diagnostic Criteria for Depression

To be diagnosed with major depression, you must meet the symptom criteria spelled out in the *Diagnostic and Statistical Manual of Mental Disorders* (DSM). This manual is published by the American Psychiatric Association and is used by mental health providers to diagnose mental conditions and by insurance companies to reimburse for treatment. To be diagnosed with major depression, you must have five or more of the following symptoms over a two-week period. At least one of the symptoms must be either a depressed mood or a loss of interest or pleasure. Symptoms can be based on your own feelings or may be based on the observations of someone else. They include:

Depressed mood most of the day, nearly every day, such as feeling sad, empty or tearful (in children and adolescents, depressed mood can appear as constant irritability);

Diminished interest or feeling no pleasure in all — or almost all — activities most of the day, nearly every day;

Significant weight loss when not dieting, weight gain, or decrease or increase in appetite nearly every day (in children, failure to gain weight as expected can be a sign of depression);

Insomnia or increased desire to sleep nearly every day;

Either restlessness or slowed behavior that can be observed by others;

Fatigue or loss of energy nearly every day;

Feelings of worthlessness, or excessive or inappropriate guilt nearly every day;

Trouble making decisions, or trouble thinking or concentrating nearly every day;

Recurrent thoughts of death or suicide, or a suicide attempt.

To be considered major depression:

Your symptoms aren't due to a mixed episode — simultaneous mania and depression that can occur in bipolar disorder;

Symptoms must be severe enough to cause noticeable problems in day-to-day activities, such as work, school, social activities or relationships with others;

Symptoms are not due to the direct effects of something else, such as drug abuse, taking a medication or having a medical condition such as hypothyroidism;

Symptoms are not caused by grieving, such as temporary sadness after the loss of a loved one.

There are several other conditions with symptoms that can include depression. It's important to get an accurate diagnosis so you can get the appropriate treatment for your particular condition. Your doctor or mental health provider's evaluation will help determine if your symptoms of depression are caused by one of the following conditions:

Adjustment Disorder

An adjustment disorder is a severe emotional reaction to a difficult event in your life. It's a type of stress-related mental illness that may affect your feelings, thoughts and behavior.

Bipolar Disorder

This type of depression is characterized by mood swings that range from highs to lows. It's sometimes difficult to distinguish between bipolar disorder and depression, but it's important to get an accurate diagnosis so that you can get the proper treatment and medications.

Cyclothymia

Cyclothymia (si-klo-THI-me-uh), also called cyclothymic disorder, is a milder form of bipolar disorder.

Dysthymia

Dysthymia (dis-THI-me-uh) is a less severe but more chronic form of depression. While it's usually not disabling, dysthymia can prevent you from functioning normally in your daily routine and from living life to its fullest.

Postpartum Depression

This is a common type of depression that occurs in new mothers. It often occurs between two weeks and six months after delivery.

Psychotic Depression

This is severe depression accompanied by psychotic symptoms, such as delusions or hallucinations.

Seasonal Affective Disorder

This type of depression is related to changes in seasons and diminished exposure to sunlight.

Etiology & Pathogenesis

Considerable progress has been made in identifying and characterizing the etiologic factors in major affective disorders, but a comprehensive and detailed understanding of the etiology of these disorders has yet to be achieved. Tremendous advances in knowledge during the past 20 years have provided excellent leads for focused scientific inquiry into the causes of these disorders; these leads, in turn, have led to the development of very specific and effective treatments. Like many other human diseases, the affective disorders are the result of interactions between the patient's genetic makeup and the environment. Evidence continues to mount that significant genetic factors are involved in these disorders, but the genetic components do not appear to be so overwhelming that the disorder is manifested without any environmental challenges. In general, the causality of a major affective episode can effectively be conceptualized by using an interactional model of two intersecting continua both with progressive intensities. One involves the patient's inherited constitutional predisposition to develop affective episodes; this interacts with the second continuum of the environmental stresses and life events to which the patient is exposed. Thus, there are those individuals with very high genetic predispositions for affective psychopathology in whom the disorder will be manifested seemingly without identifiable precipitating events. In contrast, there are patients with lower genetic predisposition in whom the disorder is manifested only when the patient is exposed to more serious precipitating life events and cumulative life stresses.

Genetic Factors

Data derived from virtually every methodologic strategy in human genetics strongly suggest significant genetic influences in the major affective disorders, but as yet the mode of genetic transmission has not been established. The degree of genetic expression varies considerably from patient to patient and in some patients marked and predictable genetic factors are present; in others genetic expression appears to be significantly less influential. The twin studies have been one of the major research strategies used by psychiatric geneticists to attempt to quantify genetic loading in various psychiatric diseases. Twin studies in affective disorders have reported concordance rates among monozygotic (MZ) twins ranging from 33.3 to 75 percent, with an average of 65 percent. In contrast, the concordance rates for dizygotic (DZ) twins range from 9 to 23 percent, averaging 15 percent. The difference in concordance rates between MZ and DZ twins strongly suggests inherited genetic vulnerability. Further, there is evidence that even the polarity of the disorder may be genetically controlled, since there is an 80 percent concordance for bipolar and 59 percent concordance for unipolar disorders in MZ twins. In an attempt to separate the "nature" and "nurture" contributions to the development of affective disorders, the adoption study strategy has also been used. Unfortunately, because of methodologic problems and the paucity of subjects studied, no definitive answers are available. There is, however, a trend indicating that adoptees with affective disorders have a greater incidence of affective illness in their biologic parents than in their adopted parents. A large number of family studies have been conducted in the affective disorders. The standard paradigm is to make independent and blind diagnoses in the first-degree relatives of affective disorder patients, anticipating that if genetic components are present, the consanguineous relatives will manifest an increased risk for affective illness. First-degree relatives of bipolar patients have a morbidity risk for bipolar disorder ranging from 2.8% to 17.7% and a risk of 0 to 22.4%for unipolar depression. The first-degree relatives of unipolar patients have a risk of 6.4% to 17% for unipolar depression and of 0.3 to 29 percent for bipolar disorder. Thus, bipolar patients have both unipolar and bipolar disorders among their blood relatives, whereas unipolar patients have increased incidence for unipolar, but not bipolar, disorders in their relatives. Modern studies of genetic transmission combine careful family pedigree studies with molecular genetics in an attempt to identify the linkage between the specific gene markers and manifestation of major affective disorder in an afflicted or informative family. At present, no clear dominant or recessive inheritance pattern has been identified. It appears that genetic heterogeneity is present, which suggests a multiple threshold model in order to account for the varying degrees of genetic variability in the affective disorders. Genetic marker surveys in informative families have been conducted, including studies which have used genetically regulated markers that are etiologically significant in affective illness, such as the concentrations of dopamine B-hydroxylase, monoamine oxidase A, monoamine oxidase B, and lithium red blood cell (RBC) plasma ratio. No marker has yet been found which segregates to the presence of affective disorder. There is however, a small subgroup of bipolar patients who do manifest a linkage of protan-deutan (red-green) color blindness and the Xg blood group with the presence of bipolar disorder. Unfortunately this very interesting genetic linkage pattern has not been present in other families similarly afflicted with major affective disorder.

In summary, the genetic studies strongly indicate the inheritance of a vulnerability to affective illness, but the genetic expression is heterogeneous and the degree of vulnerability varies significantly. There is evidence that the genetic factors are stronger in bipolar disorder than in unipolar depression. There are currently several large-scale surveys combining molecular and pedigree methodologies which are either in progress or in the final stages of implementation, and it is possible that the gene (s) coding for affective disorders will be identified and cloned in the foreseeable future.

Neurotransmitter Systems

The most consistent search for etiologic mechanisms in the affective disorders has involved studies of the various neurotransmitter systems in the brain. The original biogenic amine hypothesis focused primarily on the central nervous system (CNS) neurotransmitters norepinephrine, serotonin, and dopamine, attributing depression and mania, respectively, to the deficiency or excess of these neurotransmitters at important synaptic sites in the brain. This hypothesis has stimulated and directed research in the field for many years, and data consistent with the hypothesis continue to emerge. Urinary and cerebrospinal fluid (CSF) studies of norepinephrine, its metabolite 3-methoxy-4-hydroxyphenethyleneglycol (MHPG), and the catalytic enzyme dopamine B-hydroxylase have been consistently reported as being increased or decreased in the predictable direction during depressed and manic episodes. More recently, increases in norepinephrine have been described in both mania and depression. Alterations in serotonin and its metabolites have also been identified in patients during depressive episodes. In addition, 5-hydroxyindole acetic acid (5-HIAA), a serotonin metabolite, has been found to be reduced in the CSF of depressed patients who make frequent and aggressive suicide attempts. Deficits in other neurotransmitters such as dopamine and gamma-aminobutyric acid (GABA) have also been identified in some patients with major depression. Finally, another neurotransmitter hypothesis which has directed research in the affective disorders is the cholinergic hypothesis, which postulates increased central cholinergic tone in depression, decreased, cholinergic tone in mania, and an imbalance between the cholinergic and adrenergic neurotransmitter systems as being a central pathophysiologic mechanism in affective disorders.

Within the last 5 years, there has been a shift of research focus from the neurotransmitter biosynthetic, storage, and release mechanisms in the presynaptic neuron to the study of receptors on postsynaptic neurons. There is growing evidence that postsynaptic receptor kinetics and activity are predictibly and consistently altered during affective episodes and by the psychotropic medications known to ameliorate these disorders. Future research in the pathophysiology of the affective disorders will be concentrated on the role of postsynaptic receptor systems and the cascade of intraneuronal biochemical events in the postsynaptic neuron which follow the binding of the neurotransmitter to the receptor.

In summary, there is a general agreement in the large number of studies which have been conducted to date that the relative paucity of a neurotransmitter or the inactivation or down-regulation of postsynaptic receptors has often been correlated with depressive episodes, but the reciprocal changes which one would predict have not been consistently identified in manic episodes.

Environmental Factors

There is little systematic data available indicating what role environmental stresses and untoward life events play or what types of stressors might be etiologically significant in the development of major affective episodes. Attempts have been made, for example, to relate early childhood loss and parental separation as predisposing factors for the future development of an affective illness, but the data are inconsistent. In general, studies have shown an overall temporal relationship between stressful and negative life events and the subsequent appearance of affective episodes. Research attempting to characterize qualitative differences in the impact of life stress have been disappointing, although serious life events such as the death of a child or a spouse, job loss, marked changes in social status, and even severe assaults on self-esteem have been linked to affective episodes. While the relationship between environmental stresses and the appearance of affective episodes has not always been demonstrated, generally speaking most experts agree that a single severe or multiple severe adverse events in life can interact with the constitutional predisposition of a patient and result in the triggering of an affective episode.

In further support of the influence of environmental events are the studies which have been conducted in higher primates. In these studies, phenomena which resemble or are analogous to the depressive states in humans are seen in monkeys following both mother/infant and peer separation paradigms. Furthermore, the monkey's "despair" response to the separation paradigms can be predictably enhanced by drugs known to specifically alter central concentrations and metabolism of various relevant CNS neurotransmitters (eg, norepinephrine, dopamine).

Biologic Rhythms

The marked tendency of major affective disorders to periodic manifestation and possibly to seasonal variations has stimulated hypotheses which suggest that the dysregulation of biologic rhythms may be centrally involved in the pathophysiology of affective disorders. There are reports of dysynchronization of circadian rhythms in some bipolar patients in which these patients manifested both rapid free-running circadian rhythms (eg, 23- versus 24-hour rhythms) and a phase delay in their rhythms. There is also a specific subgroup of patients with major depression in which the depressive episodes are manifested seasonally during the wintertime. These patients, while residing in more northern latitudes, experience major depressive episodes during the winter when days are significantly shorter and periods of darkness more prolonged; they do not experience depression of this type when residing in latitudes where the environmental light/ dark cycle is not as extreme.

Because depression is common and often goes undiagnosed, some doctors and health care providers may ask questions about your mood and thoughts during routine medical visits. They may even ask you to fill out a brief questionnaire to help check for depression symptoms.

Treatments

A primary care doctor can prescribe medications to relieve depression symptoms. However, many people need to see a doctor who specializes in diagnosing and treating mental health conditions (psychiatrist). Many people with depression also benefit from seeing a psychologist or other mental health counselor. Usually the most effective treatment for depression is a combination of medication and psychotherapy. If you have severe depression, a doctor, loved one or guardian may need to guide your care until you're well enough to participate in decision making. You may need a hospital stay, or you may need to participate in an outpatient treatment program until your symptoms improve. Here's a closer look at your depression treatment options.

Medications

A number of antidepressant medications are available to treat depression. There are several different types of antidepressants. Antidepressants are generally categorized by how they affect the naturally occurring chemicals in your brain to change your mood.

Selective serotonin reuptake inhibitors (SSRIs)

Many doctors start depression treatment by prescribing an SSRI. These medications are safer and generally cause fewer bothersome side effects than do other types of antidepressants. SSRIs include fluoxetine (Prozac), paroxetine (Paxil), sertraline (Zoloft), citalopram (Celexa) and escitalopram (Lexapro). The most common side effects include decreased sexual desire and delayed orgasm. Other side effects may go away as your body adjusts to the medication. They can include digestive problems, jitteriness, restlessness, headache and insomnia.

Serotonin and norepinephrine reuptake inhibitors (SNRIs)

These medications include duloxetine (Cymbalta), venlafaxine (Effexor XR) and desvenlafaxine (Pristiq). Side effects are similar to those caused by SSRIs. These medications can cause increased sweating, dry mouth, fast heart rate and constipation.

Norepinephrine and dopamine reuptake inhibitors (NDRIs)

Bupropion (Wellbutrin) falls into this category. It's one of the few antidepressants that doesn't cause sexual side effects. At high doses, bupropion may increase your risk of having seizures.

Atypical antidepressants

These medications are called atypical because they don't fit neatly into another antidepressant category. They include trazodone (Oleptro) and mirtazapine (Remeron). Both of these antidepressants are sedating and are usually taken in the evening. In some cases, one of these medications is added to other antidepressants to help with sleep. The newest medication in this class of drugs is vilazodone (Viibryd). Vilazodone has a low risk of sexual side effects. The most common side effects associated with vilazodone are diarrhea, nausea, vomiting and insomnia.

Tricyclic antidepressants

These antidepressants have been used for years and are generally as effective as newer medications. But because they tend to have more numerous and more severe side effects, a tricyclic antidepressant generally isn't prescribed unless you've tried an SSRI first without an improvement in your depression. Side effects can include dry mouth, blurred vision, constipation, urinary retention, fast heartbeat and confusion. Tricyclic antidepressants are also known to cause weight gain.

Monoamine oxidase inhibitors (MAOIs)

MAOIs — such as tranylcypromine (Parnate) and phenelzine (Nardil) — are usually prescribed as a last resort, when other medications haven't worked. That's because MAOIs can have serious harmful side effects. They require a strict diet because of dangerous (or even deadly) interactions with foods, such as certain cheeses, pickles and wines, and some medications including decongestants. Selegiline (Emsam) is a newer MAOI that you stick on your skin as a patch rather than swallowing. It may cause fewer side effects than other MAOIs. These medications can't be combined with SSRIs.

Other medication strategies

Your doctor may suggest other medications to treat your depression. These may include stimulants, mood-stabilizing medications, antianxiety medications or antipsychotic medications. In some cases, doctor may recommend combining two or more antidepressants or other medications for better effect. This strategy is known as augmentation.

Finding the right medication

Everyone's different, so finding the right medication or medications for you will likely take some trial and error. This requires patience, as some medications need eight weeks or longer to take full effect and for side effects to ease as your body adjusts. If you have bother some side effects, don't stop taking an antidepressant without talking to your doctor first. Some antidepressants can cause withdrawal symptoms unless you slowly taper off your dose, and quitting suddenly may cause a sudden worsening of depression. Don't give up until you find an antidepressant or medication that's suitable for you, you're likely to find one that works and that doesn't have intolerable side effects.

If antidepressant treatment doesn't seem to be working, your doctor may recommend a blood test to check for specific genes that affect how your body uses antidepressants. The cytochrome P450 (CYP450) genotyping test is one example of this type of exam. Genetic testing of this kind can help predict how well your body can or can't process (metabolize) a medication. This may help identify which antidepressant might be a good choice for you. These genetic tests may not be widely available, so they're an option only for people who have access to a clinic that offers them.

If you're pregnant or breast-feeding, some antidepressants may pose an increased health risk to your unborn child or nursing child. Talk to your doctor if you become pregnant or are planning on becoming pregnant.

Although most antidepressants are generally safe, be careful when taking them. The Food and Drug Administration (FDA) now requires that all antidepressant medications carry black box warnings. These are the strictest warnings that the FDA can issue for prescription medications.

The antidepressant warnings note that in some cases, children, adolescents and young adults under 25 may have an increase in suicidal thoughts or behavior when taking antidepressants, especially in the first few weeks after starting an antidepressant or when the dose is changed. Because of this risk, people in these age groups must be closely monitored by loved ones, caregivers and health care providers while taking antidepressants. Again, make sure you understand the risks of the various antidepressants. Working together, you and your doctor can explore options to get your depression symptoms under control.

Psychotherapy

Psychological counseling is another key depression treatment. Psychotherapy is a general term for a way of treating depression by talking about your condition and related issues with a mental health provider. Psychotherapy is also known as therapy, talk therapy, counseling or psychosocial therapy.

Through these talk sessions, you learn about the causes of depression so that you can better understand it. You also learn how to identify and make changes in unhealthy behavior or thoughts, explore relationships and experiences, find better ways to cope and solve problems, and set realistic goals for your life. Psychotherapy can help you regain a sense of happiness and control in your life and help ease depression symptoms such as hopelessness and anger. It may also help you adjust to a crisis or other current difficulty. There are several types of psychotherapy that are effective for depression. Cognitive behavioral therapy is one of the most commonly used therapies. This type of therapy helps you identify negative beliefs and behaviors and replace them with healthy, positive ones. It's based on the idea that your own thoughts — not other people or situations, determine how you feel or behave. Even if an unwanted situation doesn't change, you can change the way you think and behave in a positive way. Interpersonal therapy and psychodynamic psychotherapy are other types of counseling commonly used to treat depression.

Electroconvulsive Therapy (ECT)

In ECT, electrical currents are passed through the brain. This procedure is thought to affect levels of neurotransmitters in your brain. Although many people are leery of ECT and its side effects, it typically offers immediate relief of even severe depression when other treatments don't work. It's unclear how this therapy relieves the signs and symptoms of depression. The most common side effect is confusion, which can last from a few minutes to several hours. Some people also have memory loss, which is usually temporary. ECT is usually used for people who don't get better with medications and for those at high risk of suicide. ECT may be an option if you have severe depression when you're pregnant and can't take your regular medications. It can also be an effective treatment for older adults who have severe depression and can't take antidepressants for health reasons.

Hospitalization and Residential Treatment Programs

In some people, depression is so severe that a hospital stay is needed. Inpatient hospitalization may be necessary if you aren't able to care for yourself properly or when you're in immediate danger of harming yourself or someone else. Getting psychiatric treatment at a hospital can help keep you calm and safe until your mood improves. Partial hospitalization or day treatment programs also are helpful for some people. These programs provide the support and counseling you need while you get symptoms under control.

If standard depression treatment hasn't been effective, your psychiatrist may consider whether you might benefit from a less commonly used procedure, such as:

Vagus nerve stimulation

This treatment uses electrical impulses with a surgically implanted pulse generator to affect mood centers of the brain. This may be an option if you have chronic, treatment - resistant depression.

Transcranial magnetic stimulation

These treatments use powerful magnetic fields to alter brain activity. A large electromagnetic coil is held against your scalp near your forehead to produce an electrical current in your brain. Transcranial magnetic stimulation may be an option for those who haven't responded to antidepressants

Dysthymic Disorder

Dysthymia is a mild, but chronic, form of depression. Dysthymia (dis - THI - me - uh) symptoms usually last for at least two years, and often for much longer than that. Although dysthymia symptoms may be less intense than those of depression, dysthymia can actually affect your life more seriously because it lasts for so long. With dysthymia, you may lose interest in normal daily activities, feel hopeless, lack productivity and have a low self-esteem. People with dysthymia are often thought of as being overly critical, constantly complaining and incapable of having fun.

It is a long-term mild to moderate type of mood (emotion) disorder. It is the most common type of depression and is often seen among women. Dysthymia is when you feel depressed most of the day and are depressed for more days than not for at least two years. Dysthymia affects how you feel about yourself and life in general. It can involve a depressed mood or a loss of interest or pleasure in all or almost all of your usual activities. This may greatly affect your daily activities at school, work, or at home. Dysthymia may also cause you to have problems getting along with your family, friends, and other people. When dysthymia occurs with more severe depression, you may have something called double depression. Double depression happens when you have both dysthymia and major depression. This condition has more symptoms and is harder to treat. Ask your caregiver for more information about double depression. Diagnosing and treating dysthymia as soon as possible may relieve your symptoms and improve your quality of life.

Symptoms & Signs

According to the DSM, "The essential feature of Dysthymic Disorder is a chronically depressed mood that occurs for most of the day more days than not for at least 2 years". The following specific diagnostic criteria are reproduced verbatim (except for codings and page references) from the DSM - Ⅳ TR (where 'Ⅳ TR' indicates fourth edition, text revision). Diagnostic Criteria for Dysthymic Disorder show:

A. Depressed mood most of the day, for more days than not, as indicated either by subjective account or observation by others, for at least 2 years. Note: In children and adolescents, mood can be irritable and duration must be at least 1 year.

B. Presence, while depressed, of two (or more) of the following:

1. poor appetite or overeating;

2. insomnia or hypersomnia;

3. low energy or fatigue;

4. low self-esteem;

5. poor concentration or difficulty making decisions;

6. feelings of hopelessness.

C. During the 2-year period (1 year for children or adolescents) of the disturbance, the person has never been without the symptoms in Criteria A and B for more than 2 months at a time.

Differential Diagnosis

Tests and Guides

There is no lab test that can diagnose dysthymia. Caregivers use a guide to diagnose dysthymia. You have dysthymia if you have at least two symptoms linked to your depressed mood. The symptoms must be present for at least two years, during which there has not been a period of more than one or two months where you have not had any symptoms. It should also not be caused by other problems. These symptoms must be bad enough to cause problems with your daily activities and relationships.

Psychiatric Assessment

Caregivers will ask if you have a history of psychological trauma, such as physical, sexual, or mental abuse. They will ask if you were given the care that you needed. Caregivers will ask you if you have been a victim of a crime or natural disaster, or if you have a serious injury or disease. They will ask you if you have seen other people being harmed, such as in combat. You will be asked if you drink alcohol or use drugs at present or in the past. Caregivers will ask you if you want to hurt or kill yourself or others. How you answer these questions can help caregivers decide on treatment. To help during treatment, caregivers will ask you about such things as how you feel about it and your hobbies and goals. Caregivers will also ask you about the people in your life who support you.

Prognosis

The 5-year prognosis for dysthymic disorder in old age does not seem to be good, since only 29% of dysthymic men and 39% of dysthymic women recovered from their depression during the follow-up period. One reason for the poor prognosis is the high mortality among elderly people. The question of whether mortality is higher among dysthymic persons than among the nondepressed or in the total Finnish elderly population has not been answered in this report, since we have concentrated here on describing the total prognosis and factors associated with a poor prognosis in non-demented dysthymic patients surviving the follow-up period. Comparisons of mortality figures will be made later.

The DSM-Ⅲ dysthymic disorder (American Psychiatric Association, 2009) is a chronic mild depression that has lasted at least 2 years and presents at least three of the depressive symptoms listed. According to the criteria for dysthymic disorder, possible periods of normal mood could last from a few days to a few weeks, but not more than a few months at a time. The main criteria for discriminating dysthymic disorder from major depression are based on the duration and severity of symptoms. The DSM-Ⅲ classification was used to determine depression in our first epidemiological survey, and therefore it was also used in the follow-up study. The same general practitioner made the initial,1-year follow-up and 5-year follow-up examinations. He knew the population very well, which makes the follow-up results more reliable.

The DSM-Ⅲ category of chronic depression is relatively non-specific and recommendations have been presented for subtyping chronic depression in order to make definitions more specific. The DSM-Ⅲ classification used here regards dysthymic disorder as a chronic, minor affective disorder. We suggest that the symptomatology of patients in this series is less severe than of the patients followed up for longer periods in previous reports. Previous assessments of the long-term prognosis for depression have been made among patients suffering from major types of depression, and also differ from the investigation in their follow-up methodology and definitions of the outcome. Post, Cole and Baldwin and Jolley assessed not only the psychiatric status of the patients who were alive after the follow-up period but also that of the others before their death. Our interviews and ciinical examinations concerned only the patients who were alive after the 5-year follow-up, and no attempt was made to pronounce upon the psychiatric status of those who died.

Due to the differences in the methods, no critical comparison can be made between our results and the earlier ones. The factors associated with the outcome differ between the sexes, and the number of dysthymic men is smaller than that of dysthymic women, which will have affected the power of the statistical tests in the two groups. This should be kept in mind when considering the results.

Socioeconomic factors, viz a low educational level and a wage-earning occupation, played a greater role in the prognosis for the dysthymic men than in that for the dysthymic women. On the other hand, more severe depressive symptomatology, certain symptoms and low self-perceived health played a greater role in the outcome for the dysthymic women. Social norms and values may provide a partial explanation for these sex differences. It may be more difficult to accept a wage-earning occupation and a low educational level in a male role than in a female role, because the male role stresses independence. Also, it may be more acceptable for women to show symptoms of depression than for men, and even the overall symptomatology is stronger in women. The majority of the men who had an independent occupation had been farmers, ie landowners, and not possessing property such as a farm may have affected the self-respect of the men who had been wage-earners. Ocerall physical health and functional capacity at the beginning of the follow-up were not related to the prognosis, but poor self-perceived health and pronounced depressive symptoms at the outset were associated with a poor prognosis in the women.

Other Mood Disorder

Bipolar Disorder NOS

Some individuals with bipolar disorder not otherwise specified experience hyponianic episodes without intermittent depressive symptoms. Recurrent hypomania is often socially acceptable and adaptive for the individual. Hypomanic individuals usually experience benefits from increased energy, decreased need for sleep, increased gregariousness and greater creativity without the disabling consequences of grossly inappropriate social behavior or delusional preoccupation. Most hypomanic episodes do not call for phannacological treatment, however, in specific cases a trial of lithium carbonate may he advisable. The subtle nature of many hypomanic episodes are suits in frequent misdiagnosis. Patients and clinicians alike may see such episodes as "normal" and view only the depressive episodes as pathological. Rarely, bipolar disorder not otherwise specified is used to refer to patients in whom a manic episode is superimposed on schizophrenia or delusional disorder.

Depressive Disorder NOS

Depressive disorder not otherwise specified is a diagnosis given to individuals whose depressive symptoms do not meet the criteria tor severity or duration noted in the previously described categories. Individuals may experience occasional brief and mild episodes of depression not associated with psychosocial stress or may have dysthymia with periods of normal mood that last longer than several months. The point prevalence of minor, "brief", and slibsyndromal depressive disorders is estimated to be 7-8. Recent clinical and biological studies suggest that these conditions exist on a continuum with melancholia and may respond to antidepressant treatment.

Diagnostic problems may arise with depressed individuals whose mood change is either associated with or follows a psychotic process. The rationale for putting patients in this category such as schizoaffective disorder (also poorly defined) is unclear. Historically, the diagnosis of "atypical" depressive disorder has been iriosi often used to denote individuals with inood disorder with prominent phobic and anxious features, weight gain, hypersornina, and marked interpersonal rejection sensitivity. In DSM atypical features may be coded under any of the other major mood disorders. Such individuals may respond to MAO inhibitor medication.

Summary

It is difficult to conceive of an area in psychiatry in which the clinician's attitude, knowledge, and skills are more severely tested than in the diagnosis and treatment of mood disorders. Knowledge in this area lias been accumulating at such a rate that even the most diligent physician would be hard pressed to keep up with all of the new developments in the field. As reviewed in this chapter, there is considerable evidence for a biological basis for most mood disorders. Dala supporting this hypothesis have come from genetic, biochemical, psychopharrnacological, and neuroendocrinological investigations, and the hope is that psychiatric diagnosis in this area will become a more objective process as the research efforts continue.

Although subgroups of mood disorders seem relatively distinct from one another as described, in clinical practice tliere is often considerable overlap between symptoms of different disorders as well as ambiguity about the class in which a given individual belongs. With the present slate of knowledge, predictions about course of illness and response to treatment for patients with mood disorders remain as much an art as a science. Use of the biopsychosocial model in the understanding of mood disorders illustrates the awesome complexity of central nervous system regulation of affect but holds out promise of successful methods of treatment on many different levels.

Chapter 3 Personality Disorders

Personality disorders constitute a separate diagnostic category (Axis II) in the *American Psychiatric Association's Diagnostic and Statistical Manual of Mental Disorders*. Unlike the major mental disorders (Axis I), which are characterized by periods of illness and remission, personality disorders are generally ongoing. Often, they first appear in childhood or adolescence and persist throughout a person's lifetime. Aside from their persistence, the other major characteristic of personality disorders is inflexibility. Persons affected by these disorders have rigid personality traits and coping styles, are unable to adapt to changing situations, and experience impaired social and/or occupational functioning. A further difference between personality disorders and the major clinical syndromes listed in Axis I of DSM-Ⅳ-TR is that people with personality disorders may not perceive that there is anything wrong with their behavior and are not motivated to change it. Although the DSM-Ⅳ-TR lists specific descriptions of 10 personality disorders, these conditions are often difficult to diagnose. Some characteristics of the various disorders overlap. In other cases, the complexity of human behavior makes it difficult to pinpoint a clear dividing line between pathology and normality in the assessment of personality. In still other cases, persons may have more than one personality disorder, complicating the diagnosis. There also has been relatively little research done on some of the personality disorders listed in DSM-Ⅳ-TR.

Characteristics of Personality Disorder

Personality disorders are mental illnesses that share several unique qualities. They contain symptoms that are enduring and play a major role in most, if not all, aspects of the person's life. While many disorders vacillate in terms of symptom presence and intensity, personality disorders typically remain relatively constant. To be diagnosed with a disorder in this category, a psychologist will look for the following criteria:

Symptoms have been present for an extended period of time, are inflexible and pervasive, and are not a result of alcohol or drugs or another psychiatric disorder. The history of symptoms can be traced back to adolescence or at least early adulthood.

The symptoms have caused and continue to cause significant distress or negative consequences in different aspects of the person's life.

Symptoms are seen in at least two of the following areas:

Thoughts (ways of looking at the world, thinking about self or others, and interacting);

Emotions (appropriateness, intensity, and range of emotional functioning);

Interpersonal Functioning (relationships and interpersonal skills);

Impulse Control.

Etiology and Pathophysiology

It was commonly held that the personality disorders reflected the warping effect of adverse early social environment. Now there is mounting evidence that personality is, in great measure, biologically determined. Both genetic and constitutional (ie, intrauterine and early physical developmental) factors may be important.

Genetic Factors

Although not all personality disorders have been examined, for the majority there is a severalfold increase in concordance between monozygotic twins compared with dizygotic twins.

Some of the most careful work has been with antisocial personality. Here it is noted that prevalence among men is three - to fourfold higher than in women, and that first - degree relatives of persons diagnosed as antisocial show increased prevalence of antisocial personality, alcoholism, and somatization disorder (Briquet's syndrome). The latter is characterized by intractable multiorgan system complaints in women who often have a histrionic personality. The association of these two disorders in the same pedigrees has led to suggestions that Briquet's syndrome and antisocial disorder are expressions in women and men of a common biogenetic substrate.

The operation of genetic factors in antisocial personality is further demonstrated by the finding that biologic offspring of antisocial and alcoholic parents have a higher risk of developing antisocial personality disorder even if they are raised by adoptive parents who do not have any antisocial traits. The converse has also been demonstrated: children adopted by antisocial parents tend not to develop antisocial disorder themselves unless they have antisocial personality or alcoholism in their blood relatives.

The XYY chromosomal abnormality was once thought to be related to antisocial personality disorder. More recent studies indicate that although XYY might be overrepresented in certain prison populations, the vast majority of XYY men are not antisocial.

The schizotypal, borderline, and schizoid diagnoses evolved orginally from the notion that there ought to be a "preclinical" form of schizophrenia characterized by lesser severity or fewer numbers of the cognitive and interpersonal symptons of that disorder. Thus, the schizotypal personality might, theoretically, embody earlier forms of the disturbance in thinking, perception, and attention that occur in schizophrenia; whereas the schizoid personality would represent the interpersonal awkwardness inherent in that disorder. Genetic studies have confirmed that there is some increase in schizotypal (but not schizoid) personality in relatives of diagnosed schizophrenics.

The borderline personality is genetically heterogeneous. Up to 50 percent of borderline patients have a family history of affective disorder. Borderline disorder itself, as well as other personality disorders, are also more common in first - degree relatives of borderline patients, but schizophrenia is not consistently related.

There is increased schizophrenia in the families of patients with paranoid personality. For compulsive disorder, twin studies indicate increased concordance for obsessional traits in monozygotic versus dizygotic twins. There is also some evidence that orderliness and rigidity run in families. The other personality disorders have not been studied carefully from a biogenetic standpoint.

Constitutional Factors

Although there is good evidence that infants are born with certain temperamental characteristics (eg, high versus low activity level; long versus short attention span), there is little evidence that these temperamental characteristics persist into adolescence. Infant temperament does not appear to predict later personality disorder with the exception that the "difficult child" (irritable, hard to console, irregular rhythms) tends to exhibit more behavioral disturbances. Low intelligence quotient and poor physical health as a child have been noted more frequently in the histories of persons with personality disorders.

Neurophysiologic and Neuroendocrine Correlates

Several neurophysiologic and biochemical changes may be associated with personality disorders. Abnormal slow waves and spikes have been reported in the EEGs of antisocial persons. For borderline patients, patterns suggestive of periodic limbic epileptiform discharges have sometimes been noted.

Some observers suggest that a common neurophysiologic feature of both antisocial and hysterical disorders is reduced cortical arousal to cortical stimulation, secondary to increased inhibition from lower brain regions. This may be coupled with motor disinhibition in antisocial persons and autonomic disinhibition in hysterics.

The schizotypal personality disorder has been associated with disturbance in smooth pursuit eye movement (SPEM). Since many schizophrenics are also poor trackers, it may be that schizotypals share with schizophrenics decreased neural effectiveness in "centering". Some schizophrenics and schizotypals have lowered platelet monoamine oxidase (MAO) levels. It has been suggested that lowered MAO activity could be related to inefficient degradation of certain biologically active amines, leading to accumulation of substance with psychotomimetic properties.

Cortisol escape from dexamethasone suppression and shortened rapid eye movement (REM) latency (REM latency is the time between falling asleep and first REM episode) are associated with affective disorder. Both phenomena have also been observed in borderline and obsessive - compulsive personalities, suggesting a link among the affective, borderline, and obsessive - compulsive disorders. There are no specific data on biologic correlates of the other personality disorders.

Environmental Factors

Early social environment has proved to be an inconsistent predictor of late personality disorder. For example, one study found that 30 percent of men with personality disorders who were investigated reported lack of maternal warmth as children, but so did 24 percent of controls. Multiple problems in the early environment were found in 16 percent of personality-disordered men and 10 percent of those without disorders. Being abused as a child is associated with violence in later life.

The relative weakness of both temperamental and environmental factors as predictors of future personality disorder has led to a "goodness of fit" hypothesis. This theory suggests that later behavioral disorders are more likely when there is a severe mismatch between a child's temperament and childrearing practices and environmental circumstances.

Diagnosis of Personality Disorders

The Diagnositc and Statistical Manual of the American Psychiatric Association (DSM-Ⅲ) recognizes 11 distinctive personality disorders. These are grouped into three thematic clusters. Paranoid, schizoid, and schizotypal personality disorders are characterized by oddness or eccentricity. Histrionic, narcissistic, antisocial, and borderline personality disorders share a dramatic presentation along with self-centeredness, emotionality, and erratic behavior. Anxiety and fear underlie avoidant, dependent, compulsive, and passive-aggressive personalities.

The DSM-Ⅲ diagnostic classification scheme stipulates specific inclusion and exclusion criteria for diagnosis of each disorder. Since the number of criteria for individual disorders ranges from 3 to 24, the descriptions in this chapter are highlights rather than complete expositions. The reader is referred to the DSM-Ⅲ for the detailed listing of the necessary signs and symptoms required to make the diagnosis of the various personality disorders.

Table 1 Personality disorders in ICD-10 and DSM-Ⅳ

ICD-10	DSM-Ⅳ[a]
Paranoid	Paranoid
Schizoid	Schizoid
Schizotypal[b]	Schizotypal
Dyssocial	Antisocial
Emotionally unstable, borderline type	Emotionally unstable, borderline type
Histrionic	Histrionic
Anxious	Avoidant
Dependent	Dependent
Anankastic	Obsessive-compulsive
Enduring personality change after catastrophic experience	Enduring personality change after psychiatric illness
Organic personality disorder[c]	Personality change due to general medical condition[d]
Other specific personality disorders and mixed and other personality disorders	Personality disorder not otherwise specified

a Included within an appendix to DSM-Ⅳ are proposed criteria sets for passive-aggressive (negativistic) personality disorder and depressive personality disorder.

b ICD-10 schizotypal disorder is consistent with DSM-Ⅳ schizotypal personality disorder but included within the section of Schizophrenia, schizotypal, and delusional disorders.

c Included within section of organic mental disorders.

d Included within section of mental disorders due to a general medical condition not elsewhere classified.

Schizotypal Personality Disorder

Schizotypal persons share with schizophrenics certain eccentricities of thinking, perception, speech, and interpersonal interaction; however, the degree and pervasiveness of such "schizophrenic - like" symptomatology is not sufficient to meet diagnostic criteria for schizophrenia. Odd speech (eg, vague, circumstantial, metaphorical), ideas of reference (inappropriately inferring that neutral events have some special relevance to the person), magical thinking, and suspiciousness can be prominent. Many schizotypal persons are also socially isolated, and this can lead to confusion with schizoid personality.

Borderline Personality Disorder

Borderline persons have been described as having "stable instability", characterized by chronic difficulty in regulating mood and interpersonal attachments and in maintaining a consistent self - image. Borderline persons can manifest impulsive behavior, some of it self - damaging (eg, self - mutilation, suicidal behavior). Their mood is unpredictable. Some have brief outbursts of anger, irritability, sadness, and fear. Others suffer from a chronic emptiness. Despite having chaotic interpersonal relationships punctuated by intense love and hate, borderline persons generally are intolerant of being alone. The defense mechanism of "splitting" (regarding persons and events either as "all good" or "all bad") can be prominent.

Histrionic Personality Disorder

People with a histrionic personality have seemingly intense but actually superficial relationships. They present in a dramatic, engaging, but self - centered fashion. There is an exaggerated expression of emotions, attention seeking, craving for excitement, and a tendency to overreact. While superficially warm and charming, histrionic persons are generally perceived as shallow, inconsiderate, self - indulgent, vain, demanding, dependent, and manipulative. Some make frequent suicidal threats or attempts.

Narcissistic Personality Disorder

The narcissistic person has an inflated sense of self - importance, and may be preoccupied with being unique, powerful, and gifted. The patient exaggerates his or her talents and contributions, seeks admiration, and uses others to achieve a better position, while being indifferent to their feelings and needs. A rejection can produce excessive rage, inferiority, shame, or humiliation. The narcissistic person has difficulty seeing others in a realistic light, tending either to overidealize or devalue them.

Antisocial Personality Disorder

Antisocial behavior is characterized by unconcern with the rules and expectations of society and repeated violation of the rights of others. The diagnosis is limited to adults (persons under 18 with antisocial features are classified as having conduct disorder) and requires a history of antisocial behaviors which have their onset before age 15. Such behaviors include truancy, delinquency, running away from home, lying, precocious sexuality, troubles with the law, and alcohol or drug abuse. Beyond such historical considerations, the antisocial diagnosis requires current evidence of certain deviant behaviors which include irresponsibility in work, as a parent, in financial matters, and in personal behavior (eg, recklessness, driving while intoxicated). Additionally, antisocial persons will usually commit multiple illegal acts, lie and deceive, manifest an inability to maintain a long - term attachment to a sexual partner, and exhibit irritability and agressiveness. Alcohol or other substance abuse is common.

Avoidant Personality Disorder

People who are inappropriately concerned with rejection or humiliation, and for this reason avoid close ties with others, are classified as having an avoidant personality disorder. Despite being withdrawn, they give evidence for wishing that they did have intimate relations with others. In contrast with the narcissistic individual, the avoidant person tends to manifest low self- esteem and a tendency to exaggerate his or her shortcomings.

Dependent Personality Disorder

Dependent people allow others to assume responsibility for major aspects of their life and decision making. Because they see themselves as helpless or inept, they are willing to subordinate their needs and wishes to those of others in order to avoid taking personal responsibility.

Passive- aggressive Personality Disorder

Passive - aggressive people resent responsibility, either social or work - related. Rather than expressing their opposition directly, they tend to procrastinate, dawdle, behave stubbornly, work inefficiently, and "forget". As a consequence, they fail to achieve their potential.

Compulsive Personality Disorder

This disorder, which is equivalent to the term obsessive - compulsive personality, describes people who tend to be preoccupied with rules, procedures, and detail. They are often stubbornly insistent on certain things being done a particular way, yet at other times may become indecisive to the point of ineffectiveness. Compulsives tend to value their work and possessions more than their interpersonal relationships. They have difficulties expressing warm and tender feelings toward others and are sometimes seen as stiff, cold, and awkward.

A typical, Mixed, or Other Personality Disorder

This residual DSM - Ⅲ category accommodates personality disturbances that do not fit neatly into any of the categories listed above. The most commonly used is mixed personality disorder, which indicates that an individual's behavior fulfills the criteria for more than one personality disorder, eg, passive - aggressive and dependent. Atypical personality disorder is used when a personality disorder is suspected but there is not sufficient information to make a clear classification. Other personality disorder indicates presence of a personality disturbance not specifically included in DSM - lll, eg, masochistic, impulsive, or immature personality (which are concepts from other diagnostic schemes). One increasingly recognized disorder is adult attention deficit disorder (ADD), a residual form of childhood ADD (hyperkinesis). As adults, such individuals continue to have problems in attending and manifest labile mood, explosive temper, impulsivity, stress intolerance, and inability to complete tasks. They may also manifest a paradoxical (calming) reaction to central nervous system (CNS) stimulants.

Many of these traits, however, can be problematic and even maladaptive. If one or more of them result in a clinically significant level of impairment to social or occupational functioning or personal distress, it would be appropriate to suggest that a disorder of personality is present. The World Health Organization's International Classification of Diseases (ICD-10) includes ten personality disorder diagnoses, as does the American Psychiatric Association's Diagnostic and Statistical Manual of Mental Disorders (DSM-Ⅳ). However, there are important differences between these two prominent nomenclatures (Table1). For example, ICD-10 does not include narcissistic personality disorder, DSM-Ⅳ does not include enduring personality change after catastrophic experience or enduring personality change after psychiatric illness, and ICD-10 classifies the DSM-Ⅳ schizotypal personality disorder as a form of schizophrenia rather than a personality disorder.

In DSM-Ⅳ, personality disorders (along with mental retardation) are diagnosed on a separate axis (Axis Ⅱ). ICD-10 (2) does not include a multiaxial system. There are compelling reasons for the separate axis placement. Personality disorders can provide a disposition for the onset of many of the Axis I disorders, as well as have a significant effect on their course and treatment. The reason that the authors of the multiaxial system of DSM-Ⅲ wanted to draw attention to personality disorders was precisely because of the accumulating evidence that the quality and quantity of preexisting personality disturbance may influence the predisposition, manifestation, course, and response to treatment of various Axis I conditions.

In addition, personality features are typically egosyntonic and involve characteristics that the person has come to accept as an integral part of the self. Personality traits are integral to each person's sense of self, as they include what people value, how they view themselves, and how they act most every day throughout much of their lives. Most Axis I disorders, like most medical disorders, are experienced by persons as conditions or syndromes that come upon them. Personality disorders, in contrast, will often concern the way persons consider themselves to be.

Finally, personality disorders can be related conceptually to the general personality functioning evident in all persons, the assessment of which would be of potential relevance to virtually every psychiatric patient. Some of these personality traits will be problematic to treatment, and others will be facilitative. Much of the research on the contribution of personality to the etiology of Axis I disorders has in fact concerned personality traits, such as neuroticism, introversion, and sociotropy, that are evident within general personality functioning.

The placement of personality disorders on a separate axis has been effective in increasing their recognition in clinical settings, but perhaps the pendulum has swung so far that clinicians and researchers are now confusing Axis I disorders with personality disorders. The boundaries of the anxiety, mood, and other Axis I disorders have also been expanding with each edition of the diagnostic manual. Axis I now includes diagnoses that shade imperceptibly into normal personality functioning and have an age of onset and course that are virtually indistinguishable from a personality disorder (eg, generalized social anxiety and early onset dysthymia). Some clinicians and researchers have therefore suggested that the multiaxial system be abandoned and others have even proposed that the personality disorders be deleted altogether from the diagnostic manual and replaced by early onset and chronic variants of existing Axis I disorders. A precedent for this proposal is the ICD-10 classification of DSM-Ⅳ schizotypal personality disorder as a variant of schizophrenia.

Many of the existing personality disorders could not be replaced meaningfully by an early onset variant of an Axis I disorder, notably the narcissistic, dependent, and histrionic. One potential solution might be to simply delete them. The loss of the narcissistic personality disorder might not be missed internationally, as it is already excluded from ICD-10. Clinicians with a neurophysiological orientation may also fail to miss the dependent and histrionic diagnoses, as they lack any meaningful understanding from this theoretical perspective. Another potential solution would be to include a new section of the diagnostic manual for disorders of interpersonal relatedness. DSM-Ⅳ and ICD-10 currently have sections devoted to disorders of mood, anxiety, impulse dyscontrol, eating, somatization, sleep, substance use, cognition, sex, learning, and communication but, surprisingly, no section devoted to disorders of interpersonal relatedness. Interpersonal relatedness is a fundamental component of healthy and unhealthy psychological functioning that is as important to well being as the existing sections of the diagnostic manual. A new section devoted to disorders of interpersonal relatedness would provide marital and family clinicians with a section of the manual that is more compatible with the focus of their clinical interventions and would account for much of the personality disorder symptomatology that is not well accounted for by existing Axis I diagnoses.

There are, however, significant problems with both options. Both would remove from the diagnostic manual any meaningful reference to or recognition of the existence of personality functioning, for which there is substantial and compelling empirical support. In addition, reformulating personality disorders as early onset and chronic variants of existing (or new) Axis I disorders may simply create more diagnostic problems than it solves. For example, persons have constellations of maladaptive personality traits that are not well described by just one or even multiple personality disorder diagnoses. These constellations of maladaptive personality traits will be even less well described by multiple diagnoses of "comorbid" mood, anxiety, impulse dyscontrol, delusional, disruptive behavior, and interpersonal disorders.

Psychological Testing for Personality Disorders

A qualified mental health diagnostician administers lengthy tests and personal interviews to determine the existence and virulence of a personality disorder.

The predictive power of these tests — often based on literature and scales of traits constructed by scholars — is hotly disputed. Still, they are far preferable to subjective impressions of the diagnostician which are often amenable to manipulation.

The Minnesota Multiphasic Personality Inventory. Diagnostic test composed of 567 true-or-false questions arranged in three validity scales and ten dimensional clinical scales. The latter measure hypochondriasis, depression,hysteria, psychopathic deviation, masculinity-femininity, paranoia, psychasthenia, schizophrenia, hypomania, and social introversion. There are also scales for alcoholism, post-traumatic stress disorder, and personality disorders.

The interpretation of the MMPI-Ⅱ is now fully computerized. The computer is fed with the patients' age, sex, educational level, and marital status and does the rest. The Millon Clinical Multiaxial Inventory-Ⅲ (MCMI-Ⅲ) tests for personality disorders and attendant anxiety and depression. The third edition was formulated in 1996 by Theodore Millon and Roger Davis.

Millon Clinical Multiaxial Inventory. Diagnostic test composed of 157 true-or-false items. The MCMI-Ⅲ consists of 24 clinical scales and 3 modifier scales. The modifier scales serve to identify Disclosure (a tendency to hide a pathology or to exaggerate it), Desirability (a bias towards socially desirable responses), and Debasement (endorsing only responses that are highly suggestive of pathology). Next, the Clinical Personality Patterns (scales) which represent mild to moderate pathologies of personality, are: Schizoid, Avoidant, Depressive, Dependent, Histrionic, Narcissistic, Antisocial, Aggressive (Sadistic), Compulsive, Negativistic, and Masochistic. Millon considers only the Schizotypal, Borderline, and Paranoid to be severe personality pathologies and dedicates the next three scales to them.

The last ten scales are dedicated to Axis I and other clinical syndromes: Anxiety Disorder, Somatoform Disorder, Bipolar Manic Disorder, Dysthymic Disorder, Alcohol Dependence, Drug Dependence, Posttraumatic Stress, Thought Disorder, Major Depression, and Delusional Disorder.

Scoring is easy and runs from 0 to 115 per each scale, with 85 and above signifying a pathology. The configuration of the results of all 24 scales provides serious and reliable insights into the tested subject. The Narcissistic Personality Inventory (NPI) is used to spot narcissistic traits.

The Borderline Personality Organization Scale (BPO) was designed in 1985. It sorts the responses of respondents into 30 relevant scales. It indicates the existence of identity diffusion, primitive defenses, and deficient reality testing.

To these one may add the Personality Diagnostic Questionnaire-Ⅳ, the Coolidge Axis Ⅱ Inventory, the Personality Assessment Inventory, the excellent, literature-based, Dimensional assessment of Personality Pathology, and the comprehensive Schedule of Nonadaptive and Adaptive Personality and Wisconsin Personality Disorders Inventory.

The next diagnostic aim is to understand the way the patient or client functions in relationships, copes with intimacy, and responds to triggers.

The Relationship Styles Questionnaire (RSQ) contains 30 self-reported items and identifies distinct attachment styles (secure, fearful, preoccupied, and dismissing). The Conflict Tactics Scale (CTS) (1979) is a standardized scale of the frequency and intensity of conflict resolution tactics - especially abusive stratagems - used by members of a dyad (couple).

The Multidimensional Anger Inventory (MAI) assesses the frequency of angry responses, their duration, magnitude, mode of expression, hostile outlook, and anger-provoking triggers.

The Rorschach Inkblot Test is a diagnostic test comprised of 10 ambiguous inkblots printed on 18×24 cm cards, in both black and white and color. The cards and the diagnostician's questions provoke free associations in the test subject. These are recorded verbatim together with the inkblot's spatial position and orientation. The patient can then add details and comment on his choices.

Scoring is based on the parts of the cards referred to in the subject's responses (location), the correspondence between the blot and the answers provided (determinant), the content of the responses, how unique or common they are (popularity), how coherent are the patient's narratives (organizational activity), and how well does the patient's percept fit the card (form quality).

The interpretation of the test relies on both the scores obtained and on what we know about mental health disorders. The test teaches the skilled diagnostician how the subject processes information and what is the structure and content of his internal world. These provide meaningful insights into the patient's defenses, reality test, intelligence, fantasy life, and psychosexual make-up.

The Thematic Appreciation Test (TAT) is a diagnostic test comprised of 31 cards. One card is blank and the other thirty include blurred but emotionally powerful (or even disturbing) photographs and drawings. Subjects are asked to tell a story based on the content of the cards. The TAT was developed in 1935 by Morgan and Murray.

The patient's reactions (in the form of brief narratives) are recorded by the tester verbatim. Some examiners prompt the patient to describe the aftermath or outcomes of the stories, but this is a controversial practice. The TAT is scored and interpreted simultaneously. Murray suggested to identify the hero of each narrative (the figure representing the patient); the inner states and needs of the patient, derived from his or her choices of activities or gratifications; what Murray calls the "press", the hero's environment which imposes constraints on the hero's needs and operations; and the thema, or the motivations developed by the hero in response to all of the above.

The Structured Clinical Interview (SCID-II) was formulated in 1997 by First, Gibbon, Spitzer, Williams, and Benjamin. It is based on the language of criteria for personality disorders in the the DSM-Ⅳ. Its 12 groups of questions correspond to the 12 personality disorders. The scoring is simple: either the trait is absent, subthreshold, true, or there is "inadequate information to code".

The SCID-II can be administered to third parties (a spouse, an informant, a colleague) or self-administered (in a reduced format with 119 questions). The Structured Interview for Disorders of Personality (SIDP-Ⅳ) was composed by Pfohl, Blum and Zimmerman in 1997. It also covers the self-defeating personality disorder from the DSM-Ⅲ. It is conversational and the questions are grouped into 10 topics such as Emotions or Interests and Activities. There is a version of the SIDP-Ⅳ in which the questions are grouped by personality disorder. The scoring classifies items as present, subthreshold, present, or strongly present.

Yet, even a complete battery of tests, administered by experienced professionals sometimes fails to identify personality disorders. Such patients are uncanny in their ability to deceive their evaluators.

Paranoid Personality Disorder

In fact, the central characteristic of people with PPD is a high degree of mistrustfulness and suspicion when interacting with others. Even friendly gestures are often interpreted as being manipulative or malevolent. Whether the patterns of distrust and suspicion begin in childhood or in early adulthood, they quickly come to dominate the lives of those suffering from PPD. Such people are unable or afraid to form close relationships with others.

They suspect strangers, and even people they know, of planning to harm or exploit them when there is no good evidence to support this belief. As a result of their constant concern about the lack of trustworthiness of others, patients with this disorder often have few intimate friends or close human contacts. They do not fit in and they do not make good "team players". Interactions with others are characterized by wariness and not infrequently by hostility. If they marry or become otherwise attached to someone, the relationship is often characterized by pathological jealousy and attempts to control their partner. They often assume their sexual partner is "cheating" on them.

People suffering from PPD are very difficult to deal with. They never seem to let down their defenses. They are always looking for and finding evidence that others are against them. Their fear, and the threats they perceive in the innocent statements and actions of others, often contributes to frequent complaining or unfriendly withdrawal or aloofness. They can be confrontational, aggressive and disputatious. It is not unusual for them to sue people they feel have wronged them. In addition, patients with this disorder are known for their tendency to become violent.

Despite all the unpleasant aspects of a paranoid lifestyle, however, it is still not sufficient to drive many people with PPD to seek therapy. They do not usually walk into a therapist's office on their own. They distrust mental health care providers just as they distrust nearly everyone else. If a life crisis, a family member or the judicial system succeeds in getting a patient with PPD to seek help, therapy is often a challenge. Individual counseling seems to work best but it requires a great deal of patience and skill on the part of the therapist. It is not unusual for patients to leave therapy when they perceive some malicious intent on the therapist's part. If the patient can be persuaded to cooperate — something that is not easy to achieve — low-dose medications are recommended for treating such specific problems as anxiety, but only for limited periods of time.

Symptoms and Signs

A core symptom of PPD is a generalized distrust of other people. Comments and actions that healthy people would not notice come across as full of insults and threats to someone with the disorder. Yet, generally, patients with PPD remain in touch with reality; they don't have any of the hallucinations or delusions seen in patients with psychoses. Nevertheless, their suspicions that others are intent on harming or exploiting them are so pervasive and intense that people with PPD often become very isolated. They avoid normal social interactions. And because they feel so insecure in what is a very threatening world for them, patients with PPD are capable of becoming violent. Innocuous comments, harmless jokes and other day-to-day communications are often perceived as insults.

Paranoid suspicions carry over into all realms of life. Those burdened with PPD are frequently convinced that their sexual partners are unfaithful. They may misinterpret compliments offered by employers or coworkers as hidden criticisms or attempts to get them to work harder. Complimenting a person with PPD on their clothing or car, for example, could easily be taken as an attack on their materialism or selfishness.

Because they persistently question the motivations and trustworthiness of others, patients with PPD are not inclined to share intimacies. They fear such information might be used against them. As a result, they become hostile and unfriendly, argumentative or aloof. Their unpleasantness often draws negative responses from those around them. These rebuffs become "proof" in the patient's mind that others are, indeed, hostile to them. They have little insight into the effects of their attitude and behavior on their generally unsuccessful interactions with others. Asked if they might be responsible for negative interactions that fill their lives, people with PPD are likely to place all the blame on others. A brief summary of the typical symptoms of PPD includes:

Suspiciousness and distrust of others;

Questioning hidden motives in others;

Feelings of certainty, without justification or proof, that others are intent on harming or exploiting them;

Social isolation;

Aggressiveness and hostility;

Little or no sense of humor.

History and Prognosis

Paranoid personality disorder occurs in about 0.5%-2.5% of the general population. It is seen in 2%-10% of psychiatric outpatients. It occurs more commonly in males. A large long-term Norwegian twin study found paranoid personality disorder to be modestly heritable and to share a portion of its genetic and environmental risk factors with schizoid and schizotypal personality disorder. It is often a chronic, lifelong condition; the long-term prognosis is usually not encouraging. Feelings of paranoia, however, can be controlled to a degree with successful therapy. Unfortunately, many patients suffer the major symptoms of the disorder throughout their lives.

Schizoid Personality Disorder

Schizoid personality disorder is characterized by a persistent withdrawal from social relationships and lack of emotional responsiveness in most situations. It is sometimes referred to as a "pleasure deficiency" because of the seeming inability of the person affected to experience joyful or pleasurable responses to life situations.

It is common for a person with schizoid personality disorder to avoid groups of people or appear disinterested in social situations even when they involve family. They are often perceived by others as socially inept.

A closely related trait is the absence of emotional expression. This apparent void of emotion is routinely interpreted by others as disinterested, lacking concern and insensitive to the needs of others. The person with schizoid personality disorder has particular difficulty expressing anger or hostility. In the absence of any recognizable emotion, the person portrays a dull demeanor and is easily overlooked by others. The typical person with schizoid personality disorder prefers to be viewed as "invisible" since it aids their quest to avoid social contact with others.

The person with schizoid personality disorder may be able to hold a job and meet the expectations of an employer if the responsibilities do not require more than minimal interpersonal involvement. People with this disorder may be married, but do not develop close intimate relationships with their spouse and typically show no interest in sexual relations. Their speech is typically slow and monotonous with a lethargic demeanor. Because their tendency is to turn inward, they can easily become preoccupied with their own thoughts to the exclusion of what is happening in their environment. Attempts to communicate may drift into tangents or confusing associations. They are also prone to being absent minded.

Symptoms and Signs

For decades there has been controversy about whether patients with admixtures of schizophrenic and mood symptoms were suffering from schizophrenia, an atypical variety of bipolar disorder, or a separate disorder entirely. A number of diagnostic labels have been applied to this group of patients, including (but not limited to) cycloid psychosis, atypical schizophrenia, good - prognosis schizophrenia, and remitting schizophrenia. The term "schizoaffective disorder", originated by Jacob S. Kasanin in 1933, has prevailed, although the boundaries with other disorders are still debated. In modern diagnostic practice, many of these patients are diagnosed as having psychotic mood disorders.

People with SPD are often perceived as aloof, cold, and indifferent, which causes interpersonal difficulty. Most individuals diagnosed with SPD have trouble establishing personal relationships or expressing their feelings in a meaningful way, and may remain passive in the face of unfavorable situations. Their communication with other people may be indifferent and concise at times. Because of their lack of meaningful communication with other people, those who are diagnosed with SPD are not able to develop accurate reflections of themselves with respect to how well they are getting along with others. Such reflections are important for a person's self awareness and ability to assess the impact of their own actions in social situations. R.D. Laing suggests that without being enriched by injections of interpersonal reality, there occurs an impoverishment in which one's self image becomes increasingly empty and volatilized, leading the individual himself to feel unreal.

According to Gunderson, people with SPD "feel lost" without the people they are normally around because they require a sense of security and stability. However, when the patient's personal space is violated, they feel suffocated and feel the need to free themselves and be independent. People who have SPD tend to be happiest when they are in a relationship in which the partner places few emotional or intimate demands on them; it is not people as such that they want to avoid, but both negative and positive emotions, emotional intimacy, and self disclosure.

This means that it is possible for schizoid individuals to form relationships with others based on intellectual, physical, familial, occupational, or recreational activities as long as these modes of relating do not require or force the need for emotional intimacy, which the affected individual will reject.

Donald Winnicott summarizes the schizoid need to modulate emotional interaction with others with his comment that schizoid individuals "prefer to make relationships on their own terms and not in terms of the impulses of other people", and failing to attain that, they prefer isolation.

The "Secret Schizoid"

According to Ralph Klein, there are many fundamentally schizoid individuals who present with an engaging, interactive personality style which contradicts the observable characteristic emphasized by the DSM-Ⅳ and ICD-10 definitions of the schizoid personality. Klein classifies these individuals as secret schizoids, presenting themselves as socially available, interested, engaged, and involved in interacting in the eyes of the observer, while at the same time remaining emotionally withdrawn and sequestered within the safety of the internal world.

While withdrawal or detachment from the outer world is a characteristic feature of schizoid pathology, it is sometimes overt and sometimes covert. When overt, it matches the typical description of the schizoid personality offered in the DSM-Ⅳ. However, according to Klein, it is "just as often" a covert, hidden internal state of the patient in which what meets the objective eye may not be what is present in the subjective, internal world of the patient. Klein therefore cautions that one should not miss identifying the schizoid patient because one cannot see the patient's withdrawal through the patient's defensive, compensatory, engaging interaction with external reality. Klein suggests that one need only ask the patient what his or her subjective experience is in order to detect the presence of the schizoid refusal of emotional intimacy.

Descriptions of the schizoid personality as "hidden" behind an outward appearance of emotional engagement have been recognized as far back as 1940 with Fairbairn's description of schizoid exhibitionism, in which he remarked that the schizoid individual is able to express a great deal of feeling and to make what appear to be impressive social contacts while in reality giving nothing and losing nothing; because he is only "playing a part", his own personality is not involved. According to Fairbairn, "disowns the part which he is playing and thus the schizoid individual seeks to preserve his own personality intact and immune from compromise." Further references to the secret schizoid come from Masud Khan, Jeffrey Seinfeld, and Philip Manfield, who gives a palpable description of an SPD individual who actually "enjoys" regular public speaking engagements, but experiences great difficulty in the breaks when audience members would attempt to engage him emotionally. These references expose the problems involved in relying singularly on outer observable behavior for assessing the presence of personality disorders in certain individuals.

Avoidant Attachment Style

The question of whether SPD qualifies as a full personality disorder or simply as an avoidant attachment style is a contentious one. If what has been known as schizoid personality disorder is no more than an attachment style requiring more distant emotional proximity, then many of the more problematic reactions these individuals show in interpersonal situations may be partly accounted for by the social judgments commonly imposed on those with this style. To date several sources have confirmed the synonymy of SPD and avoidant attachment style which leaves open the question of how researchers might best approach this subject in future diagnostic manuals, and in therapeutic practice. However, characteristically — and depending on the severity of the disorder — individuals do not seek social interactions merely due to lack of interest, as opposed to the avoidant personality type in which there is craving for interactions, but then fear of rejection.

Schizoid Sexuality

People with SPD are sometimes sexually apathetic, though they do not typically suffer from anorgasmia. Many schizoids have a healthy sex drive but some prefer to masturbate rather than deal with the social aspects of finding a sexual partner. Therefore, their need for sex may appear to be less than those who do not have SPD, as individuals with SPD prefer to remain alone and detached. When having sex, individuals with SPD often feel that their personal space is being violated, and they commonly feel that masturbation or sexual abstinence is preferable to the emotional closeness they must tolerate when having sex. Significantly broadening this picture are notable exceptions of SPD individuals who engage in occasional or even frequent sexual activities with others.

Harry Guntrip describes the "secret sexual affair" entered into by some married schizoid individuals as an attempt to reduce the quantity of emotional intimacy focused within a single relationship, a sentiment echoed by Karen Horney's resigned personality who may exclude sex as being too intimate for a permanent relationship, and instead satisfy his sexual needs with a stranger. Conversely he may more or less restrict a relationship to merely sexual contacts and not share other experiences with the partner." More recently, Jeffrey Seinfeld, professor of social work at New York University, has published a volume on SPD in which he details examples of "schizoid hunger" which may manifest as sexual promiscuity. Seinfeld provides an example of a schizoid woman who would covertly attend various bars to meet men for the purposes of gaining impersonal sexual gratification, an act, says Seinfeld, which alleviated her feelings of hunger and emptiness.

Salman Akhtar describes this dynamic interplay of overt versus covert sexuality and motivations of some SPD individuals with greater accuracy. Rather than following the narrow proposition that schizoid individuals are either sexual or asexual, Akhtar suggests that these forces may both be present in an individual despite their rather contradictory aims. For Akhtar, therefore, a clinically accurate picture of schizoid sexuality must include both the overt signs: "asexual, sometimes celibate; free of romantic interests; averse to sexual gossip and innuendo", along with possible covert manifestations of "secret voyeuristic and pornographic interests; vulnerable to erotomania; tendency towards compulsive masturbation and perversions", although none of these necessarily apply to all people with SPD.

Natural History and Prognosis

Schizoaffective disorder can present at any age, but it is most commonly first seen in young adulthood. Prognosis can be estimated from the relative prominence of schizophrenic and mood symptoms; more prominent and persistent schizophrenic symptoms are associated with poorer outcome, whereas more frequent and persistent mood symptoms predict more positive outcome. The presence of mood-congruent delusions and hallucinations (eg, the belief by a depressed woman that she has sinned or a manic individual's belief that he or she is the Messiah) predicts better outcome than mood-incongruent psychotic symptoms. Age of onset may also be a factor, as the functional status of adolescents diagnosed with schizoaffective disorder resembles that of schizophrenia more than it does mood disorders.

Although the causes of schizoaffective disorder are unknown, it is suspected that this diagnosis represents a heterogeneous group of patients, some with atypical forms of schizophrenia and some with very severe forms of mood disorders. There is little evidence for a distinct variety of psychotic illness. It follows then that the etiology is probably identical to that of schizophrenia in some cases or to mood disorders in others.

Estimates of the prevalence of schizoaffective disorder vary widely, but schizoaffective manic patients appear to comprise 3% - 5% of psychiatric admissions to typical clinical centers. At one point it was widely believed that schizoaffective disorder was associated with increased risk of mood disorders in relatives. This may have been because of the number of patients with psychotic mood disorders who were included in schizoaffective study populations. The current diagnostic criteria define a group of patients with a mixed genetic picture. They are more likely to have schizophrenic relatives than patients with mood disorders but more likely to have relatives with mood disorders than schizophrenic patients.

Although the causes of schizoaffective disorder are unknown, it is suspected that this diagnosis represents a heterogeneous group of patients, some with atypical forms of schizophrenia and some with very severe forms of mood disorders. There is little evidence for a distinct variety of psychotic illness. It follows then that the etiology is probably identical to that of schizophrenia in some cases or to mood disorders in others.

Histrionic Personality Disorder

Histrionic personality disorder, often abbreviated as HPD, is a type of personality disorder in which the affected individual displays an enduring pattern of attention-seeking and excessively dramatic behaviors beginning in early adulthood and present across a broad range of situations. Individuals with HPD are highly emotional, charming, energetic, manipulative, seductive, impulsive, erratic, and demanding.

Mental health professionals use the *Diagnostic and Statistical Manual of Mental Disorders* (the DSM) to diagnose mental disorders. The 2000 edition of this manual (the fourth edition text revision, also called the DSM - Ⅳ - TR) classifies HPD as a personality disorder. More specifically, HPD is classified as a Cluster B (dramatic, emotional, or erratic) personality disorder. The personality disorders which comprise Cluster B include histrionic, antisocial, borderline, and narcissistic.

HPD has a unique position among the personality disorders in that it is the only personality disorder explicitly connected to a patient's physical appearance. Researchers have found that HPD appears primarily in men and women with above - average physical appearances. Some research has suggested that the connection between HPD and physical appearance holds for women rather than for men. Both women and men with HPD express a strong need to be the center of attention. Individuals with HPD exaggerate, throw temper tantrums, and cry if they are not the center of attention. Patients with HPD are naive, gullible, have a low frustration threshold, and strong dependency needs.

Cognitive style can be defined as a way in which an individual works with and solves cognitive tasks such as reasoning, learning, thinking, understanding, making decisions, and using memory. The cognitive style of individuals with HPD is superficial and lacks detail. In their interpersonal relationships, individuals with HPD use dramatization with a goal of impressing others. The enduring pattern of their insincere and stormy relationships leads to impairment in social and occupational areas.

Symptoms and Signs

Histrionic personality disorder is characterized by a long - standing pattern of attention seeking behavior and extreme emotionality. Someone with histrionic personality disorder wants to be the center of attention in any group of people, and feel uncomfortable when they are not. While often lively, interesting and sometimes dramatic, they have difficulty when people aren't focused exclusively on them. People with this disorder may be perceived as being shallow, and may engage in sexually seductive or provocating behavior to draw attention to themselves.

Individuals with Histrionic Personality Disorder may have difficulty achieving emotional intimacy in romantic or sexual relationships. Without being aware of it, they often act out a role (eg, "victim" or "princess") in their relationships to others. They may seek to control their partner through emotional manipulation or seductiveness on one level, whereas displaying a marked dependency on them at another level.

Individuals with this disorder often have impaired relationships with same - sex friends because their sexually provocative interpersonal style may seem a threat to their friends' relationships. These individuals may also alienate friends with demands for constant attention. They often become depressed and upset when they are not the center of attention.

People with histrionic personality disorder may crave novelty, stimulation, and excitement and have a tendency to become bored with their usual routine. These individuals are often intolerant of, or frustrated by, situations that involve delayed gratification, and their actions are often directed at obtaining immediate satisfaction. Although they often initiate a job or project with great enthusiasm, their interest may lag quickly.

Longer - term relationships may be neglected to make way for the excitement of new relationships. DSM - Ⅳ - TR lists eight symptoms that form the diagnostic criteria for HPD:

Center of Attention

Patients with HPD experience discomfort when they are not the center of attention.

Sexually Seductive

Patients with HPD displays inappropriate sexually seductive or provocative behaviors towards others.

Shifting Emotions

The expression of emotions of patients with HPD tends to be shallow and to shift rapidly.

Physical Appearance

Individuals with HPD consistently employ physical appearance to gain attention for themselves.

Speech Style

The speech style of patients with HPD lacks detail. Individuals with HPD tend to generalize, and when these individuals speak, they aim to please and impress.

Dramatic Behaviors

Patients with HPD display self-dramatization and exaggerate their emotions.

Suggestibility

Other individuals or circumstances can easily influence patients with HPD.

Overestimation of Intimacy

Patients with HPD overestimate the level of intimacy in a relationship.

Natural History and Prognosis

Researchers today don't know what causes histrionic personality disorder. There are many theories, however, about the possible causes of histrionic personality disorder. Most professionals subscribe to a biopsychosocial model of causation, that is, the causes of are likely due to biological and genetic factors, social factors (such as how a person interacts in their early development with their family and friends and other children), and psychological factors (the individual's personality and temperament, shaped by their environment and learned coping skills to deal with stress). This suggests that no single factor is responsible — rather, it is the complex and likely intertwined nature of all three factors that are important. If a person has this personality disorder, research suggests that there is a slightly increased risk for this disorder to be "passed down" to their children.

DSM - Ⅳ - TR states that 2% to 16% of the clinical population and slightly less than 1% of the general population of the United States suffers from NPD. Between 50% and 75% of those diagnosed with NPD are males. Little is known about the prevalence of NPD across racial and ethnic groups.

Narcissistic Personality Disorder

Narcissistic personality disorder (NPD) is defined by the Fourth Edition Text Revision of the *Diagnostic and Statistical Manual of Mental Disorders* (DSM-Ⅳ-TR, a handbook that mental health professionals use to diagnose mental disorders) as one of ten personality disorders. As a group, these disorders are described by DSM-Ⅳ-TR as "enduring pattern(s) of inner experience and behavior" that are sufficiently rigid and deep-seated to bring a person into repeated conflicts with his or her social and occupational environment. DSM-Ⅳ-TR specifies that these dysfunctional patterns must be regarded as nonconforming or deviant by the person's culture, and cause significant emotional pain and/or difficulties in relationships and occupational performance.

To meet the diagnosis of a personality disorder, the patient's problematic behaviors must appear in two or more of the following areas:

Perception and interpretation of the self and other people;

Intensity and duration of feelings and their appropriateness to situations;

Relationships with others;

Ability to control impulses.

It is important to note that all the personality disorders are considered to have their onset in late adolescence or early adulthood. Doctors rarely give a diagnosis of personality disorder to children on the grounds that children's personalities are still in process of formation and may change considerably by the time they are in their late teens.

NPD is defined more specifically as a pattern of grandiosity (exaggerated claims to talents, importance, or specialness) in the patient's private fantasies or outward behavior; a need for constant admiration from others; and a lack of empathy for others. The term narcissistic is derived from an ancient Greek legend, the story of Echo and Narcissus. According to the legend, Echo was a woodland nymph who fell in love with Narcissus, who was an uncommonly handsome but also uncommonly vain young man. He contemptuously rejected her expressions of love. She pined away and died. The god Apollo was angered by Narcissus' pride and self-satisfaction, and condemned him to die without ever knowing human love. One day, Narcissus was feeling thirsty, saw a pool of clear water nearby, and knelt beside it in order to dip his hands in the water and drink. He saw his face reflected on the surface of the water and fell in love with the reflection. Unable to win a response from the image in the water, Narcissus eventually died beside the pool.

Havelock Ellis, a British psychologist, first used the story of Echo and Narcissus in 1898 as a capsule summary of pathological self-absorption. The words narcissist and narcissistic have been part of the vocabulary of psychology and psychiatry ever since. They have, however, been the subjects of several controversies. In order to understand NPD, the reader may find it helpful to have an outline of the different theories about narcissism in human beings, its relation to other psychiatric disorders, and its connections to the wider culture. NPD is unique among the DSM-Ⅳ - TR personality disorders in that it has been made into a symbol of the problems and discontents of contemporary Western culture as a whole.

Symptoms and Signs

The symptoms of narcissistic personality disorder revolve around a pattern of grandiosity, need for admiration, and sense of entitlement. Often individuals feel overly important and will exaggerate achievements and will accept, and often demand, praise and admiration despite worthy achievements. They may be overwhelmed with fantasies involving unlimited success, power, love, or beauty and feel that they can only be understood by others who are, like them, superior in some aspect of life.

There is a sense of entitlement, of being more deserving than others based solely on their superiority. These symptoms, however, are a result of an underlying sense of inferiority and are often seen as overcompensation. Because of this, they are often envious and even angry of others who have more, receive more respect or attention, or otherwise steal away the spotlight.

A good place to begin a discussion of the different theories about narcissism is with the observation that NPD exists as a diagnostic category only in DSM - Ⅳ - TR , which is an American diagnostic manual. The International Statistical Classification of Diseases and Related Health Problems, Tenth Revision (ICD - 10 , the European equivalent of DSM) lists only eight personality disorders. What DSM - Ⅳ - TR defines as narcissistic personality disorder, ICD - 10 lumps together with "eccentric, impulsive - type, immature, passive - aggressive, and psychoneurotic personality disorders".

DSM - Ⅳ - TR specifies nine diagnostic criteria for NPD. For the clinician to make the diagnosis, an individual must fit five or more of the following descriptions:

He or she has a grandiose sense of self - importance (exaggerates accomplishments and demands to be considered superior without real evidence of achievement).

He or she lives in a dream world of exceptional success, power, beauty, genius, or "perfect" love.

He or she thinks of him - or herself as "special" or privileged, and that he or she can only be understood by other special or high - status people.

He or she demands excessive amounts of praise or admiration from others.

He or she feels entitled to automatic deference, compliance , or favorable treatment from others.

He or she is exploitative towards others and takes advantage of them.

He or she lacks empathy and does not recognize or identify with others' feelings.

He or she is frequently envious of others or thinks that they are envious of him or her.

He or she "has an attitude" or frequently acts in haughty or arrogant ways.

In addition to these criteria, DSM - Ⅳ - TR groups NPD together with three other personality disorders in its so - called Cluster B. These four disorders are grouped together on the basis of symptom similarities, insofar as patients with these disorders appear to others as overly emotional, unstable, or self-dramatizing. The other three disorders in Cluster B are antisocial, borderline, and histrionic personality disorders.

The DSM-Ⅳ-TR clustering system does not mean that all patients can be fitted neatly into one of the three clusters. It is possible for patients to have symptoms of more than one personality disorder or to have symptoms from different clusters. In addition, patients diagnosed with any personality disorder may also meet the criteria for mood, substance abuse, or other disorders.

Prognosis

Prognosis is limited and based mainly on the individual's ability to recognize their underlying inferiority and decreased sense of self worth. With insight and long term therapy, the symptoms can be reduced in both number and intensity.

DSM-Ⅳ-TR states that 2% to 16% of the clinical population and slightly less than 1% of the general population of the United States suffers from NPD. Between 50% and 75% of those diagnosed with NPD are males. Little is known about the prevalence of NPD across racial and ethnic groups.

Antisocial Personality Disorder

Also known as psychopathy, sociopathy or dyssocial personality disorder, antisocial personality disorder (APD) is a diagnosis applied to persons who routinely behave with little or no regard for the rights, safety or feelings of others. This pattern of behavior is seen in children or young adolescents and persists into adulthood.

The most recent edition of the *Diagnostic and Statistical Manual of Mental Disorders*, (the fourth edition, text revision or DSM-Ⅳ-TR) classifies APD as one of four "Cluster B Personality Disorders" along with borderline, histrionic, and narcissistic personality disorders.

People diagnosed with APD in prison populations act as if they have no conscience. They move through society as predators, paying little attention to the consequences of their actions. They cannot understand feelings of guilt or remorse. Deceit and manipulation characterize their interpersonal relationships.

Men or women diagnosed with this personality disorder demonstrate few emotions beyond contempt for others. Their lack of empathy is often combined with an inflated sense of self-worth and a superficial charm that tends to mask an inner indifference to the needs or feelings of others. Some studies indicate people with APD can only mimic the emotions associated with committed love relationships and friendships that most people feel naturally.

People reared by parents with antisocial personality disorder or substance abuse disorders are more likely to develop APD than members of the general population. People with the disorder may be homeless, living in poverty, suffering from a concurrent substance abuse disorder, or piling up extensive criminal records, as antisocial personality disorder is associated with low socioeconomic status and urban backgrounds. Highly intelligent individuals with APD, however, may not come to the attention of the criminal justice or mental health care systems and may be underrepresented in diagnostic statistics.

Some legal experts and mental health professionals do not think that APD should be classified as a mental disorder, on the grounds that the classification appears to excuse unethical, illegal, or immoral behavior. Despite these concerns, juries in the United States have consistently demonstrated that they do not regard a diagnosis of APD as exempting a person from prosecution or punishment for crimes committed.

Furthermore, some experts disagree with the American Psychiatric Association's (APA's) categorization of antisocial personality disorder. The APA considers the term psychopathy as another, synonymous name for APD. However, some experts make a distinction between psychopathy and APD. Dr. Robert Hare, an authority on psychopathy and the originator of the Hare Psychopathy Checklist, claims that all psychopaths have APD but not all individuals diagnosed with APD are psychopaths.

Symptoms and Signs

The symptoms of antisocial personality disorder include a longstanding pattern (after the age of 15) of disregard for the rights of others. There is a failure to conform to society's norms and expectations that often results in numerous arrests or legal involvement as well as a history of deceitfulness where the individual attempts to con people or use trickery for personal profit. Impulsiveness if often present, including angry outbursts, failure to consider consequences of behaviors, irritability, and/or physical assaults.

Some argue that a major component of this disorder is the reduced ability to feel empathy for other people. This inability to see the hurts, concerns, and other feelings of people often results in a disregard for these aspects of human interaction. Finally, irresponsible behavior often accompanies this disorder as well as a lack of remorse for wrongdoings.

Studies of adopted children indicate that both genetic and environmental factors influence the development of APD. Both biological and adopted children of people diagnosed with the disorder have an increased risk of developing it. Children born to parents diagnosed with APD but adopted into other families resemble their biological more than their adoptive parents. The environment of the adoptive home, however, may lower the child's risk of developing APD.

Researchers have linked antisocial personality disorder to childhood physical or sexual abuse; neurological disorders (which are often undiagnosed); and low IQ. But, as with other personality disorders, no one has identified any specific cause or causes of antisocial personality disorder. Persons diagnosed with APD also have an increased incidence of somatization and substance-related disorders.

DSM-Ⅳ-TR adds that persons who show signs of conduct disorder with accompanying attention-deficit/hyperactivity disorder before the age of ten have a greater chance of being diagnosed with APD as adults than do other children. The manual notes that abuse or neglect combined with erratic parenting or inconsistent discipline appears to increase the risk that a child diagnosed with conduct disorder will develop APD as an adult.

The central characteristic of antisocial personality disorder is an extreme disregard for the rights of other people. Individuals with APD lie and cheat to gain money or power. Their disregard for authority often leads to arrest and imprisonment. Because they have little regard for others and may act impulsively, they are frequently involved in fights. They show loyalty to few if any other people and are likely to seek power over others in order to satisfy sexual desires or economic needs.

People with APD often become effective "con artists". Those with well-developed verbal abilities can often charm and fool their victims, including unsuspecting or inexperienced therapists. People with APD have no respect for what others regard as societal norms or legal constraints. They may quit jobs on short notice, move to another city, or end relationships without warning and without what others would consider good reason. Criminal activities typically include theft, selling illegal drugs and check fraud. Because persons with antisocial personality disorder make "looking out for number one" their highest priority, they are quick to exploit others. They commonly rationalize these actions by dismissing their victims as weak, stupid or unwary.

Natural History and Prognosis

APD usually follows a chronic and unremitting course from childhood or early adolescence into adult life. The impulsiveness that characterizes the disorder often leads to a jail sentence or an early death through accident, homicide or suicide. There is some evidence that the worst behaviors that define APD diminish by midlife; the more overtly aggressive symptoms of the disorder occur less frequently in older patients. This improvement is especially true of criminal behavior but may apply to other antisocial acts as well.

Prognosis is not very good because of two contributing factors. First, because the disorder is characterized by a failure to conform to society's norms, people with this disorder are often incarcerated because of criminal behavior. Secondly, a lack of insight into the disorder is very common. People with antisocial personality disorder typically see the world as having the problems, not him or herself, and therefore rarely seek treatment. If progress is made, it is typically over an extended period of time.

Borderline Personality Disorder

Borderline personality disorder (BPD) is a mental disorder characterized by disturbed and unstable interpersonal relationships and self-image, along with impulsive, reckless, and often self-destructive behavior.

Individuals with BPD have a history of unstable interpersonal relationships. They have difficulty interpreting reality and view significant people in their lives as either completely flawless or extremely unfair and uncaring (a phenomenon known as "splitting"). These alternating feelings of idealization and devaluation are the hallmark feature of borderline personality disorder. Because borderline patients set up such excessive and unrealistic expectations for others, they are inevitably disappointed when their expectations aren't realized.

The term "borderline" was originally used by psychologist Adolf Stern in the 1930s to describe patients whose condition bordered somewhere between psychosis and neurosis. It has also been used to describe the borderline states of consciousness these patients sometimes feel when they experience dissociative symptoms (a feeling of disconnection from oneself).

Symptoms and Signs

The major symptoms of this disorder revolve around unstable relationships, poor or negative sense of self, inconsistent moods, and significant impulsivity. There is an intense fear of abandonment with this disorder that interferes with many aspects if the individual's life. This fear often acts as a self-fulfilling prophecy as they cling to others, are very needy, feel helpless, and become overly involved and immediately attached. When the fear of abandonment becomes overwhelming, they will often push others out of their life as if trying to avoid getting rejected. The cycle most often continues as the individual will then try everything to get people back in his or her life and once again becomes clingy, needy, and helpless.

The fact that people often do leave someone who exhibits this behavior only proves to support their distorted belief that they are insignificant, worthless, and unloved. At this point in the cycle, the individual may exhibit self-harming behaviors such as suicide attempts, mock suicidal attempts (where the goal is to get rescued and lure others back into the individual's life), cutting or other self-mutilating behavior. There is often intense and sudden anger involved, directed both at self and others, as well a difficulty controlling destructive behaviors.

The handbook used by mental health professionals to diagnose mental disorders is the *Diagnostic and Statistical Manual of Mental Disorders* (DSM). The 2000 edition of this manual (fourth edition, text revised) is known as the DSM-Ⅳ-TR. Published by the American Psychiatric Association, the DSM contains diagnostic criteria, research findings, and treatment information for mental disorders. It is the primary reference for mental health professionals in the United States. BPD was first listed as a disorder in the third edition DSM-Ⅲ, which was published in 1980, and has been revised in subsequent editions. The DSM-Ⅳ-TR requires that at least five of the following criteria (or symptoms) be present in an individual for a diagnosis of borderline disorder:

Arantic efforts to avoid real or perceived abandonment;

Pattern of unstable and intense interpersonal relationships, characterized by alternating between idealization and devaluation ("love-hate" relationships);

Extreme, persistently unstable self-image and sense of self;

Impulsive behavior in at least two areas (such as spending, sex, substance abuse, reckless driving, binge eating);

Recurrent suicidal behavior, gestures, or threats, or recurring acts of self-mutilation (such as cutting or burning oneself);

Unstable mood caused by brief but intense episodes of depression, irritability, or anxiety;

Chronic feelings of emptiness;

Inappropriate and intense anger, or difficulty controlling anger displayed through temper outbursts, physical fights, and/or sarcasm;

Stress - related paranoia that passes fairly quickly and/or severe dissociative symptoms — feeling disconnected from one's self, as if one is an observer of one's own actions.

Natural History and Prognosis

The disorder usually peaks in young adulthood and frequently stabilizes after age 30. Approximately 75%-80% of borderline patients attempt or threaten suicide, and between 8%–10% are successful. If the borderline patient suffers from depressive disorder, the risk of suicide is much higher. For this reason, swift diagnosis and appropriate interventions are critical.

Prevention recommendations are scarce. The disorder may be genetic and not preventable. The only known prevention would be to ensure a safe and nurturing environment during childhood. While the disorder is chronic in nature, gradual improvements with work are definitely seen. While it is difficult for anyone to change major aspects of their personality, the symptoms of this disorder can be reduced in both number and intensity. Long term treatment is almost always required.

Obsessive-Compulsive Personality Disorder

Obsessive - compulsive personality disorder (OCPD) is a type of personality disorder marked by rigidity, control, perfectionism, and an overconcern with work at the expense of close interpersonal relationships. Persons with this disorder often have trouble relaxing because they are preoccupied with details, rules, and productivity. They are often perceived by others as stubborn, stingy, self-righteous, and uncooperative.

People suffering from OCPD have careful rules and procedures for conducting many aspects of their everyday lives. While their goal is to accomplish things in a careful, orderly manner, their desire for perfection and insistence on going "by the book" often overrides their ability to complete a task. For example, one patient with OCPD was so preoccupied with finding a mislaid shopping list that he took much more time searching for it than it would have taken him to rewrite the list from memory. This type of inflexibility typically extends to interpersonal relationships. People with OCPD are known for being highly controlling and bossy toward other people, especially subordinates. They will often insist that there is one and only one right way (their way) to fold laundry, cut grass, drive a car, or write a report. In addition, they are so insistent on following rules that they cannot allow for what most people would consider legitimate exceptions. Their attitudes toward their own superiors or supervisors depend on whether they respect these authorities. People with OCPD are often unusually courteous to superiors that they respect, but resistant to or contemptuous of those they do not respect.

While work environments may reward their conscientiousness and attention to detail, people with OCPD do not show much spontaneity or imagination. They may feel paralyzed when immediate action is necessary; they feel overwhelmed by trying to make decisions without concrete guidelines. They expect colleagues to stick to detailed rules and procedures, and often perform poorly in jobs that require flexibility and the ability to compromise. Even when people with OCPD are behind schedule, they are uncomfortable delegating work to others because the others may not do the job "properly". People with OCPD often get so lost in the finer points of a task that they cannot see the larger picture; they are frequently described as "unable to see the forest for the trees". They are often highly anxious in situations without clearly defined rules because such situations arouse their fears of making a mistake and being punished for it. An additional feature of this personality disorder is stinginess or miserliness, frequently combined with an inability to throw out worn-out or useless items. This characteristic has sometimes been described as "pack rat" behavior.

People diagnosed with OCPD come across to others as difficult and demanding. Their rigid expectations of others are also applied to themselves, however, they tend to be intolerant of their own shortcomings. Such persons feel bound to present a consistent facade of propriety and control. They feel uncomfortable with expressions of tender feelings and tend to avoid relatives or colleagues who are more emotionally expressive. This strict and ungenerous approach to life limits their ability to relax; they are seldom if ever able to release their needs for control. Even recreational activities frequently become another form of work. A person with OCPD, for example, may turn a tennis game into an opportunity to perfect his or her backhand rather than simply enjoying the exercise, the weather, or the companionship of the other players. Many OCPD sufferers bring office work along on vacations in order to avoid "wasting time", and feel a sense of relief upon returning to the structure of their work environment. Not surprisingly, this combination of traits strains their interpersonal relationships and can lead to a lonely existence.

Symptoms and Signs

The symptoms of OCPD include a pervasive overconcern with mental, emotional, and behavioral control of the self and others. Excessive conscientiousness means that people with this disorder are generally poor problem-solvers and have trouble making decisions; as a result, they are frequently highly inefficient. Their need for control is easily upset by schedule changes or minor unexpected events. While many people have some of the following characteristics, a person who meets the DSMⅣ-TR criteria for OCPD must display at least four of them:

Preoccupation with details, rules, lists, order, organization, or schedules to the point at which the major goal of the activity is lost.

Excessive concern for perfection in small details that interferes with the completion of projects.

Dedication to work and productivity that shuts out friendships and leisure-time activities, when the long hours of work cannot be explained by financial necessity.

Excessive moral rigidity and inflexibility in matters of ethics and values that cannot be accounted for by the standards of the person's religion or culture.

Hoarding things, or saving wornout or useless objects even when they have no sentimental or likely monetary value.

Insistence that tasks be completed according to one's personal preferences.

Stinginess with the self and others.

Excessive rigidity and obstinacy.

Natural History and Prognosis

Obsessive - compulsive personality disorder is estimated to occur in about 1% of the population, although rates of 3%–10% are reported among psychiatric outpatients. The disorder is usually diagnosed in late adolescence or young adulthood. In the United States, OCPD occurs almost twice as often in men as in women. Some researchers attribute this disproportion to gender stereotyping, in that men have greater permission from general Western culture to act in stubborn, withholding, and controlling ways.

Treatment

The treatment that's best for you depends on your particular personality disorder, its severity and your life situation. Often, a team approach is appropriate to make sure all of your psychiatric, medical and social needs are met. Because personality disorders tend to be chronic and can sometimes last much of your adult life, you may need long - term treatment. The team involved in treatment may include your:

Family doctor or primary care provider;

Psychiatrist;

Psychotherapist;

Pharmacist;

Family members;

Social workers.

If you have mild symptoms that are well controlled, you may need treatment from only your family doctor, a psychiatrist or a therapist. If possible, find medical and mental health providers with experience in treating personality disorders. Several treatments are available for personality disorders. They include:

Psychotherapy;

Medications;

Hospitalization.

Successful treatment depends on your active participation in your care.

Psychotherapy

Psychotherapy is the main way to treat personality disorders. Psychotherapy is a general term for the process of treating personality disorders by talking about your condition and related issues with a mental health provider. During psychotherapy, you learn about your condition and your mood, feelings, thoughts and behavior. Using the insight and knowledge you gain in psychotherapy, you can learn healthy ways to manage your symptoms. Types of psychotherapy used to treat personality disorders may include:

Cognitive behavioral therapy

This combines features of both cognitive and behavior therapies to help you identify unhealthy, negative beliefs and behaviors and replace them with healthy, positive ones. Dialectical behavior therapy. This is a type of cognitive behavioral therapy that teaches behavioral skills to help you tolerate stress, regulate your emotions and improve your relationships with others.

Psychodynamic psychotherapy

This therapy focuses on increasing your awareness of unconscious thoughts and behaviors, developing new insights into your motivations, and resolving conflicts to live a happier life.

Psychoeducation

This therapy teaches you — and sometimes family and friends — about your illness, including treatments, coping strategies and problem-solving skills.

Psychotherapy may be provided in individual sessions, in group therapy or in sessions that include family or even friends. The type of psychotherapy that's right for you depends on your individual situation.

Medications

There are no medications specifically approved by the Food and Drug Administration to treat personality disorders. However, several types of psychiatric medications may help with various personality disorder symptoms.

Antidepressant medications

Antidepressants may be useful if you have a depressed mood, anger, impulsivity, irritability or hopelessness, which may be associated with personality disorders.

Mood-stabilizing medications

As their name suggests, mood stabilizers can help even out mood swings or reduce irritability, impulsivity and aggression.

Antianxiety medications

These may help if you have anxiety, agitation or insomnia. But in some cases, they can increase impulsive behavior.

Antipsychotic medications

Also called neuroleptics, these may be helpful if your symptoms include losing touch with reality (psychosis) or in some cases if you have anxiety or anger problems.

Hospitalization and Residential Treatment Programs

In some cases, a personality disorder may be so severe that you require psychiatric hospitalization. Psychiatric hospitalization is generally recommended only when you aren't able to care for yourself properly or when you're in immediate danger of harming yourself or someone else. Psychiatric hospitalization options include 24-hour inpatient care, partial or day hospitalization, or residential treatment, which offers a supportive place to live.

Chapter 4　Eating Disorders

This chapter provides an overview of the major eating disorders: anorexia nervosa, bulimia, and obesity. Binge eating disorder is discussed as a subset of bulimia and of obesity. In reading this review, keep in mind that eating disorders are not illnesses per se but bet behavioral syndromes that develop in individuals who manifest a broad spectrum of psychological, biological and sociocultural characteristics. Recognition of the psychophysiological inipuct of associated medical complications and identihcatiun of psychiatric comorbidity are of critical importance in the diagnoses and treatment of Iliese disorders. A thorough history, including eating behavior and body image, a comprehensive psychiatric assessment, and a complete medical evaluation are essential for the successful treatment of eating disorders.

Anorexia Nervosa

Anorexia nervosa is a complex disorder manifested by physiological, behavioral, and psychological changes and characterized by morbid fear of fatness, gross distortion of body image, and unrelenting pursuit of thinness. The name is actually a misnomer, since true anorexia (loss of appetite) does not usually occur until late in its course. Although it typically begins in adolescence, the range of onset is between 10 and 30 years.

Symptoms and Signs

Individuals with anorexia nervosa go to incredible extremes to lose weight. They begin by drastically reducing caloric intake, with virtually complete avoidance of high-carbohydrate and fat-containing foods. They exercise incessantly: walking, running, swimming, cycling, dancing, and performing calisthenics. Hyperactivity is dramatic and persists even when weight loss has resulted in cachexia. Some patients alternate fasting with bulimia episodes of uncontrolled gorging without awareness of hunger or satiation. Such eating binges are often followed by selfinduced vomiting. Huge quantities of laxatives are commonly consumed. Diet pills and diuretics may also be abused in the effort to lose weight. There are two types of anorexia nervosa: patients who engage in binge eating and purging behavior are diagnosed as having the binge eating/purging type and patients who simply slarve themselves are diagnosed as having the restricting type.

The ealing behaviors of anorexics are often peculiar and may be bizarre. The diet may be exceedingly monotonous or highly eccentric. Large quantities of food may be hoarded or small amounts of food may be hidden around the house. Although they eat very little, anorexics are obsessively preoccupied with food and cooking. Food portions are carefully measured, and small meals may be eaten over many hours. Food is often stored, prepared, served, eaten, and disposed of in a specific, ritualistic fashion. Patients with anorexia nervosu are usually highly secretive and often lie to protect the privacy of their eating behaviors. Kleptomania and stealing are sometimes associated with this disorder, parcicularly among individuals who also have episodes of bulimia.

Although these features of anorexia iiervosa can occur in individuals with a variety of premorbid personality structures and traits, a fairly consistent profile of emotional and psychological manifestations common to all patients with this disorder has been described. Clinicians generally agree that the unrelenting pursuit of thinness manifests an underlying psychological struggle to maintain a sense of personal autonomy and self - control. On the surface, patients are stubbornly defiant and fiercely independent. They insist they are happy, fully aware of their condition, and completely capable of taking care of themselves. But underneath they are stricken with a paralyzing sense of helplessness and ineffectiveness, with control over ealing and body size the only mechanisms through which a sense of autonomy and mastery can be sustained. This important insight into the psychology of anorexia nervosa was discovered in 1962 by Hilde Bruch, who also described two other essential features of this disorder: a characteristic misperception of internal body cues, so that patients are unable to differentiate their own feelings and needs from those of others, and a disturbance of body image, so that patients see themselves as grotesquely fat even when exceedingly thin. These cognitive and perceptlial distortions accentuate the sense of personal ineffectiveness and reinforce the need to continue the pursuit of thinness to maintain a sense of control.

The lack of confidence in basic self - control is compounded by feelings of personal mistrust. Patients fear they will give in to overwhelming impulses and, so far as eating is concerned, gorge themselves inio obesity. Individuals with anorexia nervosa also tend to view themselves in terms of absolutes and polar opposites. Behavior is either all good or all bad: a decision is either completely right or completely wrong; and a person is either absolutely in control or totally out of control. Thus, the gain of an ounce may produce the same sense of horror as would the gain of 100 pounds. Self - mistrust and the tendency to view the world in absolutes reinforce the exaggerated need to maintain rigid control over what is and is not eaten.

Patients with anorexia nervosa often express fear about becoining adults, since that would mean either tolerating intense loneliness or entering the world of interpersonal and sexual relationships. Although desperate for contact, they are mistrustful of relationships. They are often frightened of sexuality and usually avoid sexual encounters. When they do engage in sexual activity, it is usually without enjoyment.

Low self - esteem is invariably present, with the ability to lose weight being the only thing many patients like about themselves. Patients with anorexia nervosa describe intense feelings of inner shame about their bodies in general, with their fat content a specific object of disgust.

Psychiatric Comorbidity

Two - thirds of patients with anorexia nervosa and thiee - fourths of patients who meet diagnostic criteria for both anorexia nervosa and bulimia nervosa are also diagnosed with at least one mood disorder on presentation. Of patients with anorexia nervosa, up to 60% are diagnosed with major depression and about 33% with anxiety disorders at intake. Obsessive - compulsive disorder accounts for one - half of the associated anxiety disorders, but generalized anxiety disorder, phobias, and panic disorder are also common. The lifetime risk of affective disorder in patients with anorexia nervosa is reported to range from 84% to a nearly universal 98%.

Personality disorders are diagnosed in at least 20% and as many as 80% of patients with anorexia nervosa. Patients with the restricting type of anorexia nervosa tend to exhibit Cluster C (anxious) personality disorders, such as avoidant, dependent, and compulsive, with Cluster A (odd) disorders, such as paranoid and schizoid, sometimes present. The Cluster B (dramatic) personality disorders, such as borderline, histrionic, and nurcissistic, tend to be present only in patients with anorexia nervosa binge eating/purging type. Patients with anorexia nervosa also present a lifetime risk of alcohol, amphetamme, and other substance abuse problems, which may be concurrent with the eating disorder.

In addition, starvation is known to produce psychiatric symptoms such as dysphoria, anxiety, obsessiveness, and hyperactivity, which complicate the diagnosis of comorbidity. This phenomenon further underscores the importance of ending starvation and reversing malnutrition as the essential first steps in treating anorexia nervosa.

Medical Complications

A weight loss of at least 15% of the baseline or ideal body weight is necessary to establish the diagnosis of anorexia nervosa. In addition to weight loss, a number of physical signs of anorexia nervosa can be attributed to weight loss, malnutrition, and generalized stress. Amenorrhea or oligomenorrhea, independent of weight loss and often preceding initial weight loss, is always present in women. Anorexia nervosa with premenarcheal onset often results in short stature and delayed breast development. Prolonged amenorrhea in women with anorexia nervosa may lead to the development of osteoporosis. Patients frequently complain of epigastric distress, and gastric emptying time is indeed prolonged. Vomiting, constipation, cold intolerance, headache, polyuria, and sleep disturbances are also commonly reported. In addition to emaciation, physical findings may include edema, lanugo, dehydration, low blood pressure, bradycardia, arrhythmias, diminished cardiac mass, and infantile uterus. Males with anorexia frequently have hemorrhoids and experience loss of libido.

Laboratory findings include abnormalities of vasopressin secretion, prepubertal plasma levels of follicle - stimulating hormone and luteinizing hormone, and a diminished response to gonadotropin - releasing hormone. Estrogen is at postmenopausal levels. Males have low testosterone. There is abolition or reversal of the normal circadian rhythm of plasma cortisol, the metabolic clearance rate of cortisol is reduced, and there is incomplete suppression of adrenocorticotropili and cortisol by dexamethasone. There is diminished growth hormone response to insulin - induced hypoglycemia, arginine stimulation, and levodopa. Glucose tolerance test curves may be flat. Plasma levels of triiodothyronine (T3) are reduced, and levels of plasma reverse - T3, may be elevated. Blood urea nitrogen and creatinine may be elevated, renal calculi may form, the glomenilar fillration rate may be reduced, and renal failure is possible. Hematological abnormalities may include leukopenia with a relative lymphocytosis, thrombocytopenia, and anemia. Bone marrow aspiration reveals hypocellularity with large amounts of gelatinous acid mucopolysaccharide. The erythrocyte sedimentation rate is low, and plasma fibrmogen levels are reduced. Hypercarotenemia, hypercholesterolemia, and hypomagnesemia are common findings. Hypophosphaiemia in present is an ominous sign, associated with rapid decompensation. Self - induced vomiting may produce a metabolic hypokalemic alkalosis. Electroencephalographic patterns may be abnormal, and the electrocardiogram may show flat or inverted T waves, ST depression, and increased intervals.

Refeeding edema frequently complicates the treatment of anorexia nervosa and, when severe, may increase the risk of congestive heart failure. Death, which occurs in 10% - 22% of patients, is caused by starvation and its complications (including pneumonia and other infections, cardiac arrhythmia, congestive heart failure, and renal failure) or by suicide. Patients who purge by vomiting or by abusing laxatives or diuretics are at risk for sudden death due to fluid and electrolyte imbalance.

Natural History

The onset of anorexia nervosa often follows new life situations in which the patient feels inadequate or unable to cope. Such changes may be biological, such as the onset of puberty; psychological, such as the stages of adolescence, or social, such as entering high school or college. The onset of anorexia nervosa may also follow the breakup of a relationship or the death of a relative or friend.

Typically, anorexia nervosa begins in individuals who are at normal weight or are slightly to moderately overweight. Dieting is initially supported, even actively encouraged, by Family and friends as well as, in many cases, by dance teachers and sports coaches. The patient is thus praised for the initial weight loss and takes pleasure in the achievement. Once the original weight reduction goal is attained, however, a new one is immediately set. Ostensibly, this is fur "insurance" to offset future weight gains, but weight loss in the pursuit of thiuness soon becomes an objective in itself.

Patients usually come to medical attention not because of weight loss but because of complaints such as ainenorrhea, edema, constipation, or abdominal pain. They may complain of specific "food allergies" and ask for aids of dieting such as diet pills or diuretics. Patients may also present as medical emergencies, since the complications of dieting or vomiting, such as dehydration and fluid and electrolyte imbalance, may be severe. The patient may be brought in by parents, who become worried when weight loss is extreme or are alarmed by bizarre eating habits and personality changes.

The course of anorexia nervosa is variable. There may be a single episode with complete recovery, or multiple episodes spanning many years. A single episode may also be chronic and unremitting. Complete or partial recovery may occur spontaneously in some cases or may follow treatment. Both single episodes and fluctuating courses may progress to death.

Differential Diagnosis

Anorexia nervosa must be distinguished from weight loss caused by medical illnesses such as neoplasms, tuberculosis, hypothalamic disease, and primary endocrinopathies (anterior pituitary insufficiency, Addison's disease, hyperthyroidism and diabetes mellitus). These can generally be diagnosed on the basis of thorough histories, physical examinations and laboratory studies. Patients with these medical illnesses do not present with the dread of fatness, unrelenting pursuit of thinness, and hyperactivity that characterize anorexia nervosa.

Weight loss frequently occurs in patients with depressive disorders or certain schizophrenic disorders characterized by peculiar eating habits prompted by delusions about food. Patients with other disorders also lack preoccupations with caloric intake, obsessions with body shape and size, and hyperactivity. Patients with somatization disorder may manifest weight fluctuations, vomiting, and peculiar food habits, but weight loss is usually not severe, and amenonrhea for longer than 3 months is unusual.

To establish the diagnosis of anorexia nervosa, patients should satisfy the *Dingnostic and Statistical Manual of Mental Disorders*, 4th edition (DSM - Ⅳ) diagnostic criteria listed in Table - 1. Subtyping takes into account the findings that patients with a mixture of anorexia nervosa and bulimia nervosa have a higher association of both Axis I and Axis II coinorbidity, present greater medical risks as a result of fluid and electrolyte imbalance, and may have a worse prognosis than patienis with anorexia nervosa alone.

Table 1 DSM-Ⅳ diagnostic criteria for anorexia nervosa.

A. Refusal to maintain body weight at or above a minimally normal weight for age and height (eg, weight loss leading to maintenance of body weight less than 85% of that expected, or failure to make expected weight gain during period of growth, leading lo body weight less than 85% of expected).
B. Intense fear of gaining weight or becoming fat, even though underweight.
C. Disturbance in the way in which one's body weight or shape is experienced; undue influence of body weight or shape on self-evaluation, or denial of the seriousness of the current low body weight.
D. In postmenarchal females, amenorrhea, ie, the absence of at least three consecutive menstrual cycles. (A woman is considered to have amenorrhea if her periods occur only following hormone, eg, estrogen, administration.)
Specify type:
Restricting type: During the episode of anorexia nervosa, the person does not regularly engage in binge eating or purging behavior (ie, self-induced vomiting or the misuse of laxatives or diuretics).
Binge Eating/Purging type: During the episode of anorexia nervosa, the person regularly engages in binge eating or purging behavior (ie, self-induced vomiting or the misuse of laxatives or diuretics).

Prognosis

There is marked variability in the prognosis for patients with anorexia nervosa. About 40% are completely recovered at follow-up and 30% are improved, but 20% remain unimproved or severely impaired. The mortality rate for this disorder is as high as 22% in some studies, wilh suicide reported in 2%-5% of chronic cases.

The presence of nonanorexic psychiatric impairments such as depression, anxiety, and agoraphobia is common at follow - up. Indicators of a favorable prognosis include a good piemorbid level of psycliosocial adjustment, early age at onset, less extreme weight loss, and less denial of illness at presentation. Unfavorable prognostic factors include poor premorbid level of psychosocial adjustment, low socioeconoinic status, extreme weight loss, greater denial of illness, and the presence of bulimia, vomiting, and laxative abuse. These indicators are all relative, since no single feature or set of factors can reliably predict the prognosis for any given individual.

Complete recovery in less than 2 years is unusual. The recovery rate is positively correlated with length of lime at follow - up, ie, the more time that passes before follow - up, the greater the likelihood of finding recovery. Thus, clinicians will do well to remember the words of William Gull, who described anorexia nervosa: "As regards prognosis, none of these cases, however exhausted, are really hopeless while life exists."

Epidemiology

The prevalence of anorexia nervosa among women in the United Stales and western Europe is between 0.7% and 2.1 of the population. Males constitute 10%-15% of patients with anorexia nervosa.

Etiology and Pathogenesis

A. Biological Factors

The number of hormonal changes in anorexia nervosa, as outlined above, suggests a hypothalamic - endocrine origin. However, the changes all appear to be secondary to the effects of starvation, weight loss, malnutrition and stress, and no evidence of primary hypolhalainic dysfunction has been adduced m any of the cases.

There is an increased risk for the disorder in biological siblings of patients with anorexia nervosa, and recent studies have shown a higher concordance rate for monozygotic than for dizygotic twins. However, the fact that anorexia nervosa tends to occur primarily in individuals of the upper and middle socio - economic classes, and the trend for rates to increase in socielies in accordance with exposure to Western culture, argue against an exclusive biological origin. Given that the physiological changes in anorexia nervosa (primary or secondary) definitely contribute to the pathogenesis, the clinical features must be viewed as resulting from interacting biological and psycliological factors.

Despite its high association with affective disorders, anorexia nervosa is not viewed as simply a variant of affective illness. This is so because the unrelenting pursuit of thinness and distortion of body image are not typical of afterlive disorders and because the natural course and outcome of anorexia nervosa differ from those of affective disorders.

B. Psychological Factors

A number of psychological theories have been proposed to account for anorexia nervosa. Classical psychoanalysts have emphasized the avoidance of sexuality. They view self - starvation as a rejection of the wish to be pregnanic and refusal of food as a behavioral response to fantasies of oral impregnation. Amenorrhea has been viewed as a symbolic manifestation of the wish to be pregnant. More recently, theorists have stressed impairment in the mother - child relationship as the primary cause. Such theorists view the characteristic struggle for autonomy as a manifestation of the failure to master conflicts associated with the process of separation and invalidation. The cognitive and perceptial deficits associated with anorexia nervosa, such as the distortion of body image, may also arise from impairments in early childhood development. For example, repeated invalidation of a child's perceptions by overly intrusive parents who "know too well" what a child thinks, feels, and needs can result in development of a sense of personal mistrust characteristic of patients with this disorder.

In recent years, family systems theorists have argued that anorexia nervosa is the result of dysfunctional family interactions. The function of the child who develops anorexia nervosa is to maintain the status quo, allowing the family to remain enmeshed, overinvolved, rigid, overprotective, and unable to handle conflicts openly. The child's illness may also provide the vehicle through which parents are able to fulfill their own unresolved dependency needs.

C. Cultural Factors

Anorexia nervosa occurs predominantly in upper - class families and may represent an exaggeration or caricature of class values that emphasize youth and thinness as virtues. In this regard, it is important to consider a feminist perspective on anorexia nervosa. Feminist writers such as Gloria Steinern and Naomi Wolf argue that a maledominant culture prevents women from ever being comfortable with their bodies and therefore disempowers them. Models with expressions of angst and emaciated bodies dominate fashion magazines. Men are considered desirable if they attain professional success, women must have cover girl faces and centerfold figures. Thus, Luciano Pavarotti, though large, is an international sex symbol, whereas the equally talented and equally large diva is the proverbial "fat lady who sings". Studies show that women, when asked about the shape and size of their bodies, usually respond disparagingly, eg, "my hips are too big." Men respond in terms of performance, eg, "I can run 10 miles and lift 200 pounds." Women tend to view their bodies as farther from their ideal weight than they actually are, men see themselves as closer. These differences may explain why anorexia and bu - limia nervosa occur nine times more often in females than in males.

The abundance of theories reflects the multidimensional nature of this disorder. No single theory offers a satisfactory explanation of the origin of anorexia nervosa, but each has contributed a valuable perspective on treating this puzzling and life - threatening disorder.

Treatment

Treatment approach to anorexia nervosa is summarized in the followings.

1. Assess and treat the medical complications of starvation. Determine whether purging is present, and treat for dehydration and electrolyte imbalance as necessary.

2. Decide whether hospitalization is necessary. If dizziness, light - headedness, or tainting from bradycardia or hypotension is reported, if any sign of congestive heart failure is present (including reports of dyspnea on exertion), if fluid and electrolyte balance cannot be

maintained, if excessive exercise presents a risk of congestive heart failure and cannot be monitored safely as an outpatient, if cognitive impairment from starvation precludes the utility of outpatient psychotherapy, or if the patient reports menial exhaustion from battling food and eating issues, then hospitalization is essential. Hospilalization is also indicated when reasonable outpatient efforts have failed.

3. Complete laboratory investigation. This includes full electrolyte profile including potassium, magnesium, calcium and phosphates, glucose, complete blood count, erythrocyte sedimentation rate, total protein, albumin, liver function tests, renal function tests, thyroid function tests, thyroid function test, iron, folat, B_{12}, electrocardiogram, chest X - ray, and bone density studies.

4. Restore nutritional balance through normal eating and encourage weight gain. This often involves setting up a behavior modification protocol. Low - dose neuroleptics or benzodiazepine-class anxiolytics may be used if fear of weight gain is excessive. Cyproheptadine may be useful to encourage weight gain in cases where weight loss is extreme.

5. Diagnose and treat psychiatric comorbidity. The presence of affective disorder may warrant the use of antidepressant medications. These medications may not be particularly effective when patients are significantly underweight but may be very effective when weight gain has occurred. Issues stemming from personality disorders should be addressed in psychotherapy.

6. Identify and treat underlying ideas, attitudes, and psychological conflicts. Treat with cognitive and/or psychodynamically based psychotherapy.

7. Assess the family. Utilize family therapy to facilitate support for the patient and to address family dynamics that may be contributing to the patient's development of illness.

8. Provide ongoing support. Support healthy diet and exercise habits, constructive approaches to self, family, and interpersonal problems; enhanced self - esteem, and sense of autonomy with ongoing psychotherapy.

The initial goal of treatment is to counteract the effects of starvation by promoting weight gain and restoring normal nutritional balance. In mild cases, this may be accomplished on an outpatient basis; in moderate to severe cases, an initial period of hospitalization is usually required.

Weight gain may be accomplished by hyperalimentation or total parenteral nutrition. However, because of the risks of intravenous feedings, most programs utilize behavior modification protocols based on the principles of operant conditioning. Although behavior modification may be effective in promoting initial weight gain, most outcome studies have concluded that behavior modification alone is not sufficient treatment. Lasting recovery occurs only when such methods are used in conjunction with psychotherapy, which addresses the underlying psycholoeical conflicts. Clinicians should also be advised that too rapid weight gain may cause dangerous gastric dilatation or precipitate congeslive heart failure.

Drug therapy may be useful in some cases. Some clinicians have considered the perceptual and body image disturbances characteristic of anorexia nervosa to be manifestation of psychosis, and chlorproniazine and similar drugs have facilitated weight gain in some patients. However, it is not clear whether the benefits of such medications result from their antipsychotic or their sedative effects. Anxiolytics, such as clonazepam may be helpful in reducing the overwhelming anxiety associated with eating. Recent studies suggest that the serotonin reuptake blockers fluoxetine and clomipranriine may help the depression and obsessions associated with anorexia nervosa. however, antidepressants, which have helped some patients, tend to be ineffective until weight loss has been restored. Cyproheptadine, an appetite stimulator and serotonin antagonisl, has proved helpful in the treatment of a subgroup of anorexic patients with particularly severe symptoms and a history of birth trauma.

Although psychoanalysis has not been generally eftective in the treatment of anorexia nervosa, psychodynamically oriented psychotherapies that provide slipporr to the patient and focus on issues relating to the struggle for autonomy and personal control are often successful, Cognitive behavioral therapy, which challenges irrational beliefs about food, eating and body size, and teaches patients strategies for reducing anxiety associated with behavioral change, is often effective. Family therapies, which view the symptoms of anorexia nervosa in the context of family structure and dysfunction, are also effective, particularly in the treatment of children, teenagers, and adults still living at home.

To effectively treat anorexia nervosa, biological, psychological, and behavioral changes must all be addressed. Effective treatment programs should not be welded to any single approach. Clinicians should be familiar with various methods of treatment and use them singly or in combination as called for.

Bulimia Nervosa

Bulimia nervosa is the episodic, uncontrolled binge eating of large quantities of food over a short period of time. It was originally described in the late 1950s as a pattern of behavior in some obese individuals. In the 1960s and early 1970s, it was recognized as a commonly associated feature of anorexia nervosa. Recently, it has been identified as a distinct disorder that occurs in persons of normal weight who are not obese and do not have anorexia nervosa. To establish the diagnosis of bulimia nervosa, the DSM - Ⅳ requires some form of compensatory behavior to prevent weight gain, such as purging. A number of normal - weight individuals engage in episodes of binge eating but do not engage in any compensatory behavior. The authors of DSM - Ⅳ elected not to include a separate diagnosis of binge eating disorder. However, the diagnostic and trentnieiit considerations are the same for these individuals as for those who meet the full diagnostic criteria for bulimia nervosa.

Symptoms and Signs

The essential feature of bulimia nervosa is the episodic, uncontrolled gorging of large quantities of food in short periods of time. Patients are aware of their disordered eating habits and distinguish eating binges from simple overeating. They are usually unaware of hunger during binges and do not stop eating when satiated. They express fear about not being able to stop eating voluntarily and report that binges end only when nausea or abdominal pain becomes severe, when they are interrupted or fall asleep, or when they induce vomiting.

Binges are usually preceded by depressive moods in which the patient feels sad, lonely, empty, and isolated, or by anxiety states with overwhelming tension. These feelings are usually relieved during the binges, but afterward patients typically report a return of depressive mood with disparaging self-criticism and feelings of guilt.

Binges usually occur in secret. They may last from a few minutes to several hours (typically less than 2 hours, with a median reported time of about 1 hour). Most binges are spontaneous, but some may be planned. The frequency of binges ranges from occasional (two or three times a month) to many times a day. The quantity of food consumed varies but is always large. Blilimics report consumption of 3-27 times the recommended daily allowance for calories on binge days, and some claim to spend in excess of $100 a day on binge foods. The food consumed is usually high in carbohydrates and of a texture that is easily swallowed. Patients often report eating the "junk foods" they ordinarily deny themselves but frequently eat whatever is available. Though high-carbohydrate foods are most commonly consumed, the nutritional content of binge foods varies. Although it is uncommon, some buliinics may eat huge quantities of vegetables, such as 7 pounds of carrots, at a single sitting.

Self-induced vomiting is very common but is not essential for the diagnosis. Some patients maintain normal weight by alternating binges with long periods of fasting, and many exercise excessively. (These patients are often referred to as "exercise blilimics".) Those who do vomit may use emetics such as ipecac syrup or induce vomiting by activating the gag reflex. Lesions on the back of the hand may be evidence of this. Many report that they no longer need chemical or mechanical stimulants to induce emesis, as they can simply vomit at will. Laxative abuse is coninionly associated with bulimia, the use of diuretics is not unusual, and rumination may occur.

Patients with bulimia are usually self-conscious about their behavior and often go to great lengths to conceal it. They are very concerned about their physical appearance, with self-esteem overly dependent on perception of body size and shape. Sexual adjustment may be disturbed, with behavior ranging from promiscuity to restricted sexual activity. A number of other symptoms related to poor impulse control are commonly associated with bulimia, such as alcoholism, drug abuse, stealing, self-mutilation, and suicidal gestures and attempts.

Most patients experience weight fluctuations, with weigh typically ranging from slightly underweight to slightly overweight. Other symptoms associated with bulimia include edema of hands and feet, headache, sore throat, painless or painful swelling of parotid and salivary glands, erosion of tooth enamel and severe caries, feelings of fullness, abdominal pain, and lethargy and fatigue. Light-headedness, dizziness, syncope, and seizures may occur if vomiting is severe. Menstrual irregularities are common, but amenonhea is usually not sustained.

Bulimia is usually not incapacitating except in extreme cases, where binge/purging is a virtual full-time preoccupation. When vomiting is excessive, dehydration and electrolyte imbalances can occur and may result in medical emergencies. Deaths front gastric dilatation and rupture have been reported.

Psychiatric Comorbidity

There is a high association of affective disorders with bulimia nervosa, with lifetime rates of over 80%. Major depression is most common, occurring in one - third of patients with bulimia nervosa and more than one - half of patients with mixed blilinrua nervosa and anorexia nervosa. Depression may precede, follow, of coincide with bulimia. Studies suggest that depression and bulimia operate independently, although both tend to improve with treatment. Anxiety disorders including generalized anxiety disorder, panic disorder, obsessive - compulsive disorder, social phobia, and posttraumatic stress disorder occur in nearly 60% of cases. Patients with bulimia nervosa also have a significant lifetime risk for alcohol and substance abuse, which may be concurrent with their eating disorder.

Personality disorders are commonly associated with bulimia nervosa, with rates ranging from 22% to 77% in published studies. Dramatic personality disorders including borderline personality disorder are most common, but anxious personality disorders, including avoidant personality disorder, are frequently diagnosed.

Medical Complications

The most serious medical complications of bulimia nervosa are caused by the cardiovasclilar effects of fluid and electrolyte imbalance. Purging behavior, including vomiting and laxative and diuretic abuse, may cause lifethreatening cardiac anhythinias. Ortliostatic hypotension associated with light - headed - ness and dizziness, headaches, insomnia, and fatigues denial caries and erosion of tooth enamel, and gastritis and esophagilis are common. Benign enlargement of the parotid and salivary glands occurs in about 25% of patients. The presence of a skin lesion on the back of the hand is a frequent sign of active behavior. In addition to hypokalernia, blood tests may show llypomaenesemia, disturbances in acid - base balance, and elevated serum amylase. Electrocardiogram changes such as ST segment depression and U waves may occur. Cardioinyopathy from emetine poisoning may develop in patients who use ipecac syrup to induce vomiting and may result in death. Patients who use baking soda to induce vomiting are at risk for developing lifethreatening acid - base imbalance. Patients with bulimia nervosa are at increased risk for developing seizures. They may have irregular menses or be amenorrheic.

Natural History

Bulimia typically begins in adolescence or young adulthood in individuals consciously trying to stay slim. Some report a history of anorexia nervosa and others report a history of obesity. The onset often follows changes in living situations such as leaving home, starting college, changing jobs, or becoming involved in new relationships.

The course is usually chronic, and patients often engage in such behavior for years before seeking treatment. The chronicaly of the illness may be punctuated by brief remissions in which the behavior is absent or the frequency and severity of the symptoms are reduced. Many report experiencing periods of relative improvement and other periods of worsening symptoms.

Differential Diagnosis

The DSM - Ⅳ diagnostic criteria for bulimia are listed in Table 2 that should be the diagnosis. Severe weight loss does not occur in bulimia, and amenorrhea is unusual. In diagnosing bulimia, it is necessary to rule out neurological disease, such as epileptic - equivalent seizures, central nervous system tumors, Kitiver - Bucy - like syndromes, and Kleine - Levin syndrome. Kluver - Bucy syndrome includes visual agiiosia, compulsive licking and biting, exploration of objects by mouth, inability to ignore any stimulus, placidity, hypersexuality, and hyperphagia. This syndrome is very rare and unlikely to present a problem in differential diagnosis. Kleine - Levin syndrome occurs clilefly in males and is characterized by hyperphagia and periods of hypersomnia lasting 2 - 3 weeks.

Table 2 DSM - Ⅳ diagnostic criteria for bulimia nervosa

A. Recurrent episodes of binge eating. An episode of binge eating is characterized by both of the following: (1) eating, in a discrete period of time (eg, within any 2 - hour period), an amount of food that is definitely larger than most people would eat during a similar period of time under similar circumstances, and (2) a sense of lack of control over eating during the episode (eg, a feeling that one cannot stop eating or control what or how much one is eating).
B. Recurrent inappropriate compensatory behavior to prevent weight gain, such as self - induced vomiting; misuse of laxatives, diuretics, or other medications; fasting; or excessive exercise.
C. The binge eating and inappropriate compensatory behaviors both occur, on average, at least twice a week for 3 months.

Prognosis

Blilinla nervosa is often a chronic illness characterized by multiple periods of relapse and remission. Many patients show significant improvement following brief psychotherapy and/or the administration of medication, and recovery rates (up to 85% in some series) definitely improve over time. Although outcome studies vary in their definition of recovery, and many more studies are needed, both patients and clinicians should be very encouraged by currently available data.

Epidemiology

Between 1% and 3% of young adult females in the United States meet the diagnostic criteria for bulimia nervosa. As many as 40% of young adults engage in episodic binge eating but do not meet the diagnostic criteria. Bulimia nervosa occurs in 0.2% of adolescent boys and young adult males and accounts for 10% –15% of blilimics identified in community - based studies.

The cause is not known. The episodic, uncontrolled nature of the eating behaviors has led some investigators to suggest that bulimia may be a variant of complex partial seizure disorder. However, the few electroencephalographic abnormalities reported in patients studied during the testing of this hypothesis did not correlate with treatment response to phenytoin.

The strong association between bulimia nervosa and affective disorders together with the tendency of bulimia behavior to respond to antidepressant medication has led to the hypothesis that the disorder is the result of imbalance in the doparnine, norepmephrine, and serotonin systems in the brain. Some studies have suggested that neuropeptides such as cholecystokinin, which regulate appetite and satiety in the brain, may be abnormal in patients with bulimia nervosa, but the evidence is far from conclusive.

Psychodynamic theories emphasize the symbolic nature of eating binges as representing gratification of sexual and aggressive wishes. Self - deprecation and self - induced vomiting fullowing binges may thus represent guilt - induced selt - plinishnient for fantasized transgressions.

Psychologists have also noted that the binge - vomiting cycle may represent a ritual acceptance and taking in followed by a rejection of symbolic love objects. Bulimia may thus represent an attempt to control the external environment. Patients with bulimia are noted to have low self - esteem, and the vomiting may represent a symbolic purging of bad aspects of the self. Patients with bulimia tend to be overconcerned with body image and often have impaired object relationships that are recapitulated in their eating behaviors.

As with anorexia neivosa, cultural emphasis on a thin, youthful appearance as die singular and overly valued standard of beauty may contribute to the increasing incidence of this disorder.

Sexual abuse may also be a risk factor for the development of bulimia iiervosa.

Treatment

Treatment approaches to bulimia nervosa are outlined in the followings.

Multiple studies have been published describing the efficacy of both psychotherapy and psychopharmacology in the treatment of bulimia nervosa.

1. Evaluate and treat the medical complications associated with bulimia nervosa. Replace fluid and electrolytes as necessary. Monitor electrolytes on regular basis. Refer for dental evaluation.

2. Ascertain the mechanism of purging. Educate patients regarding the medical dangers of chemical purgatives such as ipecac and baking soda as well as of diuretic and laxative abuse.

3. Hospitalize when necessary. If fluid and electrolyte balance cannot be maintained, if episodes of fainting occur, if concentration impairment makes employment or schoolwork impossible to perform, or if binge eating and purging behavior are the dominant activities in one's life, then a brief hospitalization to break the cycle and initiate treatment is necessary.

4. Diagnose and treat comorbidity. The presence of an affective disorder is an indication for treatment with an antidepressant medication if such treatment has not already been initiated on the basis of bulimic symptoms alone. Indeed, a trial of antidepressant medication is generally indicated for bulimia nervosa and is often effective even in the absence of concurrent affective disorder. Issues pertaining to personality disorders, when present, should be addressed in psychotherapy.

5. Identify and address psychoiogicai and cognitive underpinnings of bulimic behavior. Psychodynamically oriented and cognitive - behavioral treatments that address attitudes and feelings related to sell and body images are effective treatment modalities. Such treatments may

be particularly effective for many patients when combined with antidepressant medications. Support groups are also often helpful in the treatment of bulimia nervosa.

Dynamically based psychotherupies, particulary those that focus on interpersonal conflicts, eg, assertiveness, negotiation of needs, intimacy tears, etc are effective, but cognitive-behavioral therapies are by far the most studied. Such therapies focus on the thought patterns and teeling states that lead to episodes ot binge eating and purging with special emphasis on attitudes pertaining to body weight and shape. Coping strategies for handling the feelings associated with these attitudes, such as maintaining a food journal that includes both "what you are eating, and what's eating you," are suggested to the patient. Patients are expected to eat standard meals and their inational fears regarding weight gain are addressed. Obsessive preoccupation with body shape and size is challenged, as patients are helped to better tolerate painful affect, and to be more direct in interpersonal problem solving.

Psychoeducational approaches are also helpful. For example, advising patients to not fast during the day, because fasting leads to binge eating (the normal tendency to purchase more groceries, including more "junk foods", if shopping while hungry is an easily recognized example of this phenomenon), usually results in symptom reduction. Patient education and cognitive-behavioral approaches can be easily implemented in primary care settings.

Group therapies, including psychodynamic, cognitive-behavioral and self-help formats, are usually recommended. The most dramatic reports of treatment success are of studies using pharmacological therapies, with antidepressant medications being particularly effective. Tricyclic antidepressants, monoamme oxidase inhibitors and selective serotonin reuptake inhibitors such as fluoxetine, sertraline, and paroxetine have all shown efficacy in the treatment of bulimia nervosa, with responses ranging between reduction of binge eating and/or purging behavior to complete remission of symptoms. The antidepressant venlafaxine and the antiobsessional drug fluvoxamine also have proven efficacy. The antidepressant blipropion is contraindicated in anorexia nervosa and bulimia nervosa because of an increased risk of seizures. Studies show that if one antidepressant is ineffective or poorly tolerated, a trial of an alternative antidepressant may be successful. Mood-stabilizing drugs such as carbarnazepine and valproic acid are sometimes helpful (lithium is contraindicated because of the electrolyte imbalance that is commonly present in bulimia nervosa). Anxiolytics may also play a helpful role in some cases, but their potential for abuse necessitates careful monitoring.

Pica and Rumination Disorder of Infancy

Pica is the persistent (more than 1 month) ingestion of nonmitntive substances inappropriate for developmental age and unacceptable as cultural practice. Pica encompasses a wide variety of populations including toddlers who eat paint chips, pregnant women who consume starch and clay (the two largest groups), severely retarded children and adults who eat feces, and anxious adults who chew fingernails or pencils. Pica may be caused by poor nutrition, mineral deficiencies, or psychosocial deprivation. The condition is very responsive to nutritional and psychosocial intervention.

Rumination is a rare syndrome of infancy in which swallowed food is repeatedly relumed to the mouth, pleasurably sucked on or rechewed, and then swallowed again. Rumination disorder is apparently caused by severe physical and emotional neglect, since it readily responds to substitution of caretakers. The behavior may be the deprived infant's attempt at self - stimulation. Rumination behavior has also been reported in adults, where it is usually associated with stress, such as acute medical illness or surgery, losses, such as a death in the family or being fired from a job, or psychiatric illness, such as depression. Effective treatments include biofeedback and relaxation exercises. Treatment for the associated stress disorders and depression with psychotherapy and/or psychopharmacology is also effective in reducing rumination behavior.

Obesity

Simple obesity is not included among the eating disorders in DSM - Ⅳ. However, when there is evidence that psychological factors play a substantial etiological role in a specific case, this may be documented by noting "psychological factors affectinEi physical condition" in the diagnosis.

Symptoms and Signs

Despite the absence of clear- cut psychological and behavioral profiles associated with the development of obesity, there is a subgroup of obese individuals that manifests emotionally based patterns of overeating. Between 25% and 50% of participants in weight control programs report severe problems with binge eating, with women 1.5 times more likely to report this pattern than men. The eating binges are related to emotional stresses, and these individuals are more likely than nonbingers to have coexisting psychiatric disorders. DSM - Ⅳ established research criteria for diagnosing these individuals as having binge - eating disorder. This diagnosis is differentiated from bulimia nervosa only by the absence of compensatory behavior such as purging, fasting, or excessive exercising.

As many as one - third of obese patients have severe disparagement of body image. They feel that their bodies are grotesque and that others view them with hostility and contempt. Such feelings are reinforced by social attitudes, since fat people are often discriminated against and viewed by others as lazy, weak, self- destructive, and responsible for their condition. They also manifest low self- esteem and a negative self- concept.

Although many obese individuals tend to eat in response to emotional cues such as feelings of anxiety, fear, loneliness, boredom, and anger, so do many persons of normal weight. Obese individuals tend to chew less and eat more rapidly than other people, but both groups are strongly influenced by the eating behaviors of those around them.

Obese adults are usually physically less active than others, but this may be a consequence rather than a cause of obesity. Obese children are not less active than their normal - weight peers.

Dieting itself can be a significant biological and psychosocial stress factor. Dieting may cause feelings of frustration, agitation, irritability, and heightened emotional reactivity in otherwise normal persons. Thus, some of the emotional features traditionally attributed to obese persons may be a consequence of attempts to lose weight by dieting rather than a cause of their condition.

Psychiatric Comorbidity

As noted, as many as 50% of obese individuals engage in recurrent binge eating. Approximately one - fourth of obese binge eaters meet the diagnostic criteria for major depression compared with fewer than 5% of nonbingers. Obese binge eaters are twice as likely as nonbingers to have anxiety disorders, four times as likely to suffer from social phobia, and three times as likely to have drug or alcohol problems than nonbingers.

Medical Complications

It is estimated that more than 90% of cases of Type II diabetes, 70% of gallstones, 60% - 70% of coronary artery disease, 11% of breast cancers, and 10% of colon cancers are attributable to obesity.

Excess weight may cause low back pain, aggravation of osteoarthritis (particularly of the knees and ankles), and huge calluses on the feet and heels. Obesity may be associated with amenorrhea and other inenstinal disturbances. The lower ratio of body surface area to body mass leads to impaired heat loss and increased sweating. Intertrigo in tissue folds, itching, and skin disorders are common. There is often mild to moderate swelling of hands and feet.

In massively obese persons, pressure of fatty tissue on the thorax combined with pressure of intraabdoininal fat on the diaphragm may reduce respiratory capacity and produce dyspnea on exertion. This condition may progress to the so - called pickwickian syndrome, characterized by hypoventilation with hypercapilia, hypoxia, and somnolence.

Natural History

Obcsity can begin in childhood, adolescence, or adulthood. Amounts of body fat also increase with age even when weight remains constant. Obesity is usually a chronic and progressive condition. It is estimated that 300,000 deaths per year are caused by weight - related conditions, making obesity second only to cigarette smoking as the leading cause of preventable death in the United States.

Differential Diagnosis

Body mass index, or BMI, which is calculated by dividing weight in kilograms by height in meters squared, is the standard for determining obesity. A BMI under 25 is considered normal, with no weight - associated health risk. A BMI of 25–30 is considered overweight, with low to moderate health risk. Obesity is diagnosed by a BMI over 30, with high associated health risk. A BMI over 35 has a very high risk of weight - related health problems, and morbidly obese individuals (a BMI greater than 40) are at extremely high risk, with mortality rates up to 90% greater than those for normal - weight individuals.

In assessing obesity, the clinician must rule out medical illnesses such as hypothyroidism.

Prognosis

Although the prognosis for short - term weight loss has improved with the advent of new dieting and exercise strategies and the development of behavior modification prograins, the long-term prognosis for losing excess weight and keeping it off remains poor, with few patients losing more than 40 pounds and most regaining the weight they lose. It is estimated that if an obese child does not achieve nearly normal weight by the end of adolescence, the odds against doing so later are 28:1. Morbidity and mortality rates for obese individuals increase in direct proportion to increases in the BMI.

Epidemiology

It is estimated that 34% of adults in the United States are obese. The prevalence increases with age up to age 50, at which point it falls sharply in accordance with the increased mortality rate. Obesity is more common in women, particularly after age 50, because of the higher mortality rate among obese men after that age. Obesity is also more common among minorities and low - income populations. It has been estimated that about 25% of children and 20% of adolescents are significantly overweight.

Family studies of obesity show that 40% of adolescents studied at age 15 who had one obese parent were obese, whereas 80% of those with two obese parents were obese. This compares to only a 10% incidence of obesity among adolescents whose parents are of normal weight. Studies of monozygotic and dizygotic twins suggest genetic factors, but environmental influences are also present. Adoption studies have shown conflicting evidence for genetic transmission. Evidence for the heritability of soinatotypes is stronger than for obesity. This fact may be significant in that even a moderate degree of ectomorphic body habitus may protect against the development of obesity.

Etiology

Although there is great variability in weight among humans, individuals show remarkable consistency over time. Humans who agree to increase or decrease their weights for experimental purposes generally return to their starting weights when allowed to eat freely. Such observations have led to the theory that there is a biological set point for body weight in humans. This is supported by animal studies in which lesions of the ventromedial hypothalainus cause hypo and hyperphagia, respectively. To the extent that the "set point theory" is applicable to humans, many obese individuals may be dieting in opposition to biological factors that make dieting far more difficult for them than for other people.

Weight gain can occur as a result of an increase in either the number or the size of fat cells. The fat cells of adults with juvenile - onset obesity may be about the same size as those of normal - weight persons, but there may be up to five times as many. Persons with adult - onset obesity may have a normal number of larger - than - normal fat cells. In studies in which fat cell number and size were determined, individuals tended to stop losing weight when fat cell size returned to normal. Since fat cells once formed do not disappear, fat cell number may determine the lower limit of weight for persons who by dieting have worked to reduce cell size to normal.

There are two periods of cellular proliferation in normal-weight children: birth to 2 years of age and 10-14 years of age. In obese children, the period may extend well past 2 years of age, with consequent hypercellularity of fat tissue early in life. Although this may be partly under genetic control, the cellular theory of obesity thus has important implications regarding nutritional practices and weight regulation for children.

The gene governing the storage and breakdown of fat, and leptin, the protein it codes for, have been identified. Leptin has been shown to resolve obesity in genetically deficient mice, however, human trials have failed to consistently produce weight loss. There are multiple central nervous system chemical regulators of appetite, including several neuropeptides, the endogenous opiates, serotonin, dopamine, and norepinephrine. Their role in obesity, however, has not been established.

Early psychoanalylic theories of obesity held that obese individuals had unresolved dependency needs and were fixated at the oral level of psychosexual development. The symptoms of obesity were viewed as depressive equivalents, attempts to regain "lost" or frustrated nurturation and care. Recent studies have failed to demonstrate an increased incidence of psychopathological disorders in obese compared to normal-weight individuals. However, a subgroup of juvenile-onset obese subjects has gross disturbances in body image, they view their bodies as hideous and loathsome and feel that others view them with contempt. They have a negative self-concept, are very self-conscious, and have impaired social functioning. Such experiences may contribute to the development and maintenance of obesity. Furthermore, since obese individuals are often discriminated against socially and are perhaps less often the object of sexual desire than normal-weight individuals, the maintenance of obesity may in some cases reflect an unconscious wish to remain isolated to avoid conflicts relating to sexuality or emotional intimacy.

Although there is no specific family constellation that predisposes to obesity, members of families lacking in warmth and love may use food and overeating as a substitute for love. The mothers in such families are often lonely individuals whose own childhoods were marked by social, economic, or emotional deprivation. Such mothers may unconsciously wish to have fat children. Identification with their "well-fed, well-cared-for" children may compensate for earlier deprivation. Such families may also equate physical size and the state of being "well fed" with physical and emotional strength. Obese children in such families may thus actually fear weight loss by concretely interpreting it as a loss of physical strength and emotional well-being.

The higher incidence of obesity among lower socioeconomic classes has been noted. In some societies in which food is scarce, obesity may be valued as a symbol of prosperity. In affluent countries such as the United States, value is instead placed on thinness, perhaps because foods low in calories but of high nutritional value are more expensive and unaffordable to the poor.

The definition of obesity may itself be culturally determined. Since 1943, revisions in standard height and weight charts have steadily lowered the ideal weights for women. The ideal weight for an average 5 foot 4 inch woman in 1943 was approximately 130 pounds, in 1980 it was under 120 pounds. Ideal weights for men have also been lowered, though not as much, and in 1974 the ideal weight for an average 5 foot 10 inch man was actually higher than the corresponding standard in 1943. These revisions have not been based on morbidity or mortality statistics but on measurements of the heights and weights of 25 - year - old graduate students. Such standards do not take into account the fact that the percentage of body fat increases with age but instead reflect the fashion trends of the youthful, affluent college populations. For women, the steady decline in ideal weight reflects the upper - class emphasis on fashion model thinness as the standard of beauty. For men, there is greater acceptance of a wider variety of body types. Attractive men may be thin, eg, long - distance runners and basketball players, or bulky, weight lifters and football players. This broader range of acceptability may account for the less consistent downward trend in ideal weights for men listed in standard charts.

If the 1980 standards for ideal weights are accepted, and if obesity is defined as weight at least 20% above ideal, then the average American woman is by detinition obese, and the average American man is on the verge of obesity.

Treatment

Treatment Approaches to Obesity

1. Assess and treat medical complications of obesity. Patients must be monitored for hypertension, diabetes mellitus, heart disease, and fluid and electrolyte changes during weight loss.

2. Assess diet and exercise habits. Patients with binge - eating behaviors should be identified. A diet and exercise program should be prescribed in conjunction with an internist.

3. Diagnose and treat psychiatric comorbidity. Patients with affective disorders and binge - eating behaviors may be considered for treatment with antidepressant medications, particularly selective serotonin reuptake blockers.

4. Identify psychological and cognitive underpinnings of obesity. Cognitive - behavioral and dynamically oriented psychotherapies may be particularly helpful for obese individuals with affective disorders or with binge - eating patterns of behavior and for those who manifest extreme disparagement of self and body image. Support groups may also be helpful to these individuals.

5. Consider antiobesity medications. Appetite suppressants may be useful for some obese individuals who fail to respond to diet, exercise programs, and supportive psychotherapy. These medications must be reserved for significantly overweight patients (BMI>30), should be used for a short period of time, and should not be combined with serotonin reuptake blockers. Their use must be carefully monitored and they should be given only in conjunction with therapeutic modalities. Lipase inhibitors may also be helpful, but their safety and efficacy are still under investigation.

6. Consider surgical procedures as last resort. Surgical procedures such as gastric stapling, intestinal bypass, and intragastric balloons should be considered only for morbidly obese individuals who have failed all other treatment interventions.

Surgical procedures, such as intestinal bypass operations and gastric slapling are effective in producing weight loss and in improving psychosocial functioning. These surgical procedures may also produce biological change, perhaps by lowering the body weight set point. However, risks of surgery and anesthesia, which are greater in obese individuals, plus the possibility otpostoperative complications such as malabsorption syndromes following bypass procedures should limit the indications for these interventions to the treatment of massive and morbid obesity that has not responded to conservative management. Wiring the jaws shut to prevent the intake of solid food may help some individuals, particularly when used in preparation for surgery. The use of intragastric balloons, a noninvasive method of gastric restriction, may also be effective. It should be noted that surgical interventions are never curative by themselves, as many patients regain the weight they lose within 2 years of the procedures.

Anipheramines were once widely prescribed as anorexigenic agents in the treatment of obesity. However, their high potential for abuse limits their use as diet aids. Furthermore, tolerance develops easily. Anorexigenic drugs with low abuse potential include sibutramine, diethylpropion, phenterimine, and mazindol.Their effectiveness is modest and side effects, primarily anxiety and insomnia, are comparable.

The combination of the serotonin enliancer fenflurainine with the syinpalhomimetic amine phenterimine was widely prescribed in the mid 1990s. The practice of prescribing "fen-phen" was abruptly halted in 1997 with the discovery of heart valve lesions in a large number of these patients. Fenfluramine has since been withdrawn from the market, and although phentermine remains available, it should not be combined with other. serotonin-enhancing agents. Given the limited efficacy and significant risks of appetite suppressants, their use should be limited to patients who are significantly overweight (BMI greater than 30) and they should be used only for brief periods of time.

Other selective serotonin reuptake inhibitors may also be useful in the treatment of obesity, particularly with patients who engage in binge eating and who have coexisting affective disorders. Hope for the future may also lie with a new class of drugs called h-pase inhibitors, which act directly on the gastroin-testinal tract to block the absorption of fat.

Exercise regimens are recommended as part of most treatment plans. Exercise is helpful not only because of the increase in caloric expenditure but because physical activity (in otherwise sedentary individuals) is associated with decreased appetite and increased basal metabolism. This latter effect may offset the estimated 15% - 30% decrease in basal metabolic rare that occurs with caloric restriction and weight ooss from dieting. Exercise also increases the proportion of weight loss from fat as opposed to lean body tissue. Exercise combined with low-calorie diets will result in weight loss; the difficulty, of course, is in motivating patients to comply with a disciplined regimen.

Support groups such as Overeaters Anonymous and Weight Watchers may be helpful in motivaung some individuals to lose weight. In recent years, behavior moditication programs have been shown to be eftective in reducing the high dropout rate associated with most weight reduction programs, particularly when deposits of money are required and sums are refunded with regular attendance or weight loss. Behavioral programs have been shown to be effective in the short run, but weight tends to be regained. Psychoanalysis and psychoanalytically oriented psychotherapy have not traditionally been regarded as being effective in the treatment of obesity. In their classic 1983 study, Rand and Slunkard suggest a more optimistic outlook. Of 84 men and women treated by 72 psychoanalysis, 72 had weiglit losses comparable to what was achieved by other methods, even though only about 6 of obese persons who entered treatment did so because of their obesity. Analysts also reported dramatic improvements in body image perceptions in their patients. Whereas 40% of obese patients showed marked body image disturbances at the start of treatment, only 14% continued to have such problems at termination. This study suggests that psychoanalytic psychotherapy may be effective in some cases, particularly for patients with disturbances of body image and self-concept.

Chapter 5 Sexual Dysfunction, Gender Identity Disorders and Paraphilias

Sexual difficulties may begin early in a person's life, or they may develop after an individual has previously experienced enjoyable and satisfying sex. A problem may develop gradually over time, or may occur suddenly as a total or partial inability to participate in one or more stages of the sexual act. The causes of sexual difficulties can be physical, psychological, or both.

Emotional factors affecting sex include both interpersonal problems and psychological problems within the individual. Interpersonal problems include marital or relationship problems, or lack of trust and open communication between partners. Personal psychological problems include depression, sexual fears or guilt, or past sexual trauma.

The Diagnoitic and Statisticcal Manual of Mental Disorders classifies sexual disorders in three categories — sexual dysfunctions, gender identity disorders, and paraphilias.

Sexual dysfunction disorders are generally classified into four categories: sexual desire disorders, sexual arousal disorders, orgasm disorders, and sexual pain disorders.

Sexual desire disorders (decreased libido) may be caused by a decrease in the normal production of estrogen (in women) or testosterone (in both men and women). Other causes may be aging, fatigue, pregnancy, and medications — the SSRI antidepressants which include fluoxetine (Prozac), sertraline (Zoloft), and paroxetine (Paxil) are well known for reducing desire in both men and women. Psychiatric conditions, such as depression and anxiety, can also cause decreased libido.

Sexual arousal disorders were previously known as frigidity in women and impotence in men. These have now been replaced with less judgmental terms. Impotence is now known as erectile dysfunction, and frigidity is now described as any of several specific problems with desire, arousal, or anxiety. For both men and women, these conditions may appear as an aversion to, and avoidance of, sexual contact with a partner. In men, there may be partial or complete failure to attain or maintain an erection, or a lack of sexual excitement and pleasure in sexual activity.

There may be medical causes for these disorders, such as decreased blood flow or lack of vaginal lubrication. Chronic disease may also contribute to these difficulties, as well as the nature of the relationship between partners. As the success of Viagra attests, many erectile disorders in men may be primarily physical, not psychological conditions. Orgasm disorders are a persistent delay or absence of orgasm following a normal sexual excitement phase. The disorder occurs in both women and men. Again, the SSRI antidepressants are frequent culprits — these may delay the achievement of orgasm or eliminate it entirely.

Sexual pain disorders affect women almost exclusively, and are known as dyspareunia (painful intercourse) and vaginismus (an involuntary spasm of the muscles of the vaginal wall, which interferes with intercourse). Dyspareunia may be caused by insufficient lubrication (vaginal dryness) in women. There may also be abnormalities in the pelvis or the ovaries that can cause pain with intercourse. Vulvar pain disorders can also cause dyspareunia and inability to have intercourse due to pain.

Poor lubrication may result from insufficient excitement and stimulation, or from hormonal changes caused by menopause or breast-feeding. Irritation from contraceptive creams and foams may also cause dryness, as can fear and anxiety about sex. It is unclear exactly what causes vaginismus, but it is thought that past sexual trauma such as rape or abuse may play a role. Another female sexual pain disorder is called vulvodynia or vulvar vestibulitis. In this condition, women experience burning pain during sex which may be related to problems with the skin in the vulvar and vaginal areas. The cause is unknown.

Sexual dysfunctions are most common in the early adult years, with the majority of people seeking care for such conditions during their late 20s through 30s. The incidence increases again in the perimenopause and postmenopause years in women, and in the geriatric population, typically with gradual onset of symptoms that are associated most commonly with medical causes of sexual dysfunction. Sexual dysfunction is more common in people who abuse alcohol and drugs. It is also more likely in people suffering from diabetes and degenerative neurological disorders. Ongoing psychological problems, difficulty maintaining relationships, or chronic disharmony with the current sexual partner may also interfere with sexual function.

Sexual Dysfunctions

Sexual dysfunction disorders are problems that interfere with the initiation, consummation, or satisfaction with sex. They occur in both men and women and are independent of sexual orientation.

Probably nowhere in human health do the body and mind interact more than during sex. There are four generally recognized phases of sexual activity, involving both mental and physical responses and are applicable to both men and women. These phases are in sequence:

Desire or appetite, fantasies or thoughts about sex;

Excitement — physical changes to prepare the body for intercourse and accompanying sense of sexual pleasure;

Orgasm — physical response that leads to the peak of physical pleasure and release of sexual tension;

Resolution — physical relaxation accompanied by a feeling of wellbeing and satisfaction.

Sexual dysfunction disorders can occur in any of these four phases. Their cause may be physiological or psychological. More than one sexual dysfunction disorder may appear simultaneously. *The Diagnostic and Statistical Manual of Mental Disorders*, produced by the American Psychiatric Association and used by most mental health professionals in North America and Europe to diagnose mental disorders, recognizes nine specific sexual dysfunctions:

Disorders of Desire

These interfere with the initiation of sex and include hypoactive sexual desire disorder (low interest in sex) and sexual aversion disorder (objections to having the genitals touched).

Disorders of Excitement or Sexual Arousal

These are female sexual arousal disorder (when a woman fails to have physiological responses associated with arousal), and male erectile disorder (when a man fails to get an adequate erection, also referred to as "erectile dysfunction").

Disorders of the Orgasm Phase

These are female orgasmic disorder (when a woman fails to reach orgasm); and male orgasmic disorder (when a man fails to reach orgasm) and premature ejaculation (when a man reaches orgasm too soon).

Sexual Pain Disorders (Associated with Intercourse and Orgasm)

These disorders are vaginismus (the outer part of a woman's vagina spasms causing pain) and dyspareunia (pain during intercourse in either men or women).

In addition, medications or illicit drugs may cause substance-induced sexual dysfunction and sexual dysfunction may be caused by a general medical condition such as diabetes or nerve damage. If the sexual dysfunction falls into none of the above areas, it is classified as sexual dysfunction not otherwise specified.

The causes of sexual dysfunction disorders are varied, as are their symptoms. In general, symptoms either prevent the initiation of sex or the completion of the sex act, or they interfere with satisfaction derived from sex. Almost everyone has some problem with sexual functioning or fulfillment at some point in their lives, but not all problems are considered sexual dysfunction disorders. Sexual satisfaction is very personal and individual, so that what may be an annoyance for one couple may be a serious problem for another. However, estimates suggest that roughly one-fourth of the adult population may have a sexual dysfunction disorder. More women than men report having sexual dysfunction disorders, but the difference may be that women are more open and active about seeking help with sexual problems than are men.

Diagnosis begins with a sexual and medical history, and often a physical examination and laboratory tests. Treatment must be individualized based on the cause and the specific dysfunction and includes physiological treatment, psychotherapy, and education and communication counseling. Most people can be helped to resolve their problems and improve their sex life. Generally, the sooner the person receives help, the easier the problem is to resolve. Support of a partner is often critical to successful resolution of the problem.

Sexual Response Cycle

The sexual response cycle has been described by Masters and Johnson and imodified tor diagnostic purposes by Kaplan. Four basic phases are generally recognized:

A. Appetitive or Desire Phase

In this phase, one or more stimuli (eg, visual, or factory, tactile, fantasies) engender a desire to engage in sexual activity.

B. Excitement or Arousal Phase

This phase includes the individual's feelings of sexual pleasure and accompanying physiological changes. The major change in both men and women is pelvic vasocongestion with accompanying myotonia. In men, this results in penile lumescence, stimulation of Cowper's gland, drawing of the scrotum and testicles closer to the body, and penile erection. In women, pelvic congestion and inyotonia result in engorgement of the vessels of the external genilalia and die vaginal lining, sweating (transudate production) of the vagina, which produces lubrication, increased tension of the pubococcygeal muscle surrounding the vaginal orifice, development of the orgasmic platform, increased sensitivity and enlargement of the clitoris, and "ballooning" of the inner two-thirds of the vagina. Breast tissue frequently engorges, with accompanying nipple erection and sensitivity. The period of time during which a level of sexual arousal is maintained is referred to as the plateau phase.

C. Orgasmic Phase

In both men and women, generalized muscle tension is followed by muscle contractions, resulting in involuntary pelvic thrusling and heightened sexual sensations. With the release of muscle tension, there are rhytiunic contractions of the pelvic and perineal muscles. In women, contractions occur in the lower third of the vagina and in the uterus, which has been elevated in relation to the other pelvic structures (orgasmic platform). In men, contractions of the prostate, seminal vesicles, and urethra propel seminal and prostatic fluids to the exterior while the bladder sphincter closes.

D. Resolution Phase

In both sexes, vasocongestion and myotonia become less intense, and there is general body relaxation. Men experience a physiological refractory period before erection and orgasm can occur again. Vasocongeslion and myotonia subside less quickly in women, and the clitoral and perineal tissues are sensitive enough to respond almost immediately to continued stimulation.

Most sexual dysfunctions are related to disturbances in one or more phases of the sexual response cycle. The disturbance may be physiological, psychological, or both. For example, a man who feels strong desire for a partner (psychological) may find that he is not being aroused, as evidenced by an absent or partial erection (physiological). Similarly, a woman who is sexually aroused by her partner and responding physiologically may be unable to reach orgasm as she begins to worry about losing control. Specific sexual dysfunctions will be described later in this discussion.

Interventions

Levels of Intervention: the PLISSIT Model

The PLISSIT model has been proposed to characterize the stepwise approach to counseling a person wilh a sexual problem. The first level of intervention is the giving of permission — for example, to discuss sex openly, to use the language of sex without guilt, or to engage in certain sexual behaviors that are generally considered normal. In providing such permission, the clinician must take care not to insist that the patient violate any strongly held values. The clinician may also provide limited information about sexual development, male - female differences, genital anatomy, etc. Specific suggestions may be provided that will enhance sexual pleasure or funclion, such as varying time or location of sexual activity, using certain sexual techniques, approaching a partner more effectively, or rejecting a partner in a supportive way. It may be important to ask the patient specifically about the use of safe sex procedures, to explain such procedures to them, and to recommend HIV testing, particularly if he or she is in a new relationship or is involved with multiple partners.

Many times, a sexual concern can be dealt with by utilizing only the first three levels of counseling. However, if a dysfunction is clearly present, intensive therapy should be undertaken by someone who is skilled in the techniques of sex therapy, in which cases all four levels of intervention are usually involved. In cases in which a dystunction is shown to have a medical basis, appropriate medical treatment may be provided as well.

Basic Considerations in Sex Therapy

Modern sex therapy was developed in the late 1960s with the pioneering work of Masters and Johnson, who demonstrated the value of behavioral therapy techniques in alleviating sexual symptoms.

Treatment was done in an intense, 2 - week format, using male and female cotherapists. Later, Kaplan showed that the same techniques could be effective in the more traditional 1 - hour- per- week therapy format using a single therapist. Whereas the treatment format of Masters and Johnson has the advantage of focusing on the sexual problem in a protected environment, the more spaced format has the advantage of flexibility for both patient and therapist while also integrating the ongoing treatment into the patient's normal lifestyle.

Basic Premises of Sex Therapy

A central precept of the Masters and Johnson technique is that the sexual response is a natural function that is barring any medical disturbance to the normal cycle, sexual responses will occur under appropriate psychosocial or tactile stimulation, unless something else in the intrapsychic or interpersonal environment blocks these responses. Kaplan referred to these factors as the immediate causes of sexual dysfunction. These may include things such as performance anxiety, absence of fantasy, inability to immerse oneself in a sexual situation (or "spectatoring"), or difficulties in seducing or arousing one's partner.

Deeper causes, such as psychodynamic issues, relationship problems, or early conditioning, may also be involved in the etiology of sexual dysfunctions. However, a short - term behavioral approach focused on the immediate causes of the dysfunction is often more successful and more economical than longer - term insight - oriented therapy. In most cases, the therapist must approach the presenting problem at more than one level of intervention. For example, concomitant problems in the couple's relationship often demand the simutineous attention to communication and control issues or the need to deal with a partner's fear of intimacy or fear of separation.

Table 1 outlines examples of both immediate and deeper causes of sexual dysfunction, many of which will be described more fully throughout the chapter.

There may be no direct correspondence between specific deeper causes and specilic dysfunctions. which become the final common pathway for a number of possible precipitating factors. For example, a woman's history of incest may be reflected sexually in hypoactive desire (or sexual aversion), anorgasinia, vaginismus, or a combination of these, or she may show no sexual pathology at all.

A. The Couple as the Patient

Another central premise on which the Masters and Johnson techniques were developed is the conviction that the couple is the patient. Thus, although one person may present with a sexual symptom, it is usually important that within treatment one partner is not blamed for the problem. Treatment should elicit the cooperation and support of the other partner and the sexual problem should be evaluated and treated as a relationship issue. Indeed, the other partner may display sexual symptoms (eg, absence of desire) in the course of treating the presenting problem, particularly if the original symptom was in some way functional for the partner.

Table 1 Etiology of sexual dysfunctions

Ⅰ Immediate causes	Ⅱ Deeper causes
A. Performance anxiety — fear of inadequate	A. Intrapsychic issues
B. Spectatoring — critically monitoring ones own sexual performance	1. Early conditioning 2. Sexual trauma
C. Inadequate communication with partner regarding sex	3. Depression 4. Anxiety
D. Fantasy	5. Guilt
1. Absence of fantasy	6. Fear of intimacy or separation
2. Distracting thoughts	B. Relationship issues
3. Antifantasy — fantasies incompatible with sexual arousal	1. Lack of trust 2. Power and control issues
	3. Anger at partner
	C. Sociocultural factors
	1. Attitudes and values
	2. Religious beliefs
	D. Educational and cognitive factors
	1.Sexual myths (gender roles, age and appearance, proper sexual activity, performance expectations)
	2. Sexual ignorance

Of course, there may be times when the person which presents with a sexual symptom has no partner, or the partner may refuse to participate in treatrnent. In such instances it is usually best to do what one can with the individual patient while explaining clearly the therapist's conviction that treatment done in the context of the relationship is more likely to be effective. Some sexual dysfunctions, such as a global anorgasmia, premature ejaculation, or vaginismus, can at least initially be treated through the use of individual therapy and/or masturbation exercises.

B. Education and Reassurance — Reframing One's Concept of Sexuality

Another extremely important aspect of sex therapy is the need to educate patients about various aspects of sexuality or to help restructure their conception of what sexuality is, or what it can be. This does not mean that a therapist imposes his or her ideas of what sex should be on the patient. If both members of a couple are satisfied with their level of activity or with their sexual repertoire, the therapist should not advocate personal beliefs concerning enhanced sexual practices. However, when two partners are incompatible in their approach to sex, or if advancing age, disability, or illness affects certain aspect of sex ablility. It can be seen as a recreational activity as fun. It can be s seen as the expression of caring and aftection. It can be seen simply as a release of sexual energy. It can be any combination of these four things at different times for the same couple.

The reproductive focus of sexuality in our culture also often leads to an excessive focus on gen itals, genital contact, and orgasm as goals of a fulfilling sexual response. Men and women often differ in this regard, as women more typically prefer a slower, whole - body approach to a sexual encounter than do men. Excessive focus on genitals, intercourse, orgasm, and performance only tends to heighten the level of anxiety in the man who experiences erectile problems or the wom an who suffers from vaginismus or hypoactive desire. One of the major accomplishments of sex therapy can be a broadening of the couple's approach, so that sexual practices become more varied and creative, anxiety about specific practices diminished, and the needs of both members of the couple are met.

A third aspect of reframing may be helping the couple to become more immersed in a sexual experience: leaving their daily cares outside the bedroom, being comfortable with a variety of sexual fantasies, and being involved in experiencing sex, rather than watching themselves perform or what Masters and Johnson called "spectatoring". Fantasy is difficult or incomfortable for some people to experience, as they may have paraphitic fantasies about partners other than the one to whom they are making love at the moment, or they may feel pressure from their partner to disclose their fantasies. People often need to be assured that in most cases, sexual fantasies, even unusual ones, are natural and that they can be kept private.

C. Respecting the Patient's Values

One of the most important qualities of a sex therapist is his or her ability tlo deal with sexual values and attitudes: both the therapist's and the patient's. Many programs for health professionals in sexliality education require trainers to participate in a values clarification or Sexual Attitude Reassessment (SAR) workshop, which may also be required for certification.

By taking a few days to openly and confidentially discuss their sexual attitudes and experiences with a group of peers, clinicians can clarily their own sexual values while developing an understanding of and a respect for the values and attitudes of others. By gaining an appreciation of the range of sexual values, they are less likely to impose their own values on the patient while finding it easier to work within the patient's own value system. The SAR experience can also increase the ability of the clinician to comnuinicate more easily about sexual matters and to use the language of sexuality with less apprehension or anxiety.

The patient's experiences and values may be different sharply from those of the clinician, and it is important that the clinician work effectively within the patient's framework. Couples who are not married will appear for treatment of a sexual dysfunction. An orgasmic woman or a male experiencing premature ejaculation may be unwilling to maslurbate, when mastlurbatory exercises would appear to be an important component of the treatment of choice. The sexual fulfillment of a lesbian couple may involve the kind of manual stimulation of the genitals that many hetero sexual individuals consider foreplay. In these and other instances, the clinician must be open, understanding, and flexible if the needs of the patient are to be met.

Whatever techniques may be used in treating these dysfunctions, there can be no substitute for the therapists' comfort level, skill, creativity, flexibilify, humor, sensitivity, patience, and warmth in making this process work. The couple presenting with a sexual problem should be able to leave therapy feeling good about sex, however they may define it, and they need to feel good about themselves as sexual people. In this frequently uncomfortable area, the sensitive, prepared professional can both provide relief and faciliate growth, often with relatively little of the right kind of help and support.

D. Qualifications of a Sex Therapist

There are two or three professional organizations that certify individuals in sex therapy. These organizations have developed standards of training and practice that health professionals are expected to meet if they are to be certified. Since certification us a sex therapist is typically not a legal requirement for the practice of sex therapy, many well-trained sex therapists are not certified as such. However, a referring clinician should be aware of the qualifications normally expected of a competent sex therapist.

A sex therapist should first be qualified in a recognized health care field, such as medicine, psychology, social work, or psychiatric nursing. It is helpful if the therapist already possesses good skills as an individual or couples therapist, as these skills are important to the effective treatment of sexual dystunction.

The therapist should have a thorough knowledge of the sexual response cycle, the effects of illness, medication, and substances such as alcohol on sexual function, and the effects of intrapsychic and cultural factors on sexual attitudes and function. The therapist's approach to the multidimensional nature of the sexual response must be balanced so that an awareness of all possible causes of a dysfunction is maintained. This awareness should be evident in the comprehensive approach to evaluation and in the therapist's willingness to consult with and refer to professionals in other relevant specialties, as may be necessary. For example, an erectile dysfunction can result from a combination of any number of neurological, endocrinolog ical, circulatory, or behavioral factors. It may often be necessary to refer a patient for a medical workup, treatment of a substance abuse problem, or individual therapy before an appropriate treatment plan can be developed for the presenting sexual problem.

The behavioral and cognitive techniques that are the hallmark of modern sex therapy also require special skill. These techniques and their applications will be discussed in some detail later.

Evalualion of Sexual Problem

The evalualion of a presenting sexual problem involves identifying both the immediate and deeper causes of the problem and developing an initial treatment plan. In keeping with the central idea that "the couple is the patient", equivalent histories are taken from both members of the couple. Detailed descriptions of evaluation procedures are beyond the scope of this discussion. However, it may be of value to highlight some of the key issues that should be ad-dressed in conducting the initial interviews.

Some therapists obtain background information from the patient in the form of pencil-and-pape tests or questionnaires. Formal testing may include general assessments (eg, MMPI-, SCL-90), assessments of sexual function (eg, LoPiccolo's Sexual Interaction Inventory, Derogatis Sexual Function Inventory), or inventories of relationship status (eg, Dyadic Ad-justment Inventory). Questionnaires may gather pertinent data such as ages and number of children, household occupants, religious background, names ot physicians and time of last physical examination, illnesses, surgeries, and present medications, a brief description of the presenting problem, and the patient's expectations for therapy.

The first two parts of the psychosexual evaluation are the description of the chief complaint and what Kaplan calls the sexual status examination. These are important, as they help determine the relative contributions of medical and psychosocial factors and enable the therapist to identify the immediate causes of the sexual problem.

Description of the Chief Complaint

This phase of the evalualion should include a description of the problem, its history, and why the patient sotiglit help at the present time. It is here that clear communication and definition of terms need to be established. What does the patient mean by "having sex" or "making love"or "partial erection" or "pain during intercourse?" Does "having sex" mean (only) vaginal in tercourse? Is the "partial erection" sufficient for pene tration? Is the pain experienced during intercourse deep in the vagina or at the entrance? And so on. A reluctance to communicate in de tail may prevent an adequate definition of the problem. The clinician should take care not to assume that the patient means one thing when something quite different mighl be meant.

A critical aspect of the description of the chief complaint is the determination of whether the symptoms are global or situational: that is, under what conditions the symptoms occur. This will help the clinician to determine (1) whether a medical examination might aid in a complete diagnosis and (2) the extent to which the symptoms are relationship related. For example, if a patient presents with an erectile problem, the clinician should attempt to determine whether the patient experiences erections in masturbalion or on awakening, and whether the onset of symptoms was sudden or gradual. The more global the symptoms and the more gradual the onset, the more likely it is that the problem has a medical etiology. If the erectile problem occurs primarily in the context of the patient's current relationship, it is important to know whether the problem began at the beginning of the relationship or whether it was related to a specitic event or situation that occurred since the relationship began (eg, moving in together, marriage). Does the problem occur with all partners, or perhaps with certain kinds of partners, such as those for whom the patient has strong feelings?

Sexual Status Examination

The sexual status examination is the patient's account of a recent or typical sexual encounter. The clinician can play an important role in helping patients feel more comfortable discussing their sexual activity in detail, pointing out its importance to the clinician's understanding of the problem. This is the clinician's way of determining the often subtle immediate causes of symptoms, and it should be done during each session in order to elucidate both progress and problems. The sexual status examination should assess all three phases of the sexual response cycle desire, aronsal, and orgasm. The clinician should determine the conditions under which the sexual encounter took place (eg, time of day, location, ambiance), who initiated it, what took place, what problems occurred, if any, how each partner responded to problems, and how the encounter ended. The clinician should also attempt to determine what thoughts or feelings accompanied any problems experienced during the encounter, which may be reassessed during individual interviews, as necessary.

When appropriate, it may be useful to do a detailed account of inas turbatory practices, dreams, or fantasies, as these may provide keys to the immediate causes of sexual symptoms while also aiding in the development of suitable behavioral assignments. The case of George, presented earlier, illustrates the value of doing a sexual status examination on a reported fantasy. Knowledge about a patient's masturbalory practices was helpful in developing suitable initial assignments.

Medical and Psychiatric Histories

The medical history should concentrate on illnesses, surgeries, and medications that are likely to cause or exacerbate sexual dysflinction, such as diabetes, vaginal infections, or circulatory problems. Assessment of drug use should include smoking, alcohol, illicit drugs, and both pre scription and over - the - counter medications. For example, over - the - counter antihistamines may inhibit vaginal lubrication. If appropriate, the couple should he asked about menstrual cy cling, the couple's sexual practices during menstruation, contraceptive use, and plans for hav ing children. At times, a couple will have stopped using contraception because "we're not having sex anyway." Unless they are trying to get pregnant, the clinician should encourage the couple to begin or resume whatever contraceptive practices they may wish to use.

This will minimize another possible source of anxiety regarding sexual success while helping the couple learn to integrate contraceptive use comfortably into their sexual encounters.

The psychiatric history focuses on previous or existing emotional problems and treatment, as well as a brief family history of psychiatric problems. In most cases, existing psychiatric problems, such as substance abuse or psychosis, should be stabilized before sex therapy is attempted. If a patient is in ongoing individual therapy, the sex therapist should establish consent and communication with the other therapist. Financial considerations may necessitate suspension of individual therapy while sex therapy is in progress.

Family and Sexual Histories

The family history concentrates on relationships in the home during childhood and adolescence, with special attention to the patient's perception of the intimate relationships of parents or other caregive's. This is followed by the sexual history, which includes a description of sexual learning and modeling as well as accounts of sexual experiences, both with and without partners. Patiepts should specifically be asked about any unwanted sexual experiences including, but not limited to rape, incest, or other traumatic sexual encounters. The response of both the patient and the family to these experiences should be assessed, as well as any treatment related to these events and the patient's current feelings about them. These questions should be asked of men as well as women, as it is not unusual for men to have experienced an event that they may not have previously identified as a sexual trauma. Such incidents may include incest, sexual contact with older individuals. Over exposure to nudity or sexuality in the home, and threats of castration.

Relationship History and Status

Relationship history and status are usually assessed gradually throughout the evaluation, although specific questions may remain at the end. Depending on the nature and age of the relationship, the clinician should determine how the relalionship began, how the partners feel aboat each other (both positive and negative feelings are important), how the relationship may be different from previous relationships, whether there are any problems with intimacy, whether communication and control issues exist, and whether there are plans for cohabitation, children, marriage, etc.

Individual Sessions

Each member of the couple should be seen alone for at least part of a session, with an invitation for further individual sessions as needed and the agreement that any information presented as confidential will be maintained as such. The clinician may introduce these sessions with the assurance that any well - functioning couple has "secrets" that they may not feel comfortable sharing with their partner, but that such information may be useful to the therapist. Both partners are asked whether there is anything about the relationship or about their own development that they are not comfortable disclosing in the partner's presence, but that may he important for the clinician to know. The clinician may also ask about the nature of the person's fantasies and how comfortable he or she is with fantasy. At this session it is also important to ask about any other ongoing sexual relationships. The clinician may point out that such relationships, although the patient's business, may impede the therapeutic process, and that for the duration of therapy it is best that they be discontinued. It is in response to this question that a patient experiencing erectile problems with lack of desire may admit good performance will another partner, signifying problems in the primary relationship that need to be addressed. At times, the sudden anandonment of a sexual affair will lead to an almost instantaneous "cure" by encouraging a focus on the primary partner.

Considerations in Overall Assessment

In evaluating the presenting problem, it oftlen becomes clear that the meaning symptom is secondliry to a more primary sexual problem, and the therapy must take both into nccount. For example, lack of desire in a male may be secondary to an erectile problem. Vaginismus is frequently secondary to an underlying hypoaclive desire or sexual aversion. A good understanding of the conditions under which symptoms present themselves as well as the history of the presenting problem will clarify the real nature of the problem and enable the clinician to develop an appropriate treatment plan.

When it appears that there may be a medical etiology to a sexualy dysfunction, the patient should be referred to a physician who is knowledgeable about current diagnostic and treatment techniques, respectful of the psychusocial aspects of sexual dysfunction, and comfortable dealing with sexual issues. It is of utmost importance that the various professionals involved in a case communicate clearly about the patient's.

Treatment Techniques

Direct advice, guidance, information, reassurance, or instruction may suffice to overcome the milder, simpler, and more transient cases of impotence and frigidity. The correction of faulty attitudes and irrational beliefs is often an essential forerunner to specific techniques of lovemaking. One should endeavor to impart nonmoralistic insights into all matters pertaining to sex. It is often helpful to prescribe nontechnical but authoritative literature.

Graded Sexual Assignments

Gunther (1998) evolved a simple but effective procedure for promoting sexual adequacy and responsiveness in those cases where anxiety partially inhibits sexual performance. A cooperative sexual partner is indispensable to the successes of the technique. The patient is instructed not to make any sexual responses that engender feelings of tension or anxiety but to proceed only to the point where pleasurable reactions predominate. The partner is informed that she must never press him to go beyond this point, and that she must be prepared for several amorous and intimate encounters that will not culminate in coitus. The theory is that by maintaining sexual arousal in the ascendant over anxiety, the latter will decrease from one amorous session to the next. Thus, positive sexual feelings and responses will be facilitated and will, in turn, further inhibit residual anxieties. In this manner, conditioned inhibition of anxiety is presumed to increase until the anxiety reactions are completely eliminated.

The Role of Desensitization Procedures in Overcoming Frigidity

Treatment of chronic frigidity by systematic desensitization was first reported Lazarus (1963). Desensitization has also been successfully applied to groups of impotent men and frigid women. The preferred size of desensitization groups is between four and eight members. The sessions are conducted at the pace of the slowest (most anxious) individual. If one group member obviously delays the progress of the other patients, he is given a few individual sessions to expedite matters. The typical hierarchy applied to the frigid women consisted of the following progression: embracing, kissing, being fondled, mild petting, undressing, foreplay in the nude, awareness of husband's erection, moving into position for insertion, intromission, changing positions during coitus.

In the treatment of vaginismus (as well as in those cases suffering from generalized fears of penetration), desensitization, first in imagination, followed at home by gradual dilation of the vaginal orifice, has proved highly successful. The patient, under conditions of deep relaxation, is asked to imagine her inserting a graded series of objects into the vagina. When she is no longer anxious about the imagined situation, she is asked to use real objects. One might commence with the tip of a cotton bud, or the tip of the patient's little finger, followed by the gradual insertion of two or more fingers, internal sanitary pads, various lubricated cylinders, and eventually by the gradual introduction of the penis, culminating with vigorous coital movement. Masters and Johnson consider it necessary for husband and wife to cooperate in all phases of dilatation therapy.

Assertive Training for Impotent Men

Many impotent men appear to have servile attitudes toward women and respond to them with undue deference and humility. Their sexual passivity and timidity are often part of a generally nonassertive outlook, and their attendant inhibitions are usually not limited to their sex life. These men feel threatened when required to assume dominance in a male - female relationship. Therapy is aimed at augmenting a wide range of expressive impulses, so that formerly inhibited sexual inclinations may find overt expression. This is achieved first by explaining to the patient how ineffectual forms of behavior produce many negative emotional repercussions. The unattractive and exceedingly distasteful features of obsequious behavior are also emphasized. The patient is then told how to apply principles of assertiveness to various interpersonal situations. For instance, he is requested to "express his true feelings; stand up for his rights," and to keep detailed notes of all his significant attempts (whether successful or unsuccessful) at assertive behavior. His feelings and responses are then fully discussed with the therapist, who endeavors to shape the patient's behavior by means of positive reinforcement and constructive criticism.

Aversion- Relief Therapy in the Treatment of a Sexually Unresponsive Woman

Here patient is given aversive stimuli such as electric shock. When the electrical impulses became intolerable, she was required to turn her attention toward several photographs of nude men on the desk in front of her. Upon looking at the pictures, the shock is immediately terminated (producing definite signs of relief). She receives intermittent shocks when averting her gaze from the pictures. A slightly modified method can be at a later stage. The therapist says, "Shock! " and administered a very strong burst of electricity to the patient's palm if she did not proceed to look at the pictures within eight seconds. She is told that she could avoid the shock by looking at the pictures in good time.

The Treatment of Premature Ejaculation

Premature ejaculation is sometimes a symptom of anxiety. The amelioration of anxiety by such techniques as relaxation, desensitization, and assertive training has therefore proved helpful in certain instances. In general, however, it should be noted that psychotherapeutic efforts have not proved especially effective in altering the premature response pattern. Nevertheless, some essentially simple tricks may occasionally meet with gratifying success. For instance, some individuals have managed to delay orgasm and ejaculation merely by dwelling on nonerotic thoughts and images while engaged in sexual intercourse. Others have found it more effective to indulge in self - inflicted pain during coitus (eg, pinching one's leg, biting one's tongue). Masters and Johnson (1970), however, are not in favor of distraction techniques. The use of depressant drugs (eg, alcohol or barbiturates) may also impede premature ejaculation in some individuals. The reduction of tactile stimulation (eg, by wearing one or more condoms, or by applying anesthetic ointments to the glans penis) is also often recommended. All of the foregoing procedures are of limited value (Lazarus, 1978).

Two very effective techniques for the treatment of premature ejaculation are the pause (Semans, 1956) and the squeeze (Masters and Johnson, 1970) procedures. The pause technique consists of the female stimulating the male manually until he feels the physical sensations immediately preceding orgasm. At this point, the wife stops stimulating him until the sensations subside, then begins stimulating the penis again, and stops just before ejaculation. As this procedure is repeated, the male begins to develop ejaculatory control. The next step consists of repeating the procedure with the penis lubricated, so that the intravaginal environment is more closely approximated.

Masters and Johnson (1970) have developed a modification of this procedure in which the wife manually stimulates the penis until it becomes erect. She then squeezes the penis at the coronal ridge for three to four seconds, which causes the man to lose the urge to ejaculate and to lose 10% - 30% of his erection. The wife waits fifteen to thirty seconds, then repeats the procedure. After practicing for a few days, the couple repeats the procedure with intravaginal containment of the penis, but no thrusting, to produce stimulation. The next steps are intravaginal containment with slow movement, and than fast movement, using the squeeze as before.

Bibliotherapy

Bibliotherapy refers to treatment for mental and physical health problems in which written material plays a central role. It is often applied within treatment formats with minimal or absent therapist contact, such as self - help manuals, brief skills training, or education. It is cost effective and considered a succesful adjunct to psychotherapy for SDs, particularly orgasmic disorders. Growing research also indicates that sexual dysfunction, as compared to other psychological disorders, is particularly amenable to a bibliotherapy.

It is recommended to see a physician, counselor, therapist or other health care and human service provider when first addressing these concerns due to the multiple factors influencing the development of sexual problems (eg, depression, anxiety and physical illness).

Pharmacological and Medical Intervention

Modern medicine is also capable of treating various sexual dysfunctions. Although many pharmacological treatments may be utilized in place of psychotherapy, it is important to recognize the limitations. Pharmacological treatment focuses primarily on restoring physiological sexual responses while leaving other important psychological and psychosocial concerns, such as poor couple communication, negative attitudes and inaccurate beliefs about sex. It is therefore recommended that these interventions be utilized as adjuncts to psychotherapy for sexual dysfunction.The following are a list of treatments which have shown effectiveness:

Desire & Arousal Disorders;

Ejaculatory Inhibition.

Gender Identity Disorders

Gender identity disorders are a relatively new category of psychiatric disturbance that continues to be subject to confusion and controversy. Cross-gender behavior has been described since antiquity and entered the medical literature as a distinct condition in the nineteenth century. However, gender disorders were not added to the DSM until the third edition in 1980, first as psychosexual disorders and then, in DSM-Ⅲ-R, as disorders first evident in infancy, childhood, or adolescence. In DSM-Ⅳ, sexual and gender identity disorders have all been grouped together in the same section. The gender identity disorders are essentially disturbances in an individual's sense of masculinity or femininity, which interact with social conceptualizations of gender and sexual orientation. DSM-Ⅳ diagnostic criteria for substance induced sexual dysfunction:

A. Clinically significant sexual dysfunction that results in marked distress or interpersonal difficulty.

B. There is evidence from the history, physical examination, or laboratory findings of substance intoxication, and the symptoms in Criterion A developed during, or within a month of, significant substance intoxication.

C. The disturbance is not better accounted for by a sexual dysfunction that is not substance-induced. Evidence that the symptoms are better accounted for by a sexual dysfunction that is not substance-induced might include: the symptoms precede the onset of the substance abuse or dependence: persist for a substantial period of time (eg, about a month) after the cessation of acute withdrawal or severe intoxication: are substantially in excess of what would be expected given the character, duration, or amount of substance used: or there is other evidence suggesting the existence of an independent non - substance - induced sexual dyslunction (eg, a history of recurrent non-substance-related episodes).

Definitions

Sex is defined on the basis of the physical appearance of the genitals (gonadal sex or sex phenotype) or in some cases on the basis of the chromosomes (genotype). Socially, sex is partitioned into two complementary categories: male or female. Newboms with intersex conditions, such as herinaphroditisrn, are assigned to one sex for rearing.

Gender refers to the individual's status as male or female (or in some rare cases intersex) including personal experience and social and legal identification. Gender is phenoinenologically broader than genilal anatomy. Gender identity is the private experience of gender role as male or female in self-awareness and beliavior. Gender role refers to the public manifestation of gender identity, everything a person says or does (including sexual behavior) that indicates a status as either male or female. The definitional content of gender statuses varies among groups. Gender includes components of erotic or sexual orientation. For most individuals, gender identity and role are integrated (as gender identity/role) with a unity and persistence.

Gender identity disorders can occur when a person does not experience a unity and persistence of the personal experience of gender identity and the social expression of gender role. Gender dysplioria is the pathological state of dissatisfaction and subjective incongruity between the sex phenotype (genilal anatomy and secondary sexual characteristics) and the gender identity and role. Gender dysphoria is expressed as a body image disorder, for which the treatment has been a combination of psychotherapy and the alteration of the body through medical and surgical procedures.

Transsexualism as a diagnostic label was dropped from DSM - Ⅳ but is still used as a descriptive term in the professional and popular literature. Properly considered, transsexualism refers to a process of sex reassignment. Labeling a person as a iranssexual might also reflect the status of having completed sex reassignment, as a resolution of an underlying gender dysphoria or gender identity disorder. However, many individuals with gender identity disorders never seek or complete sex reassignment. So the synonymous use of the term transsexualism for gender identity disorder can be misleading.

Gender identity disorders in children and in adolescents and adults are described together in DSM-Ⅳ, although the diagnostic criteria and nature of the syndrome vary greatly, and they are assigned different code numbers. For clarity of discussion, these two categories of gender identity disorders are separated in the following sections.

Gender identity disorder (GID) or transsexualism is defined by strong, persistent feelings of identification with the opposite gender and discomfort with one's own assigned sex. People with GID desire to live as members of the opposite sex and often dress and use mannerisms associated with the other gender. For instance, a person identified as a boy may feel and act like a girl. This is distinct from homosexuality in that homosexuals nearly always identify with their apparent sex or gender.

Identity issues may manifest in a variety of different ways. For example, some people with normal genitals and secondary sex characteristics of one gender privately identify more with the other gender. Some may cross - dress, and some may actually seek sex - change surgery. Others are born with ambiguous genitalia, which can raise identity issues.

Many individuals with gender identity disorder become socially isolated, whether by choice or through ostracization, which can contribute to low self - esteem and may lead to school aversion or even dropping out. Peer ostracism and teasing are especially common consequences for boys with the disorder.

Boys with gender identity disorder often show marked feminine mannerisms and speech patterns. The disturbance can be so pervasive that the mental lives of some individuals revolve only around activities that lessen gender distress. They are often preoccupied with appearance, especially early in the transition to living in the opposite sex role. Relationships with parents also may be seriously impaired. Some males with gender identity disorder resort to self - treatment with hormones and may (very rarely) perform their own castration or penectomy. Especially in urban centers, some males with the disorder may engage in prostitution, placing them at a high risk for human immunodeficiency virus (HIV) infection. Suicide attempts and substance - related disorders are common.

Children with gender identity disorder may manifest coexisting separation anxiety disorder, generalized anxiety disorder and symptoms of depression. Adolescents are particularly at risk for depression and suicidal ideation and suicide attempts. Adults may display anxiety and depressive symptoms. Some adult males have a history of transvestic fetishism as well as other paraphilias. Associated personality disorders are more common among males than among females being evaluated at adult gender clinics.

Gender Identity Disorders in Children

Psychologists believe human sexual identities are made up of three separate components. The first shows the direction of a child's sexual orientation, whether he or she is heterosexual (straight), homosexual (gay), or bisexual. The second is the child's style of behavior, whether a female is a "tomboy" or homemaker - type and a male is a "macho guy" or a "ensitive boy". The third component is what psychologists call the core gender identity. According to an article in the May 12, 2001 issue of *New Scientist*, it is the most difficult to ascertain but is essentially the deep inner feeling a child has about whether he or she is a male or female.

In most people, the three components point in the same direction but in some people, the components are more mixed. For example, a gay woman (lesbian) might look and act either feminine or masculine (butch), but she still deeply feels she is a female. Scientists are uncertain about where the inner feeling of maleness or femaleness comes from. Some believe it is physical, from the body, while others believe it is mental, from the hypothalamus region of the brain. There is also debate on whether the determination is shaped by hormones, particularly testosterone and estrogen, or by genes assigned at conception.

Gender identity emerges by the age of two or three and is influenced by a combination of biological and sociological factors reinforced at puberty. Once established, it is generally fixed for life.

Aside from sex differences, other biological contrasts between males and females are already evident in childhood. Girls mature faster than boys, are physically healthier, and are more advanced in developing oral and written linguistic skills. Boys are generally more advanced at envisioning and manipulating objects. They are more aggressive and more physically active, preferring noisy, boisterous forms of play that require larger groups and more space than the play of girls the same age.

In spite of conscious attempts to reduce sex role stereotyping in the final decades of the twentieth century and in the early 2000s, boys and girls are still treated differently by adults from the time they are born. The way adults play with infants has been found to differ based on gender. Girls are treated more gently and approached more verbally than boys. As children grow older, many parents, teachers, and other authority figures still tend to encourage independence, competition, aggressiveness, and exploration more in boys and expression, nurturance, motherhood and childrearing, and obedience more in girls.

Symptoms and Signs

This is especially important as another new study, "Childhood Gender Nonconformity: A Risk Indicator for Childhood Abuse and Posttraumatic Stress in Youth," found that these children were at risk for "childhood sexual, physical, and psychological abuse and PTSD."

Many of these children also present with serious psychological symptoms, including anxiety, depression, or suicidal ideation. Many also engage in self - harm behaviors. It is important that this study notes that these symptoms do not seem to be primarily psychiatric. Instead, they found that their "psychological functioning improves with medical intervention and suggests that the patients' psychiatric symptoms might be secondary to a medical incongruence between mind and body".

Ideally, it would seem like treatment with reversible gonadotropin - releasing hormone (GnRH) analogs to suppress puberty should occur before secondary sexual characteristics have fully developed. They also provide some clues that might indicate a child has gender identity disorder, including:

Preference for female clothing and underwear (boys);

Always sitting to void (boys);

Exclusive play with female toys when given a choice (boys);

Desire for long hair (boys);

Preference for male underwear (girls);

Breast binding (girls);

Refusal to wear female swimsuits (girls);

Psychiatric decompensation at the onset of menstruation (girls).

If symptoms of gender dysphoria persist or intensity as the child starts puberty, then they should be referred to a specialist who treats teens with gender identity disorder and medical treatment should be considered.

Unfortunately, there aren't that many clinics that specialize in this type of treatment. Among those that do are the Gender Management Service (GeMS) Clinic at Children's Hospital Boston and the Disorders of Sexual Development Clinic at UCSF Benioff Children's Hospital.

Keep in mind that some gender questioning and gender role exploration can be normal. The prevalence of true gender identity disorder is much lower than rates of reported cross-gender behavior. That may indicate that "a lot of children seem to be experimenting with cross-gender behavior, but very few are following through to request gender change as they mature." At least that is the conclusion of a commentary in the same issue of Pediatrics, "Gender Identity Disorder: An Emerging Problem for Pediatricians."

Still, the bottom line, according to the American Academy of Pediatrics, is that "Study authors advocate for early evaluation of children exhibiting GID, but treatment with medications should not be started until they reach puberty. Pediatricians and parents should consult with experienced mental health professionals for children and adolescents experiencing gender-related issues. When patients are sufficiently physically mature to receive medical treatment, they should be referred to a medical specialist or program treating GID."

Natural History

Overt behaviors may be evident as early as age 2-3 and many characteristics subside by age 8 with or without any treatment. Extreme gender-noncon-formist behavior can lead to social ostracization from the peer group and to teasing. Distress associated with social impairment is the most common complaint. This can lead to sequelae of poor self-concept and depression. There may also be problems in interactions within the family.

Gender identity disorders of childhood are infrequently diagnosed or referred for treatment. The actural incidence is unknown and may vary according to social standards of sex role stereotyping. There is no association with any single pattern of child rearing or family dynamics. Family dynamics may influence the severity of the presenting problems, particularly in cases in which there are conflicts belween parents, pathological encouragement of gender-atypical behavior, or extreme rejection of it.

There is a growing amount of scientific research that suggests gender identity develops at a very early age. Several studies show that infants can discriminate between male and female faces and associate faces and voices according to gender by the time they reach one year old. However, gender-labeling tasks, such as toy identification, do not occur until about age two. Gender identity and awareness of sex differences generally emerge in the first three to four years of a child's life. However, children begin to demonstrate a preference for their own sex starting at about age two.

Gender identification is often associated with the choice and use of toys in this age group, according to a number of studies done in the 1970s, 1980s, and 1990s. Sex differences in toy play have been found in children as young as one year old. By age two, children begin to spontaneously choose their types of toys based on gender. Several of these studies show that by age one, boys display a more assertive reaction than girls to toy disputes. By age two, the reaction of boys is more aggressive.

Most two-year-olds know whether they are boys or girls and can identify adults as males or females. By age three, most children know that men have a penis and women have breasts. Also at age three, children begin to apply gender labels and stereotypes, identifying gentle, empathic characteristics with females and strong, aggressive characteristics with males. Even in the twenty-first century, most young children develop stereotypes regarding gender roles, associating nurses, teachers, and secretaries as females and police officers, firefighters, and construction workers as males.

Preschoolers develop an increasing sense of self-awareness about their bodies and gender differences. Fears about the body and body mutilation, especially of the genitals, are often major sources of fear in preschoolers. As children become more aware of gender differences, preschoolers often develop intense feelings of vulnerability and anxiety regarding their bodies.

By the age of six years, children are spending about 11 times as much time with members of their own sex as with children of the opposite sex. This pattern begins to change as the child approaches puberty, however.

By the teenage years, most children have an established sexual orientation of heterosexual, homosexual, or bisexual. They have also established their style of behavior and core sexual identity. However, a very small fraction have not.

While most children follow a predictable pattern in the acquisition of gender identity, some develop a gender identity inconsistent with their biological sex, a condition variously known as gender confusion, gender identity disorder, or transsexualism, which affects about one in 20,000 males and one in 50,000 females. Researchers have found that both early socialization and hormonal factors may play a role in the development of gender identity disorder. Children with gender identity disorder usually feel from their earliest years that they are trapped in the wrong body and begin to show signs of gender confusion between the ages of two and four. They prefer playmates of the opposite sex at an age when most children prefer to spend time in the company of same-sex peers. They also show a preference for the clothing and typical activities of the opposite sex; transsexual boys like to play house and play with dolls. Girls with gender identity disorder are bored by ordinary female pastimes and prefer the rougher types of play typically associated with boys, such as contact sports.

Both male and female transsexuals believe and repeatedly insist that they actually are, or will grow up to be, members of the opposite sex. Girls cut their hair short, favor boys' clothing, and have negative feelings about maturing physically as they near adolescence. In childhood, girls with gender identity disorder experience less overall social rejection than boys, as it is more socially acceptable for a girl to be a tomboy than for a boy to be perceived as feminine. About five times more boys than girls are referred to therapists for this condition. Teenagers with gender identity disorder suffer social isolation and are vulnerable to depression and suicide. They have difficulty developing peer relationships with members of their own sex as well as romantic relationships with the opposite sex. They may also become alienated from their parents.

Treatment

Cross - gendered interests and behaviors can be troublesome for children and upsetting for parents. Parents worry about what the likely outcomes will be. Boys severely stigmatized by peers may develop pour self - concepts and litter act in self - destructive ways that may have serious health consequences (including increased risk of suicide or AIDS). Therefore, psychological intervention is helpful for the children and their families. Treatment is not likely to change the outcome in terms of sexual orientation but may help the adjustment of the individuals in the firnuly system.

Treatment usually involves an evaluation of the child and the family system. The parents are then given assistance in developing positive ways to help the child reduce the expression of the gender - atypical behavior or mininuze the negative social consequences of such behavior. Depending on the family issues, the parents may be seen individually, as a couple, or in a support group with other parents of children with gender problems. In some cases, the child might participate in behavioral treatment to help modify problematic gender behavior. Child therapy may also be helpful if there are significant family problems or significant anger or depression. Otherwise, the cliild may not be seen regularly except for follow - up evaluations.

Gender Identity Disorder in Adolescents or Adults

Symptoms and Signs

There are two components of Gender Identity Disorder, both of which must be present to make the diagnosis. They must be evidence of astrong and persistent gross - gender identification, which is the desire to be, or the insistence that one is of the other sex. This cross-gender identification must not merely be a desire for anyperceived cultural advantages of being the other sex. there must also be evidence of persistent discomfort about one assigned sex or asense of inappropriateness in the gender role of that sex. The diagnosis is not made if the individual has a concurrent physicalintersex condition (eg, androgen insensitivity syndrome or congenitaladrenal hyperplasia). To make the diagnosis, there must beevidence of clinically significant distress or impairment in social, occupational, or other important areas of functioning.

In boys, the cross gender identification is manifested by a marked preoccupation with traditionally feminine activities. They may have a preference for dressing in girls' or womens' clothes or may improvise such items from available materials when genuine articles areunavailable. Towels, aprons, and scarves are often used to representlong hair or skirts. There is a strong attraction for the stereotypical games and pastimes of girls. They particularly enjoy playing house, drawing pictures of beautiful girls and princesses, and watching television or videos of their favorite female - type dolls, such as Barbie, are often their favorite toys, and girls are their preferred playmates. When playing house, these boys role - play female figures. Most commonly mother roles, and often are quite preoccupied with female fantasy figures. They avoid rough - and - tumble play and competitive sports and have little interest in cars and trucks or other no-aggressive but stereotypical boy's toys. They may express a wish tobe a girl and assert that they will grow up to be a woman. They may insist on sitting to urinate and pretend not to have a penis by pushing it in between their legs. More rarely, boys with Gender Identity Disorder may state that they find their penis or testes disgusting, that they want to remove them, or that they have, or wish to have, avagina.

Girls with Gender Identity Disorder display intense negative reactionsto parental expectations or attempts to have them wear dresses or other feminine attire. Some may refuse to attend school or social events where such clothes may be required. They prefer boy's clothing and short hair, are often misidentified by strangers as boys, and may ask to be called a boy's name, their fantasy heroes are most often powerful male figures, such as Batman or Superman. These girls prefer boys as playmates, with whom they share interests in contact sports, rough-and-tumble play and traditional boyhood games. They show little interest in dolls or any form of feminine dress up or role-play activity. A girl with this disorder may occasionally refuse to urinatein a sitting position. She may claim that she has or will grow a penisand may not want to grow breasts or menstruate. She may assert that she will grow up to be a man. Such girls typically reveal marked cross-gender identification in role-play, dreams and fantasies.

Adults with Gender Identity Disorder are preoccupied with their wish to live as a member of the other sex. This preoccupation may be manifested as an intense desire to adopt the social role of the other sex or to acquire the physical appearance of the other sex through hormonal orsurgical manipulation. Adults with this disorder are uncomfortable being regarded by others as, or functioning in society as, a member of their designated sex. To varying degrees, they adopt the behavior, dress, and mannerisms of the other sex. In private, these individuals may spend much time cross-dressed and working on the appearance of being the other sex. Many attempt to pass in public as the other sex. With cross-dressing and hormonal treatment (and for males, electrolysis), many individuals with this disorder may passconvincingly as the other sex. The sexual activity of these individuals with same-sex partners is generally constrained by the preference that their partners neither see nor touch their genitals. For some males who present later in life (often following marriage), sexual activity with a woman is accompanied by the fantasy of being lesbian lovers or that his partner is a man and he is a woman.

In adolescents, the clinical features may resemble either those of children or those of adults, depending on the individual developmental level, and the criteria should be applied accordingly. In younger adolescents, it may be more difficult to arrive at an accurate diagnosis because of the adolescent guardedness. This may be increased if the adolescent feels ambivalent about cross-gender identification or feels that it is unacceptable to the family. The adolescent may be referred because the parents or teachers areconcerned about social isolation or peer teasing and rejection. In such circumstances, the diagnosis should be reserved for those adolescents who appear quite cross-gender identified in their dress and who engagein behaviors that suggest significant cross-gender identification (eg, shaving legs in males). Clarifying the diagnosis in children and adolescents may require monitoring over an extended period of time.

Distress or disability in individuals with Gender Identity Disorder is manifested differently across the life cycle, in young children, distress is manifested by the stated unhappiness about their assigned sex. Preoccupation with cross - gender wishes often interferes with ordinary activities. In older children, failure to developage - appropriate same sex peer relationships and skills often leads to isolation and distress, and some children may refuse to attend school because of the teasing or pressure to dress in at tire stereotypical of their assigned sex. In adolescents and adults, preoccupation withcross - gender wishes often interferes with ordinary activities. Relationship difficulties are common and functioning at school or at work may be impaired. These are the proposed criteria for adults and teenagers for the upcoming DSM - V.

A. A marked incongruence between one's experienced/expressed gender and assigned gender, of at least 6 months duration, as manifested by 2 or more of the following indicators:

A marked incongruence between one's experienced/expressed gender and primary and/or secondary sex characteristics (or, in young adolescents, the anticipated secondary sex characteristics);

A strong desire to be rid of one's primary and/or secondary sex characteristics because of a marked incongruence with one's experienced/expressed gender (or, in young adolescents, a desire to prevent the development of the anticipated secondary sex characteristics);

A strong desire for the primary and/or secondary sex characteristics of the other gender;

A strong desire to be of the other gender (or some alternative gender different from one's assigned gender);

A strong desire to be treated as the other gender (or some alternative gender different from one's assigned gender);

A strong conviction that one has the typical feelings and reactions of the other gender (or some alternative gender different from one's assigned gender).

B. The condition is associated with clinically significant distress or impairment in social, occupational, or other important areas of functioning, or with a significantly increased risk of suffering, such as distress or disability.

Post - transition, ie, the individual has transitioned to full - time living in the desired gender (with or without legalization of gender change) and has undergone (or is undergoing) at least one cross - sex medical procedure or treatment regimen, namely, regular cross - sex hormone treatment or gender reassignment surgery confirming the desired gender (eg, penectomy, vaginoplasty in a natal male, mastectomy, phalloplasty in a natal female).

Etiology and Prognosis

The cause of gender identity disorders in adolescents and adults is not known. Patients typically report the onset of their awareness of gender dysphoria in early childhood. In many cases, however, they did not exhibit cross - gendered behaviors that were noticed by others. Few mature individuals with this disorder have a documented history of gender identity of childhood. In other cases, the onset of the disorder would appear to be in adolescence or adnithood, sometimes after marrying and raising a family.

There are several different patterns for gender identity disorders, which may reflect different etiologies and prognoses. However, research is still preliminary and there is no consensus about any typology. One group of males reports a period of identification as male homosexuals; some of these were effeminate boys. Another group of males had what appeared to be conventional, even macho, masculine heterosexual histories, although they may have reported underlying gender dysphoria. Still another group of males had a history of heterosexual transvestisin that evolved into a gender identity disorder later in adulthood. Females with gender identity disorder often describe tomboyish histories' and sexual interests in females, although usually not to the extreme that would bring them to professional attention. Asexual individuals seeking sex reassignment also report childhood histories of gender dysphoria, even though they did not exhibit cross - gendered behaviors that aroused the suspicions of others or resulted in referral for evaluation.

Once diagnosed, gender identity disorders of adolescence and adulthood are usually chronic until the individual is rehabilitated in the desired gender identity and role. However, there may be periods of remission, and rehabilitation may not in all cases extend to surgical sex reassignment. Following reassignment, the frequency of satisfaction is very high with remission of most pathology associated with gender dysplioria.

Treatment

Treatment of gender identity disorders is complex and is rarely successful when the goal is to reverse the disorder.

Children

Improve existing role models or, in their absence, provide one from the family or elsewhere. Caregivers are helped to encourage sex - appropriate behavior and attitudes. Any associated mental disorder should be addressed.

Adolescents

Are difficult to treat due to the coexistence of normal identity crises and gender identity confusion. Acting out is common, and adolescents rarely have a strong motivation to alter their stereotypic cross-gender roles.

Adults

(1) Psychotherapy, with the goal of helping patients to become comfortable with the gender identity they desire. Also explores sex - reassignment surgery and the indications and contraindications for such procedures.

(2) Sex-reassignment surgery. This is definitive and irreversible. Patients must go through a 3 to 12 month trial of cross dressing and receive hormone treatment. 70%-80% of patients are dissatisfied with the results. A reported 2% commit suicide.

(3) Hormonal treatments. In this case patients are treated with hormones in time of surgery.

Paraphilias

Paraphilias are psychosexual disorders characterized by recurrent, intense sexual fantasies, urges, or behaviors involving atypical or unacceptable sexual content. They are the sexual equivalents of obsessions and compulsions, focusing on aspects of human sexuality that do not have the goal of mutual sexual arolisal with a partner. The term "paraphilia" comes from the Greek for love (philia) that is "aside" (para) in the sense of being altered or modified, a deviation in the object of attraction. Paraphilia has replaced the older terms of sexual perversion or deviation.

Symptoms and Signs

The paraphilias all involve "recurrent intense sexually arousing fantasies, sexual urges, or behaviors" that have been present for more than 6 months, according to DSM - Ⅳ criteria. These urges and fantasies are not the transitory or variant sexual scenarios imagined by the sexually adventurous. They do not change readily, are difficult to keep out of sexual consciousness, and have a power that at times makes it difficult to resist acting them out. Paraphilias are manifested in imagery, which may exist as a sexual problem or be associated with erection or orgasm in masturbation or other sexual behavior. Because acting out some paraphilias may involve illegal acts, many individuals with paraphilias are reluctant to acknowledge public acts or acts with a partner.

The paraphtlias are named for the sexual content that is the primary focus of the sexual fantasy. There are over 40 named paraphilias, although only the more common ones for which people seek psychiatric help are listed in DSM - Ⅳ. This content may be independent of sexual orientation. Although some paraphitias usually occur only in hetrosexuals, for most a person may be heferosexual, homosexual, or bisexual. Some paraphilias are distinguished by a preoccupation with objects as essential for maximal sexual arousal primarily items of clothing or materials, as in felishism, or by wearing the clothing of the sex as in transvestic felishism. Other paraphilias derive their excitement from the lack of a mutual relationship with the partner, for example, exhibitionism, voyeurism, or frotteurism. Sexual inasochism and sadism focus on humiliation and suffering. In pedophilia the fanlasized partners are prepubescent children. Tliese paraphilias are discussed in detail in the following sections.

Some paraphilic fantasies are very elaborate and may involve content from several different general paraphilic themes. Thus, for example, sadistic pedophilia involves fantasies of the humiliation and suffering of prepubescent children. Paraphilias may be acted out through masturbation accompanied by the paiaphilic fantasy, sometimes incorporating relevant props. Some paraphilias are acted out with partners. The paraphilic ritual provides indications of the underlying sexual fantasy, although the ritual may act out only some select portion of the fantasy. The paraphilia is diagnosed, insofar as possible, based on the elaborated fantasy, not just the behavior. Thus, a man who mastlirbates his exposed penis while watching unsuspecting children and having fantasies about sadistic acts with the children would be diagnosed with sadistic pedophilia (a sexual disorder not otherwise specified in DSM - lV), not with the separate diagnoses of voyeurism, exhibitionism, sadism, and pedophilia, unless these fantasies recurrently occurred independently of each other. Sometimes two or more independent paraphilias may exist in the same individual, with no overlap or shared content. Each of the independent paraphilias must have been independently and recurrently present in fantasies for at least 6 months to meet diagnostic requirements for two or more paraphilic diagnoses.

The content of common paraphilic fantasies may occur occasionally in the sexual imagery of individuals with generally conventional sexlialities. Or an individual may engage in occasional behaviors or acts involving atypical sexual content. This behavior may be playful and experimental, particularly with a consenting partner. It may be regressed in situations of stress associated with organic impairment. The criteria of recurrent and intense sexual urges, fantasies, or behaviors over at least 6 months must be met before a paraphilia can be diagnosed. For a patient with a paraphilia, the atypical sexual imagery is often necessary for sexual arousal, sometimes to the extent of being intrusive during conventional sexual activity. In some cases, particularly with aging and experience, the paraphilic fantasies may evoke more of a feeling of relief from tension or produce feelings of calm and comfort rather than sexual arousal.

Paraphilias are diagnosed almost exclusively in females, although they may also occur in females. Usually the onset is reported in the sexual fantasies of adolescence. Critical events or early indicators of paraphilic arousal may be reported as early as age 3 - 5. In other cases, the recognition of paraphilic interests is delayed into adulthood. Paraphilias may be associated with sexual dysfunclion, since the sexual arousal is associated with a fantasy scenario rather than the partner. There is usually impairment in sexual or social relationships. Paraphilic imagery and behavior may seriously distract the individual from work and everyday activities. Paraphilic behavior may also be embarrassing or illegal if acted out with a nonconsenting partner.

Individuals with paraphilias may not report feeling distress and may justify their sexual interests as variant sexlialities. Olivers feel shame or guilt about their sexual interests and can be depressed. Referral for treatment is usually a result of problems with partners or potential for legal charges.

Etiology

The incidence of paraphilias is not known but is believed to be low. The incidence of specific paraphilias varies in different societies and historical periods. Paraphilias have been identified mostly in men but also exist in women.

The cause of paraphilias is not known, however the content of many paraphilic fantasies seems to be associated with childhood experiences. Although the expression of paraphilic fantasies typically begins in adolescence, the disorder does not seem to be caused by adolescent or adult experiences except perhaps in rare cases of severe trauma.

Treatment

Unfortunately many paraphilic individuals are poorly motivated to undergo treatment. Also, at least with the present state of knowledge, there is no "cure" for these abnormalities. Motivated patients can, however, be helped to control their urges thereby reducing their own distress and reducing the likelihood of harming themselves and/or other people.

Paraphilias are generally chronic conditions that some individuals can learn to control. The treatment for the different paraphilias is similar, although some adjustments are made in association with the differing contents. Compulsive paraphilic acting out that poses a risk to others or is not well controlled may be treated in inpatient settings. Medications that reduce testosterone may be used to decrease the intensity of the sexual urges and facilitate self-control. Individual psychotherapy and group treatment can examine issues concerning the origin of the paraphilia and its effects on an individual's personality development and life-style. Cognitive and behavioral techniques are favored; psychodynamic approaches are not generally believed to be effective. Techniques for reducing inappropriate sexual arousal and controlling undesirable sexual behavior are developed. Patients attempt to increase socially acceptable heterosexual or homosexual sexual arousal and may participate in training to improve social skills and help develop relationships. Cognitive distortions are challenged, and understanding of societal and victims' points of view is enhanced. The patient must learn to identify and avoid risk situations. Relapse prevention planning is part of the therapeutic process, and patients may need to be maintained in long-term follow-up.

Treatments can be broadly grouped into psychological and pharmacological (medications) approaches. As with other psychiatric disorders, a combination of the two is usually more effective than either alone.

A number of psychological techniques have been used but currently cognitive behavioral methods, including relapse prevention strategies, appear the most effective. Pharmacological treatments have included sex-drive reducing hormones such as Provera, Androcur and Lupron, though SSRI's (Serotonin Reuptake Inhibitors), such as Prozac and Paxil, have shown some promise.

Exhibitionism

In exhibitionism, the sexually arousing fantasies involve exposing the genitals to an unsuspecting stranger. Almost always, this involves a heterosexual male exposing his penis to an adolescent or adult woman. However, this disorder may be underreported in women. There is no attempt at further sexual activity with the target female. Erection or masturbation may occur during the act, or the episode may be recalled later for sexual arousal and masturbation. Usually the fantasy focuses on the reaction of the female (surprise, shock, disgust, or interest), but there may be other fantasies of the female becoming sexually aroused or approaching the male for sexual activily.

In some cases there may be rape fantasies, which should be diagnosed as a paraphilia not otherwise specified (rapisin or raptophilia). Exposure to children may be indicative of pedophilia rather than exhibitionism. In both of these examples, the exposure is a prelude in lantasy to other sexual activities, which the individual has not acted out, rather than being the goal and end point of sexual tuntasy and activity.

Exhibitionism tends to be highly compulsive in younger men, with frequent episodes starting in the teens, but then decreasing in severity in older men.

Voyeurism

Voyeurism is the counterpart of exhibitionism, in which the man repeatedly watches unsuspecting persons undressing or engaging in sexual activity. Usually the target is female, and the man masturbates while watching. What distinguishes this as a disorder is the recurrent fantasies and compulsive pattern of behavior lasting at least 6 months. Men with this disorder spend large amounts of time going around or waiting for an opportunity to observe a target woman. Voyeurisin may be reported as exhibitionism when the target woman sees the man masturbating and thinks he is exposing himself to her. Voyeuristic acts may also be part of stalking for rape or a sexual obsession with a specific woman; these would be diagnosed as sexual disorders not otherwise specified.

Frotteurism

Frotteurism involves unsuspecting or nonconsenting partners: the sexual fantasy or arousal focuses on surreptitious touching or rubbing. Typically, the man may touch or fondle erogenous zones of the target female such as buttocks, breasts, thighs, or genitalia. Other men rub their penis, usually with an erection, against the buttocks or crotch of an unsuspecting woman. Males are rarely targets for men with this disorder.

When children are the targets, the diagnosis is usually pedophilia. It is the furtive nature of the contact that is the stimulus for sexual excitement in frotteurism. Touching as an overture to more involved sexual contact is not frotteurism, nor is touching associated with poor judgment, as in mental retardation, deficient social skills, or problems with impulse control.

Pedophilia

Pedophilia, according to DSM-Ⅳ, involves "over a period of at least 6 months, recurrent intense sexually arousing fantasies, sexual urges, or behaviors involving sexual activity with a prepubescent child or children (generally age 13 years or younger)." The person must be at least 16 years old and more than 5 years older than the child. Although most pedophiles are males, there is a growing literature regarding sexual behavior between women and children.

The sexual attraction of the pedophile should be specified as to males, females, or both. Attraction to girls is more common than attraction to boys. However, pedophiles who are attracted to boys tend to have had more involvement with different children than those attracted to girls. Pedophiles attracted to both sexes usually prefer younger children. Pedophiles typically have highly specific age ranges and physical characteristics that define the children whom they tind arousing. There is great variety in the types of sexualized activities they engage in with children. Some pedophilic relationships involve close emontional bonding.

Pedophilia is also coded as exclusive type, for individuals who are attracted only to children, or nonexclusive. Most male pedophiles who are attracted to boys are not interested in mature males and thus would not be considered homosexual. Nonexclusive pedophiles are usually heterosexual in terms of their adult sexual interests. Nonexclusive pedophilia may be also coded if limited to incest. Nonexclusive pedophilia also might be found in examples of regressed behavior, particularly if the sexual fantasies or behavior are manifested with reference to only one child and situation. Nonexclusive or regressed pedophilic behavior may be more likely to occur during times of stress. However, a diagnosis of pedophilia requires at least 6 months of recurrent sexually arousing fantasies, urges, or behaviors: isolated sexual activity with children is not sufficient evidence for diagnosis.

Some cases of pedophilia are associated with histories of having been sexually abused as a child. Pedophilia can also coexist with sexual sadism or hist murder, although this is rare. In most cases, pedophiles attempt to develop otherwise positive relationships with children.

Although adolescents may be defined as children according to the law, a primary and exclusive sexual attraction to adolescents in an adult would be ephebophilia, a paraphilia not otherwise specified.

Sexual Masochism

DSM-Ⅳ defines sexual masochism as intense sexually arousing fantasies, sexual urges, or behaviors, recurrent over a period of at least 6 mouths, "involving the act (real, not simulated) of being humiliated, beaten, bound, or otherwise made to suffer." In addition, there should be clinically significant distress or impairment. Most masochism, as found in heterosexual or homosexual sadomasochistic scenes, involves consensual simulated acts and thus would not be considered disordered. Suffering as the unintentional result of sexual activity is also not considered masochistic.

Masochistic fantasies are common but are not often enacted in reality in the repetitive way characteristic of paraphilic masochism. Masochism is one of the more common paraphilias for which women seek treatment. Masochistic sexual practices can be life threatening, including maslurbatory activities such as asphyxiophilia, which may involve strangulation and self-torture for sexual arolisal.

Sexual Sadism

Sexual sadism, according to DSM-Ⅳ, involves "over a period of at least 6 months, recurrent intense sexually arousing fantasies, sexual urges, or behaviors involving acts (real, not simulated) in which the psychological or physical suffering (including humiliation) of the victim is sexually exciting to the person." In addition, there should be clinically significant distress or impairment.

Acting out sexual sadism with consenting partners usually involves only simulated acts. However, the sadist may be distressed and seek treatment because of the concern that he will lose control and actually injure the partner. Although sadism exists as a disorder in women, in heterosexual practices women are more often acting out the fantasies of their masochistic partners rather than expressing their own paraphilic sadistic fantasies. In extreme cases, sexual sadism may be acted out with nonconsensual partners in rape or lust murder.

Chapter 6 Childhood Mental Disorders

Nearly 5 million children in the world have some type of serious mental illness (one that significantly interferes with daily life). In any given year, 20% of American children will be diagnosed with a mental illness.

The term "mental illness" is not entirely accurate, because there are many "physical" factors — including heredity and brain chemistry that might be involved in the development of a mental disorder. As such, many mental disorders can be effectively treated with medication, psychotherapy (a type of counseling), or a combination of both.

Children are precious, as parents we worry about their health. When our children have issues and crises, these issues and crises affect us just as much, if not more, than it affects them. We fear that which might bring them fear; we hurt when we see them hurt; and sometimes, we cry just seeing them cry. Writer Elizabeth Stone once said "Making the decision to have a child is momentous. It is to decide forever to have your heart go walking around outside your body." So, when it seems like something is not quite right with your children — perhaps they seem more afraid than other kids, or they seem to get a lot angrier than their playmates do over certain things, this odd or "off" behavior can be experienced as terrifying. In fact, a child's difficulty can be just the starting point for your parental worry and concern. You might not know what to do to help your child, or where to go for help. Possibly, you may worry because you don't even know if your child's problem is something you should be concerned about in the first place.

We've created this survey of childhood mental and emotional disorders to help worried parents better understand the various ways that mental illness can effect children, what it looks like and how it can be helped. Children's mental and emotional disorders are problems that affect not only their behavior, emotions, moods, or thoughts, but can also affect the entire family as well. These problems are often similar to other types of health problems that your child might have, and can generally be treated with medications or psychotherapy (or a combination of both).

We are going to be using the term "childhood disorders" with some frequency. Many childhood disorders are often labeled as developmental disorders or learning disorders, so you may have heard those terms as well. Generally, when we speak about childhood disorders, we are referring to mental and emotional problems that most often occur and are diagnosed when children are school aged or younger. Usually, symptoms start during infancy or in early childhood, although some of the disorders may develop throughout adolescence.

The diagnostic criteria for the childhood disorders specifically require that symptoms first appear at some point during childhood. Adults may find themselves relating to some of the symptoms characteristic of one or more childhood disorders, but unless those adults first experienced their symptoms as children themselves, whatever it is that they may have will not be a childhood disorder, but instead, some other adult diagnosis.

Though by definition, no disorder discussed in this document may begin in adulthood, it is possible for a childhood disorder to begin at a young age but continue to be problematic on into adulthood. Conversely, some childhood disorders tend to resolve by the time children enter adulthood. Or, prior to adulthood, children may developed a set of coping skills that allow them to compensate for their disorder(s) so that they can go on to lead a happy and productive life. This latter outcome is especially likely when the right type of professional intervention has been obtained (and followed consistently) from an early age.

There are a great diversity of childhood disorder forms and causes. Some of these disorders are primarily disorders of the brain, while others are more behavioral in nature. Brain - based disorders are caused by neurochemical problems or structural abnormalities of the brain. They can be innate (ie, appearing at or shortly after birth); or they may result from a physical stress such as illness or injury, or an emotional stress, such as trauma or loss. Behavioral problems, on the other hand, are outward signs of difficulty displayed at home, at school, or among friends in an otherwise physically healthy child. Like brain - based problems, behavioral problems may also result from physical or emotional stress. Note that the division between brain - based and behavioral disorders is somewhat arbitrary in many cases. Brain - based disorders such as ADHD clearly impact a child's behavior in school and at home, and vice versa, many disorders previously thought to be primarily behavioral in nature have turned out to have a biological component to them.

Some of the childhood disorders we will discuss in this article can be cured or otherwise resolved, while others end up becoming chronic (long - term) problems that resist the best state - of - the - art interventions. The disorders we will discuss also vary in terms of prevalence and severity. Prevalence refers to a ratio, or percentage, of how often a disease or disorder occurs within a group of people in a population at a given time. Recently, the American Psychological Association has noted an increase in the prevalence of childhood mental illnesses as a whole. Estimates of the current prevalence suggest that between 17.6% and 22% of children have symptoms of one or more childhood disorders; and that 15% of American children suffer from a mental illness that is severe enough to cause some level of functional impairment.

Analyzing information about large group of British residents followed for five decades from the week of their birth, researchers found that family income was about one - fourth lower on average by age 50 among those who experienced serious psychological problems during childhood than among those who did not experience such problems.

In addition, childhood psychological problems were associated later in life with being less conscientious, having a lower likelihood of being married and having less - stable personal relationships, according to findings being published in the Proceedings of the National

Academies of Sciences.

Alissa's findings demonstrate that childhood psychological problems can have significant negative impacts over the course of an individuals life, much more so than childhood physical health problems, said Alissa, one of the study's authors and a senior economist at the RAND Corporation, a nonprofit research organization. "The findings suggest that increasing efforts to address these problems early in children may have large economic payoffs later in life."

The other two authors of the study are Alissa Goodman and Robert Joyce of the Institute for Fiscal Studies in London.

Researchers found that the impacts of psychological disorders during childhood are far more important individually and collectively over a lifetime than childhood physical health problems. To illustrate, while family income at age 50 is reduced by 25 % or more due to childhood mental problems, the reduction in family income on average is 9 percent due to major childhood physical health problems and only 3 percent due to minor childhood physical health problems. A central reason for the larger impact of childhood mental health problems is their effects take place much earlier in childhood and persist, researchers say.

An earlier study coauthored by Smith showed that childhood psychological problems had a major impact on adult socioeconomic standing, costing 2.1 U.S. dollar trillion over the lifetimes of all affected Americans. The results found for the American sample closely parallel those found for the British sample. Another source of concern is that in both America and Britain childhood mental problems appear to be increasing over time. The latest study was conducted by analyzing information collected as part of the National Child Development Study, which has followed the lives of a single group of 17,634 children who were born in Britain during the first week of March in 1958. Information has been collected from the group periodically, including surveys about childhood physical and psychological health through physician-led examinations, extensive parental questionnaires and teacher reports. The study includes detailed information about participants' parents, including socio-economic details and family circumstances such as whether there was instability in the home.

Researchers found that the negative economic impact of childhood psychological problems were apparent early in adulthood, with household income 19% percent lower among 23-year-olds who had psychological problems as a child as compared to those who did not.

Some of the smaller family income is caused by a lower likelihood that those who had childhood psychological problems will live with a partner as an adult. By age 50, people who had childhood psychological problems had a 6% lower probability of being married or cohabitating and an 11 percent lower chance of working.

The National Child Development Study includes assessments of participants' cognitive functioning and personality traits at age 50, allowing researchers to estimate the impact of childhood psychological problems in those areas.

Children with mental health issues showed reduced cognitive abilities as adults, possibly because their psychological problems make it difficult for them to concentrate and remember, researchers say. Childhood mental health problems also had a negative impact at age 50 on agreeableness and conscientiousness, two key measures of personality.

Despite how common they may be, childhood disorders are not part of the normal developmental process that children are expected to go through. The diagnostic criteria for childhood mental disorders requires that children's behavior and/or development deviates from normal age-appropriate behavior and/or development, so understanding normal child development is important. For this reason, you might want to read over our extensive material concerning normal childhood development. Understanding normal developmental milestones for different ages puts you in a better position to understand why disordered behavior is considered abnormal.

Common childhood mental illnesses and developmental disorders include Depression, Bipolar Disorder and Anxiety Disorders, Autism and similar Pervasive Developmental Disorders, Attention Deficit and Hyperactivity Disorder, Learning Disabilities, Adjustment Disorders, Oppositional Defiant Disorder, and Conduct Disorder. The first three of these disorders are not strictly childhood disorders, but instead, affect both children and adults. Since we've already discussed these disorders in detail elsewhere, we will not go into much detail about them here.

In order to obtain treatment, it is important that children are appropriately and accurately diagnosed. Diagnosis is the term used to describe the process that a professional goes through when figuring out whether children have a particular disorder. Professionals make diagnoses by comparing observations and measurements of children's behavior against published criteria that must be present in order for a diagnosis to be made.

In the United States, diagnostic criteria for mental disorders are published in the Diagnostic and Statistical Manual of Mental Disorders, an important tool that clinicians use to diagnose both child and adult psychological disorders. The most current volume, (the DSM Ⅳ-TR), provides comprehensive diagnostic criteria based on the best available clinical and research literature findings regarding mental illness (as of the publication date). It is a standard way of measuring and classifying mental disorders, and is used extensively by psychologists, psychiatrists, social workers, mental health counselors and other mental health professionals.

An important organizing principle of the DSM is the fact that individuals are assessed across five separate "axes" (dimensions) in order to develop a more complete understanding of their functioning. Each axis describes a different aspect of functioning. Axes Ⅰ and Ⅱ are used to describe mental disorders, per se, with Axis Ⅱ specifically devoted to describing developmental disorders (which by definition occur from a young age). Importantly, not all child disorders are classified as developmental disorders. Instead, many are categorized as Axis Ⅰ disorders, which can be any disorder that is not developmental in nature, a disorder that is primarily a medical problem (in which case it would be described on Axis Ⅲ), or a social problem (in which case it would be described on Axis Ⅳ). Most of the disorders discussed in this paper are Axis I disorders, except for Mental Retardation, which is classified as an Axis Ⅱ disorder.

The DSM is mostly concerned with adult mental problems. Child mental problems are described and contained within a single large chapter, and considered separately from adult disorders, even when adult disorders exist, which are similar in nature. For instance, childhood feeding disorders are not discussed within the eating disorders chapter of the DSM, but instead within the "ghetto" of the child disorders chapter. While there are good conceptual reasons for thinking about childhood feeding disorders in separate terms from "adult" eating disorders like anorexia (which typically have their onset in adolescence), the extent of separation between child and adult disorders seems arbitrary to us, and appears to be due more to the politics which have shaped DSM's structure than based on actual scientific evidence. As the division between child and adult disorders is necessarily ambiguous in many ways (it is easy to differentiate between an infant and an adult, how easy is it to differentiate between a late adolescent and an adult?), perhaps future revisions of this centrally important work will come to be organized differently.

For the time being, childhood disorders occupy a separate space within DSM. Within the childhood disorders chapter of the DSM, problems are further subdivided based on similarities of dysfunction. You may notice that this is also how we have chosen to organize this article. Disorders that share qualities in common have been grouped together under their broader heading, as is the case in DSM.

Interestingly, there is growing evidence that a similar process happens when a person experiences psychological trauma. Unfortunately, this type of inflammation can be destructive.

Risk of Childhood Adversity

Previous studies have linked depression and inflammation, particularly in individuals who have experienced early childhood adversity, but overall, findings have been inconsistent. Researchers Gregory Miller and Steve Cole designed a longitudinal study in an effort to resolve these discrepancies, and their findings are now published in a study in *Biological Psychiatry*.

They recruited a large group of female adolescents who were healthy, but at high risk for experiencing depression. The volunteers were then followed for 2 years, undergoing interviews and giving blood samples to measure their levels of C-reactive protein and interleukin-6, two types of inflammatory markers. Their exposure to childhood adversity was also assessed.

The researchers found that when individuals who suffered from early childhood adversity became depressed, their depression was accompanied by an inflammatory response. In addition, among subjects with previous adversity, high levels of interleukin-6 forecasted risk of depression six months later. In subjects without childhood adversity, there was no such coupling of depression and inflammation.

Dr. Miller commented on their findings: "What's important about this study is that it identifies a group of people who are prone to have depression and inflammation at the same time. That group of people experienced major stress in childhood, often related to poverty, having a parent with a severe illness, or lasting separation from family. As a result, these individuals may experience depressions that are especially difficult to treat."

Another important aspect to their findings is that the inflammatory response among the high - adversity individuals was still detectable six months later, even if their depression had abated, meaning that the inflammation is chronic rather than acute. "Because chronic inflammation is involved in other health problems, like diabetes and heart disease, it also means they have greater - than - average risk for these problems. They, along with their doctors, should keep an eye out for those problems," added Dr. Miller. "This study provides important additional support for the notion that inflammation is an important and often under - appreciated factor that compromises resilience after major life stresses. It provides evidence that these inflammatory states persist for long periods of time and have important functional correlates," said Dr. John Krystal, Editor of *Biological Psychiatry*.

Data from the Economic and Social Research Council (ESRC) show that 40,000 UK households over a number of years more than 2,000 young people aged between 10 to 15 years have been asked how satisfied they are with their lives. The findings indicate there is little difference between the average life satisfaction score of those children living in the household with the bottom fifth income and those children living in households in the top fifth income bracket. "Despite the seemingly high levels of happiness amongst young people in the UK, our children's well - being has remained about the same since in 2007, which rated Britain's children as some of the most unhappy in the developed world. Understanding Society research suggests that a focus on just improving income and material deprivation does not necessarily represent real improvements in quality of life as they are perceived by children themselves."

The results also show that young people are less materialistic than adults in their assessment of happiness. A much greater influence on a child's happiness is whether they live with both parents and the happiness of their parents' relationship, and in particular their mother. In families where the child's mother is unhappy in her relationship, only 55 per cent of young people say they are "completely happy" with their family situation, compared with 73 per cent young people whose mothers are "perfectly happy" in their relationships.

Understanding Society also asked parents and children living at home questions about family relationships, including partners, and their level of happiness with these relationships. The answers from 11,825 adults and 1,268 young people (aged 10 - 15) were analysed and compared. Together these findings reveal the complex influences of different family relationships on a child's happiness: 60% of the children said they were "completely satisfied" with their family situation, children in lone - parent families were less likely to report themselves completely happy with their situation having older siblings is not related to children's happiness with their family, but having younger siblings in the household is associated with lower levels of satisfaction and this effect is greater the more younger siblings present in the household children who quarrel more than once a week with their parents, and don't discuss important matters with them have only a 28 % chance of rating themselves completely happy with their families, children who eat an evening meal with their family at least three times a week are more likely to report being completely happy with their family situation than children who never eat with their family, watching TV are completely unrelated to a young person's happiness with their family situation.

Families are a big part of every child's life, and our research highlights just how much family relationships matter for children's well-being. Over the years, as we follow the lives of the families in Understanding Society, we'll build up an even better picture of how children's lives are affected by all kinds of factors. Understanding Society is really set to become a fantastic resource for anyone interested in the well-being of children.

Emotional stress or trauma in the parent-child relationship tends to be a cause of child psychopathology. First seen in infants, separation anxiety in root of parental-child stress may lay the foundations for future disorders in children. There is a direct correlation between maternal stress and child stress that is factored in both throughout adolescences development. In a situation where the mother is absent, any primary caregiver to the child could be seen as the "maternal" relationship. Essentially, the child would bond with the primary caregiver, exuding some personality traits of the caregiver.

In studies of child in two age groups of pregnancy to five years, and fifteen years and twenty years, Raposa and colleagues (2011) studied the impact of psychopathology in the child-maternal relationship and how not only the mothers stress affected the child, but the child's stress affected the mother. Historically, it was believed that mothers who suffered from post partum depression might be the reason their child suffers from mental disorders both earlier and later in development. However this correlation was found to not only reflect maternal depression on child psychopathology, but also child psychopathology could reflect on maternal depression.

Children with a predisposition to psychopathology may cause higher stress in the relationship with their mother, and mothers who suffer from psychopathology may also cause higher stress in the relationship with their child. Child psychopathology creates stress in parenting which may increase the severity of the psychopathology within the child. Together, these factors push and pull the relationship thus causing higher levels of depression, ADHD, defiant disorder, learning disabilities, and pervasive developmental disorder in both the mother and the child. The outline and summary of this study is found below: "In looking at child-related stress, the number of past child mental health diagnoses significantly predicted a higher number of acute stressors for mothers as well as more chronic stress in the mother-child relationship at age 15. These increased levels of maternal stress and mother-child relationship stress at age 15 then predicted higher levels of maternal depression when the youth were 20 years old."

Looking more closely at the data, the authors found that it was the chronic stress in the mother-child relationship and the child-related acute stressors that were the linchpins between child psychopathology and maternal depression. The stress is what fueled the fires between mother and child mental health. Going one step further, the researchers found that youth with a history of more than one diagnosis as well as youth that had externalizing disorders (eg, conduct disorder) had the highest number of child-related stressors and the highest levels of mother-child stress. Again, all of the findings held up when other potentially stressful variables, such as economic worries and past maternal depression, were controlled for.

Additionally, siblings — both older and younger and of both genders, can be factored in to the etiology and development of child psychopathology. In a longitudinal study of maternal depression and older male child depression and antisocial behaviors on younger siblings adolescent mental health outcome, the study factored in ineffective parenting and sibling conflicts such as sibling rivalry. Younger female siblings were more directly affected by maternal depression and older brother depression and antisocial behaviors when the indirect effects were not place, in comparison to younger male siblings who showed no such comparison. However, if an older brother were antisocial, the younger child — female or male would exude higher antisocial behaviors. In the presence of a sibling conflict, antisocial behavior was more influential on younger male children than younger female children. Female children were more sensitive to pathological familial environments, thus showing that in a high-stress environment with both maternal depression and older-male sibling depression and antisocial behavior, there is a higher risk of female children developing psychopathological disorders. This was a small study, and more research needs to be done especially with older female children, paternal relationships, maternal-paternal-child stress relationships, and/or caregiver-child stress relationships if the child is orphaned or not being raised by the biological child to reach a conclusive child-parent stress model on the effects of familial and environmental pathology on the child's development.

Happy Children Make Happy Adults

The child-parent stress and development is only one hypothesis for the etiology of child psychopathology. Other experts believe that child temperament is a large factor in the development of child psychopathology. High susceptibility to child psychopathology is marked by low levels of effortful control and high levels of emotionality and neuroticism. Parental divorce is often a large factor in childhood depression and other psychopathological disorders. That is not to say that divorce will lead to psychopathological disorders, there are also other factors such as temperament, trauma, and other negative life events (e.g. death, sudden moving of home, physical or sexual abuse), genetics, environment, and nurture that correlate to the onset of a disorder.

Found in "The Role of Temperament in the Etiology of Child Psychopathology", a model for the etiology of child psychopathology proposed that the four things that are important to the development of psychopathological disorders is: (1) biological factors: hormones, genetics, neurotransmitters; (2) psychological: self-esteem, coping skills, cognitive issues; (3) social factors: family rearing, negative learning experiences, and stress; (4) child's temperament. Using an array of neurological scans and exams, psychological assessment tests, family medical history, and observing the child in daily factors can help the physician find the etiology of the psychopathological disorder to help release the child of the symptoms through therapy, medication use, social skills training, and life style changes.

Child psychopathology can cause separation anxiety from parents, attention deficit disorders in children, sleep disorders in children, aggression with both peers and adults, night terrors, extreme anxiety, antisocial behavior, depression symptoms, aloof attitude, sensitive emotions, and rebellious behavior that are not in line of typical childhood development. Aggression is found to manifest in children before five years of age, and early stress and aggression in the parental - child relationship correlates with the manifestation of aggression. Aggression in children causes problematic peer relationships, difficulty adjusting, and coping problems. Children who fail to overcome acceptable ways of coping and emotion expression are put on tract for psychopathological disorders and violent and antisocial behaviors into adolescence and adulthood. There is a higher rate of substance abuse in these children with coping and aggression issues, and causes a cycle of emotional instability and manifestation psychopathological disorders.

Much is known about the associations between a troubled childhood and mental health problems, but little research has examined the affect of a positive childhood. For the first time, researchers from the University of Cambridge and the MRC Unit for Lifelong Health and Ageing have analysed the link between a positive adolescence and well-being in midlife.

Using information from 2776 individuals who participated in the 1946 British birth cohort study, the scientists tested associations between having a positive childhood and well-being in adulthood.

A "positive" childhood was based on teacher evaluations of students' levels of happiness, friendship and energy at the ages of 13 and 15. A student was given a positive point for each of the following four items — whether the child was "very popular with other children", "unusually happy and contented", "makes friends extremely easily" and "extremely energetic, never tired". Teachers also rated conduct problems (restlessness, daydreaming, disobedience, lying, etc) and emotional problems (anxiety, fearfulness, diffidence, avoidance of attention, etc).

The researchers then linked these ratings to the individuals' mental health, work experience, relationships and social activities several decades later. They found that teenagers rated positively by their teachers were significantly more likely than those who received no positive ratings to have higher levels of well-being later in life, including a higher work satisfaction, more frequent contact with family and friends, and more regular engagement in social and leisure activities.

Happy children were also much less likely than others to develop mental disorders throughout their lives, 60% less likely than young teens that had no positive ratings.

The study not only failed to find a link between being a happy child and an increased likelihood of becoming married, they found that the people who had been happy children were actually more likely to get divorced. One possible factor suggested by the researchers is that happier people have higher self-esteem or self-efficacy and are therefore more willing and able to leave an unhappy marriage.

"The benefits to individuals, families and to society of good mental health, positive relationships and satisfying work are likely to be substantial," said Professor Felicia Huppert, one of the authors of the paper and Director of the Well-being Institute at the University of Cambridge. "The findings support the view that even at this time of great financial hardship, policymakers should prioritise the well-being of our children so they have the best possible start in life."Dr Marcus Richards, co-author of the paper from the MRC Unit for Lifelong Health and Ageing, said "Most longitudinal studies focus on the negative impact of early mental problems, but the 1946 birth cohort also shows clear and very long-lasting positive consequences of mental well-being in childhood."

Child Psychopathology

Child psychopathology is the manifestation of psychological disorders in children and adolescents. Oppositional defiant disorder, attention-deficit hyperactivity disorder, and pervasive developmental disorder are examples of child psychopathology. The full list of formal diagnostic codes and classification of mental health disorders can be found in the DSM-Ⅳ-TR; this is the same manual which covers adult psychopathology, but it has certain diagnoses specific to children and adolescents. Counselors, social workers, psychologists and psychiatrists who work with mentally ill children are informed by research in developmental psychology, developmental psychopathology, clinical child psychology, and family systems. The first section of the DSM Ⅳ-TR Disorders usually first diagnosed in infancy, childhood or adolescence includes diagnoses from mental retardation to selective autism. In addition, the DC 0-3 or Diagnostic Classification 0-3 is used to assess mental health problems in infants.

Attention Deficit Disorder

Have you ever had trouble concentrating, found it hard to sit still, interrupted others during a conversation or acted impulsively without thinking things through? Can you recall times when you daydreamed or had difficulty focusing on the task at hand? Most of us can picture acting this way from time to time. But for some people, these and other exasperating behaviors are uncontrollable, persistently plaguing their day-to-day existence and interfering with their ability to form lasting friendships or succeed in school, at home and with a career.

ADHD, also known as hyperkinetic disorder (HKD) outside of the United States, is estimated to affect 3%-9% of children, and afflicts boys more often than girls. Although difficult to assess in infancy and toddlerhood, signs of ADHD may begin to appear as early as age two or three, but the symptom picture changes as adolescence approaches. Many symptoms, particularly hyperactivity, diminish in early adulthood, but impulsivity and problems focusing attention remain with up to 50% of individuals with ADHD throughout their adult life.

Children with ADHD have short attention spans, becoming easily bored and/or frustrated with tasks. Although they may be quite intelligent, their lack of focus frequently results in poor grades and difficulties in school. Children with ADHD act impulsively, taking action first and thinking later. They are constantly moving, running, climbing, squirming, and fidgeting, but often have trouble with gross and fine motor skills and, as a result, may be physically clumsy and awkward. In social settings, they are sometimes shunned due to their impulsive and intrusive behavior.

Unlike a broken bone or cancer, attention deficit hyperactivity disorder (ADHD, also sometimes referred to as just plain attention deficit disorder or ADD) does not show physical signs that can be detected by a blood or other lab test. The typical ADHD symptoms often overlap with those of other physical and psychological disorders.

The causes remain unknown, but ADHD can be diagnosed and effectively treated. Many resources are available to support families in managing ADHD behaviors when they occur.

ADHD, also known as attention deficit disorder (ADD) or hyperkinetic disorder, has been around a lot longer than most people realize. In fact, a condition that appears to be similar to ADHD was described by Hippocrates, who lived from 460 to 370 BC. The name Attention Deficit Disorder was first introduced in 1980 in DSM-Ⅲ, the third edition of the "Diagnostic and Statistical Manual of Mental Disorders", used in psychiatry. In 1994 the definition was altered to include three groups within ADHD: the predominantly hyperactive-impulsive type; the predominantly inattentive type; and the combined type. ADHD usually appears in childhood but can be diagnosed in adults. Recent steps forward in our understanding of ADHD include:

An estimated 3 to 5 per cent of children are affected — approximately 2 million children in the US. In a classroom of 25 to 30 children, it is likely that at least one will have ADHD.

ADHD is among the most common mental disorders among children. It is one of the top reasons for referral to a pediatrician, family physician, pediatric neurologist, child psychiatrist or psychologist. ADHD is best diagnosed by a child psychologist or other child specialist in ADHD.

ADHD is about three times more common among boys than girls.

The symptoms of ADHD do not always go away — up to 60 per cent of child patients retain their symptoms into adulthood. Many adults with ADHD have never been diagnosed, so may not be aware they have the disorder. They may have been wrongly diagnosed with depression, anxiety, bipolar disorder or a learning disability.

ADHD has been identified in every nation and culture that has been studied.

ADHD is difficult for everyone involved to deal with. As well as the difficulty of living with the symptoms, wider society may face challenges. Some experts have linked ADHD with an increased risk of accidents, drug abuse, failure at school, antisocial behavior and criminal activity. But others view ADHD in a positive light, arguing that it is simply a different method of learning involving greater risk-taking and creativity.

Diagnosis

The first step in determining if a child has ADHD is to consult with a pediatrician. The pediatrician can make an initial evaluation of the child's developmental maturity compared to other children in his or her age group. The physician should also perform a comprehensive physical examination to rule out any organic causes of ADHD symptoms, such as an overactive thyroid or vision or hearing problems.

If no organic problem can be found, a psychologist, psychiatrist, neurologist, neuropsychologist, or learning specialist is typically consulted to perform a comprehensive ADHD assessment. A complete medical, family, social, psychiatric, and educational history is compiled from existing medical and school records and from interviews with parents and teachers. Interviews may also be conducted with the child, depending on his or her age. Along with these interviews, several clinical questionnaires may also be used, such as the Conners Rating Scales (Teacher's Questionnaire and Parent's Questionnaire), Child Behavior Checklist (CBCL), and the Achenbach Child Behavior Rating Scales. These inventories provide valuable information on the child's behavior in different settings and situations. In addition, the Wender Utah Rating Scale has been adapted for use in diagnosing ADHD in adults.

It is important to note that mental disorders such as depression and anxiety disorder can cause symptoms similar to ADHD. (Depression can cause attention problems, and anxiety can cause symptoms similar to hyperactivity.) A complete and comprehensive psychological assessment is critical to differentiate ADHD from other possible mood and behavioral disorders. Bipolar disorder, for example, may be misdiagnosed as ADHD. Public schools are required by federal law to offer free ADHD testing upon request. A pediatrician can also provide a referral to a psychologist or pediatric specialist for ADHD assessment. Parents should check with their insurance plans to see if these services are covered.

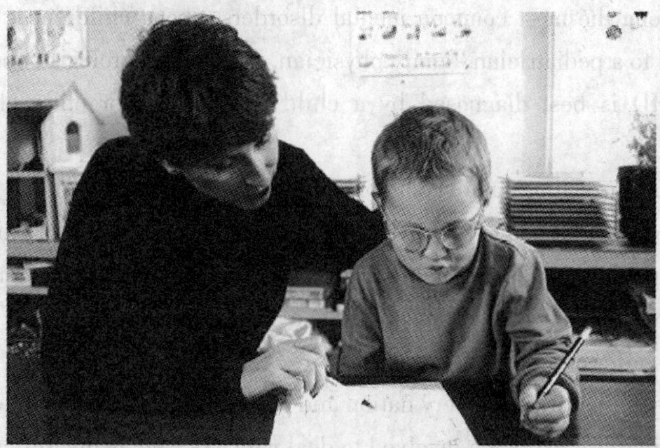

A special education teacher helps a student with attention-deficit/hyperactivity disorder with his math assignment.

DSM-Ⅳ Criteria

The DSM-Ⅳ allows for diagnosis of the predominantly inattentive subtype of ADHD (under code 314.00) if the individual presents six or more of the following symptoms of inattention for at least six months to a point that is disruptive and inappropriate for developmental level:

Often does not give close attention to details or makes careless mistakes in schoolwork, work, or other activities.

Often has trouble keeping attention on tasks or play activities.

Often does not seem to listen when spoken to directly.

Often does not follow instructions and fails to finish schoolwork, chores, or duties in the workplace (not due to oppositional behavior or failure to understand instructions).

Often has trouble organizing activities.

Often avoids, dislikes, or doesn't want to do things that take a lot of mental effort for a long period (such as schoolwork or homework).

Often loses things needed for tasks and activities (e.g. toys, school assignments, pencils, books, or tools).

Is often easily distracted.

Is often forgetful in daily activities.

An ADD diagnosis is contingent upon the symptoms of impairment presenting themselves in two or more settings (eg, at school or work and at home). There must also be clear evidence of clinically significant impairment in social, academic, or occupational functioning. Lastly, the symptoms must not occur exclusively during the course of a pervasive developmental disorder, schizophrenia, or other psychotic disorder, and are not better accounted for by another mental disorder (eg, mood disorder, anxiety disorder, dissociative disorder, personality disorder). Examples of observed symptoms are showed as following table 1.

Table 1 Examples of observed symptoms

Life Period	Example
Children	Failing to pay close attention to details or making careless mistakes when doing schoolwork or other activities
	Trouble keeping attention focused during play or tasks
	Appearing not to listen when spoken to (often being accused of "daydreaming")
	Failing to follow instructions or finish tasks
	Avoiding tasks that require a high amount of mental effort and organization, such as school projects
	Excessive distractibility
	Forgetfulness
	Procrastination, inability to begin an activity
	Frequently losing items required to facilitate tasks or activities, such as school supplies
Adults	Often making careless mistakes when having to work on uninteresting or difficult projects

Treatment

Therapy that addresses both psychological and social issues (called psychosocial therapy), usually combined with medications, is the treatment approach of choice to alleviate ADHD symptoms. Assuming a proper diagnosis of ADHD and co - morbid depression has been made, the clinician should use a biopsychosocial approach to offer individualized treatments that target specific functional deficits in the patient as well as environmental factors likely to be contributing to the child's psychopathology. More complicated cases will often require a broader array of pharmacological and psychosocial.

Pharmacotherapy

Stimulants pharmacotherapy is generally considered the first - line treatment for uncomplicated ADHD, and there is also good evidence for the efficacy of atomoxetine, tricyclic antidepressants, and bupropion in such youths. A randomized controlled trial (RCT) of desipramine versus placebo in youths with ADHD has suggested that co-morbid depression may predict a better ADHD response to desipramine. However, tricyclic antidepressants are rarely used today because of their cardiovascular risks, need for plasma level and electrocardiogram (ECG) monitoring, and lack of efficacy for pediatric depression in multiple RCTs. Findings from the Multimodal Treatment Study of ADHD have suggested that children with co-morbid ADHD and anxiety are responsive to stimulant pharmacotherapy, but it is unclear how these findings relate to youths with ADHD and co-morbid depressive disorders. Two RCTs of ADHD youths with co-morbid anxiety or depressive symptoms have yielded contradictory findings regarding whether internalizing symptoms lessen response to methylphenidate. No study to date has directly compared treatment responses in ADHD youths with and without depression. Thus, it is still not clear how co-morbid depressive disorders impact the response of children with ADHD to pharmacological treatments of their ADHD.

There is increasing evidence for the efficacy of selective serotoninergic reuptake inhibitors (SSRIs) in treating pediatric MDD in general (Cheung et al. 2006; Birmaher et al. 2007). Investigators in several recent trials of SSRIs in youths with MDD have conducted post hoc analyses of the effects of co - morbid ADHD on depressive response, once again with contradictory findings. The Treatment of Adolescent Depression Study (TADS) reported that co-morbid disorders were a significant moderator of lowered antidepressant response, but did not specifically report on the moderating effects of co-morbid ADHD.

To date, a few studies have examined the effects of pharmacological treatments, specifically in youths with both depressive disorders or symptoms and ADHD, as summarized in Table 1. Most studies are limited by their small sample sizes, and lack of placebo arms or randomized controlled designs, but provide preliminary evidence that monotherapy with bupropion, or combination therapies with stimulants, SSRIs, and atomoxetine may be reasonable alternative treatments for ADHD and co-morbid depression. Only one study of youths with ADHD and co-morbid MDD, a study of atomoxetine monotherapy, used a placebo - controlled design and showed significantly better improvement for ADHD, although not for depressive symptoms on active drug. Although no subjects taking atomoxetine in this trial experienced emerging suicidality on active drug, a recent change in the label of atomoxetine reports suicidality as a rare adverse event.

On the basis of the available empirical evidence, a consensus panel of experts in the Texas Children's Medication Algorithm Project (CMAP) recently revised their pharmacotherapy algorithms for ADHD and co-morbid depression. These algorithms offer a rational approach to treating this co-morbid group. The CMAP panel recommends the use of validated depressive and ADHD instruments to monitor treatment response. They first recommend a single medication to target whichever is the more severe disorder, before resorting to medication combinations, because improvements in one disorder may coincide with improvements in the other. Changes in medications should be made one at a time. Regardless of the treatment selected, clinicians should educate families about the potential risk of worsening moods, suicidality, and iatrogenic mania and the need to monitor closely for such emerging problems. Clinicians should reconsider the child's underlying diagnoses and choices about treatment when adverse and unexpected responses to pharmacotherapy occur.

If ADHD is judged the bigger problem, the CMAP algorithm suggests an initial trial of a stimulant medication. Should the patient's depressive and ADHD symptoms persist on a stimulant alone, then the stimulant could be changed to an SSRI. If ADHD symptoms improve but not depressive symptoms, then a concomitant SSRI could be added. Alternatively, when the depressive disorder is judged the bigger problem, CMAP recommends consecutive trials of at least two separate SSRIs before resorting to bupropion or a tricyclic antidepressant as a third-line treatment. If ADHD symptoms persist despite improvement of depressive symptoms on an SSRI alone, then concomitant stimulant could be added.

A recent study of the feasibility of the CMAP depression algorithm suggests that such an approach works reasonably well for comorbid ADHD and depression in a community setting. Of the 15 patients enrolled in the study with ADHD and a co-morbid depressive disorder, 9 were prescribed a stimulant first. Of these, only 2 had an SSRI added later for residual depressive symptoms. Another 2 initially received an SSRI alone, and 4 had the combination of an SSRI and a stimulant at entry into the study, with mixed success. This study provides preliminary evidence that these algorithms may be effective in treating ADHD and co-morbid depression, but that patients receiving treatment for ADHD and co-morbid depression need close follow up and may sometimes have to go beyond the first stage of the treatment algorithm.

Psychosocial Therapies

Behavior modification therapy uses a reward system to reinforce good behavior and task completion and can be implemented both in the classroom and at home. A tangible reward such as a sticker may be given to the child every time he completes a task or behaves in an acceptable manner. A chart may be used to display the stickers and visually illustrate the child's progress. When a certain number of stickers are collected, the child may trade them in for a bigger reward such as a trip to the zoo or a day at the beach. The reward system stays in place until the good behavior becomes ingrained.

A variation of this technique, cognitive-behavioral therapy, may work for some children to decrease impulsive behavior by getting the child to recognize the connection between thoughts and behavior, and to change behavior by changing negative thinking patterns.

Individual psychotherapy can help an ADHD child build self-esteem and provide a place to discuss worries and anxieties.

Recent stu dies indicate that medications approved by the U.S. Food and Drug Administration (FDA) in the treatment of ADHD tend to work well in individuals with the predominantly inattentive type. These medications include two classes of drugs, stimulants and non - stimulants. Drugs for ADHD are divided into first - line medications and second - line medications. First - line medications include several of the stimulants, and tend to have a higher response rate and effect size than second - line medications. Some of the most common stimulants are Methylphenidate (Ritalin, Concerta), Adderall and Vyvanse. Second - line medications are usually anti - depressant medications such as Zoloft, Prozac, and Wellbutrin. These medications can help with fidgeting, inattentiveness, irritability, and trouble sleeping. Some of the symptoms the medications target are also found with ADD patients.

Although ADHD has most often been treated with medication there are questions as to the efficacy of these medications. Medications do not cure ADHD, they are used solely to treat the symptoms associated with this disorder. The symptoms will come back once the medication stops. Also, medication works better for some patients while it barely works for others.

The use of these medications is often the first treatment choice and is based on a bio - medical model of ADHD which views the disorder as a result of deficiencies in brain processing most likely resulting from defective genes. Many studies have shown the use of psychostimulants to be an effective treatment for ADHD, as well as ADD, however these studies have shown a number of methodological flaws. Firstly they measure behavior changes from the perspective of the parents, or teachers involved and assume that this change in behavior is helping the child without ever consulting with the child. This has led to a questioning of who the medication is actually helping, and if the medication is being used simply to eliminate unwanted childhood behaviors rather than to actually help the child. Although most studies focus on children with ADHD the side effects and potential misuse of stimulant medications is identical for ADHD as many of the same medications are used .

Conduct Disorder

Conduct disorder (CD) is one of the most difficult and intractable mental health problems in children and adolescents. CD involves a number of problematic behaviors, including oppositional and defiant behaviors and antisocial activities (eg, lying, stealing, running away, physical violence, sexually coercive behaviors).

A preventable predisposing factor for the development of all mental health disorders in children and adolescents has been found in a cross - sectional survey involving second - hand smoke exposure in youth who are not themselves cigarette smokers. The study adjusted for poverty, race/ethnicity, sex, asthma, hay fever, and maternal smoking; serum cotinine level was positively associated with CD, especially for non- Hispanic white males.

Research studying brain function of adolescent males with CD has found possible differences. These differences resemble the differences found in persons with addiction as compared with normally developing controls regarding brain structure and function. These differences may, in part, result in deficits in the perception of emotions and impairment in affect regulation, as well as a lack of development of empathy despite intellectual capacity for those cognitive functions. In addition, these youth exhibit a decreased dopamine response to reward and increased risk - taking behaviors related to abnormally disrupted frontal activity in the anterior cingulate cortex (ACC), orbitofrontal cortices (OFC), and dorsolateral prefrontal cortex (DLPFC) that worsens over time due to dysphoria activation of brain stress systems and increases in corticotropin releasing factor (CRF).

Areas deep in the brain, especially the amygdala and insula, appear to exhibit abnormal function reflected in overall decreases in resting state connectivity and smaller overall size. This decrease in brain structure and functionality is also seen in youth with other diagnoses such as in cases of child abuse and neglect, causing reactive attachment disorder and temper dysregulation as well as schizophrenia, which makes careful attention to the differential of rule-breaking behaviors important for accurate diagnosis.

This disorder is marked by chronic conflict with parents, teachers, and peers and can result in damage to property and physical injury to the patient and others. These patterns of behavior are consistent over time. Formal classification with the Diagnostic and Statistical Manual of Mental Disorders, DSM - Ⅳ defines the essential characteristics as "a persistent pattern of behavior in which the basic rights of others or major age-appropriate social norms are violated".

Behaviors used to classify CD fall into the 4 main categories of (1) aggression toward people and animals; (2) destruction of property without aggression toward people or animals; (3) deceitfulness, lying, and theft; and (4) serious violations of rules.

CD usually appears in early or middle childhood as oppositional defiant behavior. Nearly one half of children with early oppositional defiant behavior have an affective disorder, CD, or both by adolescence. Thus, careful diagnosis to exclude irritability due to another unrecognized internalizing disorder is important in childhood cases. Evaluation of parent - child interactions and teacher - child interactions is also critical. Even in a stable home environment, a small number of preschool - aged children display significant irritability and aggression that results in disruption severe enough to be classified as CD.

The DSM - Ⅳ specifies that CD can be diagnosed in children younger than 10 years if they demonstrate even one of the criterion antisocial behaviors. Diagnosis after 10 years of age requires the presence of 3 of the criteria behaviors from the categories of (1) aggression toward people and animals; (2) nonaggressive destruction of property; (3) deceitfulness, lying, and theft; and (4) serious violations of rules.

Oppositional defiant disorder (ODD) is discriminated from CD based on the defiance of rules and argumentative verbal interactions involved in ODD; CD involves more deliberate aggression, destruction, deceit, and serious rule violations, such as staying out all night or chronic school truancy. The DSM - Ⅳ defines the 2 major subtypes of CD as childhood - onset type and adolescent - onset type. The childhood - onset type is defined by the presence of 1 criterion characteristic of CD before an individual is aged 10 years; these individuals are typically boys displaying high levels of aggressive behavior. These individuals often also meet criteria for attention deficit/hyperactivity disorder (ADHD). Poor peer and family relationships are present, and these problems tend to persist through adolescence into adult years. These children are more likely to develop adult antisocial personality disorder than individuals with the adolescent-onset type.

Adolescent-onset type is defined by the absence of any criterion characteristic of CD before an individual is aged 10 years. These individuals tend to be less aggressive and have more normative peer relationships. They often display their conduct behaviors in the company of a peer group engaged in these behaviors, such as a gang. These patients are less likely to fit criteria for ADHD; however, the diagnosis of ADHD is still possible. These individuals are also far less likely to develop adult antisocial personality disorder. While boys are identified more often, the estimated sex ratio of this type of CD approaches 50% for girls and boys in some communities. The prognosis for an individual with adolescent-onset type is much better than for a person with the childhood-onset type. CD is highly resistant to treatment. It follows a clear developmental path with indicators that can be present as early as the preschool period. Treatment is more successful when initiated early and must include medical, mental health, and educational components as well as family support. Close communication between home and school is particularly important at younger ages.

DSM-Ⅳ Criteria

DSM-IV Diagnostic Criteria for Conduct Disorder

A.

A repetitive and persistent pattern of behavior in which the basic rights of others or major age-appropriate societal norms or rules are violated, as manifested by the presence of three (or more) of the following criteria in the past 12 months, with at least one criterion present in the past six months:

Aggression to people and/or animals

1. Often bullies, threatens or intimidates others.
2. Often initiates physical fights.
3. Has used a weapon that can cause serious physical harm to others (eg, a bat, brick, broken bottle, knife, gun).
4. Has been physically cruel to people.
5. Has been physically cruel to animals.
6. Has stolen while confronting a victim (eg, mugging, purse snatching, extortion, armed robbery).
7. Has forced someone into sexual activity.

Destruction of property

1. Has deliberately engaged in fire setting with the intention of causing serious damage.
2. Has deliberately destroyed others' property (other than by fire setting).

Deceitfulness or theft

1. Has broken into someone else's house, building or car.
2. Often lies to obtain goods or favors or to avoid obligations (ie, "cons" others).
3. Has stolen items of nontrivial value without confronting the victim (eg, shoplifting, but without breaking and entering; forgery).

Serious violations of rules

1. Often stays out at night despite parental prohibitions, beginning before age 13 years.
2. Has run away from home overnight at least twice while living in a parental or parental surrogate home (or once without returning for a lengthy period).
3. Is often truant from school, beginning before age 13 years.

B.

The disturbance in behavior causes clinically significant impairment in social, academic or occupational functioning.

C.

If the individual is age 18 years or older, criteria are not met for antisocial personality disorder.

Specify severity:

Mild: few if any conduct problems in excess of those required to make the diagnosis, and conduct problems cause only minor harm to others.

Moderate: number of conduct problems and effect on others intermediate between "mild" and "severe".

Severe: many conduct problems in excess of those required to make the diagnosis, or conduct problems cause considerable harm to others.

Patients with conduct disorder typically do not perceive their behavior as problematic. Similarly, parents and teachers often do not consider longstanding conduct disorder when attributing causes to children's behavior. Therefore, symptoms of conduct disorder are not usually a presenting concern in the office. The following cases illustrate typical ways that condust disorder may present in family practice.

Ilustrative Cases

Tim is a six - year - old boy brought to the family medicine clinic for an initial visit. On entering the examination room, the physician observed Tim spinning in circles on the stool while his mother pled, "If I have to tell you one more time to sit down ..." Tim was not permitted to begin first grade until his immunizations were updated. His mother explained that Tim had visited several physicians for immunization but was so disruptive that the physicians and nurses always gave up. She hoped that with a new physician, Tim might comply. The mother described a several - year history of aggressive and destructive behavior, as well as four school suspensions during kindergarten. He often becomes "uncontrollable" at home and has broken dishes and furniture. Last year, Tim was playing with the gas stove and started a small fire. Tim frequently pulls the family dog around by its tail. Tim's older sisters watched him in the past but have refused to do so since he threw a can of soup at one of them. Tim's father is a long - haul truck driver who sees Tim every three to four weeks.

Sharon, a 15 - year - old girl, was brought to the office by her mother. Her mother explained that Sharon was suspended from school for assaulting a teacher and needed a "doctor's evaluation" before she could return to class. The history reveals that this is Sharon's 10th school suspension during the past three years. She has previously been suspended for fighting, carrying a knife to school, smoking marijuana and stealing money from other students' lockers. When asked about her behavior at home, Sharon reports that her mother frequently "gets on my nerves" and, at those times, Sharon leaves the house for several days. The family history indicates that Sharon's father was incarcerated for auto theft and assault. Sharon's mother frequently leaves Sharon and her eight - year - old brother unsupervised overnight.

Pharmacotherapy

Pharmacotherapy may be considered as an adjunct treatment for conduct disorder and comorbid conditions. While there are no formally approved medications for conduct disorder, pharmacotherapy may help specific symptoms. Further studies are needed to evaluate the role of pharmacotherapy for conduct disorder. By improving attention and increasing inhibitory activity, medication may improve children's capacity to benefit from other psychosocial intervention. The majority of published studies involve patients with conduct disorder and comorbid conditions, such as ADHD or major depression. Stimulants, anti - depressants, lithium, anticonvulsants and clonidine (Catapres) have all been used in the treatment of conduct disorder.

Stimulants

Dextroamphetamine (Dexedrine) and methylphenidate (Ritalin) are the most promising agents used in the treatment of conduct disorder. However, there is no consensus concerning stimulant efficacy in conduct disorder. Stimulants evaluated in relatively small studies have been shown to be effective in reducing aggression, primarily in patients with ADHD as a comorbidity, when compared with placebo.

Antidepressants

One small, open - label trial evaluating the efficacy and toxicity of bupropion (Well - butrin) in attention - deficit disorder (ADD) and conduct disorder demonstrated parental - rated and self - rated improvement in conduct. This study suggested that bupropion was safe and effective for use in this population. However, controlled double - blind studies are needed for further evaluation. Fluoxetine (Prozac) also was associated with a significant reduction in impulsive - aggressive behavior in adults with personality disorder. While some controversy exists, there is concern about the cardiotoxic effects of tricyclic antidepressants in children. The selective serotonin reuptake inhibitors (SSRIs) may be particularly helpful in treating children with conduct disorder and comorbid major depression.

Lithium and Anticonvulsants

Lithium is a psychoactive agent with anti - aggressive properties. Results of several studies have demonstrated reduction of aggression. However, lithium requires regular blood level monitoring to assess possible toxicity. Lithium levels should be checked twice weekly until clinical status and levels are stable, with monthly checks thereafter. Monitoring and the toxicity associated with lithium treatment may limit the use of this agent. Anticonvulsants have also been used to reduce aggression. The side effect profile and monitoring requirements provide similar limitations to the anticonvulsants.

Clonidine

Several studies have demonstrated a significant reduction in impulsivity and aggressive outbursts with clonidine. Side effects include drowsiness, low blood pressure, bradycardia and depression. The first three effects may be limited by reducing the dosage. Patients taking clonidine should be closely monitored for symptoms of depression and oversedation.

Psychological Treatment

Of the psychological therapies, parent management training (PMT) is the method demonstrated to have the most impact on the child's coercive pattern of behavior. PMT refers to procedures in which parents have been trained to alter their child's behavior in the home. PMT is based on research demonstrating that conduct problems inadvertently are developed and sustained by maladaptive parent - child interactions. While this conflictual interaction often is triggered by the irritable temperament in the child, a major component of this pattern is ineffective parenting. This includes the parent directly paying attention to disruptive and deviant behaviors but using unclear vague commands and directions and inconsistently applied harsh punishment. A pattern of failing to pay attention to appropriate behaviors, when they occur, is also present.

PMT alters the pattern of ineffective parenting by encouraging the parent to practice prosocial behavior (positive, specific feedback for desirable behavior), employ the use of natural and logical consequences, and use effective, brief, nonaversive punishments on a limited basis when specific encouragement and consequences are not applicable.

PMT educators and therapists teach the child's parents to use specific procedures at home to alter interactions with their child. Parents are trained to carefully identify and observe behaviors and to reinforce desired behaviors. Training sessions provide opportunities to see how procedures work and to practice and refine their use of techniques.

In treating groups of preschool children who had severe oppositional and aggressive behavior, some evidence-based parenting therapies exist. In these clinical random assignment studies, when therapists adhered to a manual of techniques and parents made changes in parenting skills (which were documented), the outcome included immediate posttreatment improvement and evidence of improvement 1-3 years after treatment. One study reflected gains 10 years later. Treatment effects have been stronger with younger children but have also co-varied with the severity of the problems. Children with the most severe problems are more resistant to improvement. A parental training program for early intervention with preschoolers at risk for conduct problems was shown in one study to improve dispositional variables post-intervention and at one-year follow-up.

More recent research suggests that the severity of the problem, rather than the age of the child, is predictive of treatment failure. Severe conduct problems in adolescents are the most resistant to this type of treatment, when compared with younger children. However, with appropriate treatment programs, some improvement has been documented in all age ranges and all levels of severity. Treatment needs to be highly structured with specific goals and the use of established behavioral techniques to improve communication and problem solving skills, as well as the reinforcement of prosocial behaviors and the implementation of clear discipline for inappropriate behaviors.

Group treatment has had both benefits and drawbacks for children with conduct disorder (CD). While some evidence exists that group social skills or problem-solving treatment has some benefit in children aged 12 years and younger, concerns exist about group treatment of adolescents diagnosed with CD. With younger children, combined treatment in which parents attend a PMT group while the children attend a social skills group consistently has exhibited good effect. However, research demonstrates that treatment of adolescents with CD conducted in groups of individuals with CD tends to worsen the behavior, particularly if the group participants engage in discussions of oppositional and illegal behaviors.

Thus, group treatment should be enacted with great care and consideration of group goals and possible negative adverse effects. More drastic solutions (eg, boot camps) consistently have demonstrated initial good outcome but worsening outcome in the long term, with higher rates of arrests and serious crimes found in boot camp graduates. Poor long-term outcome following this treatment is believed to be due, in part, to group mutual reinforcement and discussion of criminal activity and to the lack of family or community change in many of these programs.

Thus, the adolescents are released back into the same environment, in which little support for the newly acquired skills and behavior is present.

In general, individual psychotherapy as a single treatment has not proven effective for conduct problems. However, individual therapy sessions certainly can facilitate compliance with an overall program that emphasizes changes in the family, the school, and in social settings. Thus, individual counseling may help a child who is trying to adhere to a more comprehensive intervention program.

The multisystemic treatment package is a comprehensive model of treatment of CD that includes behavioral PMT, social skills training, academic support, pharmacologic treatment of ADHD or depression symptoms, and individual counseling as needed. Initial outcome data for this type of comprehensive approach have been encouraging. Multisystemic therapy has been proven to be helpful for children and adolescents with CD, especially when parent management has been attempted unsuccessfully.

Referral for Specialized Treatment

While mild and early - stage cases of conduct disorder may be effectively managed by family physicians, many children and adolescents with conduct disorder will require specialized mental health treatment. Typically, patients with conduct disorder are not distressed by their behavior; furthermore, there are almost always major family issues and dysfunctions that contribute to or limit treatment of the patient's problem. Therefore, family therapy is the treatment of choice. In addition to behavior management, effective therapy requires parental consistency and reduction of marital or intergenerational conflict. Empowering parents to take charge of discipline and rule setting is often difficult because of adults' own self - focus or concurrent psychopathology. In managed health care systems, primary care clinicians are often the gatekeepers to mental health care. By accurately diagnosing these children and determining the degree of risk to self or others, while noting resources available in the patient's natural environment, family physicians can more effectively advocate the appropriate level of service these patients require.

When adult caregivers are unavailable or unable to provide the degree of structure and supervision required, residential treatment may be necessary. Family physicians who prescribe medication for conduct disorder or comorbid conditions should maintain regular contact with other professionals treating the child.

Autistic Disorder

Autistic disorder, a pervasive developmental disorder resulting in social, language, or sensorimotor deficits, occurs in approximately seven of 10,000 persons. Early detection and intervention significantly improve outcome, with about one third of autistic persons achieving some degree of independent living. Indications for developmental evaluation include no babbling, pointing, or use of other gestures by 12 months of age, no single words by 16 months of age, no two - word spontaneous phrases by 24 months of age, and loss of previously learned language or social skills at any age. The differential diagnosis includes other psychiatric and pervasive developmental disorders, deafness, and profound hearing loss. Autism is frequently associated with fragile X syndrome and tuberous sclerosis, and may be caused by lead poisoning and metabolic disorders. Common comorbidities include mental retardation, seizure disorder, and psychiatric disorders such as depression and anxiety. Behavior modification programs are helpful and are usually administered by multidisciplinary teams; targeted medication is used to address behavior concerns. Many different treatment approaches can be used, some of which are unproven and have little scientific support. Parents may be encouraged to investigate national resources and local support networks.

Recognition of the disorder called autism may have its origin in Itard's 1801 description of the "wild boy of Aveyron", a violent child with no language skills who related to other people as if they were objects. It was not until 1943 that Kanner identified a complex set of characteristics (eg, aberrations in social development, verbal and nonverbal communication, symbolic thinking) for a syndrome he labeled "autism".

Although Kanner theorized that a single, biologically based defect was responsible for the development of autistic disorders, treatment in the 1950s and 1960s was dominated by the psychodynamic theory of the etiology of autism that charged that pathologic parenting was responsible for the withdrawal of children from their environment. Following the 1970s discovery of neuroreceptors, endogenous neurohormones, and the stereospecific binding sites of neuropeptides to neurons, clinicians have discounted the psychodynamic theory of autism and repostulated Kanner's original supposition that biologically based deficits are responsible for the Etiology.

Autistic disorder is a pervasive developmental disorder defined behaviorally as a syndrome consisting of abnormal development of social skills (withdrawal, lack of interest in peers), limitations in the use of interactive language (speech as well as nonverbal communication), and sensorimotor deficits (inconsistent responses to environmental stimuli). In this article, the more generic terms autism and autistic refer to the broad spectrum of pervasive developmental disorders that exhibit autistic features as their primary presenting behaviors. The term autistic disorder is used to describe the specific developmental disorder that occurs at them.

Epidemiology

In general, pervasive developmental disorders are estimated to occur at a rate of 63 per 10,000 persons. While the reported incidence of autistic disorder ranges from about five per 10,0004 to 20 per 10,000 persons, a recent meta-analysis reports the median rate for 11 surveys conducted since 1989 to be seven per 10,000 persons. Male-to-female ratios vary with IQ scores from 2:1 in severely handicapped persons to 4:1 in moderately handicapped persons. The occurrence rate in siblings is suspected to be from 3 to 7 percent, representing a 50- to 100-fold increase in risk.

Etiology

No single cause has been identified for the development of autism. Genetic origins are suggested by studies of twins. In addition, an increased frequency of occurrence is noted in patients with genetic conditions such as fragile X syndrome and tuberous sclerosis. Some reports have suggested a possible association with Down syndrome.

In addition to the implication of neurotransmitters, such as serotonin, in the development and expression of autism, many other disorders may result in brain dysfunction. Possible contributing factors in the development of autism include infections, errors in metabolism, immunology, lead poisoning, and fetal alcohol syndrome.

Concerns have been raised in recent years that immunizations, particularly measles, mumps, and rubella (MMR) vaccine, may precipitate autism. In addition to reports from several parents who first detected autism in their children following an MMR vaccination at 12 to 15 months of age, an anecdotal study reported similar suspicions on the part of physicians who provided care for 12 autistic patients. Subsequent studies in the United Kingdom reference and the United States have failed to show an association between any vaccine and the development of autism. Information about ongoing studies being conducted by the Centers for Disease Control and Prevention and the National Institutes of Health (NIH) is available at their Web sites.

DSM-Ⅳ Criteria

The following is from Diagnostic and Statistical Manual of Mental Disorders: DSM-Ⅳ

(I) A total of six (or more) items from (A), (B), and (C), with at least two from (A), and one each from (B) and (C).

(A) qualitative impairment in social interaction, as manifested by at least two of the following:

1. marked impairments in the use of multiple nonverbal behaviors such as eye-to-eye gaze, facial expression, body posture, and gestures to regulate social interaction;

2. failure to develop peer relationships appropriate to developmental level;

3. a lack of spontaneous seeking to share enjoyment, interests, or achievements with other people, (eg, by a lack of showing, bringing, or pointing out objects of interest to other people);

4. lack of social or emotional reciprocity (note: in the description, it gives the following as examples: not actively participating in simple social play or games, preferring solitary activities, or involving others in activities only as tools or "mechanical" aids).

(B) qualitative impairments in communication as manifested by at least one of the following:

1. delay in, or total lack of, the development of spoken language (not accompanied by an attempt to compensate through alternative modes of communication such as gesture or mime);

2. in individuals with adequate speech, marked impairment in the ability to initiate or sustain a conversation with others;

3. stereotyped and repetitive use of language or idiosyncratic language;

4. lack of varied, spontaneous make-believe play or social imitative play appropriate to developmental level.

(C) restricted repetitive and stereotyped patterns of behavior, interests and activities, as manifested by at least two of the following:

1. encompassing preoccupation with one or more stereotyped and restricted patterns of interest that is abnormal either in intensity or focus;

2. apparently inflexible adherence to specific, nonfunctional routines or rituals;

3. stereotyped and repetitive motor mannerisms (e.g hand or finger flapping or twisting, or complex whole-body movements);

4. persistent preoccupation with parts of objects.

(Ⅱ) Delays or abnormal functioning in at least one of the following areas, with onset prior to age 3 years:

(A) social interaction;

(B) language as used in social communication;

(C) symbolic or imaginative play.

(Ⅲ) The disturbance is not better accounted for by Rett's Disorder or Childhood Disintegrative Disorder.

Special Education

Special education is central to the treatment of autistic disorder. Although parents may choose to use various experimental treatments, including medication, they should concurrently use intensive individual special education by an educator familiar with instructing children who have autistic disorder or a related condition. Intensive behavioral interventions, instituted as early as possible, are indicated for every child in whom autistic disorder is suspected.

The Education for All Handicapped Children Act of 1975 requires free and appropriate public education for all children, regardless of the extent and severity of their handicaps. Amendments to *the Education of the Handicapped Act of 1986* extended the requirement for free and appropriate education to children aged 3-5 years.

Pediatricians and parents cannot assume, however, that their community's school will provide satisfactory education for a child with autistic disorder or a related condition. *The Individuals with Disabilities Education Act* authorized states to determine how to provide educational services to children younger than 3 years. Pediatricians and parents need to determine the best way to proceed with local agencies. Therapies that are reported to help some individuals with autism include the following:

Assisted communication — Using keyboards, letter boards, word boards, and other devices (eg, the Picture Exchange Communication System), with the assistance of a therapist;

Auditory integration training — A procedure in which the individual listens to specially prepared sounds through headphones;

Sensory integration therapy — A treatment for motor and sensory motor problems typically administered by occupational therapists;

Exercise and physical therapy — Exercise is often therapeutic for individuals with autistic disorder; a regular program of activity prescribed by a physical therapist may be helpful.

In addition, social skills training helps some children with autism spectrum disorder, including those with comorbid anxiety disorders. Children with autism spectrum disorder and comorbid attention deficit hyperactivity disorder may not benefit from social skills training.

In a 2 - year randomized, controlled trial, children who received the Early Start Denver Model (ESDM), a comprehensive developmental behavioral intervention for improving outcomes of toddlers diagnosed with autism spectrum disorder, showed significant improvements in IQ, adaptive behavior, and autism diagnosis compared with children who received intervention commonly available in the community. A follow - up electroencephalographic study showed normalized patterns of brain activity in the ESDM group.

In contrast, a 12 - week study of parent - delivered ESDM intervention found no effect on child outcomes compared with usual community treatment. However, starting intervention at an earlier age and providing a greater number of intervention hours both related to the degree of improvement in children's behavior.

Many people with autism have sleep problems. These are usually treated by staying on a routine, including a set bedtime and time to get up. Your doctor may try medicines as a last resort.

Stories about alternative therapies, such as secretin and auditory integration training, have circulated in the media and other information sources. When you are thinking about any type of treatment, find out about the source of the information and about whether the studies are scientifically sound. Accounts of individual success are not sufficient evidence to support using a treatment. Look for large, controlled studies to validate claims.

Experts have not yet identified a way to prevent autism. Public concern over stories linking autism and childhood vaccines has persisted. But numerous studies have failed to show any evidence of a link between autism and the measles - mumps - rubella (MMR) vaccine. If you avoid having your children immunized, you put them and others in your community at risk for developing serious diseases, which can cause serious harm or even death.

Separation Anxiety Disorder

Separation anxiety disorder is a medical condition that is characterized by significant distress when a person is away from parents, another caregiver, or home. Unlike the occasional, mild worries that children may feel at times of separation, separation anxiety disorder can dramatically affect a person's life by limiting the ability to engage in ordinary activities. Children with the disorder become extremely upset whenever they separate from their primary caregiver, whether that person is a parent, relative, nanny, or other caregiver. Unlike children who are simply shy, children with separation anxiety disorder may become severely anxious and agitated even when just anticipating being away from their home or primary caregiver.

Separation anxiety disorder affects approximately two to five percent of children. These children, who often have additional anxiety disorders, frequently have other family members with anxiety disorders. The tendency to develop separation anxiety disorder involves complex genetic and environmental factors.

Depression

About 11 percent of adolescents have a depressive disorder by age 18 according to the National Comorbidity Survey - Adolescent Supplement (NCS - A). Girls are more likely than boys to experience depression. The risk for depression increases as a child gets older. According to the World Health Organization, major depressive disorder is the leading cause of disability among Americans age 15 to 44. Because normal behaviors vary from one childhood stage to another, it can be difficult to tell whether a child who shows changes in behavior is just going through a temporary "phase" or is suffering from depression.

People believed that children could not get depression. Teens with depression were often dismissed as being moody or difficult.

It wasn't known that having depression can increase a person's risk for heart disease, diabetes, and other diseases.

Today's most commonly used type of antidepressant medications did not exist. Selective serotonin reuptake inhibitors (SSRIs) resulted from the work of the late Nobel Laureate and NIH researcher Julius Axelrod, who defined the action of brain chemicals (neurotransmitters) in mood disorders.

We now know that youth who have depression may show signs that are slightly different from the typical adult symptoms of depression. Children who are depressed may complain of feeling sick, refuse to go to school, cling to a parent or caregiver, or worry excessively that a parent may die. Older children and teens may sulk, get into trouble at school, be negative or grouchy, or feel misunderstood.

Findings from NIMH - funded, large - scale effectiveness trials are helping doctors and their patients make better individual treatment decisions. For example, the Treatment for Adolescents with Depression Study (TADS) found that combination treatment of medication and psychotherapy works best for most teens with depression. The Treatment of SSRI - resistant Depression in Adolescents (TORDIA) study found that teens who did not respond to a first antidepressant medication are more likely to get better if they switch to a treatment that includes both medication and psychotherapy.

The Treatment of Adolescent Suicide Attempters (TASA) study found that a new treatment approach that includes medication plus a specialized psychotherapy designed specifically to reduce suicidal thinking and behavior may reduce suicide attempts in severely depressed teens.

Depressed teens with coexisting disorders such as substance abuse problems are less likely to respond to treatment for depression. Studies focusing on conditions that frequently co - occur and how they affect one another may lead to more targeted screening tools and interventions.

With medication, psychotherapy, or combined treatment, most youth with depression can be effectively treated. Youth are more likely to respond to treatment if they receive it early in the course of their illness.

Although antidepressants are generally safe, the U.S. Food and Drug Administration has placed a "black box" warning label — the most serious type of warning — on all antidepressant medications. The warning says there is an increased risk of suicidal thinking or attempts in youth taking antidepressants. Youth and young adults should be closely monitored especially during initial weeks of treatment.

Studies focusing on depression in teens and children are pinpointing factors that appear to influence risk, treatment response, and recovery. Given the chronic nature of depression, effective intervention early in life may help reduce future burden and disability.

Multi - generational studies have revealed a link between depression that runs in families and changes in brain structure and function, some of which may precede the onset of depression. This research is helping to identify biomarkers and other early indicators that may lead to better treatment or prevention.

Advanced brain imaging techniques are helping scientists identify specific brain circuits that are involved in depression and yielding new ways to study the effectiveness of treatments.

DSM-Ⅳ Criteria

The diagnostic criteria and key defining features of major depressive disorder in children and adolescents are the same as they are for adults. However, recognition and diagnosis of the disorder may be more difficult in youth for several reasons. The way symptoms are expressed varies with the developmental stage of the youngster. In addition, children and young adolescents with depression may have difficulty in properly identifying and describing their internal emotional or mood states. For example, instead of communicating how bad they feel, they may act out and be irritable toward others, which may be interpreted simply as misbehavior or disobedience. Research has found that parents are even less likely to identify major depression in their adolescents than are the adolescents themselves.

The symptoms of depression in children vary. It is often undiagnosed and untreated because they are passed off as normal emotional and psychological changes that occur during growth. Early medical studies focused on "masked" depression, where a child's depressed mood was evidenced by acting out or angry behavior. While this does occur, particularly in younger children, many children display sadness or low mood similar to adults who are depressed. The primary symptoms of depression revolve around sadness, a feeling of hopelessness, and mood changes. Signs and symptoms of depression in children include:

Irritability or anger;

Continuous feelings of sadness and hopelessness;

Social withdrawal;

Increased sensitivity to rejection;

Changes in appetite — either increased or decreased;

Changes in sleep — sleeplessness or excessive sleep;

Vocal outbursts or crying;

Difficulty concentrating;

Fatigue and low energy;

Physical complaints (such as stomachaches, headaches) that don't respond to treatment;

Reduced ability to function during events and activities at home or with friends, in school, extracurricular activities, and in other hobbies or interests;

Feelings of worthlessness or guilt;

Impaired thinking or concentration;

Thoughts of death or suicide.

Not all children have all of these symptoms. In fact, most will display different symptoms at different times and in different settings. Although some children may continue to function reasonably well in structured environments, most kids with significant depression will suffer a noticeable change in social activities, loss of interest in school and poor academic performance, or a change in appearance. Children may also begin using drugs or alcohol, especially if they are over the age of 12.

Although relatively rare in youths under 12, young children do attempt suicide — and may do so impulsively when they are upset or angry. Girls are more likely to attempt suicide, but boys are more likely to actually kill themselves when they make an attempt. Children with a family history of violence, alcohol abuse, or physical or sexual abuse are at greater risk for suicide, as are those with depressive symptoms.

Depression can arise from a combination of genetic vulnerability, suboptimal early developmental experiences, and exposure to stresses. How children respond to different stressors is different depending on the child's personality and situation. Most children become silent and do not open up to the parents about what is wrong and what is bothering them. Symptoms go unnoticed because of a tendency of depression to have an insidious onset in children, and because symptoms may fluctuate in intensity. There are several theories of depression that exist to define the causes of this mental illness and to explain what is going on in the mind of a depressed person, whether that individual is an adult or a child.

Models of Vulnerability

Cognitive Theory of Depression. According to cognitive theory, thinking negatively greatly affected the likelihood of developing a depression and maintaining it during stressful events in a person's life. Individuals who think negatively are more vulnerable towards depression because they perceive the environment, their future and themselves in a negative, depressive context. This negative way of thinking guides child's or adult's perception, interpretation, and memory of personally relevant experiences, thereby resulting in a negatively biased construal of their personal world, and ultimately, the development of depressive symptoms.

Parent and Child Model of Socialization

Parent and Child Model of Socialization is another model used by clinicians. The model was applied to development of depressive symptoms. It was expected that when parents used intrusive support frequently, children engaging in negative self-evaluative processes would be more vulnerable to depressive symptoms that children engaging in positive self-evaluative processes. The results of the study performed on the model suggest that both parents and children contribute to the development of depressive symptoms. Parents use of control with children had been identified as a central dimension of socialization model. Two forms of control are: psychological — parents attempt to oversee and regulate children's psychological and emotional development through constraining verbal expression and invalidating feelings; and behavioral — parents try to regulate children's behavior by using limit setting and positive reinforcement

Psychological control appears to have negative consequences for children because it communicates to them that they are incompetent and intrudes their individuality. Behavioral control causes positive consequences because it provides guidance in meeting standards and shows support of the parents. The term intrusive support, used in the study, identifies with those two forms of control and yet it is defined as monitoring and helping children when they do not request help. The study was done to investigate the hypothesis that when parents frequently used intrusive support, children engaging in negative self - evaluative processes would be more vulnerable to depressive symptoms than would children engaging in positive self - evaluative processes. The results showed that hypothesis was right to assume. The findings also showed the importance of use of the model for studying of the depression disorder and relevance of the model to the current research in the area of depression.

Tripartite Model of Depression and Anxiety

The Tripartite Model of Depression and Anxiety was developed. They theorized that depression is specifically characterized by anhedonia or low positive effect (PA), anxiety is specifically characterized by physiological hyperarousal (PH), and general negative affect (NA) is a non specific factor that relates to both depression and anxiety. The study was performed to examine whether the model could discriminate youth with depressive disorders from youth with externalizing symptoms. The results found corroborated the hypothesis. It was shown that the model can be used to differentiate between the depressive conditions from anxious syndromes.

The model that represented anxiety (NA), depression (PA) and fear (PH) as distinct factors provided best fit for data from the child and parent report for 216 clinically anxious children. Results supported the expected pattern of relations of NA and PA with current symptoms of depression and anxiety in a community sample. NA was significantly associated with symptoms of both depression and anxiety, whereas PA was mostly strongly associated with symptoms of depression. Thus, the model was shown to be a useful tool for differentiation between anxiety and depression symptoms in children. Children with a depressive disorder diagnosis may be identified by using the factors of the tripartite model. Specifically, children with a depressive disorder were distinguishable from other youth psychiatric patients on the basis of low PA and high NA. Low PA was found to distinguish inpatient children with depression from those with anxiety.

Stressors

Stressors in everyday life take place and affect an individual's emotional state. Such stressors as school problems, problems with peers, family, loses, medical illness affect children.

Stressors lead to feelings such as sadness, crabbiness, being bored, and not enjoying anything; lead to behaviors such as withdrawal, decreased activity, irritability with others; and lead to thoughts such as pessimism, negativity, low self-esteem, and hopelessness. All the factors come together to evolve into clinical depression with physical problems: trouble sleeping, poor concentration, low energy, agitation and appetite problems. Clinical depression may go a step further to evolve into more severe depression and depletion of brain chemicals.

Family Instability

Certain types of family organizations are closely related to the development and maintenance of symptoms in children. According to family systems theory, when the married couple has conflict and can not solve it in a constructive way, they are likely to involve their children in the conflict to release some anxiety and tension between them. Child is physiologically vulnerable to everything going on between his parents. Tension and conflict in the family induces emotional arousal in the child, triggering physiological and psychological responses. The results of the study conducted in investigation of the relationship between parents' marital stability, triangulation and the level of depression in children showed that children of marital dissatisfied fathers were more likely to have depressive symptoms than those of dissatisfied mothers.

When fathers felt unstable in the marriage and, experienced triangulation in their families at the same time, their children were likely to have depressive symptoms. When fathers felt stable but unsatisfied in their marriage, their children were also more prone to develop depressive symptoms. The finding that the mothers' scores do not affect children as the fathers' do was consistent with the results found in that other studies comparing fathers' and mother's influences on children. It may be explained by the roles in the family in bringing up children and taking care of the family financially, and by the difference of gender in solving a marital conflict. Mothers are often thought of as primary care-takers of the family, fathers are the providers. It is quite common to believe that mothers are more emotionally involved with their children and more emotionally available to them. They consciously separate their roles as mothers and wives, and therefore the independence between roles takes place. When men feel dissatisfied and unstable in their marriage, they may concentrate their energy on the outside of their family, on their friends and society and abandon their role as providers. There is evidence that intense marital conflict is related to a husband's withdrawal during conflict interaction. When man withdraws from a unstable marriage, he withdraws from the mother and the child at the same time, his role as a father is greatly affected by the level of marital satisfaction. Men are also more likely to express an unusual overt behavior such as being aggressive, angry, argumentative, unaffectionate and withdrawn. Women on the other hand, will tend to be more internally hurt, more likely to have depression. Thus, for a child it is easier to identify their father's over behavior and be disturbed by it, rather that their mothers depressive symptoms, such as being sad and crying. When mothers experience marital instability, they become more involved with their children than previously.

Depressed Parents

The study mentioned above, also leads to a theory that depressed children are more likely to live with depressed parents. In single parent families the stress is always present because of the family situation. One parent performs dual roles for the child and that is stressful for both of them. The single mother is a provider for the family and also a care - taker. But the first role is of primary concern because that role was not her role originally, that is why the mother has to work harder at it. At that time the second role of the mother as a care - taker is partially abandon because of the lack of time left to spend with a child. The mother may express overt changes in behavior, such as anger and frustration, to show hew feelings of helplessness. In this case the child can sense the depression and unhappiness of the mother because there is no father figure to be more influential than the mother.

Treatment

Cognitive Therapy

Once the depression disorder is diagnosed there are several ways to approach the treatment. Cognitive behavioral therapy is one therapy most used for treating depression. Treatment consists of identifying copying strategies for kids and their parents. The therapist helps kids to identify cognitive distortions. Beck's cognitive theory suggests that depressed children's negative self - perceptions reflect cognitive distortions about the self and about the environment. Cognitive theories assume that errors in depressive judgment result form negative bias introduced by the negative self schemas of depressed persons. Aaron T. Beck and his colleagues initially developed cognitive therapy as treatment for depression. Cognitive behavioral treatment or CBT of depression involves the application of specific strategies directed at the following three domains: cognition, behavior and physiology. In the cognitive domain, patients are taught to correct their negative thinking. In behavioral domain, patients learn activity scheduling, social skills and assertiveness. In physiological domain patients are taught relaxation techniques, meditation and pleasant imagery to calm themselves. Numerous studies conducted showed that cognitive therapy was more effective than tricyclic antidepressant therapy.

Family Therapy

Numerous studies have shown the importance and effectiveness of family intervention, family participation in the treatment, parents' demonstration of positive control over the child, and lower stress level within the family. Five negative outcomes have been shown to appear if the family is not participating in the intervention. First, among children with depression, greater family stress has been found to be associated with a longer initial episode and lower social competence at 3 - year follow up. Second, depressed children whose homes were characterized by high levels of parental criticism or emotional over involvement demonstrated significantly lower recovery rates at the end of the first year after hospitalization than did children whose parents scored low on those variables. Third, during depressive episodes, children demonstrate more negative and guilt - inducing behavior in laboratory - based family interactional tasks when compared to non depressed psychiatric and control participants, underscoring the high level of stress experienced by families of depressed children. Fourth, maternal and child depressive symptoms may be temporarily linked such that symptoms in one member of the dyad potentiate symptoms in the other. Fifth, although studies of depressed adults indicate strong family histories of depression in the first degree relatives, familial loading appears to be even more substantial in children and adolescents with major depression. Parental depression, conflict in the family, criticism of a child, dysfunction, family stress contribute to child depression which in turn also fuels family stress and dysfunction. A therapist works with both the parents and the child to identify the negative thoughts and behaviors influencing depression of both and tries to turn those into a positive influence to correct the disorders.

There is emerging support for the value of psychoeducational family programs. The sessions are taught by the professionals in the field of depression greatly increase awareness and knowledge of parents in the area of child depression. The parents are taught to identify the symptoms, how to approach a depressed child, how to help him, information about mood disorders, interpersonal skills, stress reduction, medication and medication side effects. The effect of various stressor in a child's life is also examined in the context of different environments such as school, home, community. Participants of the programs get to meet other parents and their children to discuss common issues such as symptoms, social skills, approaches to accepting depression disorder. Other therapeutic strategies include a nonblaming reforming of the goals of treatment from a focus on the child's symptoms to a focus on the quality of parent-child relationships, building alliances between the therapist and both parents and child, promoting attachment between the parents and the child, and competencies within the child.

Pharmacotherapy

Use of different antidepressants such as clomipramine, tricyclic antidepressants (amitriptyline, desipramine, notriptyline), selective serotonin inhibitors (Prozac, Zoloft, Lexapro) showed a reduction in depression for certain children. Mood stabilizers and possibly antipsychotic or anticonvulsant drugs have been also used successfully (Kalb & Raymond, 2003). In the study exploring the effectiveness of antidepressants in treating depression it was found that fluoxetine was superior to a placebo in the acute phase of major depressive disorder in child and adolescent outpatients with severe, persistent depression. After 5 weeks follow up with the outpatients the superiority of fluoxetine was not seen. There were no significant differences between patients in both placebo and fluoxetine groups on measures of general psychiatric symptoms, global functioning or self-reported depressive symptom measurements. In the second study performed to evaluate tricyclic antidepressant amitriptyline, it was found that there were no significant differences between the control and measurement groups, so there was no evidence recorded that tricyclic antidepressant amitriptyline is effective to use in treatment for depression. The findings suggest that there are no an effective antidepressant to treat depression successfully. Different depressed children respond differently to various antidepressants and some may get better and some may not. It is very common for clinicians to prescribe serotonin selective reuptake inhibitors or SSRIs such as fluoxetine, sertraline, paroxetine, fluvoxamine rather than tricyclic antidepressants such as amytriptyline, imipramine, desipramine, due to better tolerance and fewer side effects. Ultimately, depression is a prevalent mental disorder in children and adolescents that requires a comprehensive, multidisciplinary treatment plan to prevent its persistence or reoccurrence into adulthood. If prescribed, antidepressants should always be used in combination with other treatment strategies such as cognitive - behavioral therapy, family intervention, family education and various prevention strategies.

In children and adolescents, the recurrence rate of depressive episodes first occurring in childhood or adolescence is 70 percent by five years, which is similar to the recurrence rate in adults. Young people experiencing a moderate to severe depression may be more likely to have a manic episode in their adulthood (Hazel, 2003). Bottom line is that children with symptoms of depression are likely to develop depression in the adulthood if not treated, than children without the symptoms.

Prevention of Depression in Children

According to the models of depression, the same skills that would reduce depression could be used to inoculate children against it. Prevention of depression includes early detection of the symptoms and immediate treatment. In 1994, on the children at risk for depression by virtue of subthreshold depressive symptoms or a high degree of family conflict at home. Immediately after treatment the 69 treated children showed lower levels of depressive symptoms and better classroom behavior compared to 73 children in the nontreated condition. Moreover, the treated children continued to report fewer depressive symptoms at a 2 - year follow - up assessment, with the number of treated children who reported symptoms of depression in the moderate to severe range reduced by one - half. Another approach to prevent depression in children was tested by Beardslee in 1992, who identified the children at high risk for depression as having a parent with a serious mood disorder. The psychoeducational session was attended by the parent and the child and was aimed on helping parents to convey to their children an understanding of the parent's mood disorder, and assisting the child in identifying questions and concerns for the parent to address. Compared to the participants in the control group with lecture to the parents only, parents in psychoeducational session reported greater satisfaction, more behavior and attitude changes, increased understanding of disorder by the child, improved communication between the parent and the child.

Child Maltreatment

In 1993, the U.S. Advisory Board on Child Abuse and Neglect declared a child protection emergency. Between 1985 and 1993, there was a 50 percent increase in reported cases of child abuse. Three million cases of child abuse are reported in the United States each year. Treatment of the abuser has had only limited success and child protection agencies are overwhelmed. Recently, efforts have begun to focus on the primary prevention of child abuse. Primary prevention of child abuse is defined as any intervention that prevents child abuse before it occurs. Primary prevention must be implemented on many levels before it can be successful. Strategies on the societal level include increasing the "value" of children, increasing the economic self-sufficiency of families, discouraging corporal punishment and other forms of violence, making health care more accessible and affordable, expanding and improving coordination of social services, improving the identification and treatment of psychologic problems, and alcohol and drug abuse, providing more affordable child care and preventing the birth of unwanted children. Strategies on the familial level include helping parents meet their basic needs, identifying problems of substance abuse and spouse abuse, and educating parents about child behavior, discipline, safety and development.

Child abuse or maltreatment includes physical abuse, sexual abuse, psychologic abuse, and general, medical and educational neglect. The National Center on Child Abuse and Neglect has established a set of working definitions of the various types of abuse; however, the specific acts that constitute the various forms of abuse are defined under state law and, thus, vary from one jurisdiction to another. For this reason, child abuse is a legal finding, not a diagnosis.

Primary prevention is defined as both the prevention of disease before it occurs and the reduction of its incidence. In the context of child abuse, primary prevention is defined as any intervention designed for the purpose of preventing child abuse before it occurs. This definition encompasses what some authorities have defined as secondary prevention.

Family physicians should be aware of the risk factors for child abuse and possible interventions that could prevent it. This article reviews possible causes of child abuse and current intervention strategies.

Epidemiology

Between 1985 and 1993, the number of cases of child abuse in the United States increased by 50 percent. In 1993, three million children in the United States were reported to have been abused. Thirty-five percent of these cases of child abuse were confirmed.

Data from various reporting sources, however, indicate that improved reporting could lead to a significant increase in the number of cases of child abuse substantiated by child protection agencies. The lack of substantiation does not indicate that maltreatment did not occur, only that it could not be substantiated. The fact remains that each year, 160,000 children suffer severe or life-threatening injury and 1,000 to 2,000 children die as a result of abuse. Of these deaths, 80 percent involve children younger than five years of age, and 40 percent involve children younger than one year of age. One out of every 20 homicide victims is a child. Homicide is the fourth leading cause of death in children from one to four years of age and the third leading cause of death in children from five to 14 years of age. Neonaticide (ie, the murder of a baby during the first 24 hours of life) accounts for 45 percent of children killed during the first year of life.

It is generally accepted that deaths from maltreatment are underreported and that some deaths classified as the result of accident and sudden infant death syndrome might be reclassified as the result of child abuse if comprehensive investigations were more routinely conducted. Most child abuse takes place in the home and is instituted by persons known to and trusted by the child. Although widely publicized, abuse in day-care and foster-care settings accounts for only a minority of confirmed cases of child abuse. In 1996, only 2 percent of all confirmed cases of child abuse occurred in these settings.

Child abuse is 15 times more likely to occur in families where spousal abuse occurs. Children are three times more likely to be abused by their fathers than by their mothers. No differences have been found in the incidence of child abuse in rural versus urban settings.

Consequences

Not only do children suffer acutely from the physical and mental cruelty of child abuse, they endure many long-term consequences, including delays in reaching developmental milestones, refusal to attend school and separation anxiety disorders. Other consequences include an increased likelihood of future substance abuse, aggressive behaviors, high-risk health behaviors, criminal activity, somatization, depressive and affective disorders, personality disorders, post-traumatic stress disorder, panic attacks, schizophrenia and abuse of their own children and spouse. Recent research has shown that a loving, caring and stimulating environment during the first three years of a child's life is important for proper brain development. This finding implies that children who receive maltreatment in these early years may actually have suboptimal brain development.

Research regarding the causes of child abuse has recently undergone a paradigm shift. The results of research initiated by the National Research Council's Panel on Research on Child Abuse and Neglect signal the first important step away from simple cause-and-effect models. As was recognized by researchers for the National Research Council's panel, the simple cause-and-effect models have certain limitations, mainly related to their narrow focus on the parents. These models limit themselves by asking only about the isolated set of personal characteristics that might cause parents to abuse or neglect their children. Moreover, these models also fail to account for the occurrence of different forms of abuse in one child. At the same time, these models had very little explanatory power in weighing the value of various risk factors involved in child abuse. As a result, they were not very accurate in predicting future cases of child abuse.

To replace the old static model, the panel has substituted what it calls an "ecologic" model. This model considers the origin of all forms of child abuse to be a complex interactive process. This ecologic model views child abuse within a system of risk and protective factors interacting across four levels: (1) the individual, (2) the family, (3) the community and (4) the society. However, some factors are more closely linked with some forms of abuse than others.8 The factors thought to contribute to the development of physical and emotional abuse and neglect of children are discussed below.

Primary Prevention Strategies

The U.S. Advisory Board on Child Abuse and Neglect has stated that only a universal system of early intervention, grounded in the creation of caring communities, could provide an effective foundation for confronting the child abuse crisis. It is generally held that successful strategies for preventing child abuse require intervention at all levels of society. However, no consensus has formed regarding which programs or services should be offered to prevent child abuse. In part, this is because research on the prevention of child abuse is limited by the complexity of the problem, the difficulty in measuring and interpreting the outcomes, and the lack of attention to the interaction among variables in determining risk status for subsequent abuse. Although a broad range of programs has been developed and implemented by public and private agencies at many levels, little evidence supports the effectiveness of these programs.

A 1994 retrospective review of 1,526 studies on the primary prevention of child abuse found that only 30 studies were methodologically sound. Of the 11 studies dealing primarily with physical abuse and neglect, only two showed a decrease in child abuse as measured by a reduction in hospital admissions, emergency department visits or reports to child protective services. Although there is a need for better designed research to evaluate the effectiveness of prevention strategies, recommendations for preventive interventions are based on what we currently know about the causes of child abuse.

Social Interventions

Primary prevention strategies based on risk factors that have a low predictive value are not as likely to be effective as more broadly based social programs. In addition, programs focused on a societal level rather than on the individual level prevent the stigmatization of a group or an individual.

Social strategies for preventing child abuse that are proposed but unproven include increasing the value society places on children, increasing the economic self - sufficiency of families, enhancing communities and their resources, discouraging excessive use of corporal punishment and other forms of violence, making health care more accessible and affordable, expanding and improving coordination of social services, improving treatment for alcohol and drug abuse, improving the identification and treatment of mental health problems, increasing the availability of affordable child care and preventing the births of unwanted children through sex education, family planning, abortion, anonymous delivery and adoption.

Families

Strategies targeted at the individual can also be considered strategies for helping the family.

Until parents' basic needs are met, they may find it difficult to meet the needs of their children. The first thing parents need is assistance in meeting their basic requirements for food, shelter, clothing, safety and medical care. Only when these needs are met can higher needs be addressed.

The next step should be to identify and treat parents who abuse alcohol or drugs, and identify and counsel parents who suffer from spousal abuse. Identifying and treating parents with psychologic problems is also important. Other issues that need attention include financial concerns, and employment and legal problems. Providing an empathetic ear and being a source of referral for help with these issues may take physicians a long way toward nurturing needy parents.

The next higher level of need includes education about time management and budgeting skills, stress management, coping and parenting skills such as appropriate discipline, knowledge of child development, nutrition and feeding problems, and safety issues.

In the United States, some of the specific methods of delivering services to families include long-term home visitation, short-term home visitation, early and extended postpartum mother/child contact, rooming in, intensive physician contact, drop-in centers, child classroom education, parent training and free access to health care.

Of these methods, only long-term home visitation (up to two years) has been found to be effective in reducing the incidence of child abuse as measured by hospital admissions, emergency department visits and reports to child protective services. Indeed, many organizations are now embracing the concept of home visitation as a method of preventing child abuse by identifying family needs and providing the appropriate services. Results of one study on home visitation showed benefits or improvements in several areas: parents' attitudes toward their children, interactions between parents and children, and reduction in the incidence of child abuse. However, without an infrastructure of support services such as health care, social services and child care, home visitors will be unable to deliver needed services.

What Can Physicians Do?

It is clear that many of the causes of child abuse center on the needs and problems of the parents. Therefore, in order to prevent child abuse, we must first help and support the parents. Parents with multiple emotional, medical, financial and social needs find it difficult to meet the needs of their children. It is imperative that physicians develop a supportive attitude toward parents to ultimately help the children.

Effective prevention of child abuse and neglect can best be achieved using strategies designed to help parents protect and nurture their children. These strategies include giving parents the necessary support, resources and skills. The physician should obtain help from social workers, home health agencies, financial counselors, psychologists, local mental health facilities, alcohol and drug treatment centers and parenting centers, as appropriate. To that end, physicians should become familiar with the resources available in their community. It is useful to keep a list of such agencies with telephone numbers and addresses readily available in patient education files to distribute to patients. Physicians should be aware of the many public and private agencies already available for information and referral. The National Committee to Prevent Child Abuse has a nationwide network that provide leadership in the prevention of child abuse.

Although child abuse is a pervasive and complex problem with many causes, we should not take a defeatist attitude toward its prevention. Despite the absence of strong evidence to guide our preventive efforts, physicians can do many things to try to prevent abuse. At the very least, showing increased concern for the parents or caregivers and increasing our attempts to enhance their skills as parents or caregivers may help save our most vulnerable patients from the nightmare of abuse and neglect.

Studies have shown that busy physicians may spend as little as one minute discussing anticipatory guidance with parents. One proposed strategy for improvement in this area is to provide group parenting classes to discuss such issues. Topics for discussion include safety issues, nutrition and feeding concerns, discipline and normal child development. Classes should be divided into two groups: one for the parents of infants and one for the parents of toddlers, since these two groups will require a different focus. Providing child care during these classes may be necessary to ensure attendance.

Questions for Parents in Assessing the Risk of Child Abuse:

What is it like for you taking care of this baby?

Who helps you with your children?

Do you get time to yourself?

What do you do when the child's behavior drives you crazy?

Do you have trouble with your child at mealtime or bedtime?

Are your children in day care?

How are things between you and your partner?

It is important to address issues that are of concern to the parents. It is also important to try to give very specific and concrete suggestions to parents instead of talking in broad generalities. For example, physicians could suggest that parents use an egg timer to help children anticipate and be more compliant with bedtime or use time-out as an alternative to spanking a child for bad behavior. Parents should be reminded of and taught to distinguish between childish behavior and willful disobedience, and to discipline only those actions that are in the child's control according to his or her stage of development.

The physician who is concerned for the welfare of children should be an advocate for more accessible, affordable and high-quality child and health care in the local community. Studies have shown that countries with the most generous social services have the lowest rate of child homicide. Physicians should lobby for greater availability of drug and alcohol treatment programs, more shelters for the homeless, more accessible mental health care and more shelters for abused women and children. These programs and those that provide parenting skills, support groups and respite care for parents and care-givers should be available in every community.

Many practical strategies can help the busy physician try to prevent child abuse. Spending less time examining an obviously well child and more time discussing psychosocial issues with that child's parent is one recommendation. Questions to ask parents that might help physicians assess the risk of child abuse are mentioned above. If psychosocial problems are uncovered, the physician might schedule more frequent visits to allow for further discussions. Other strategies include inviting fathers for an office visit and encouraging the parents to rely on the support of families and friends

Chapter 7 Introduction to Psychiatric Treatment

Mental illness is classified today according to the Diagnostic and Statistical Manual of Mental Disorders, Fourth Edition (DSM Ⅳ), published by the American Psychiatric Association (1994). The DSM uses a multiaxial or multidimensional approach to diagnosing because rarely do other factors in a person's life not impact their mental health. It assesses five dimensions as described below:

Axis Ⅰ: Clinical Syndromes

This is what we typically think of as the diagnosis (eg, depression, schizophrenia, social phobia).

Axis Ⅱ: Developmental Disorders and Personality Disorders

Developmental disorders include autism and mental retardation, disorders which are typically first evident in childhood.

Personality disorders are clinical syndromes which have a more long lasting symptoms and encompass the individual's way of interacting with the world. They include Paranoid, Antisocial, and Borderline Personality Disorders.

Axis Ⅲ: Physical Conditions Which Play a Role in the Development, Continuance, or Exacerbation of Axis Ⅰ and Ⅱ Disorders

Physical conditions such as brain injury or HIV/AIDS that can result in symptoms of mental illness are included here.

Axis Ⅳ: Severity of Psychosocial Stressors

Events in a persons life, such as death of a loved one, starting a new job, college, unemployment, and even marriage can impact the disorders listed in Axis Ⅰ and Ⅱ. These events are both listed and rated for this axis.

Axis Ⅴ: Highest Level of Functioning

On the final axis, the clinician rates the person's level of functioning both at the present time and the highest level within the previous year. This helps the clinician understand how the above four axes are affecting the person and what type of changes could be expected.

As the preceding chapters have attempted to show, a multifactorial approach is necessary to explain the etiology and pathogenesis of psychiatric illness. Similarly, the most useful treatment approaches are developed with the framework of the biopsychosocial model.

Psychiatric treatment may comprise one or many modalities and may be rendered in a number of settings depending on both the needs and the circumstances: physical, economic, geographic of each individual patient. Weekly outpatient behavior modification treatment would be appropriate for an otherwise happy and successful advertising executive who wishes to be cured of fear of flying, whereas involuntary inpatient treatment along with pharmacotherapy and, later, social service interventions would be mandatory for the psychotic. Furthermore, different treatment approaches may be useful at different times over the course of any individual patient's illness. For example, a young person undergoing a major depressive episode may not be able to respond to or tolerate exploratory psychotherapy without prior antidepressant drug therapy and supportive treatment. In this chapter, the settings in which mental illness may be treated are described as well as the individuals who deliver such treatment.

Psychiatric Disorders

The DSM Ⅳ (American Psychiatric Association, 1994) identifies 15 general areas of adult mental illness. We'll discuss each one briefly. For more information about a specific category, open Psychiatric Disorders on the Main Menu and follow the links provided.

1. Delirium, Dementia, Amnestic, and Other Cognitive Disorders

The primary symptoms of these disorders include significant negative changes in the way a person thinks and/or remembers. All of these disorders have either a medical or substance related cause and are therefore not discussed in detail in this chapter.

2. Mental Disorders Due to a Medical Condition

Like those above, all disorders in this category are directly related to a medical condition. If symptoms of anxiety, depression, etc are a direct result of a medical condition, this is the classification used.

3. Substance Related Disorders

There are two disorders listed in this category: Substance Abuse and Substance Dependence. Both involve the ingestion of a substance (alcohol, drug, chemical) which alters either cognitions, emotions, or behavior.

Abuse refers to the use of the substance to the point that it has a negative impact on the person's life. This can mean receiving a DUI for drinking and driving, being arrested for public intoxication, missing work or school, getting into fights, or struggling with relationships because of the substance.

Dependence refers to what we typically think of as "addicted". This occurs when (a) the use of the substance is increased in order to get the same effect because the person has developed a tolerance, (b) the substance is taken more frequently and in more dangerous situations such as drinking and driving, or (c) the person continues to take the substance despite negative results and/or the desire to quit, or (d) withdrawal symptoms are present when the substance is stopped, such as delirium tremors (DTs), amnesia, anxiety, headaches, etc.

4. Schizophrenia and Other Psychotic Disorders

The major symptom of these disorders is psychosis, or delusions and hallucinations. The major disorders include schizophrenia and schizoaffective disorder.

Schizophrenia is probably the most recognized term in the study of psychopathology, and it is probably the most misunderstood. First of all, it does not mean that the person has multiple personalities. The prefix "schiz" does mean split, but it refers to a splitting from reality. The predominant features of schizophrenia include hallucinations and delusions and disorganized speech and behavior, inappropriate affect, and avolition. There is no known cure for schizophrenia and is without doubt the most debilitating of all the mental illnesses.

Schizoaffective Disorder is characterized by a combination of the psychotic symptoms such as in Schizophrenia and the mood symptoms common in Major Depression and/or Bipolar Disorder. The symptoms are typically not as severe although when combined together in this disorder, they can be quite debilitating as well.

5. Mood Disorders

The disorders in this category include those where the primary symptom is a disturbance in mood. The disorders include Major Depression, Dysthymic Disorder, Bipolar Disorder, and Cyclothymia.

Major Depression (also known as depression or clinical depression) is characterized by depressed mood, diminished interest in activities previously enjoyed, weight disturbance, sleep disturbance, loss of energy, difficulty concentrating, and often includes feelings of hopelessness and thoughts of suicide.

Dysthymia is often considered a lesser, but more persistent form of depression. Many of the symptoms are similar except to a lesser degree. Also, dysthymia, as opposed to Major Depression is more steady rather than periods of normal feelings and extreme lows.

Bipolar Disorder (previously known as Manic-Depression) is characterized by periods of extreme highs (called mania) and extreme lows as in Major Depression. Bipolar Disorder is subtyped either I (extreme or hypermanic episodes) or II (moderate or hypomanic episodes).

Like Dysthymia and Major Depression, Cyclothymia is considered a lesser form of Bipolar Disorder.

6. Anxiety Disorders

Anxiety Disorders categorize a large number of disorders where the primary feature is abnormal or inappropriate anxiety. The disorders in this category include Panic Disorder, Agoraphobia, Specific Phobia, Social Phobia, Obsessive-Compulsive Disorder, Posttraumatic Stress Disorder, and Generalized Anxiety Disorder.

Panic Disorder is characterized by a series of panic attacks. A panic attack is an inappropriate intense feeling of fear or discomfort including many of the following symptoms: heart palpitations, trembling, shortness of breath, chest pain, dizziness. These symptoms are so severe that the person may actually believe he or she is having a heart attack. In fact, many, if not most of the diagnoses of Panic Disorder are made by a physician in a hospital emergency room.

Agoraphobia literally means fear of the marketplace. It refers to a series of symptoms where the person fears, and often avoids, situations where escape or help might not be available, such as shopping centers, grocery stores, or other public place. Agoraphobia is often a part of panic disorder if the panic attacks are severe enough to result in an avoidance of these types of places.

Specific or Simple Phobia and Social Phobia represents an intense fear and often an avoidance of a specific situation, person, place, or thing. To be diagnosed with a phobia, the person must have suffered significant negative consequences because of this fear and it must be disruptive to their everyday life.

Obsessive - Compulsive Disorder is characterized by obsessions (thoughts which seem uncontrollable) and compulsions (behaviors which act to reduce the obsession). Most people think of compulsive hand washers or people with an intense fear of dirt or of being infected. These obsessions and compulsions are disruptive to the person's everyday life, with sometimes hours being spent each day repeating things which were completed successfully already such as checking, counting, cleaning, or bathing.

Posttraumatic Stress Disorder (PTSD) occurs only after a person is exposed to a traumatic event where their life or someone else's life is threatened. The most common examples are war, natural disasters, major accidents, and severe child abuse. Once exposed to an incident such as this, the disorder develops into an intense fear of related situations, avoidance of these situations, reoccurring nightmares, flashbacks, and heightened anxiety to the point that it significantly disrupts their everyday life.

Generalized Anxiety Disorder is diagnosed when a person has extreme anxiety in nearly every part of their life. It is not associated with just open places (as in agoraphobia), specific situations (as in specific phobia), or a traumatic event (as in PTSD). The anxiety must be significant enough to disrupt the person's everyday life for a diagnosis to be made.

7. Somatoform Disorders

Disorders in this category include those where the symptoms suggest a medical condition but where no medical condition can be found by a physician. Major disorders in this category include Somatization Disorder, Pain Disorder, Hypochondriasis.

Somatization Disorder refers to generalized or vague symptoms such as stomach aches, sexual pain, gastrointestinal problems, and neurological symptoms which have no found medical cause.

Pain Disorder refers to significant pain over an extended period of time without medical support.

Hypochondriasis is a disorder characterized by significant and persistent fear that one has a serious or life-threatening illness despite medical reassurance that this is not true.

8. Factitious Disorder

Factitious Disorder is characterized by the intentionally produced or feigned symptoms in order to assume the "sick role". These people will often ingest medication and/or toxins to produce symptoms and there is often a great secondary gain in being placed in the sick role and being either supported, taken care of, or otherwise shown pity and given special rights.

9. Dissociative Disorders

The main symptom cluster for dissociative disorders include a disruption in consciousness, memory, identity, or perception. In other words, one of these areas is not working correctly causing significant distress within the individual. The major diagnoses in this category include Dissociative Amnesia, Dissociative Fugue, Depersonalization Disorder, and Dissociative Identity Disorder.

Dissociative Amnesia is characterized by memory gaps related to traumatic or stressful events which are too extreme to be accounted for by normal forgetting. A traumatic event is typically a precursor to this disorder and memory is often restored.

Dissociative Fugue represents an illness where an individual, after an extremely traumatic event, abruptly moves to a new location and assumes a new identity. This disorder is very rare and typically runs its course within a month.

Depersonalization Disorder, occurring after an extreme stressor, includes feelings of unreality, that your body does not belong to you, or that you are constantly in a dreamlike state.

Dissociative Identity Disorder (DID) is most widely known as Multiple Personality Disorder or MPD. DID is the presence of two or more distinct personalities within an individual. These personalities must each take control of the individual at varying times and there is typically a gap in memory between personalities or "alters". This disorder is quite rare and a significant trauma such as extended sexual abuse is usually the precursor.

10. Sexual Dysfunctions, Paraphilias, and Gender Identity Disorders

These disorders are all related to sexuality, either in terms of functioning (Sexual Dysfunctions), distressing and often irresistible sexual urges (Paraphilias), and gender confusion or identity (Gender Identity Disorder). It should be noted that for these, as well as many other categories, a medical reason should always be ruled out before making a psychological diagnosis.

Sexual Dysfunctions include Hypoactive Sexual Desire Disorder (deficiency or absence of sexual fantasies and desire for sexual activity), Sexual Aversion Disorder (persistent or recurring aversion to or avoidance of sexual activity), Sexual Arousal and Male Erectile Disorder (Inability to attain or maintain until completion of sexual activity adequate lubrication [in women] or erection [in men] in response to sexual excitement), Orgasmic Disorder (male) (female) (delay or absence of orgasm following normal excitement and sexual activity), and Premature Ejaculation (ejaculation with minimal sexual stimulation before or shortly after penetration and before the person wishes it).

Paraphilias include Exhibitionism (the intense urge to expose oneself to an unsuspecting stranger), Voyeurism (the intense urge to watch an unsuspecting person in various states of undress or sexual activity), Fetishism (intense sexual fantasies, urges, and behaviors involving an inanimate object), Pedophilia (sexually arousing fantasies. urges, and behavior involving a prepubescent child), Sexual Masochism (intense sexual fantasies, urges, and behavior involving the act of being beaten, humiliated, and/or bound), and Sexual Sadism (intense sexual fantasies, urges, and behavior involving the infliction of pain and/or humiliation on another person).

The final category, Gender Identity Disorder, is characterized by a strong and persistent identification with the opposite sex and the belief that one is actually the opposite sex due to an extreme discomfort in one's present sexual identity.

11. Eating Disorders

Eating disorders are characterized by disturbances in eating behavior. There are two types: Anorexia Nervosa and Bulimia Nervosa.

Anorexia is characterized by failure to maintain body weight of at least 85% of what is expected, fear of losing control over your weight or of becoming "fat". There is typically a distorted body image, where the individual sees themselves as overweight despite overwhelming evidence to the contrary.

The key characteristics of Bulimia include bingeing (the intake of large quantities of food) and purging (elimination of the food through artificial means such as forced vomiting, excessive use of laxatives, periods of fasting, or excessive exercise).

12. Sleep Disorders

All sleep disorders involve abnormalities in sleep in one of two categories, dysomnias and parasomnias.

Dysomnias are related to the amount, quality and/or timing of sleep. Examples of sleep disorders include insomnia (inability or reduced ability to sleep), hypersomnia (excessive sleepiness and prolonged sleep without physical justification), and narcolepsy (irresistible attacks of sleep).

Parasomnias refer to sleep disturbances related to behavioral or physiological events related to sleep. Disorders in this subcategory include nightmare disorder (occurance of extremely frightening dreams which result in awakening and resulting distress), sleep terror disorder (similar to nightmare disorder but the fear is more intense and the person is often unresponsive during the episode), and sleepwalking disorder (walking or performing tasks during sleep without recollection once awakened).

13. Impulse Control Disorders

Disorders in this category include the failure or extreme difficulty in controlling impulses despite the negative consequences.

Specific disorders include Intermittent Explosive Disorder (failure to resist aggressive impulses resulting in serious assaults or destruction of property), Kleptomania (stealing objects which are not needed), Pyromania (fire starting for pleasure or relief of tension), Pathological Gambling (maladaptive gambling behavior), and trichotillomania (pulling out of one's own hair).

14. Adjustment Disorders

This category consists of an inappropriate or inadequate adjustment to a life stressor. Adjustment disorders can include depressive symptoms, anxiety symptoms, and/or conduct or behavioral symptoms.

15. Personality Disorders

Personality Disorders are characterized by an enduring pattern of thinking, feeling, and behaving which is significantly different from the person's culture and results in negative consequences. This pattern must be longstanding and inflexible for a diagnosis to be made.

There are ten types of personality disorders, all of which result in significant distress and/or negative consequences within the individual: Paranoid (includes a pattern of distrust and suspiciousness, Schizoid (pattern of detachment from social norms and a restriction of emotions), Schizotypal (pattern of discomfort in close relationships and eccentric thoughts and behaviors), Antisocial (pattern of disregard for the rights of others, including violation of these rights and the failure to feel empathy), Borderline (pattern of instability in personal relationships, including frequent bouts of clinginess and affection and anger and resentment, often cycling between these two extremes rapidly), Histrionic (pattern of excessive emotional behavior and attention seeking), Narcissistic (pattern of grandiosity, exaggerated self-worth, and need for admiration), Avoidant (pattern of feelings of social inadequacies, low self-esteem, and hypersensitivity to criticism), and Obsessive-Compulsive (pattern of obsessive cleanliness, perfection, and control).

Settings in Which Mental Health May Be Offered

Mental health services are traditionally delivered in hospitals, outpatient office settings, day treatment programs, and emergency rooms. In some cases, psychiatrists and oilier mental health professionals may work with, and in, other agencies such as penal institutions, law courts, schools at all levels, places of employment, and even in the patient's home.

Individuals requiring or requesting treatment may present in a variety of ways at a number of different "entry points" into the mental health care delivery system. New patients may present at the private offices of general physicians or specialists, mental health professionals, community-based crisis intervention centers, community mental health centers, or hospital emergency rooms. Specially trained professionals at these sites evaluate the current status and needs of each individual patient and make recommendations or referrals for further treatment. When patients are dangerous to themselves or others or are unable to care for themselves and do not understand their need for treatment, such a recommendation may be made mandatory by court order.

Inpatient Settings

Psychiatric hospitalization may be necessary for a variety of patients who cannot be treated effectively or safely as outpatients. Some patients require specialized diagnostic procedures (eg, for close observation of symptoms, specialized endocrine or sleep studies) that can be performed safely and properly only in a hospital, others may require almost constant nursing attention (eg, physically ill patients who develop dangerous side effects to medications, agitated patients who require seclusion) that can be provided only on an inpatient basis. Psychiatric patients are also admitted for their own protection or the protection of others, as in the case of suicidal or homicidal patients or patients who are so disorganized, depressed, or demented that they cannot care for themselves. Such patients are observed closely, protected, restricted, and confined and are usually treated for the specific mental disorder underlying their behavior. In some cases, individuals accused of criminal activity are admitted to a hospital for forensic psychiatric evaluation of criminal responsibility or competence to stand trial. Hospitals may also be used inappropriately and unnecessarily when less intensive services would suffice, and some patients may even "manipulate the system" to obtain admission (eg, the homeless individual who uses the hospital as a shelter or the individual with antisocial personality disorder who is in trouble on the streets and "escapes" into the psychiatric unit).

Hospital settings offer a wide variety of treatment options, including medical treatments group, individual, and family psychotherapy, social worker services, and occupational and recreational activity therapies. Ideally, the treatment plan is tailored to meet the medical, social, and psychological needs of each individual patient.

In the United States, inpatient psychiatric care may be delivered in state and county mental hospitals, private mental hospitals, general hospitals (often in specialized psychiatric units), Veterans Administration hospitals, and military hospitals. Improvements in the efficacy of somatic treatments that resulted in shortening the period of acute symptoms in many patients shifted the emphasis from long-term to short-term care and away from reliance on state and county hospital systems. Furthermore, since hospitalization can lead to stigmatization loss of self-esteem, dependency, and regressed behavior, the trend is toward minimizing hospital stays and utilizing less restrictive treatment settings (eg, day treatment) in innovative and more intensive ways. Progress in this area is encouraged by governmental agencies (Medicaid and Medicare) and private third-paity payers, who are reluctant to pay for inpatient services for any but the sickest of patients. Current managed care practices have encouraged the trend away from hospital admissions, favoring less expensive services provided in lieu of hospital days.

Outpatient Care

Outpatient services are provided in freestanding clinics, clinics attached to hospitals, community mental health centers, and private offices. Almost unknown in the nineteenth and early twentieth centuries, outpatient services now account for the majority of psychiatric utilization. In the 1950s the split between outpatient and inpatient care was approximately 25%/75%. Today, that ratio has been reversed.

Outpatient treatment is appropriate for patients with a wide variety of psychiatric illnesses varying from problems of living and adjustment disorders to those with psychotic and mood disorders. As alluded to above, the trend over the past 30-40 years has been to move away from inpatient care toward outpatient treatment. Traditionally, outpatient care has consisted of seeing a therapist in group or individual treatment for no more than 1 or 2 hours a week. Although many people who function well at home and at work benefit from such limited treatment, there are many others with more severe mental disorders who need a more intense level of care but who do not require 24-hour supervision as is provided in a traditional inpatient selling.

In the past, prior to the era of managed care, many patients who could not function within the limited framework of traditional outpatient treatment were hospitalized; (1) it was often easier to hospitalize a patient than to provide the complex and time-consuming kind of support that an outpatient in crisis may require; (2) third-party payers often paid for in-patient care more readily than intense outpatient care; and (3) few resources had been developed to provide intermediate alternatives to the choice between traditional outpatient and costly and restrictive inpatient care.

However, as managed care companies limit payment for inpatient treatment to only the sickest patients, innovations in outpatient care are developing. Less seriously impaired individuals may be seen in intensive outpatient treatment, where contact with the patient is "titrated" to the patient's condition. Patients who are more impaired may be treated in a partial hospital setting.

Partial Hospitalization

In partial hospitalization programs, patients receive much the same range of services provided in traditional inpatient settings but are, in most cases, allowed to go home at night. (Rarely, patients work or study by day but stay at the hospital at night.) Such care may be offered to hospitalized patients to help them readjust to life outside the hospital or to fairly ill patients who need supervision but who can safely be at home nights and weekends. This form of treatment is much less expensive than full-time hospitalization.

Chronically ill patients sometimes receive similar care in "day treatment" and "psychiatric rehabilitation" programs designed to provide structure, training in social skills, vocational training, and other treatment over longer periods of time.

Residential Treatment Programs

Residential treatment programs offer treatment in structured nonhospital settings. Some offer graduated services ranging from completely supervised homes with 24-hour supervision and a full range of structured activities and treatments to less supervised arrangements in which patients combine treatment with other activities such as volunteer or paid work. Such facilities slowly move the patient in the direction of semi-independent or fully independent living.

Residential self-help communities are usually sponsored by nongovernmental agencies for the purpose of helping individuals with some specific difficulty, often chemical dependency. Examples include Oxford House and the Salvation Army (both created for persons with drug and alcohol problems). Residents in these communities often maintain ties with the community after leaving the residence.

Substitute homes provide shelter and limited treatment to patients who either do not require or would not benefit from other kinds of residential treatment programs. Persons living in such homes often are unable to live alone and unsupervised and have either no family support or families who cannot continue to provide care. Treatment is usually confined to supervision of activities of daily living, medication, informal counseling (usually provided by a layperson who manages the home), and sometimes transportation to therapists' offices or in-house medication management provided by a psychiatrist on contract to the home. Examples include adult foster care homes, hoard and care homes, family care homes, and mental hygiene homes. There is increasing reliance on "supported housing," typically apartments scattered throughout a community with no live-in staff but supportive services as required.

Other examples of substitute housing include "crash pads" for people withdrawing from drugs or in crisis and in need of a sate place. Similarly, temporary shelters for abused women and even the homeless may be regarded as part of the mental health care system.

Emergency and Crisis Intervention

Crisis intervention services are offered by hospital and nonhospital facilities and provide episodic acute intervention in life-threatening or extreme circumstances involving patients with mental illness or others in crisis. In such settings, including private homes, patients are evaluated, sometimes over several hours and, when feasible attempts are made to help resolve the crisis. In many cases, these facilities serve as entry points into the mental health system whereby patients may be referred for further inpatient or outpatient care. In some crisis intervention settings, a patient may be seen frequently on a short-term basis until the crisis has subsided.

Also important are services such as suicide and drug prevention hotlines that offer telephone support and refer patients in crisis.

Community Outreach Services

In some communities, mental health professionals provide services to patients where they live and congregate. These community outreach services are utilized most commonly within the community mental health system, and are targeted to improve care for the chronically mentally ill. The best studied of these are assertive community treatment (ACT) teams. Services may include home visits to assess living conditions, improve medication compliance, and provide support. Mobile teams may identify and offer services to patients on the streets and other public places. Although such services are expensive, they have been shown to improve health status und reduce the. use of hospital services.

Social Support Services

Social Support services are offered by most mental health and community social service, agencies to bolster the patient's natural support system (eg, family, church, neighborhood) or to provide a substitute system it natural supports are lacking. The effect of these services may be to alter the acute course of illness to prevent chronicity.

Nonresidential self-help organizations are the "out-patient" parallel to the residential self-help services described above and are often founded by individuals who have survived a problem and have handed together to help others who have had similar life experiences. Examples are Alcoholics Anonymous, Narcotics Anonymous, Schizophrenics Anonymous, Recovery, the Manic Depressive/Depressive Association colostomy clubs, the Epilepsy Society, and burn recovery groups. A new "recovery movement" emphasizes the potential for patients to be "well" and integrated into their communities. This optimism counters decades of stigma and pessimism.

Miscellaneous agencies provide services, counseling, and assistance to a variety of individuals in need. Although not formally part of the mental health care system, these organizations often provide enough psychosocial assistance to prevent or avert crises. Examples include the Visiting Nurse Association, Homeniakers Services, Big Brothers, Planned Parenthood, Traveler's Aid and consumer credit agencies.

Mental Health Professionals

There are many different kinds of professional mental health care providers. Most have certain skills in common and provide similar services (eg, psychotherapy). Some have areas of specialized training and practice. A variety of treatments are available for those who experience difficulty in coping with their problems. There are two general categories of treatment: psychotherapy and biologically centered treatment. The over 200 types of psychotherapy use psychological techniques to treat emotional or behavioral problems and may deal with individuals or groups, children or adults. Therapists choose an approach (or approaches) consistent with their training and the problems and goal (s) of their clients. Biomedical therapy focuses on somatic (body) treatment and usually employs medications. The training of psychotherapists varies widely. Examples of disciplines studied and degrees earned are given in Table 1 .

Table 1 Training of Psychotherapists

Discipline	Degree
Psychologist	PhD (Doctor of Philosophy) or PsyD (Doctor of Psychology)
Psychiatrist	MD (Doctor of Medicine)
Social worker	MSW (Master of Social Work)
Psychiatric nurse	BSN (Bachelor of Science in Nursing) or MA (Master of Arts)
Counselor	MA (Master of Arts in Counseling)

Psychiatrists are physicians doctors of medicine or osteopathy who have completed a 4-year residency training program in general psychiatry. Psychiatrists are named to apply both biomedical and psychosocial diagnostic and therapeutic skills to the management of patients with physical and mental disorders. They are trained in techniques of psychotherapy and are skilled at both diagnosis and psychosocial formulation (psychodynamic, behavioral. or both). They are the only members of the mental health care team trained and licensed to prescribe medication and (along with nurses) to perform complete physical examinations.

Clinical psychologists are mental health professionals with doctorates like Doctor of Philosophy (PhD), Doctor of Education (EdD), Doctor of Psychology (PsyD), or master's degrees who may be licensed as independent practitioners in psychotherapy and psychological assessment; some masters-level professionals have licenses restricting their practice to marriage and family counseling. These professionals attend graduate schools and have clinical placements and internships in which they learn psychotherapy, diagnosis, and psychological testing under supervision. When licensed, they may diagnose and treat patients with mental disorders.

Psychologists often have specialized training in administering psychological tests and performing behavior and cognitive therapies. They also have more extensive research training than most physicians. As with physicians, the services of psychologists are now being reimbursed by insurance. In addition, psychologists are beginning to gain admitting privileges to some hospital inpatient services, permitting them to admit a patient jointly with a physician.

Clinical social workers are doctoral (PhD) or (more frequently) master's - level psychotherapists, caseworkers, and marriage, family, and child therapists trained in accredited schools of social work and social welfare and accredited by the National Association of Social Work as having completed a specified program of supervised clinical training. They are licensed by many states as independent practitioners, and increasingly they are being reimbursed by health insurance payers. Social workers are skilled at psychosocial therapies, are knowledgeable about community and social welfare resources, and have a special interest in families.

Clinical nurse specialists are registered nurses who may take special training in psychiatric nursing. They may be licensed as independent practitioners, but more often work in organized ambulatory health care settings and in hospitals. Nurses have specie skills in the biomedical as well as the psychosocial aspects of mental health care.

Occupational, activities' and recreational/expressive therapists are registered practitioners from a variety of educational backgrounds with specialized training in using art, music, dance, drama, play, and vocational activities to help patients express their feelings and thoughts, learn new behavior, and develop or recover emotionally and socially valuable skills.

Pastoral counselors are clergy with specialized training in counseling patients with emotional disorders. Case managers are individuals with diverse training and experience who provide advocacy and support to patients, usually outside of an office setting. They often link patients with needed services, but they may also provide direct support and counseling themselves.

Other mental health care providers include clinical sociologists, clinical pharmacists, and specialists in other related clinical disciplines who have developed clinical skills related to their core academic or professional training and apply them in clinical settings.

Psychoanalysts are graduates of psychoanalytic institutes, including Freudian, neo - Freudian, and Jungian training centers, who have completed a course of study, a personal analysis, and supervised training analyses. Although most are psychiatrists, other professionals have been trained as lay analysts. Training takes many additional years after completion of other professional mental health training.

Multidisciplinary teams of mental health professionals function in psychiatric and general hospital and ambulatory settings. The inpatient team has a traditional hierarchy and division of labor, with the psychiatrist leading the team; the nurse managing day-to-day ward activities and medications and monitoring patients: the psychologist performing psychological tests or leading patient therapy groups; the social worker finding a place for the patient to go on discharge, arranging for the financing of hospital and posthospital care, and often performing family therapy; and the occupational therapist organizing activities for the patient during the hospital stay. This traditional organization is still the mode, although in some settings the inpatient team has evolved with less differentiated functions and roles and a less hierarchical organization.

The outpatient team tends to be less hierarchical, though certain functions are still performed by different disciplines (eg, psychiatrists manage medication and psychologists give tests and conduct behavior treatments).

Chapter 8 Psychotherapy

Introduction to Psychotherapy

Treatment of mental illnesses can take various forms. They can include medication, talk-therapy, a combination of both, and can last only one session or take many years to complete. Many different types of treatment are available, but most agree that the core components of psychotherapy remain the same. Psychotherapy consists of the following:

1. A positive, healthy relationship between a client or patient and a trained psychotherapist;
2. Recognizable mental health issues, whether diagnosable or not;
3. Agreement on the basic goals of treatment;
4. Working together as a team to achieve these goals.

With these commonalities in mind, this chapter will summarize the different types of psychotherapy, including treatment approaches and modalities and will describe the different professionals who perform psychotherapy.

Types of Psychotherapy

When describing "talk" therapy or psychotherapy, there are several factors that are common among most types. First and foremost is empathy. It is a requirement for a successful practitioner to be able to understand his or her client's feelings, thoughts, and behaviors. Second, being non-judgmental is vital if the relationship and treatment are going to work. Everybody makes mistakes, everybody does stuff they aren't proud of. If your therapist judges you, then you don't feel safe talking about similar issues again. Finally, expertise. The therapist must have experience with issues similar to yours, be abreast of the research, and be adequately trained.

Aside from these commonalties, therapists approach clients from slightly different angles, although the ultimate goal remains the same: to help the client reduce negative symptoms, gain insight into why these symptoms occurred and work through those issues, and reduce the emergence of the symptoms in the future. The three main branches include Cognitive, Behavioral, and Dynamic.

Therapists who lean toward the cognitive branch will look at dysfunctions and difficulties as arising from irrational or faulty thinking. In other words, we perceive the world in a certain way (which may or may not be accurate) and this results in acting and feeling a certain way. Those who follow more behavioral models look at problems as arising from our behaviors which we have learned to perform over years of reinforcement. The dynamic or psychodynamic camp stem more from the teaching of Sigmund Freud and look more at issues beginning in early childhood which then motivate us as adults at an unconscious level.

Cognitive approaches appear to work better with most types of depression, and behavioral treatments tend to work better with phobias. Other than these two, no differences in terms of outcome have been found to exist. Most mental health professionals nowadays are more eclectic in that they study how to treat people using different approaches. These professionals are sometimes referred to as integrationists.

Treatment Modalities

Therapy is most often thought of as a one - on - one relationship between a client or patient and a therapist. This is probably the most common example, but therapy can also take different forms. Often times group therapy is utilized, where individuals suffering from similar illnesses or having similar issues meet together with one or two therapists. Group sizes differ, ranging from three or four to upwards of 15 or 20, but the goals remain the same. The power of group is due to the need in all of us to belong, feel, understood, and know that there is hope. All of these things make group as powerful as it is. Imagine feeling alone, scared, misunderstood, unsupported, and unsure of the future; then imagine entering a group of people with similar issues who have demonstrated success, who can understand the feelings you have, who support and encourage you, and who accept you as an important part of the group. It can be overwhelming in a very positive way and continues to be the second most utilized treatment after individual therapy.

Therapy can also take place in smaller groups consisting of a couple or a family. In this type of treatment, the issues to be worked on are centered around the relationship. There is often an educational component, like other forms of therapy, such as communication training, and couples and families are encouraged to work together as a team rather than against each other. The therapist's job is to facilitate healthy interaction, encourage the couple or family to gain insight into their own behaviors, and to teach the members to listen to and respect each other.

Sometimes therapy can include more than one treatment modality. A good example of this is the individual who suffers from depression, social anxiety, and low self - esteem. For this person, individual therapy may be used to reduce depressive symptoms, work some on self - esteem and therefore reduce fears about social situations. Once successfully completed, this person may be transferred to a group therapy setting where he or she can practice social skills, feel a part of a supportive group, therefore improving self - esteem and further reducing depression.

The treatment approach and modality are always considered, along with many other factors, in order to provide the best possible treatment for any particular person. Sometimes more than one is used, sometimes a combination of many of them, but together the goal remains to improve the life of the client.

Therapy Providers

We all know that medical illnesses are treated by medical professionals, namely physicians. But what we sometimes fail to realize is that there are many different types of physicians and there are many non - physicians who treat medical illnesses. The same holds true for mental illness. Although medication for mental illness is prescribed by a medical doctor, typically a psychiatrist, the vast majority of psychotherapy is performed by non - physician professionals. These mental health professionals typically have a minimum of a Master's Degree and complete internships, residencies, and state and federal testing just like all direct - care providers. Below is a description of the four most common mental health providers, including required education and training, and the populations with whom they typically work.

Psychologist

A doctoral degree which means a minimum of four years of graduate training beyond the bachelors degree is required in most states, as well as one year of internship and at least one year of post - graduate residency. Typically psychologists complete core coursework in therapy, assessment, and research and are required to pass competency exams and complete a dissertation prior to receiving their degree.

To be licensed, psychologists must pass a national and state examination. Some states grant different licenses for school, counseling, and clinical psychologists. School psychologists usually work in Social Worker.

Social workers must hold a bachelors degree in social work although many complete a Master's program (two years beyond their bachelor degree) leading to the Master of Social Work degree. Social workers are often referred to as the liaison between the patient or client and the community.

According to the *Occupational Outlook Handbook* (1998 –1999), "Social work is a profession for those with a strong desire to help people. Social workers help people deal with their relationships with others; solve their personal, family, and community problems; and grow and develop as they learn to cope with or shape the social and environmental forces affecting daily life. Social workers often encounter clients facing a life - threatening disease or a social problem requiring a quick solution. These situations may include inadequate housing, unemployment, lack of job skills, financial distress, serious illness or disability, substance abuse, unwanted pregnancy, or antisocial behavior. They also assist families that have serious conflicts, including those involving child or spousal abuse."

Mental Health Counselor

Mental health counselors typically have a Masters degree in psychology, social work, counseling, mental health counseling or related field and pass a state exam in order to be licensed. Mental health counselors can practice independently in some states, although most are employed in clinics and hospitals. They perform individual, couples/family, and group therapy, and may assist psychologists with testing and other forms of treatment.

Marriage and Family Therapist

Like mental health counselors, a Master's degree is typically the minimal requirement for marriage and family therapists. They receive special training in the dynamics of families and relationships and often treat couples who are having marital or relationship difficulties and families struggling with dysfunctional interactions. Many marriage and family therapists are provided more general training, allowing them to perform individual and group therapy as well for a variety of mental health related issues.

Behavior Therapy and Cognitive Therapy

This is the golden age of cognitive therapy. Its popularity among society and die professional community is growing by leaps and bounds. And in a survey of graduate and internship training directors in psychology, over half indicated that a cognitive - behavioral approach was their program's major theoretical orientation. Interest in cognitive - behavioral approaches has been spurred by the positive outcome that results from careful and replicable research, the increasing sophistication of the consumer - client - patient who demands effective treatment and the increased emphasis on cost containment of managed health care.

Cognitive Behavior Therapy (CBT), is a form of psychotherapy in which the therapist and the client work together as a team to identify and solve problems. Therapists use the Cognitive Model to help clients overcome their difficulties by changing their thinking, behavior, and emotional responses. Cognitive therapy has been found to be effective in more than 1000 outcome studies for a myriad of psychiatric disorders, including depression, anxiety disorders, eating disorders, and substance abuse, among others, and it is currently being tested for personality disorders. It has also been demonstrated to be effective as an adjunctive treatment to medication for serious mental disorders such as bipolar disorder and schizophrenia. Cognitive therapy has been extended to and studied for adolescents and children, couples, and families. Its efficacy has also been established in the treatment of certain medical disorders, such as irritable bowel syndrome, chronic fatigue syndrome, hypertension, fibromyalgia, post - myocardial infarction depression, noncardiac chest pain, cancer, diabetes, migraine, and other chronic pain disorders.

Although there are many types of behavior and cognitive therapies, they have in common several elements that form an underlying core and theoretical rationale. For this reason, the terms behavior therapy, cognitive therapy, and cognitive - behavioral therapy are viewed as roughly interchangeable. The approach of the behavior of cognitive therapist involves an implicit five- step procedure.

1. The individual is evaluated for "symptoms" of behavioral dysfunction, which may be noted by direct observation (eg. overeating, stuttering, crying), by the verbalization of thoughts and feelings (eg, suicidal thoughts, depression), and by clinical measurements (eg, blood pressure, heart rate). The behavioral - cognitive therapist does not conceptualize a problem in terms of a psychiatric diagnosis (eg, schizophrenia), but instead defines it in term's of specific

behaviors that affect the individual's functioning (eg. hallucinating in public).

2. The therapist and client, working collaboratively, determine the goals of the treatment. These often focus on specific behaviors to be changed, ie, target behaviors.

3. In addition to defining the problem in behavioral terms, the therapist develops a hypothesis about the underlying beliefs and/or environmental events that maintain or minimize these behaviors.

Steps 1 and 3 are referred to as developing a case formulation or conducting a behavioral analysis. Careful documentation and quantification are of great importance in determining factors that influence or trigger the undesired behaviors and in evaluating the effectiveness of the interventions. Since clients are often unaware of sequences of events that lead to a specific type of behavior, direct observation of clients in their environments is some-times a necessary part of behavioral analysis.

Clients can often be trained in the skills of self-observation and in recording of events so that the behavioral analysis is more accurate. Data derived from the analysis are used by the therapist to formulate a clinical hypothesis (the case formulation) about what stimulates (precedes) and what maintains (reinforces) the undesired actions, thoughts, feelings, or physiological changes. Newer formulations also include proposals about the nature of tire cognitions (beliefs, attitudes) that may underlie and play a causal role in problematic behaviors and symptoms.

4. Using methods supported by theories and findings from the literature, the clinician tests the hypothesis of cause and effect by altering the behavior, the underlying cognitions, or the environment (or all three) and observing the effects of the alteration on the client's dysfunctional actions, thoughts, and feelings.

5. From systematic observation and documentation of behavioral changes, the clinician either revises the hypothesis or continues with treatment until the goals of therapy are reached, ie, the target behaviors are changed. It is important to stress that behavior therapy is based on a way of thinking about people and problems and is not a set of techniques. Testing one hypothesis often leads to the development of another hypothesis, which in turn must be tested. Systematic data collecting, used to monitor the outcome of treatment, which can be conceptualized as a clinical experimental study with an N=1, is a central component of therapy (see Barlow et al, 1984).

Other Characteristics Shared by Behavior and Cognitive Therapies

In addition to sharing the empirical, scientific approach outlined above, behavior and cognitive therapies have other characteristics in common:

1. Therapy involves action as well as discussion. It is often directive, structured, and brief or time limited.

2. The client must be a responsible participant in the therapy and capable of achieving personal change.

3. The present (there and now) determinants of behavior are emphasized rather than the historic (then and there) determinants.

4. It is assumed that human behavior follows natural laws.

5. It is assumed that people's behavior reflects their adaptation to the environment and not necessarily underlying pathological disorders.

6. It is assumed that behavior can be changed directly without changing personality dynamics.

7. Paraprofessionals, lay people significant to the client, and even the clients themselves can carry out treatment.

8. The treatment often involves "homework".

Only in rare instances is treatment confined to 1 or 2 hours a week with the therapist. Rehearsal, practice, and other activities are generally carried out by the client between sessions.

Historical Context

In his experiments on learned and unlearned (conditioned and unconditioned) behavior, Ivan Pavlov (1849–1936) trained dogs to salivate at the sound of a bell by repeatedly pairing a conditioned stimulus (bell) with an unconditioned stimulus (food powder) that naturally causes an unconditioned response (salivation). Similarly, John B. Watson (1878–1958) taught a 1-year-old boy to be afraid of a white rat by pairing the child's approach to the rat with a loud noise. The boy then generalized his fear to other white furry objects. This study suggested the process whereby phobias might develop and gave impetus to later work on aversive conditioning and counterconditioning.

For their research using classical conditioning, Pavlov and Watson are credited with beginning the systematic study of the effects of environment on behavior. Operant (instrumental) conditioning has also had a major effect on behavioral theory as applied to clinical problems. In the 1950s, behavioral modification began to attract attention, largely because of the work of B. F. Skinner (1904–1990). Skinner used operant conditioning principles which hold that behavior is a function of its consequences (reinforcers) to change the behaviors of psycholic patients who were in the wards of state hospitals. Techniques such as extinction and positive reinforcement, as well as programmatic efforts such as token economies (all described in subsequent sections), are examples of applied operant conditioning principles. Recent applications of operant principles to clinical problems include Robert J. dialectical behavior therapy for the treatment of borderline personality disorder. The therapist following Linehan's protocol conducts repeated behavioral analyses of problem behaviors (eg, self-destructive wrist cutting) in an attempt to develop hypotheses about the function of the problem behaviors.

Throughout the 1950s and 1960s, behavior modification focused on stimulus (S) and response (R), while factors mediating the stimulus-response (S-R) connection were largely ignored. However, with the accumulation of empirical clinical data, it soon became clear that the variance in how someone responded to a situation could not always be predicted by the stimulus that preceded it or the consequence that followed it.

To improve their ability to understand, predict, and control behavior, therapists and researchers (eg, Albert Bandura, Julian Rotter) began exploring cognitive variables such as expectancy (predictions of future happenings), attributions (inferred characteristics of people or events), and mental images (ideas). Whereas traditional behavior therapy focused on observable S - R connections, cognitive behavior therapy took into account the importance of mediating factors within the organism (S-O-R). Since the 1970s cognitive variables have been given a central role in the understanding of processes that influence behavior (eg, self-instruction, cognitive therapy for depression, imagery techniques).

Cognitive therapy which is farther along the continuum from behavior therapy to cognitive behaviorism focuses more on the individual's interpretations of internal and external events and views them as crucial in understanding behavior. The purely cognitive view holds that dysfunctional thoughts may be influenced by dealing with the individual's thoughts directly. Most cognitive-behavioral therapists now utilize principles from both the behavioral (Pavlovian, Skinnerian) and cognitive theories.

Techniques

Although the exact number of cognitive-behavioral intervention strategies is not known, it is estimated to be in the hundreds. Several approaches have been selected to illustrate various techniques, but by no means should these be considered all — inclusive or even representative of this quickly expanding field. Any attempt to classify these treatments into behavioral or cognitive categories is frustrating for all but the most naive, since the methods in the field have so intertwined behavioral and cognitive perspectives. However, the techniques have been presented in a progression from those relying more on observable behavior to those relying more on private and subjective cognitions.

Positive Reinforcement and Extinction

Reinforcement and extinction are discussed first since they represent an early attempt to apply behavioral principles to treatment of seriously disturbed patients. It is a well-known learning principle that the probability a specific behavior will occur is increased when the behavior is followed by certain pleasurable consequences (reinforcers). For example, in a now classic study, it was demonstrated that certain verbal responses of a patient would be increased by an approving from the therapist. When a behavior is no longer reinforced and is ignored, the probability of its occurring is decreased. For example, ignoring a patient's request for special treatment should lead to the elimination of these requests.

A clinical example from the literature will illustrate not only the effectiveness of positive reinforcement but also the care with which behavioral data are used for determining improvement:

39-year-old woman with a diagnosis of schizophrenia exhibited self-destructive behaviors such as burning herself and her clothing with cigarettes at a baseline rate of once a day. Because she liked to smoke (ie, would frequently indulge in this behavior), hospital staff members were instructed to inspect the patient fur bums every hour and to give the patient half of a cigarette (reinforcer) and praise her for her appearance (secondary social reinforcer) if she were found to be burn - free. If she burned herself during the hour, she received no further cigarettes that day. Burns decreased from one a day to one approximately every 4 days (0.24 burns a day), and during the last 2 weeks of her hospitalization she remained burn - free.

Among the learning theory concepts that are important in applying positive reinforcement and extinction are the concepts of shaping, prompting, and modeling. Since it may take some time for a specific behavior (eg. speech in a mute patient) to be elicited the desired behavior must be shaped by the therapist's reinforcing successive approximations of the wanted behavior (eg. progressively rewarding lip movement, then vocalizations, then isolated words, and finally sentences). Desired behaviors may also be prompted (eg. shaping the lips of the patient) or modeled (eg, saying words in front of the patient). In institutional settings such as inpatient psychiatric wards or prisons, behaviors can be reinforced indirectly by issuing tokens (secondary reinforcers) that can be "traded in" for primary reinforcers or for other reinforcers such as watching television. This token economy approach is based on the premise that dysfunctional behavior exists because it has been reinforced. Even professional staff members inadvertently reinforce undesired behavior by attending to (and thereby reinforcing) unwanted behavior such as head banging or delusional speech. Token economies represent an effort to provide an environment that systematically reinforces the desired behavior and extinguishes self - defeating dysfunction at activities.

Tokens (such as poker chips or points) offer several advantages over direct reinforcers: (1) They are readily available and can be handed over immediately after the desired behavior. (2) Tokens may be saved and redeemed later when the desire arises for goods or services, so that satiation is not a problem. (3) The number of tokens issued for a specific behavior may be increased or decreased depending on how consistently the new behaviors are evidenced.

The staff must be trained to recognize desired behavior, to administer tokens, and to ignore dysfunctional actions. They must consistently apply the reinforcement and extinction principles. One or two staff members who do not apply these principles reliably and readily can undermine the efforts of the others.

A study spanning a 6 - year period including a postinstitutionalization follow - up indicated that 89% of the patients in a token economy unit had improved while on the ward, whereas improvement was seen in only 46% of patients receiving milieu therapy alone. Eighteen months following discharge, 92% of patients treated in the token economy unit and 71% of those treated in the milieu therapy unit were living in the community. A little - emphasized but important result of token economies is the improved morale and efficiency of the staff, who see progress and feel a sense of accomplishment with a difficult population.

Aversive Procedures

Much of our everyday behavior reflects avoidance of aversive consequences built into various components of our personal and institutional lives disapproval from friends, failing grades, imprisonment, etc. The application of this principle to clinical problems is aversive therapy. Aversive procedures are useful clinically either when dysfunctional or inappropriate behavior is naturally reinforcing to the individual (eg, addictions, deviant sexual behavior) or when behavior is self-destructive and needs to he brought under control quickly.

There are three main aversive procedures: classical conditioning, punishment, and avoidance training. The aversive stimuli used clinically are numerous, but usually involve electric shock, chemicals, or vivid descriptions of noxious scenes.

In classical conditioning procedures, the stimuli leading to unwanted behavior (eg, sight and smell of one's favorite alcoholic beverage) are paired with a noxious stimulus (eg, shock). After the unconditioned stimulus (shock) is repeatedly associated with the conditioned stimulus (alcohol), patients develop the same feeling toward the alcohol as they feel toward the shock (tear). Since learned responses are more generalizable in lifelike settings, clinicians have had barlike settings constructed in inpatient alcohol units. Here patients are exposed to the sights, sounds, and smells of a bar, but these stimuli are paired with shocks. The goal of such treatment is avoidance of bars by the patients once they have been discharged.

In punishment procedures, a specific behavior, drinking alcohol is followed by a noxious stimulus or punishment. In the bar setting just described, punishment was used as a component of the treatment. Patients who had poured a favorite alcoholic beverage received a strong electric shock to the little finger (punishment) when they started to take the drink. The shock continued until the patient spit out the alcohol (negative reinforcement or escape conditioning). Thus, the patient was punished for undesired behavior (drinking) and then reinforced for desired behavior (spitting out the alcohol).

In avoidance training procedures, patients can escape the noxious stimulus if they avoid the undesired behavior. This is the theory behind the use of disulfiram. If the patient drinks even a small amount of alcohol while a dose of disulfiram is still in the body, severe nausea and vomiting will occur. The patient can avoid these unpleasant effects by not drinking.

The effectiveness of aversive principles for the treatment of self-destructive behaviors is well documented. For example, Lovaas and Simmons (1969) reported a case in which a 16-year-old mentally retarded girl bit her hands (and had previously bitten them to the extent that one finger had to be amputated), ripped her nails out with her teeth, and severely banged her head. Five 1-second shocks following these behaviors eliminated the problem.

In general, aversive techniques are most effective when used in conjunction with other forms of treatment and with procedures that reinforce the patient for desired behavior. When using aversive techniques, the clinician must always consider ethical factors and keep in mind that aversive techniques are more susceptible to abuse than other procedures.

Exposure

Modern exposure treatments had their origins in systematic desensitization, developed by Joseph Wolpe (1958). Wolpe, a psychiatrist trained in South Africa around the time of the second World War, noted that patients he treated for "war neurosis" using traditional psychoanalytically based methods did not appear to benefit much from treatment. His extensive readings, including Pavlov's writings, Jacobson's (1938) *Progressive Relaxation*, and others, led him to develop a new treatment for fears and phobias, which he named "systematic desensitization". In systematic desensitization, Wolpe developed a "hierarchy" or list of situations that were frightening to the patient, ordered from least to most fear-evoking. After training his patients to use Jacobson's relaxation methods, Wolpe systematically carried out brief pairings of relaxation and fear-evoking situations, beginning with the least-fear-evoking situations and moving gradually up to more frightening ones. During the pairings, the patient was instructed to use the relaxation strategies, then to imagine the fear-evoking stimulus briefly until the fear increased, then to relax again, then to imagine the fear-evoking situation again, and so on, over and over, with repeated pairings of fear-evoking images and relaxation until the patient could imagine (and confront, in vivo, or "in real life") the fear-evoking cues without experiencing fear.

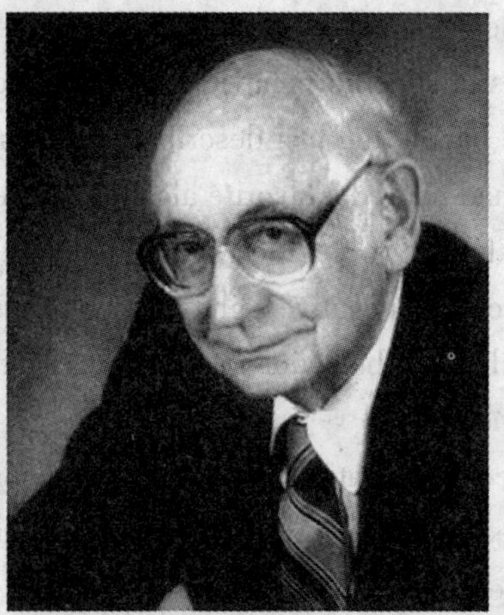

Joseph Wolpe (1958–1997)

Joseph Wolpe — a psychotherapist who helped revolutionize the treatment of mental disorders — have been added to the holdings of the USC libraries. The South African-born American psychiatrist helped usher in behavior therapy with his treatment to desensitize phobia patients by exposing them incrementally to images of their fears. In addition to establishing the Association for Advancement of Behavior Therapy and founding the Journal of Behavior Therapy and Experimental Psychiatry, he helped to develop assertiveness training as an approach to combating depression and other emotional problems.

But Wolpe is probably best known for urging his colleagues to view psychotherapy as an applied science in which the effectiveness of treatment is evaluated through controlled experiments.

"Today it's hard to appreciate the kind of intellectual courage that Wolpe displayed by going against the zeitgeist of 1950s psychiatry and clinical psychology," said Gerald C. Davison, a professor of psychology in the College of Letters, Arts and Sciences. "Editors of top-tier clinical journals now adhere to the kind of hard-headed empiricism that Wolpe urged on his peers more than 40 years ago."

Wolpe's materials are available to scholars and researchers through the library's department of special collections. Wolpe is credited with helping to develop a new type of therapy in the 1950s and 1960s. The techniques of behavior therapy — relaxation techniques, guided imagery and other scientifically validated exercises — were based on theories of learning derived from the classical conditioning research carried out by Ivan Pavlov and from the work of B. F. Skinner, John B. Watson and Andrew Salter.

A specialist in the study and treatment of neurosis, Wolpe produced scientific data that phobias are based on learned behavior, as opposed to repressed conflict, and can therefore be "cured" in far fewer sessions than needed in traditional psychotherapy. Wolpe's influence can be felt in today's managed care, which favors short-term, empirically supported treatments over long-term psychotherapy, said Davison, a longtime colleague of Wolpe's.

Trained as a physician at Johannesburg's University of Wit-watersrand, Wolpe developed an interest in mental health as a medical officer in the South African army during World War II. He was dissatisfied with the effects of electroshock therapy and other common treatments for shell shock. Behavior therapy is based upon theoretical principles first developed in animal experiments. Wolpe, for example, found that cats could be cured of experimentally induced "neuroses".

Based on this animal research, he developed a modality of treatment called "systematic desensitization" for people with phobias. In this procedure, fearful patients are exposed, while relaxed, to images of what they are afraid of, beginning with the least distressing scene and moving gradually to the most fearsome. "Systematic desensitization markedly reduces or completely eliminates unrealistic fears in most patients in fewer than a dozen sessions," Davison said. Wolpe set forth his findings in the landmark 1958 book *Psychotherapy by Reciprocal Inhibition* — one of the first scholarly challenges to the notion that scientific evaluation is irrelevant to psychotherapy — and contended that phobias are most effectively treated by confronting them directly.

In 1965, Wolpe established a behavior therapy unit at Temple University in Philadelphia. With a small group of scientifically oriented clinicians, he established the Association for Advancement of Behavior Therapy and founded the scholarly journal *Behavior Therapy and Experimental Psychiatry* and edited it from its inception in 1970 until his death last year. He also developed two measuring systems still in use today — the subjective anxiety scale and the fear survey schedule.

In addition to *Psychotherapy by Reciprocal Inhibition* (1958), major publications by Joseph Wolpe include *Behavior Therapy Techniques: Guide to the Treatment of Neuroses*;

Theme and Variations: A Behavior Therapy Casebook; The Practice of Behavior Therapy; and *Life without Fear: Anxiety and Its Cure*; as well as 700 journal articles.

Major awards he received include the American Psychological Association's Distinguished Scientific Award, a Psi Chi National Distinguished Member Award and a Lifetime Achievement Award and Special Award from the Association for Advancement of Behavior Therapy. After retiring from Temple University, Wolpe served as a distinguished professor in the Graduate School of Education and Psychology at Pepperdine University. Stella, his wife of 40 years, died shortly after the couple moved to Southern California in 1988; Wolpe married Eva Gyarmati, a retired insurance underwriting manager, in 1996. He died of lung cancer in Los Angeles on Dec. 4, 1997.

Deeply committed to preserving her husband's professional legacy, Eva Wolpe decided to give her husband's books and papers to USC — partly because of Davison's long-standing interest in her husband's work and partly because of "the scientific orientation and high quality of the university's clinical psychology program". She was influenced, as well, by ties between the university and members of her extended family, which includes six USC alumni and a current student. Granddaughter Alyssa Weinstein will be a sophomore at the university next fall. "I hope the students and scholars reading his archives will be motivated to continue his research and find solutions to yet-unsolved problems," Eva Wolpe said.

Victoria Steele, head of special collections at Doheny Memorial Library, said the Wolpe archives consist of about 25 boxes of correspondence, research files and other documentation, copies of Wolpe's books in their multiple translations, as well as video- and audiotapes of his lectures and some of his sessions with clients who agreed in advance to disclosure. Highlights of the Wolpe archives include:

Wolpe's reports on his pioneering "systematic desensitization" studies with cats.

Audiotapes of a successful 16-session treatment with an intensely phobic client who was socially paralyzed by fear of fainting in public.

Wolpe's correspondence with Skinner and other luminaries of the behavior therapy field.

Videotapes of an extensive 1994 interview with Wolpe, an interview conducted by Davison, whose research in cognitive behavior therapy has been strongly influenced by Wolpe's work.

Wolpe's new method was quite effective, and lie collected data on and published the results from a series of 210 cases effectively treated in this manner. Wolpe's view was that the therapy worked via the mechanism of "reciprocal inhibition", that is, the relaxation and the anxiety reciprocally inhibited one another to produce the therapeutic result. Later research did not support Wolpe's view that systematic desensitization was the therapeutic mechanism, and the current view is that systematic desensitization and a variety of methods derived later for treatment of fears and phobias are all effective because they involve therapeutic exposure to the feared situation.

Exposure treatment involves exposure of clients to the stimuli that evoke discomfort until they become accustomed to them. The types of procedures vary, ranging from those evoking little anxiety (as in the slow - graded, imagined process of desensitization) to those immersing the client in the feared situation (process of flooding).

Marks (1981) has done extensive work in both developing the theory and refilling the clinical practice of exposure treatments. Based on past systematic research, he outlined the conditions most suitable for exposure therapy: agoraphobia, social phobias, illness phobias, simple ("specific") phobias, obsessive thoughts, compulsive rituals, obsessive - compulsive disorder, and types of sexual dysfunction.

For treatment of agoraphobia, Marks suggests choosing to work on simple but important activities at first. Initially, a reassuring person should accompany the agoraphobic person into the feared situations (eg, driving on a freeway). Exposure can then be attempted alone but at less anxiety - provoking times (eg, not at rush hour). Prolonged exposures (1 - 2 hours) seem to be more effective than short exposures. The client is required to record behaviors in a diary.

A married 40 - year - old woman had been agoraphobic for 15 years. Lately, she had been unable to leave the house without her husband, fearing that if she went outside alone she would have a panic attack, would become overwhelmed and go crazy, screaming hysterically in the street, out of control, embarrassing and humiliating herself. She chose as her goal (target behavior) the ability to cross a busy street alone. Treatment began with crossing a street with the therapist. After they had done this several times, the therapist stood apart and then moved farther away as the client crossed the street. By the end of the first 1.5 - hour treatment session, the woman was able to cross the street alone.

She felt pleased with her accomplishment and much calmer. She was given homework assignments consisting of crossing streets near her home. By the end of the eighth treatment, the woman was crossing streets and shopping alone without anxiety.

In a theoretical research propose that all effective exposure treatments for fears and phobias are effective because they promote cognitive change by providing patients with information that contradicts the beliefs underlying their fears. Thus, the agoraphobic described above is anxious before treatment because of her belief that she will lose control. The exposure treatment teaches her that if she goes outside alone, the catastrophes she fears do not occur. Exposure treatments for panic disorder developed by David Barlow and his colleagues extend the treatment of panic and agoraphobia to include not just exposure to the external situations these patients fear, but also exposure ("interoceptive exposure") to the feared internal sensations (eg, dizziness, pounding heart rate). Exposure treatment for obsessive - compulsives includes both exposure to the situations these patients fear (eg, touching items the patient believes are contaminated) and blocking of the rituals (eg, hand washing) the patient typically uses to neutralize the fear; this treatment is called exposure and response prevention.

Exposure therapies for treatment of anxiety disorders have been studied extensively in randomized controlled trials. Results are impressive. In general terms, exposure treatments are consistently more effective than wait - list controls, and a few recent studies have shown them to be superior to alternative psychotherapies for treatment of anxiety disorders.

Self-talk

Self - talk is widely used and appears to be the most thoroughly researched cognitive - behavioral intervention that addresses childhood difficulties focusing on problem behaviors, hyperactivity, and impulsivity (Kendall, 1991). It is common for children to repeat instructions to themselves as they attempt new tasks. For example, while crossing the street unaccompanied for the first time, a child may engage in a running monologue of the parents' instructions: "Stop at the corner. Wait for the light to change from red to green, and make sure the 'walk' sign is on. Now look both ways to make sure no traffic is coming." These instructions may be repeated aloud, in a whisper, or silently. Adults too may attempt to learn new tasks in this way, eg, in taking up golf or tennis or assembling a bicycle.

People may be taught to use such self - talk in the form of evaluative statements, suggestions, reminders of sequential steps, and encouragement to help them relax, to improve performance of cognitive and physical activities, to increase motivation, and to become more aware and alert. Such self - talk is obviously related to the processes of covert modeling and cognitive therapy.

Various techniques may be used for teaching self-talk in therapy, but the general approach is demonstrated by Howard R program of self - talk for children, which has been successful in treatment of problems related to hyperactivity, aggression disruption, and cheating. There are five basic step after the problem has been identified and the behavior to be learned has been defined: (1) The child observes as an adult model performs the behavior. While the child is watching, the model describes the behavior aloud. (2) The child performs the same task while the model gives instructions. (3) The child performs the task while giving instructions aloud. (4) The child whispers the instructions while performing the task. (5) The child performs the task without audible speech.

In using self-talk techniques, it is often important first to identify and modify the child's current maladaptive self - statements. To do this, the therapist helps the child to recognize critical self-references (eg, "I am so stupid, I can't do this homework"), monitor them and then generate alternative self - statements that serve to encourage more adaptive coping (eg, less anxiety, hopelessness).

Cognitive Therapy

The underlying premise of cognitive therapy is that affect and behavior are largely functions of how people constructure their world. According to one cognitive theory, everyone has "filters" through which the world is interpreted (eg, seeing the glass half-full versus seeing it half-empty). These constructs are called "schemas." When these constructs become distorted and dysfunctional, clients experience helplessness, anxiety, and depression. Aaron T. Beck, a psychiatrist at the University of Pennsylvania developed cognitive therapy for depression when he noted, in his clinical work, the prominent stream of negative cognitions reported by depressed patients. The goals of cognitive therapy are to make clients aware of their cognitive distortions and to effect change through correction of these distortions. Common distortions (errors in information processing) that make people depressed include selective abstractions (missing the significance of a total situation by selecting a detail out of context), arbitrary inferences (jumping to a conclusion with missing or contradictory evidence), overgeneralizations (unjustified generalizations on the basis of one incident), and magnifications (exaggerating or elaborating on specifics).

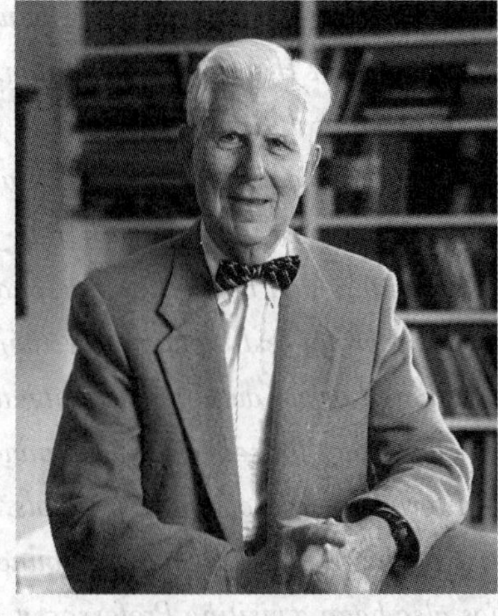

Aaron T. Beck

Aaron Temkin Beck, M.D. is the father of Cognitive Therapy, having created and refined cognitive therapy over the course of his research and clinical career. He has published more than 550 scholarly articles and 18 books and has developed widely-used assessment scales. He has received many prestigious awards including the 2006 Albert Lasker Clinical Medical Research Award for developing cognitive therapy, which fundamentally changed the way that psychopathology is viewed and its treatment is conducted. He has been listed as one of the "10 individuals who shaped the face of American Psychiatry" and one of the 5 most influential psychotherapists of all time. However, he did not pursue this interest until later in his professional career. At Brown University, he was associate editor of the Brown Daily Herald and received a number of honors and awards, including Phi Beta Kappa, the Francis Wayland Scholarship, the Bennet Essay Award, and the Gaston Prize for Oratory. After graduating magna Cum laude in 1942, he embarked on a career in medicine at Yale Medical School graduating in 1946. He served a rotating internship, followed by a residency in pathology at the Rhode Island Hospital. Although initially interested in psychiatry, he found the approaches at Medical School to be nihilistic and unrewarding and decided on a career in neurology, attracted by the high degree of precision that characterized this discipline. During his residency in neurology at the Cushing Veterans Administration Hospital in Framingham, MA, a required rotation in psychiatry intrigued him with some of the more recent developments in the field. He decided to explore further developments in psychotherapy. He spent two years as a fellow at Austin Riggs Center at Stockbridge where he acquired substantial experience in conducting long-term psychotherapy. The Korean War shifted Beck's area of work to the Valley Forge Army Hospital where he was

Assistant Chief of Neuropsychiatry.

Beck joined the Department of Psychiatry of the University of Pennsylvania in 1954 and is currently University Professor Emeritus of Psychiatry. He initially conducted research into the psychoanalytic theories of depression, but when these hypotheses were disconfirmed, he developed a different theoretical - clinical approach that he labeled cognitive therapy. Since 1959 he has directed funded research investigations of the psychopathology of depression, suicide, anxiety disorders, panic disorders, alcoholism, drug abuse, and personality disorders and of cognitive therapy of these disorders. His work was supported by a 10 - year M.E.R.I.T. Award from the National Institute of Mental Health and grants from the Centers for Disease Control for a study to determine the efficacy and effectiveness of a short - term cognitive therapy intervention for suicide attempters. His most recent work has focused on reducing suicide attempts among chronic suicide attempters and borderline personality disorder patients. He has also directed an international working group testing cognitive therapy of schizophrenia. He has published over 450 articles and authored or co - authored seventeen books.

Beck has been a member or consultant for several review panels of the National Institute of Mental Health, served on the editorial boards of many journals, and lectured throughout the world. He was a visiting scientist of the Medical Research Council at Oxford and is a visiting fellow of Wolfson College. He has also been a visiting Professor at Harvard, Yale, and Columbia, and is a member of The Institute of Medicine. He has received awards from numerous professional organizations and is the only person to have received research awards from both The American Psychiatric Association and The American Psychological Association. He is also the recipient of the Heinz Award for "The Human Condition" and The Sarnat Award from The Institute of Medicine. Beck has been awarded two honorary degrees, a Doctor of Medical Science from Brown University and a Doctor of Humane Letters from Assumption College. He has been listed as one of the "10 individuals who shaped the face of American Psychiatry" and one of the 5 most influential psychotherapists of all time.

The numerous strategies used in cognitive therapy are designed to help the client become aware of negative automatic thoughts (eg, "If I can't be perfect, then no one will love me"), to recognize connections among thoughts, mood, and behavior, and to replace distorted thoughts with more realistic interpretations.

The following discussions between patient and therapist are examples from Beck et al (1979):

P: The only way I could ever be happy is if I could be a great writer.

T: What level of writing would you have to reach?

P: I would have to be as good as (a specific poet).

T: Did this poet achieve great happiness?

P: No. I guess not. She killed herself.

A central component of the therapy is "homework". Patient and therapist work together to devise assignments the patient can do outside the therapy session to forward the work of the therapy. Often assignments include monitoring and recording emotions and situations associated with negative automatic thoughts, behavioral experiments designed to test the accuracy of some of the client's negative beliefs, and activities designed to practice and strengthen newer, more adaptive beliefs.

Source: Reproduced, with permission, from Beck et al: *Cognitive Therapy of Depression.*

Another central component of the therapy is the identification of recurrent or common themes, often stated as beliefs the person holds about him or herself or others, that make the person vulnerable to depression:

T: Your automatic thought was, "Your children shouldn't fight and act up." And because they do, "I must be a rotten mother." Why shouldn't your children act up?

P: They shouldn't act up because ... I am so nice to them.

T: What do you mean?

P: Well, if you're nice, bad things shouldn't happen to you.

The therapy focuses explicitly on reducing depressive symptoms and accomplishing other concrete, here-and-now goals that the patient and therapist set collaboratively at the beginning of the therapy. The outcome of the therapy is monitored frequently, ideally weekly, and adjustments are made when the patient is not responding as expected. In contrast to the more traditional psychotherapies, in cognitive therapy the clinician is active and directive, and the focus is on "here and now" problems.

The efficacy of cognitive therapy for depression has been studied in numerous randomized controlled trials. Results show that cognitive therapy is as effective as antidepressant medications for treating depression. Studies comparing cognitive therapy with other psychotherapies have not shown cognitive therapy to be superior to other psychotherapies; however, it is important to remember that few psychotherapies for depression have been subjected to a randomized controlled trial. Some recent evidence indicates that severely depressed patients benefit most from combined psychotherapy and pharmacotherapy. Studies report that patients treated with cognitive therapy relapse less often than patients treated with pharmacotherapy.

Positive Imagery

Jie (2009) pioneered the research, theory, and clinical applications of positive imagery. The idea is simple: engaging in positive imagery tends to elevate one's moods and affects, tends to increase enjoyment, and can decrease the frequency and intensity of potentially debilitating and self-defeating thoughts and feelings. The key idea is that imagery need not be explicitly related to one's difficulties or embody modeled "answers"; it just needs to be pleasant. This approach has been effective in the treatment of pain, anxiety, severe depression, and phobic behavior.

The client presented for psychotherapy with the following pattern of severe anxiety and depression on awakening each morning, she began to worry about her job, finances, and children. By the time she went to work, she was a "nervous wreck". She often returned home early because of "sickness", and more recently she began missing days of work. Though exhausted at the end of day, she had trouble falling asleep. Anxious about her situation and concerned and sad about the way things were going, she tossed and turned all night.

The treatment plan for modifying various aspects of the client's experiences, habits, and situation included the use of positive imagery. Four times a day (upon awakening and before lunch, dinner, and going to bed), the client spent at least 15 minutes with her eyes closed, thinking of the most pleasant scenes she could imagine. According to her reports during subsequent weeks of therapy, the imagery varied widely and included scenes of vacations she had taken or would like to take, funny scenes, and sexual fantasies. Some imagery was far from realistic (eg, she pictured herself floating high above the clouds). She found that these positive scenes were helpful in "setting the tone" for her days and nights: breaking the momentum generated by her depressive, anxious, and obsessive thoughts; relearning what it felt like to enjoy herself, and freeing her from the depression of what she described as those days when my women seemed to snowball and come down.

Misconception about Behavior - Oriented Therapy

Popular misconceptions and concerns about the use of behavior - oriented therapies are listed and briefly described below.

1. Behavior Therapy is manipulative and controlling. Because behavioral techniques are often powerful, direct approaches to changing behavior, they are criticized for controlling the individual's behavior. Behavior therapists respond to this concern by pointing to the way in which the behavior therapist and patient work closely together as a collaborative team, the way in which the methods of the therapy are completely transparent ("out on the table," understood by both patient and therapist not mysterious, understood only by the therapist), the way in which much of the therapy is self - directed (eg, homework done outside the session by the patient), and the way in which a central goal of the therapy is to empower patients by teaching them the. skills needed to overcome or manage difficulties.

2. Behavior therapy is superficial and "symptom substitution" will occur: Proponents of the theory that many undesired behaviors are symptoms of (or epiphenomena associated with) an underlying disease argue that if only symptoms are addressed, new symptoms will appear at a later date because the underlying problem (ie, disease) has been left untreated. Extensive empirical data from published reports fail to support any indication of new symptoms occurring after the target behaviors have been removed. In fact, effective treatment of specific target behaviors has often resulted in improvement in oilier aspects of the clients' lives.

3. Behavior therapist ignore feeling and treat humans as robots. This criticism of behavior therapy derives in part from the way cognitive and behavior therapies emphasize the use of techniques and interventions to address clinical problems very directly even aggressively in

contrast to more traditional therapies, which place greater emphasis on the patient - therapist relationship. Cognitive - behavioral therapists in recent years have begun to recognize the importance of the therapeutic relationship. It is also important to remember that without a strong, trusting relationship with the therapist, patients in cognitive and behavior therapies are unlikely to be willing to carry out the technical interventions of the therapy. A good example of this is exposure therapy, which is frequently quite stressful and difficult for the patient. The effective behavior therapist knows how to use the power of a warm, strong, trusting therapeutic relationship to strengthen the therapy.

4. Cognitive - behavior therapy denies the importance of resistance. Perhaps because behavior therapy and cognitive therapy stood, in their early development, in such contrast to psycho - dynamic approaches that analyzed resistance, many therapists may have mistakenly assumed that behavioral and cognitive therapy ignored this phenomenon. However, because resistance is manifested in observable behavior and is reflected in client cognitions, behavior therapy and cognitive therapy have developed a variety of specific procedures for addressing resistance, which they often describe using the term "non - compliance". "Recommended strategies for forestalling client resistance include offering a clear rationale for treatment procedures, emphasizing the gradual nature of change, using Socratic dialogue and hypothesis - testing techniques and conducting thorough task analyses of the patient's problems, skills, and goals that can guide the therapist in the selection of appropriate procedures and homework assignments".

5. Behavioral - cognitive techniques are practiced only by psychologist and paraprofessionals, not by psychiatrists. This statement has some validity, although several of the well - known pioneers in these fields are psychiatrists. Behavioral techniques can often be implemented by paraprofessionals and the clients themselves. This is seen by many as an advantage, since professional time can be devoted to developing treatment strategies and performing thorough behavioral analyses. Unfortunately, most residency programs for psychiatrists do not include training in basic behavioral science. This is a regrettable situation, since research in behavioral science has led to a number of specific treatment programs and has provided a method of approaching problems that has great clinical value. With the increasing importance of evidence - based approaches to treatment in psychiatry, training opportunities for psychiatrists in cognitive and behavior therapies are likely to increase.

Recent Trends in Behavioral - Cognitive Therapy

Several trends have emerged:

1. With the increase in emphasis on effective and cost - effective treatment, cognitive - behavioral methods will flourish, in an article on the future of behavior therapy, state that the press for more efficient treatments will lead to an improvement in the dissemination of behavioral techniques. They note that "stripped - down versions" of behavior therapy via computers are already tinder way. Treatment manuals describing detailed assessment and

application of theory and technique are also predicted to increase.

2. New cognitive and behavior therapies will continue to be developed to address additional clinical problems. Of growing interest to clinicians is the new field of behavioral medicine, which involves the use of behavioral and cognitive principles and techniques in the treatment of medical problems such as heart disease, obesity, irritable bowel syndrome, diabetes, cancer, and chronic pain. Cognitive and behavior therapists are also beginning to develop methods to treat the personality disorders. New developments in treatment for children include the application of cognitive and behavior therapies to the treatment of attention - deficit hyperactivity disorder, learning disabilities, depression, and childhood aggression.

3. Application of cognitive and behavior therapies to heterogeneous, complex disorders and populations will receive increasing attention. A recent important debate in the literature points to the fact that the randomized clinical trials typically used to demonstrate the efficacy of psychotherapies, including cognitive and behavior therapies, typically study homogeneous populations of patients with one or two disorders, not the heterogeneous samples of patients with multiple comorbidities typically seen in clinical practice. To address this weakness, researchers will begin and have begun, to study the efficacy of their methods with more complex patients and problems (work with borderline personality disorder). The study of more complex populations is likely to increase the importance of individualized case formulation, a method in which the clinician uses the theory to develop an idiosyncratic formulation of the case and then uses that formulation to guide treatment decisions as the therapy proceeds.

4. Although the effectiveness of cognitive therapy has been well documented, much is still unknown about how and why cognitive and behavioral therapy works. Researchers in file field are working to learn more about the process whereby cognitive - behavioral therapies have achieved their results. For example, Freda M. (2002) found evidence for the importance of a common factor the working alliance as being the only significant predictor of both the reduction of depressive symptomatology and the improvement in global functioning in a cognitive therapy.

5. There will he more integration of cognitive - behavioral approaches with other systems of psychotherapy. Beck and, in a paper on the future of cognitive therapy, predicted that the movement toward psychotherapy integration will continue at an accelerated puce and that cognitive - behavioral techniques have much to contribute to future integration therapies. The fact that most clinicians practicing today were not originally trained in the cognitive and behavior therapies, coupled with the increasing evidence of the effectiveness of these therapies, increases the pressure to find modes of integrating therapies.

6. There is growing attention to strengthening the effectiveness of cognitive and behavior therapies. Although cognitive and behavior therapies have been shown to be effective in the treatment of a number of clinical problems, not all patients can comply with the therapies or benefit from them. Thus, for example, the response rate to cognitive therapy for depression is typically about 60% with 40% of patients failing to show a full response to the treatment. Thus, researchers are working hard to develop new, more effective therapies and to strengthen the

therapies already in place.

7. Cognitive and behavior therapists will devote increasing attention to dissemination of their methods. Cognitive and behavior therapists are becoming increasingly aware of the fact that although data from randomized trials show many new cognitive and behavior therapies are quite effective, clinicians are slow to adopt these new methods. Increasingly, researchers and others are emphasizing the need to actively work to disseminate the new methods to consumers, clinicians, insurance companies, policymakers, and others. Laypersons have formed organizations such as the Anxiety Disorders Association of America and the Obsessive Compulsive Foundation, which educate their constituents about effective treatments for these disorders, many of which include the behavior and cognitive therapies described here. In addition, there is a growing number of self - help texts and work - books employing cognitive - behavioral techniques that can be used alone or in conjunction with professional therapy.

Psychoanalysis and Long - term Dynamic Psychotherapy

Sigmund Freud said the psychoanalysis was three things:

1. A theory of how the mind works. Psychoanalysis attempts to understand and explain the normal and the abnormal functioning of the human mind at all ages. Many of the central psychoanalytic concepts, the unconscious, psychic determinism, infantile sexuality and the theory of drives, the Oedipus complex, ambivalence, anxiety, the defense mechanisms, psychic conflict, the structure of the mind or of the psychic apparatus form a body of scientific knowledge that has now become part of our intellectual heritage in 1947. Ernst Kris summarized psychoanalysis as a theory of the mind most tersely: Psychoanalysis is however, more than a theory of the mind and behavior.

2. An investigative or research method. The technique of free association by the patient (analysand) makes it possible for the analyst to gain access to the data and processes of mental life, conscious or otherwise and rational or not. The data thus retrieved are rendered coherent and intelligible according to the theory of psychoanalysis. As Ransohoff in 2010, it is the phenomenal data of psychoanalysis that may be irrationals the method and the theory are rational.

3. A specific form of therapy of mental illness. Psychoanalysis uses free association to obtain data in the form of thoughts, feelings, memories, fantasies and dreams and then proceeds to order and comprehend the data within the framework of psychoanalytic theory, through interpretation of psychic data.

Dynamic psychotherapy, also called psychodynamic therapy, psychoanalytic psychotherapy, or psychoanalytically oriented psychotherapy, is intensive psychological therapy based on psychoanalytic theory but without the specific technique of free association. A variety of techniques are employed, including interpretation, to treat patients not considered suitable candidates for psychoanalysis.

Both psychoanalysis and the psychoanalylic psychotherapy described in this chapter are "open ended", protracted therapies that may continue for many years. At the start of therapy, the analyst, or therapist, and the analysand, or patient, agree to explore the patient's psychological problems for whatever period of time is necessary to achieve an acceptable result. This is in contrast to short-term or brief time-limited psychotherapy, which usually consists of 12 or 20 weekly or twice-weekly sessions of 50 minutes each. The critical distinction between psychoanalysis and short-term therapy is not the difference in duration, important as that is, but the fact that time-limited psychotherapy is not open ended from the first session the patient is conscious of the agreed termination date and knows that what has to be done must be achieved by that date. One consequence is that the patient may be tempted, consciously or not, to withhold painful areas from therapeutic scrutiny to be "saved by the bell" as it were. If open-ended therapy is to be completed successfully, whatever is not talked about now or next week will come out later, because treatment continues until all of the relevant psychological issues and problems are explored and resolved to the extent possible, however long it takes. Long-term and open-ended therapy is thus much more than an extended form of short-term (time-limited) therapy; they differ in very significant ways.

Psychoanalysis

Psychoanalysis is a process of examination in continuity of the internal working of the mind on a day-to-day basis. On each successive day, the analyst and the patient can mail where they left off and go from there. Ideally, this process would go forward 7 days a week for an hour each day. (This became the "50-minute hour" to allow time for analysts to order their thoughts, make notes, and get ready for the next patient.) However, to free weekends, the analytic work week, in practice, is the traditional five working days, and Freud often complained of the "Monday crust": the sealing over of open mental surfaces during the weekend, so that the first task on Monday would be to reestablish the continuity of daily exploration. Because of the limited availability of qualified analysts and the need to accommodate more patients, analyses are now often conducted 4 days a week. Most analysts do not consider fewer than 4 days a week proper psychoanalysis, because the vital element of continuity does not survive longer or more frequent interruptions. Ideally, each session is scheduled at the same time each day so that the analysis can blend into the rhythm of the patient's life.

In classical psychoanalysis, the patient is recumbent on a couch with the analyst behind and out of the patient's line of vision. Intrusions, such as telephone calls, are avoided except in emergencies. The patient tries to say whatever comes to mind, no matter how seemingly remote, irrelevant, trivial, repugnant, anxiety provoking, or shamful (the "fundamental rule"). The patient agrees to refrain from motor activity so that all available energy can be channeled into the effort to verbalize mental content. The analyst decides when and how to interject questions and comments: no attempt is made to sustain a conversational dialogue. The analyst must unswervingly focus attention on the effort to track the shifting subject matter of the patient's discourse and keep personal concerns, prejudices, values, and judgments out of the analytic field. The purpose is to gain and maintain full access to the contents of the patient's mind, conscious and unconscious, now and in the remote past, and even to infancy if that can be achieved. Dreams, fantasies, wishes, fears, thoughts, and feelings of all kinds are discussed in the analysis. What is experienced by people practicing or undergoing psychotherapy is that "one thing leads to another". The patient focuses on his or her mental processes and free associates in what is apparently a random manner. The analyst apprehends what the patient verbalizes by a counterpart process of "free-floating attention" without preconceptions about what is important or what the relationships are between various items of content.

It is within this "regressive" analytic process that the patient's mental life, including its conflictual matter, slowly begins to emerge around the analyst. Long-forgotten (repressed) feelings, traumas, and reaction patterns, along with active or discarded defensive or adaptive strategies, all eventually "come out again" in the interaction with the analyst, and what results is called the transference. The psychic past is reenacted in the analytic present. It is recognized and interpreted via the inappropriateness of the patient's present (transference) reactions and feelings to the reality of the ongoing interaction with the analyst. The complete revival of the past in the present is called the "regressive transference neurosis". Through the systematic interpretation of these complex transference phenomena, unresolved problems from the past are reworked, more adaptive solutions are found and maladaptive, neurotic solutions are discarded. In the course of analysis, patients "rewrite" their autobiographies and along the way shed the neurotic symptoms and the problems that first brought them to treatment.

Success in psychoanalysis relies essentially on skillful interpretation leading to enlarging insights. The analyst helps the patient see connections between unconscious wishes and beliefs and conscious speech and behavior. Slowly, patients begin to understand their own mental scheme of things. Symbolic meanings and mental connections begin to take on plausible configurations that "make sense". The insights gained are then "worked through" repeatedly as they reappear in other contexts as long as the analysis continues.

Balck described five essential psychotheiapeutic techniques: abreaction (catharsis), suggestion, manipulation, clarification, and interpretation. Different combinations of these techniques characterize the different psychoanalytically based psychotherapies. Within psychoanalysis proper, interpretation is the central technique and the others are deployed only to enhance interpretation. There is a vast literature on the nature of interpretation: the issues of tact and timing in making interpretations; what makes interpretations "mutative" (eg, able to affect change), the special nature of interpretations of the transference relationship; interpretations in the here and now as opposed to reconstructive interpretations of past (including infantile) matter; and the role of interpretation and insight in relation to behavioral change. This essentially is what is involved in the proper conduct of psychoanalysis.

Indications and Contraindications of Patients Who Come for Psychiatric Evaluation

Psychoanalysis has been called the treatment of choice for that narrow middle group that is sick enough to need it and well enough to tolerate it. Most psychiatric patients have symptoms or problems in living that can be resolved to their satisfaction with therapies that are less intensive or less prolonged than analysis (including expressive and supportive psychotherapies and crisis-oriented and brief dynamic therapies). Patients with acute reactive illnesses, situational maladjustments, and various circumscribed symptom-neurotic and character-neurotic stales do not need the thoroughgoing life and character reconstruction that psychoanalysis offers. Other patients whose illnesses are severe enough to require psychoactive drug management cannot always tolerate the anxiety-provoking stresses of psychoanalysis. For patients with fragile or vulnerable "ego strength" (including a tenuous hold on reality), psychoanalysis can be psychologically disorganizing, with dangers of regressive, even psychotic swings, severe acting out, flight from treatment, or suicidal pressures. Such patients, including borderline and narcissistic patients, those with character, addictive, or severe sexual disorders, those with character neuroses, and even some with severe and refractory symptom neuroses, are often deemed too ill for psychoanalysis and need to be treated by other dynamic (more supportive) psychotherapies.

There is controversy within the field between those who advocate "narrowing" and those who advocate "widening" the scope of indications for psychoanalysis. From the perspective of a proponent of "narrowing", only about 5% of patients who come for psychiatric evaluation and treatment are suitable candidates for psychoanalysis. These are patient with classical symptom neuroses and moderate character neuroses set within the context of a "strong ego organization", they are not only amenable to psychoanalysis but are able to tolerate it as well.

Benefits

Given the limited role of psychoanalysis in the treatment of neurotic disorders, it is proper to question both its social value and its scientific importance. Psychoanalysis is valuable and important in three areas: research, education, and treatment. As a research investigative technique, psychoanalysis affords access to the innermost workings of the mind and to knowledge of psychological development, character formation, and normal and abnormal metal processes. Knowledge about mental functioning derived from psychoanalytic research forms the basis of the theory of psychoanalysis as a comprehensive theory of the mind. From this theory have evolved the specific therapeutic applications of both psychoanalysis and the psychoanalytically based dynamic psychotherapies.

As an educational tool, the personal analysis of the therapist, required for those who seek certification as psychoanalytic practitioners and often sought by those who seek enhanced professional effectiveness as dynamic psychotherapists is necessary to provide successive generations of clinicians best qualified to offer these therapeutic resources to patients who need them.

As specific treatment for that small number of patients for whom it is indicated, psychoanalysis offers the best hope not always realized for the thoroughgoing resolution of neurotic problems and for fundamental character reconstruction. Since individuals in analysis are often in positions of responsibility, making decisions that affect others, the social value of the technique is apparent.

Limitations

Those who would widen the scope of indications for psychoanalysis believe that because the therapeutic goal of psychoanalysis is fundamental personality reorganization, the results, when successful, are more complete and enduring than can be achieved with less ambitious forms of therapy. Over the years, psychoanalysis has therefore been extended and modified to treat broader categories of patients, including children and adolescents, an extension that has by now become the established discipline of child and adolescent analysis groups, delinquents patients with psychosomatic disorders, overtly psychotic patients, narcissistic characters and others' and patients with borderline personality disorders. The movement to extend the indications for analysis to more kinds of mental disorders was reviewed in 1954 in a widely cited article on the widening scope of psychoanalysis. Anna Freud (1954), in discussing that paper, undertook to spearhead the opposing trend toward narrowing the indications for analysis back to classically neurotic adults and children. Glover in 1954 divided patients for whom psychoanalysis might be the treatment of choice into three categories: the ideally suitable, the moderately suitable, and those for whom psychoanalysis was the last hope albeit a forlorn one. The patients in the third category had severe personality disorders and were to be offered analysis as a "heroic measure" (this was in the days before adjunctive pharmacotherapy was available). The concept of intensive psychoanalytic treatment for patients much sicker than those usually seen in outpatient practice was a major rationale for the psychoanalytic sanatorium (such as the Menninger Foundation), where treatment could be conducted in a protected milieu with total life management.

Psychodynamic Psychotherapy

The psychoanalytically based dynamic psychotherapies are available for that much larger population of psychiatic patients who are not candidates for psychoanalysis proper. Psychodynamic psychotherapy, created in the United States, is now practiced worldwide. It was developed between World Wars Ⅰ and Ⅱ and refined as a coherent body of theory and technique in the decade after World War Ⅱ when psychoanalytic theory became the dominant psychological perspective of psychiatrists in the United Stales. The dynamic psychotherapies arose in pragmatic response to the treatment needs of the vast majority of patients who were not suitable candidates for psychoanalysis proper.

The dynamic psychoanalytically based psychotherapies have been divided conceptually into two types: expressive and supportive. The treatment aim of the expressive type is to uncover (or make conscious) psychological conflict through analysis of the patient's defenses and resistances and, in this way, to resolve conflict through interpretation, insight, and change motivated by insight, the treatment aim of the supportive type is to diminish the force of external (situational) or internal pressures by a variety of ego - strengthening techniques. Supportive therapies thus increase the patient's capacity to suppress mentally painful conflict and its dysphoric or symptomatic expression, thereby effecting behavioral change and symptomatic relief through means other than interpretation and insight.

As useful as this expressive - supportive division is for heuristic, prescriptive, and prognostic purposes, it is also a misleading oversimplification All psychiatric treatment that helps patients is supportive even when most uncompromisingly expressive, as in psychoanalysis. What could be more supportive than an open - ended psychoanalysis offered daily for as long as necessary, in which the patient is encouraged to express any kind or amount of verbal content, with the entire enterprise consisting of two people whose energies and intellect are focused exclusively on the problems and concerns of the one? Any treatment, no matter how supportive in the sense of strengthening defenses and suppressing unwanted conflict and symptom expression, must also be expressive of some aspect of the patient's concerns. The important question, is not expressive versus supportive but rather expressive of what and when and how in regard to the patient's mental and emotional life and support of what and when and how, in regard to that same mental and emotional life. Indeed, in every therapeutic decision to foster the expression of some aspect of mental conflict and distress in whatever way, there is a tacit decision to avoid (ie, suppress) some other aspect of mental conflict and distress.

Whatever one thinks of these arguments, at the practical level of ongoing psychotherapy there has always been a useful distinction between therapeutic interventions that have a preponderantly expressive effect and those that have a preponderantly supportive effect. Christopher in 2011 has presented in a systematic way every aspect of the psychotherapeutic process: (1) the beginning of the process and the establishment of the therapeutic situation and the "therapeutic contract"; (2) the patient's role and activity; (3) the therapist's role and activity in the therapeutic process; (4) the handling of the transference; (5) the handling of manifestations of resistance, regression, and psychic conflict; (6) the role of insight and working through in bringing about change; (7) the emotional involvements of the therapist (the "countertransference"); (8) the adjuvant role of psychoactive drugs; and (9) the process of natural termination. All of the foregoing are discussed by Christopher from the contrasting perspectives of expressive and supportive psychotherapeutic approaches.

Techniques and Patient Selection

The dynamic psychotherapies expressive or supportive are quite similar to each other in procedural form and greatly different from the formal structure of the psychoanalytic interview. In psychoanalysis the patient does most of die talking while the analyst chooses when and how to intervene; in psychotherapy the format is more like a conversation: the patient sits in a chair facing the therapist, with the expectation of feedback and reciprocal exchange. In psychoanalysis the patient tries to say everything that comes to mind without editorial revision or censorship; in psychotherapy the patient agrees to present problems and distress for consideration only to the extent that he or she is able and willing. No "fundamental rule" is violated by a decision to withhold specific items of mental content, either temporarily or permanently.

The frequency of weekly sessions with the therapist is more flexible in psychotherapy, ranging from one to three or four sessions a week, with once or twice a week most common. Unless some form of time - limited therapy is elected, the duration is open ended, as with psychoanalysis. Although in practice psychotherapy is usually briefer in duration than psychoanalysis (1–2 years versus 3–5 years), it can continue for just as long and may even (unlike psychoanalysis) continue for the life of the patient. Such "therapeutic Lifers" have consciously undertaken, out of need, to continue a supportive relationship with the therapist similar to the lifelong medical maintenance regimens required by diabetic patients, cardiac patients, and others with chronic and incurable but manageable disorders. In terms of total time spent in therapy, the dynamic psycholherapies usually consume 50–200 hours, in contrast to 600–1000 hours in analysis. The treatment hour is usually 50 minutes. But in some sustained, essentially supportive psychotherapies, particularly with schizoid individuals and others fearful of interpersonal intimacy, sessions are in some instances curtailed to no more than 30 minutes each. In both expressive and supportive therapies, at times of acute crisis or emergency, sessionsmay be extended as long as necessary, up to 2 hours or more. Occasionally in the psychotherapies, emergency weekend or evening sessions are held. Supportive treatment sessions may be scheduled less frequently than once a week, and the time may come, if the patient is seeing the therapist only once a month, when the sessions should be characterized as follow- up visits or "reporting in" rather than a continuing psychotherapeutic process.

In the psychotherapies (again in contrast to psychoanalysis), there is greater use of adjuvant drug management, coordination of care with the patient's family physician, telephone contacts, and involvement of third parties (family, employers, teachers, etc). All of these extra-session activities are more frequent die more supportive and the less expressive the particular psychotherapy is intended to be. Within this overall common structure, then, how do the technical interventions differ between the more expressive and the more supportive psychotherapies?

A. Expressive Psychotherapy: Essentially in expressive psychotherapy, the patient is free to bring up problems and anxieties in his or her own way, the therapeutic emphasis is on interpretation and insight, and the objective is to bring about beneficial change by resolution of as much psychic conflict as possible. This is accomplished by uncovering unconscious conflicts and through understanding, achieving mastery. These are to some extent the techniques of psychoanalysis but without free association, dream analysis, or deep discovery of infantile sources of current pain.

Expressive psychotherapy is the treatment of choice for persons with enough ego strength, intelligence, and anxiety tolerance to participate in therapy and with serious but relatively circumscribed neurotic conflicts and symptoms ie, individuals who need help but not the greater commitment implied by a decision to enter analysis. If such patients will assume responsibility for their character traits and their problems in living and are willing to look introspectively at the irrational aspects of their interpersonal relationships, significant help and change can be effected without the full - scale reconstructive effort required to uncover the infantile developmental roots of the neurotic personality development. For example, the issue is whether a patient with severe marital problems can be helped to resolve the problems without the need to recreate the earlier prototype, the infantile conflicts with the mother, repressed behind the childhood amnesia. In psychoanalysis, the aim is to pursue conflicts back to their infantile roots so they can be carefully analyzed; in analytically oriented expressive psychotherapy the aim is to recognize (and only partially to analyze) those same conflicts and use that recognition in therapy. Insight is achieved but only to the "depth" of the problem being addressed it never penetrates to the unconscious infantile origins of the patient's original conflicts.

Expressive therapy is indicated for patients with problems similar to those treated in psychoanalysis, patients with classical symptom neuroses (dysthymic disorder, anxiety disorders), and with the character neuroses (personality disorders). Character neuroses that cause problems in living (eg, rigidly compulsive or chronically depressive characters) and symptom neuroses (eg, characterized by irrational compulsions or bouts of depression) can at times blend into each other, or one may give way to the other.

The distinction between those who need psychoanalysis and those who can be treated by less intensive therapy is well illustrated by the example of psychotherapeutic work with a patient suffering from posttraumatic stress disorder. The therapeutic work would be limited to a defined sector of the individual's life and problems and directed toward the stresses precipitating the breakdown and enough of their underlying causes to permit resolution of the current conflict. Thus, in the case of the survivor of an accident, grief - stricken over the death of a companion and feeling guilty for having luckily survived, the events surrounding the death, ambivalent (love? hate?) feelings about the companion, and perhaps even a parallel between the adult friendship and conflictual sibling relationships of childhood might all come within the scope of the expressive therapeutic work. Therapy in this example probably would not explore earlier conflicts in the infantile relationship with the parents.

However, expressive psychotherapy need not be confined to a specific area of difficulty. It could include concern with characterological problems and symptoms and their maladaptive roles in the patient's life, but with the object of working only at the level of the individual's willingness and capacity to assume responsibility for their modification in the present without the need for the concomitant uncovering of their infantile roots in the past. Such treatment can be long term and can undertake to explore and modify the entire range of the patient's life adjustments, attitudes, and reactions.

In expressive psychotherapy conflict resolution and symptomatic relief are made possible by the relative "autonomy" of the present - day neurotic problem from its earlier infantile prototype, though clearly a developmental line can be traced from one to the other. Success depends on the ability of the patient and therapist to resolve the conflict in the "here and now", without the necessity of exploring its roots in infancy or its development from earlier neurotic relationships. Because such relative autonomy of conflict is common, there is a very large population of psychoneurotic patients who can use expressive dynamic psychotherapy. Because it is accepted dogma among psychiatrists that expressive (uncovering, interpretive) treatment is "better". because presumably it leads to changes that are more stable and more able to withstand adverse environmental pressures, the therapeutic tendency is fostered among practitioners of dynamic psychotherapy to, in the words of a popular training aphorism "be as expressive as you can be and as supportive as you have to be."

B. Supportive Psychotherapy: It is easier to agree on and expound the indications for expressive psychotherapy than to explain when supportive psychotherapy is called for and how it should be managed. Expressive psychotherapy is similar to foreshortened analysis, and most interested people understand something about analysis, even if they do not agree on when it should be used. Supportive psychotherapy, on the other hand, employs all manner of techniques and can be used in the management of all classes of patients not candidates for analysis or expressive psychotherapy.

In its early days psychoanalysis was acclaimed as the first successful scientific psychotherapy, in contrast to all preexisting therapies, which were viewed only as different types of suggestion therapy and therefore inherently unpredictable and unstable. Hypnosis was the prototype of such suggestive therapies. This view was expressed by Freud many times and was emphasized forceful by Edward Glover in 1931. As employed by nonanalytically trained practitioners, supportive psychotherapy often involves heavy doses of common-sense reassurance, to the extent that this, along with suggestion, came to be considered characteristic of the supportive approach. This perception is misleading and oversimplified. Explicit reassurance is seldom comforting to patients with problems severe enough to bring them to a therapist and the effort to give reassurance may only convince the patient that the therapist simply does not understand the nature of the difficulty or does not want to hear about it.

What does supportive therapy actually consist of? One of the earliest efforts to explain supportive psychotherapy was made by Peter F. who identified three kinds of interventions that lie felt "strengthened the defenses", in contrast with expressive approaches that undertook to uncover and interpret defenses as a step toward eventual integration. These explicitly supportive interventions are (1) to consistently encourage adaptive (and discourage maladaptive) combinations of impulse and defense expression, both behaviorally and symptomatically; (2) to deliberately refrain from interpreting defenses and character configurations, no matter how rigid or maladaptive, that are deemed essential to maintain functioning, and (3) to partially uncover some aspect of neurotic conflict (eg, within a troubled marriage or work situation) in an effort to reduce inner conflict that might be creating unwanted symptom (eg, anxiety, depression, phobic avoidances). In this way the balance of psychic forces is altered, rendering repression of the core of neurotic conflict easier to accomplish. An example would be not exploring in detail how the origin of a troubled marital or work situation relates to earlier ingrained patterns of interpersonal difficulty.

Differentiating the five therapeutic techniques listed, abreaction, suggestion, manipulation, clarification, and interpretation: it can be said that psychoanalysis uses mostly interpretation, with other techniques employed only when necessary to facilitate and enhance it; expressive psychotherapy uses interpretation to a large extent but also uses clarification as well as the other techniques; and supportive psychotherapy uses all five techniques in whatever proportions see in to be called tor by the specific needs of the patient.

Techniques of Supportive Psychotherapy

The principal therapeutic ingredient of supportive psychotherapy is the evocation and firm establishment of a positive dependent emotional attachment to the therapist. Within this bond, the patient's emotional needs and wishes are allowed to achieve varying degrees of overt or covert symbolic gratification. In supportive therapy, the meanings and sources of the bond between the patient and the therapist are for the most part not interpreted or "analyzed".

This dependent emotional attachment seems, in turn, to be an essential precondition to the proper functioning of various other supportive mechanisms. It is also the basis of the so-called "transference cure". The willingness and capacity of the patient to reach therapeutic goals, change behavior and modes of living, and give up symptoms "for the therapist" as the quid pro quo for the emotional gratifications received within the benevolent dependent attachment. On this base, then, other supportive devices are employed as indicated by the clinical needs of particular patients. If the dependent need for continued emotional gratification cannot be transferred or somehow either terminated or made therapeutically sustaining, it can be incorporated into a continuing and even an unending therapeutic relationship.

These chronic maintenance supportive therapies may be employed over long periods in the management of vulnerable patients whose hold on reality is tenuous. Patients with comparable dependent tendencies but greater psychological resources (eg, a greater capacity to identify with the therapist) are often able to terminate treatment, perhaps after a period of "weaning" as first advocated by Alexander and French (1946). These are patients who can identify successfully with the therapist and the therapies approach toward and mastery of conflict pressures and who thus can learn to go forward on their own.

Intermediate between those patients who can be helped to achieve reasonable psychological autonomy by identification with the therapist and those for whom continued (perhaps lifelong) therapy is necessary are those whose attachments and the emotional gratifications derived there from can be "transferred" within the patient's now-improved life situation. The transfer is usually made to the spouse, and the success of transfer depends not only on the effectiveness of the psychotherapeutic work within ongoing treatment but also on the capacity and willingness of the spouse (or other significant person) to carry the transferred emotional burden indefinitely. Obviously, some patients will be more fortunate than others in the matter of availability of someone willing and able to accept such a burden.

Another useful supportive mechanism is to foster the displacement of the patient's neurotic behavior into the therapeutic relationship so that its ill effects can be ameliorated in "real life". A typical example would be to encourage an unduly dependent and submissive patient to be more assertive outside treatment by allowing greater (covert) submissiveness to the therapist, which is experienced by the patient as requiring the altered (more assertive) external behaviors as the price of continuation of the dependent gratifications within the treatment. The success of this maneuver depends on life circumstance, the reinforcing positive feedback, and enhanced self - esteem. Beneficial change stabilizes when the new behaviors bring real reward and gratification rather than neurotically anticipated disaster.

What has just been described are varieties of the "transference cure", whereby the patient "does what the therapist wants" in exchange for the satisfaction of emotional needs. The "transference cure" occurs when the patient makes changes not "for therapist" but "against the therapist", in the face of what are perceived as the therapist's contrary expectations, usually as an act of triumph over the therapist in the overt or covert treatment struggle. Such "cures", of course, must somehow be buttressed against their potential instability by enduring, beneficial real-life consequences.

The "corrective emotional experience" is a concept Alexander and French invoked almost as the all - explanatory construct to elucidate the mechanism of action of supportive psychotherapy. Basically, this consists of deliberately responding to the patient's expressed emotional needs in a way that is different from what he or she has been led, by accumulated life experiences, to expect, with the effect of jarring entrenched patterns of neurotic (ultimately self-defeating) interactions. The concept can in a sense be applied to the entire range of supportive therapeutic techniques, since everything that goes on in psychotherapy is intended to function in some sense as a corrective emotional experience. However, the term is more useful if it is restricted to treatments whose central mechanism consists of interaction with a kindly, understanding, reality - oriented therapist able to absorb the patient's onslaughts and importunities in a spirit of benevolent neutrality without becoming entangled in the kind of interacting neurotic relationships the patient has used to maintain a life of suffering in the years before treatment was sought.

Reality testing and reeducation are related, but differ in subtle ways from the corrective emotional experience in the conduct of supportive psychotherapy. Reality testing and reeducation consist of helping patients with difficulties in this area distinguish internally derived expectations and fantasy from the external reality of the situation. Again, broadly speaking, they have a role in any type of psychotherapy including psychoanalysis, but direct educational efforts by the therapist are more characteristic of psychotherapy when the therapeutic emphasis is in greater part supportive. The therapist gives advice, explains, and instructs to the patient about what types of behavior are tolerable and expected in the community. The must do this in a way that is perceived as nonjudgmental and to the extent that the therapeutic intervention is coercive, that it is guided solely by the patient's well-being and best interests.

No purpose is served by trying to make a clear distinction between such educational activities and the steady provision of a corrective emotional experience. In both instances, the patient is taught the techniques of reality - oriented problem solving and reality - corrected emotional responses on the basis of the "borrowed strength" derived from psychological identification with the therapist in the role of helper and healer. Again, the stabilization of progress during and after treatment depends on positive reinforcement from the environment along with some measure of transfer of the attachments to the spouse or other stable life companion.

Another form of supportive psychotherapy involves the kind of life manipulation required by very ill patients who come to hospital, residential care, and day hospital settings, eg, the alcoholic, the drug addict, the acting - out or suicidal patient. In such cases, a major aspect of treatment involves the planned disengagement, temporarily or even at times permanently, from noxious life situations. For other patients, the opposite is true: success can be achieved only if psychotherapy is conducted while contact with the patient's accustomed environment is maintained. With these patients, if the usual interacting life situation cannot be properly maintained, for whatever reason, the chances for an optimal result diminish at times sharply.

Still another helping mechanism that can play a major role in supportive psychotherapy is the "collusive bargain". The "bargain" the therapist makes with the patient is to exempt specific problems, symptoms and areas of personality malfunction from therapeutic scrutiny leaving more or less consequential islands of maintained psychopathology in return for the patient's willingness to make substantial changes in other areas. This is similar to the "transference cure" in the sense that the patient makes changes "for the therapist" in return for a specific reward the shielding from therapeutic interference of a particularly tenacious or rewarding symptom or behavior. The success of such a maneuver depends on the value of the symptom or behavior to the patient as well as the patient's ability to detach the symptom or behavior from other problems or symptoms, which patient and therapist can then address. For example, a homosexual patient with conflicts about professional achievement may decide with a therapist to discuss the professional life issues and to ignore or deemphasize the life - style issues. Since the symptom or behavior "allowed" to the patient in this compromise solution is experienced as at least in some ways rewarding or gratifying, these particular therapeutic outcomes have a built - in stability.

Another technique available to patients who need supportive therapy is transfer of the attachment or dependency either to fortunate life circumstances (eg, wealth or social cultural advantage) or to alternative psychological supports. These may be selected by the patients, sometimes with the concurrence of the therapist. Alcoholics Anonymous and similar self - help groups are examples. In turning to external material or alternative psychological support for continuing emotional dependencies and gratifications, patients can sometimes save a failing or stalled therapeutic situation, they can stabilize even if they can not always enhance their level of psychological functioning.

It should be clear from the foregoing that there are many ways in which psychotherapy can support and maintain improved psychological functioning and, additionally, that ways can be built to maintain such improvement in a stable and enduring fashion. These techniques can be combined in various ways to meet the needs of specific patients: to form a basis for therapeutic "trades", to replace maladaptive impulse - defense configurations with more adaptive (healthy) ones, to decide what to talk about and explore, and to decide specifically what to talk about. Success in these endeavors may improve the patient's life situation, may help in the transfer of emotional attachments or in undertaking or disengaging from ongoing life context, and may provide positive reinforcements that result in enhanced self - esteem and more comfortable and rewarding life experiences.

Given this great variety of techniques available for supportive psychotherapy, it should be obvious that a high degree of skill and extensive experience are required by the therapist. This is contrary to the common misconception that more skill in psychodynamics is required to conduct expressive psychotherapy and that the supportive psychotherapists dispense mostly common sense, good will and kindly reassurance. Actually, neither kind of psychotherapy involves less knowledge or skill than the oilier, though supportive psychotherapy calls for greater flexibility and permits or even requires a wider deployment of "extras" in regard to the two - person treatment situation, such as the use of adjuvant psychoactive drug management, contacts with third panics (including other treating physicians), and telephone or other contacts with the patient outside of scheduled sessions.

Indications

Supportive psychotherapy is the treatment of choice for a more diverse range of patients than expressive psychotherapy. It is indicated for some patients "not sick enough" for analysis and for the great majority of very ill patients considered too sick for analysis or any intensive expressive approach. The first category includes many patients who may be caught up in disruptive responses (anxiety, depressive affect, rage) to traumatic or otherwise disturbing situations: some grief reactions, acute anxiety states, adjustment disorders, etc. In some cases, expressive - interpretive activity is also indicated, but often there may be just a need to slow up to take stock, to reassess the clinical situation and the therapeutic options and to reintegrate, over time, to the best of one's coping or mastery potential. Supportive therapy in such cases usually is of shorter duration than expressive psychotherapy or psychoanalysis.

A larger category of patients for whom supportive psychotherapy is indicated consists of those much sicker individuals who require sustaining psychotherapeutic relationships, perhaps for life and who respond slowly to the therapist's best efforts. Stability of psychological functioning at the best achievable level is often the modest therapeutic goal, though at times the hope for cure should be pursued because greater success is sometimes possible. This group includes most patients with psychosis or severe personality disorders, severe addictions, alcoholism, sexual disorders, and acting - out, delinquent, and antisocial characters. In almost all of these cases, some degree of expressive therapeutic work can usually be done, but with difficulty, because these patients have poor impulse control and low tolerance for anxiety and are vulnerable to regressive (psychotic or suicidal) swings in psychological functioning and integrity. The eruption of a florid psychotic state is a potential danger that often cannot be ignored. Attempts at "widening the scope" of expressive therapy (including psychoanalysis) in an effort to do something for these much sicker patients (see section on indications and contraindications for psychoanalysis) have met with poor results.

Other School and Paradigms

The discussion of psychotherapies in this chapter has been within the framework of psychoanalytic (psychodynamic) theories of mental functioning. Other kinds of psychotherapies have been developed within different theoretical models of how the mind works, such as the behavioral model based on a learning theory paradigm and the existentialist - humanist model based on a phenomenological - existentialist view of mental life and function. The therapies that derive from these schools differ radically in concept and in practice from those described in this chapter, and they are discussed elsewhere in this book.

Psychoanalysis Today

In today's era of empirically validated treatments and brief structured interventions. The evidence that exists for the effectiveness of psychoanalysis as a treatment for psychological disorder is reviewed. The evidence base is significant and growing, but less than might meet criteria for an empirically based therapy. The author goes on to argue that the absence of evidence may be symptomatic of the epistemic difficulties that psychoanalysis faces in the context of 21st century psychiatry, and examines some of the philosophical problems faced by psychoanalysis as a model of the mind. Finally some changes necessary in order to ensure a future for psychoanalysis and psychoanalytic therapies within psychiatry are suggested.

Psychoanalysis today is an embattled discipline. What hope is there in the era of empirically validated treatments, which prizes brief structured interventions, for a therapeutic approach which defines itself by freedom from constraint and preconception, and counts treatment length not in terms of number of sessions but in terms of years? Can psychoanalysis ever demonstrate its effectiveness, let alone cost - effectiveness? After all, is psychoanalysis not a qualitatively different form of therapy which must surely require a qualitatively different kind of metric to reflect variations in its outcome? Symptom change as a sole indicator of therapeutic benefit must indeed be considered crude in relation to the complex interpersonal processes which evolve over the many hundreds of sessions of the average 3–5 times weekly psychoanalytic treatment. Most psychoanalysts are sceptical about outcome investigations.

Surprisingly, given this unpropitious backdrop, there is, in fact, some suggestive evidence for the effectiveness of psychoanalysis as a treatment for psychological disorder. The evidence in relation to psychoanalytic outcomes was recently overviewed, and suggestions for enriching this literature with ongoing naturalistic follow-along investigations were offered. But the absence of evidence is only part of the problem. Indeed, it may be symptomatic of the scientific difficulties that psychoanalysis faces in the 21st century. I will review the evidence base of psychoanalytic treatments and go on to examine in more detail the problems faced by psychoanalysis as a body of ideas rather than as a mode of treatment.

Data Gathering and Psychoanalysis

Psychoanalysts emulating the founder of the discipline take special pride in discovery. This has led to an abundance of psychoanalytic ideas. Yet this very overabundance of clinically rooted concepts is beginning to threaten the clinical enterprise. The plethora of clinical strategies and techniques that are not all mutually compatible creates almost insurmountable problems in the transmission of psychoanalytic knowledge and skills. Sadly, this also leads to resistance to the systematization of psychoanalytic knowledge, since those whose frame of reference depends on ambiguity and polymorphy can be threatened by the systematization of clinical reasoning. The source of the problem of theoretical diversity lies in psychoanalytic methods of data-gathering. As is well known, data is not the plural of anecdote. Psychoanalytic practice has profound limitations as a form of research. Psychoanalytic theory precludes the possibility that psychoanalysts can be adequate observers of their clinical work. The discovery of the pervasiveness of countertransference has totally discredited Freud's clinician-researcher model. In the absence of a genuine research tradition, academic disciplines will appropriately distance themselves from psychoanalytic study, in much the same way that they hold journalism at arm's length.

Progress in disciplines concerned with the mind has been remarkable. Excluding information from these disciplines is a high risk strategy at a time when interdisciplinary collaboration is perceived as the driving force of knowledge acquisition. Modern science is almost exclusively interdisciplinary. Many major universities have been restructured to facilitate interdisciplinary work. The impetus is for the abolition of discipline based departments and the reconfiguring of medical faculties in terms of interdisciplinary research groupings (scientists working on similar problems regardless of their discipline of origin). It is likely that many basic questions that psychoanalysts have not been able adequately to answer, such as how psychological therapy cures, will only be illuminated by interdisciplinary (neuroscientific) research.

The last 30 years' advances in all the neurosciences have negated the reasons for the earlier psychoanalytic disregard of this field. Neuroscientists are no longer just concerned with cognitive disabilities or so-called organic disorders. Recent reviews of neuroscientific work confirm that many of Freud's original observations, not least the pervasive influence of non-conscious processes and the organizing function of emotions for thinking, have found confirmation in laboratory studies. If Freud were alive today, he would be keenly interested in new knowledge about brain functioning, such as how neural nets develop in relation to the quality of early relationships, the location of specific capacities with functional scans, the discoveries of molecular genetics and behavioral genomics and he would surely not have abandoned his cherished Project for a Scientific Psychology, the abortive work in which he attempted to develop a neural model of behavior. Genetics has progressed particularly rapidly, and mechanisms that underpin and sustain a complex gene-environment interaction belie early assumptions about constitutional disabilities. In fact, for the past 15–20 years the field of neuroscience has been wide open for input from those with an adequate understanding of environmental determinants of development and adaptation.

It may be that the difficulty in pinpointing the curative factors in psychoanalytic treatment is directly related to the limitations of the uniquely clinical basis for psychoanalytic inquiry. The impact of psychoanalysis cannot be fully appreciated from clinical material alone. The repetition of patterns of emotional arousal in association with the interpretive process elaborates and strengthens structures of meaning and emotional response. This may have far-reaching effects, I would argue, even on the functioning of the brain and the expression of genetic potential. A range of studies have already suggested that the impact of psychotherapy can be seen in alterations in brain activity, using brain imaging techniques. These studies as a group provide a rationale for the hope that intensive psychoanalytic treatment might meaningfully affect biological as well as psychological vulnerability. This field is in its infancy but is progressing so fast that it seems highly likely that many future psychoanalytic discoveries about the mind will be made in conjunction and collaboration with biological science.

How Psychoanalysis will Benefit from Interdisciplinary Dialogue

Whilst clinical psychoanalysis needs little help in getting to know an individual's subjectivity in the most detailed way possible, when we wish to generalize to a comprehensive model of the human mind, the discipline can no longer exist on its own. A general psychoanalytic model of mind, if it is to be credible, should be aligned with the wider knowledge of mind gained from a range of disciplines. This is already happening, albeit informally. Psychoanalysts cannot help incorporating advances about discoveries relevant to mental function because these are invariably contained in all our intuitive, common sense, folk psychologies or theories of the mind. Folk psychology develops alongside scientific discovery. The impact of psychoanalysis on psychiatric disorder over the course of the 20th century offers the best evidence for this. Our culture's acceptances of Freudian discoveries have made it more difficult for individuals to claim dramatic dysfunctions such as blindness, anesthesia, and paralysis. Medicine has advanced to a point where individuals must accept that the absence of a pathophysiological account for a bodily dysfunction implies emotional determinants, thus the disguise function of the physical symptom is lost and the point prevalence of conversion hysteria plummets. Just as common-sense knowledge of medicine and psychology impacts on our patients, so it must unconsciously influence the nature of psychoanalysts' theoretical musings. Thus, scientific advances infiltrate psychoanalytic theory by the backdoor of the analyst's preconscious.

Mitchell, by contrast, claimed that "no experiment or series of experiments will ever be able to serve as a final and conclusive arbiter of something as complex and elastic as the psychoanalytic theory". Indeed, Mitchell writes that "ultimately it is the community of psychoanalytic practitioners who provide the crucial testing - ground in the crucible of daily clinical work". As we have seen, the community has been singularly unsuccessful in definitively eliminating theories, in part because of the loose definitions adopted to define underlying concepts. This is inevitable if the mechanisms or processes that underpin the surface function described are not well understood. The meaning of the construct has to be sensed or intuited. In psychoanalysis, communication, whether in writing or clinical discourse, occurs in terms of its impact upon the reader. As Phillips puts it, paraphrasing Emerson, in psychoanalytic writing there is an attempt to return the reader to his own thoughts whatever their majesty, to evoke by provocation. According to this way of doing it, thoroughness is not inciting. No amount of "evidence" or research will convince the unamused that a joke is funny. In psychoanalysis we accept that something has been understood when the discourse about it is inciting. Elusiveness and ambiguity are not only permissible, they may be critical to accurately depict the complexity of human experience. It is here, in the specification of the mental mechanisms whose effects psychoanalytic writings describe and whose nature they allude to, that systematic research using psychoanalytic methods as well as methods from other disciplines will turn out to be so useful. Gill, in his discussion of the possible validation of psychoanalytic concepts, adopted a similar approach and suggested that Mitchell underestimated the potential contribution of systematic, not necessarily experimental, research on the psychoanalytic situation.

The above does not constitute an attempt to suggest that psychoanalytic concepts can be tested or validated by the methods of another science. Rather, systematic observations could be used to investigate the psychological processes underpinning clinical phenomena, which psychoanalysts currently use the metaphoric language of metapsychology to approximate. Inter-disciplinary research cannot test psychoanalytic theory, it cannot demonstrate that particular psychoanalytic ideas are true or false. What it can do is to elaborate the mental mechanisms that are at work in generating the phenomena that psychoanalytic writings describe. It is here, in the specification of the mental mechanisms whose effects psychoanalytic writings describe and whose nature they allude to, that systematic research using psychoanalytic methods as well as methods from other disciplines will be useful. This in turn will help to systematize the knowledge base of psychoanalysis so that integration with the new sciences of the mind becomes increasingly easier. Not only will psychoanalysts be able more readily to show that their treatment works, but they will have new possibilities of communicating with other scientists about their discoveries. It is to this set of opportunities that I would now like to turn. The integration of psychoanalytic ideas with modern science is unlikely to interest investigators from other disciplines unless psychoanalysis can actually contribute to directing or to informing data collection in these disciplines. For psychoanalysis to be taken seriously as a scientific study of the mind, it has to engage in systematic laboratory studies, epidemiological surveys or qualitative exploration in the social sciences.

Of course, methods for such systematic research are still in their infancy. The validation of theory poses a formidable challenge. Even apparently easily operationalisable constructs such as defense mechanisms have rarely been formulated with the kind of exactness required by research studies. Extra - clinical investigations, however, may help to constrain theorizing; for example our growing knowledge of infants' actual capacities may enable us to limit speculation concerning the impact of infancy on adult function. The projective processes of infancy are unlikely to work in the adultomorphic way described by Bion and Klein, but this does not mean that these descriptions do not contain important truths about adult mental function, simply that infancy is used metaphorically in these theorizations about mental process. It uses the more readily operationalizable notion of "marked mirroring" to denote the mother's capacity to reflect the infant's affect, while also communicating that the affect she is expressing is not hers but the infant's. Mothers who can "mark" their emotional expression (add a special set of attributes, such as playfulness, to their expression of the child's affect that makes it clearly different from their own expression of that affect) appear to be able to soothe their baby considerably more rapidly. This may not be all that it meant by containment, but it seems to be linked to his hypotheses concerning the subsequent problems faced by individuals whose caregivers were unable to provide this mirroring encounter with emotion regulation. Restricting theory building to the clinical domain is foolhardy in the extreme.

To summarize, psychoanalysis could benefit from integrating its working theories with research findings from other fields by elaborating the psychoanalytic psychological models of the mechanisms involved in key mental processes. This in turn would help to systematize the psychoanalytic knowledge base, so that integration with the new sciences of the mind becomes increasingly easier. Not only will we be able more readily to show that our treatment works, but we will have new possibilities of communicating with other scientists about our discoveries. The integration of psychoanalytic ideas with modern science is unlikely to interest investigators from other disciplines unless psychoanalysis can actually contribute to directing or to informing data collection in these disciplines. Merely reviewing ideas in developmental science or neuroscience for their proximity to psychoanalytic hypotheses has scant relevance to them. For psychoanalysis to take its place at the high table of the scientific study of the mind, it has to show its mettle in the battlefield of systematic laboratory studies, epidemiological surveys or qualitative exploration in the social sciences.

The Evidence Base for Psychoanalytic Treatment

The evidence base for psychoanalytic therapy remains thin. There is little doubt that the absence of solid and persuasive evidence for the efficacy of psychoanalysis is the consequence of the self - imposed isolation of psychoanalysis from the empirical sciences. Few would dispute the assertion that psychoanalytic theory is in a perilous state. The psychoanalytic clinical situation might have yielded all that it can offer to advance our understanding of mind. Yet importing extra - clinical data is often fiercely resisted and those psychoanalysts who have attempted to do so have commonly been subjected to subtle and not so subtle derision.

Psychoanalysts have been encouraged by the body of research that supports brief dynamic psychotherapy. A meta - analysis of 26 such studies has yielded effect sizes comparable to other approaches. It may even be slightly superior to some other therapies if long term follow-up is included in the design. One of the best designed randomized controlled trials (RCTs), the Sheffield Psychotherapy Project, found evidence for the effectiveness of a 16 session psychodynamic treatment based on Hobson's model in the treatment of major depression. There is evidence for the effectiveness of psychodynamic therapy as an adjunct to drug dependence programs. There is ongoing work on a brief psychodynamic treatment for panic disorder. There is evidence for the use of brief psychodynamic approaches in work with older people.

There are psychotherapy process studies which offer qualified support for the psychoanalytic case. For example, psychoanalytic interpretations given to clients which are judged to be accurate are reported to be associated with relatively good outcome. There is even tentative evidence from the reanalysis of therapy tapes from the National Institute of Mental Health (NIMH) Treatment of Depression Collaborative Research Program that the more the process of a brief therapy (eg, Cognitive-Behavioral Therapy, CBT) resembles that of a psychodynamic approach, the more likely it is to be effective.

Evidence is available to support therapeutic interventions which are clear derivatives of psychoanalysis. However, most analysts would consider that the aims and methods of short-term once a week psychotherapy are not comparable to "full analysis". What do we know about the value of intensive and long-term psychodynamic treatment? Here the evidence base becomes somewhat patchy.

The Boston Psychotherapy Study compared long term psychoanalytic therapy (two or more times a week) with supportive therapy for clients with schizophrenia in a randomized controlled design. There were some treatment specific outcomes, but on the whole clients who received psychoanalytic therapy fared no better than those who received supportive treatment. In a more recent randomized controlled study, individuals with a diagnosis of borderline personality disorder were assigned to a psychoanalytically oriented day-hospital treatment or treatment as usual. The psychoanalytic arm of the treatment included therapy groups three times a week as well as individual therapy once or twice a week over an 18 month period. There were considerable gains in this group relative to the controls and these differences were not only maintained in the 18 months following discharge, but increased, even though the day hospital group received less treatment than the control group. The cost-effectiveness of these treatments is surprisingly impressive, with the cost of psychoanalytic partial hospital treatment comparable to treatment as usual for these patients, and the costs of the treatment mostly recovered in terms of savings in service use within 18 months of the end of treatment. Trials with similar patient groups using comparisons of outpatient psychoanalytic therapy treatments with extended baselines have yielded relatively good outcomes as did comparisons with treatment as usual. Several prospective follow-along studies using a pre-post design have suggested substantial improvements in patients given psychoanalytic therapies for personality disorders. Uncontrolled studies, however, particularly those with relatively small sample sizes and clinical populations whose condition is known to fluctuate wildly, cannot yield data of consequence concerning what type of treatment is likely to be effective for whom.

A further controlled trial of intensive psychoanalytic treatment of children with chronically poorly controlled diabetes reported significant gains in diabetic control in the treated group which was maintained at one year follow-up. Experimental single case studies carried out with the same population supported the causal relationship between interpretive work and improvement in diabetic control and physical growth. The work also suggests that four or five times weekly sessions may generate more marked improvements in children with specific learning difficulties than a less intensive psychoanalytic intervention.

One of the most interesting studies to emerge recently was the Stockholm Outcome of Psychotherapy and Psychoanalysis Project. The study followed 756 persons who received national insurance funded treatment for up to three years in psychoanalysis or in psychoanalytic psychotherapy. The groups were matched on many clinical variables. Four or five times weekly analysis had similar outcomes at termination when compared with one to two sessions per week psychotherapy. However, in measurements of symptomatic outcome using the Short Check List-90 (SCL-90), improvement on three year follow-up was substantially greater for individuals who received psychoanalysis than those in psychoanalytic psychotherapy. In fact, during the follow-up period, psychotherapy patients did not change, but those who had had psychoanalysis continued to improve, almost to a point where their scores were indistinguishable from those obtained from a non-clinical Swedish sample.

A large scale follow-up study of a representatively selected group of psychoanalytically and psychotherapeutically treated individuals was recently reported from the German Psychoanalytic Association's collaborative investigation. A selection of patients whose treatments had taken place in a designated time period were interviewed by independent assessors and outcomes assessed by both standardized and interviewer coded instruments. While the group had been quite impaired at the time of referral according to retrospective assessments, on follow-up over 80% showed good outcomes. Follow-up data was favorable in relation to both anxiety and depression and savings were also demonstrated in relation to the use of hospital and outpatient medical treatment of physical symptoms replicating earlier German investigations. This carefully conducted study also provided important qualitative data in relation to the experience of psychoanalytic treatment and the relatively common disjunction of psychological changes at the level of self-understanding, and interpersonal-relational and work-related domains.

Another large pre-post study of psychoanalytic treatments has examined the clinical records of 763 children who were evaluated and treated at the Anna Freud Centre, under the close supervision of Freud's daughter. Children with certain disorders (eg, depression, autism, conduct disorder) appeared to benefit only marginally from psychoanalysis or psychoanalytic psychotherapy. Interestingly, children with severe emotional disorders (three or more Axis I diagnoses) did surprisingly well in psychoanalysis, although they did poorly in once or twice a week psychoanalytic psychotherapy. Younger children derived greatest benefit from intensive treatment. Adolescents appeared not to benefit from the increased frequency of sessions. The importance of the study is perhaps less in demonstrating that psychoanalysis is effective, although some of the effects on very severely disturbed children were quite remarkable, but more in identifying groups for whom the additional effort involved in intensive treatment appeared not to be warranted.

The Research Committee of the International Psychoanalytic Association has recently prepared a comprehensive review of North American and European outcome studies of psychoanalytic treatment. The Committee concluded that existing studies failed to unequivocally demonstrate that psychoanalysis is efficacious relative to either an alternative treatment or an active placebo, and identified a range of methodological and design problems in the fifty or so studies described in the report. Nevertheless, the report is encouraging to psychoanalysts. A number of studies testing psychoanalysis with "state of the art" methodology are ongoing and are likely to produce more compelling evidence over the next years. Despite the limitations of the completed studies, evidence across a significant number of pre - post investigations suggested that psychoanalysis appears to be consistently helpful to patients with milder (neurotic) disorders and somewhat less consistently so for other, more severe groups. Across a range of uncontrolled or poorly controlled cohort studies, mostly carried out in Europe, longer intensive treatments tended to have better outcomes than shorter, non-intensive treatments. The impact of psychoanalysis was apparent beyond symptomatology, in measures of work functioning and reductions in health care costs.

The limitations of the Evidence Base Approach

There are limitations concerning the nature of the evidence base for all psychotherapies. These limitations are well-known and their implications go well beyond the evaluation of the current status of psychoanalysis. The outcomes literature concerns RCTs administered over relatively brief periods (three to six months) with short follow-ups and a failure to control for inter-current treatments over these periods. Most evidence-based treatment reviews have been uniquely based on RCTs. RCTs in psychosocial treatments are often regarded as inadequate because of their low external validity or generalizability. In brief, they are not relevant to clinical practice, a hotly debated issue in the field of psychotherapy and psychiatric research. There are a number of well publicized reasons: (1) the unrepresentativeness of healthcare professionals participating; (2) the unrepresentativeness of participants screened for inclusion to maximize homogeneity; (3) the possible use of atypical treatments designed for a single disorder; (4) limiting the measurement of outcome to the symptom that is the focus of the study and is easily measurable.

Belief in the supremacy of RCTs opens the door to treatments which, even if effective, one may not wish to entertain. A recent report in the British Medical Journal on the effects of remote, retro - active intercessory prayer on the outcome of patients with bloodstream infection is salutary. Penny E randomized 3,393 adult patients whose bloodstream infection was detected in the hospital between 1990 and 1996. A list of the first names of the patients in the intervention group was given to a person who said a short prayer for the wellbeing and recovery of the group as a whole. It was argued that as God is unlikely to be limited by linear time, an intervention carried out 4–10 years after the patients' infection and hospitalization was as likely to be effective as one carried out during the infection. Staggeringly, there were significant results on two of the three outcome measures. Length of hospital stay and duration of fever were both shorter in the intervention group. Mortality was also lower in the intervention group but the difference was not statistically significant. As two other independent studies also support intercessory prayer by the American Psychological Association's criteria for empirically based treatments, this intervention should be accepted except for the heterogeneity of the medical conditions for which the treatment was used. This finding highlights the risk associated with an atheoretical stance to evidence based practice that reifies and idealises a research design. RCTs unquestionably have the potential to yield clinically relevant data in the absence of an adequate understanding of the underlying process. When James Lind in 1753 determined that lemons and limes cured scurvy, he knew nothing about ascorbic acid, nor did he understand the concept of a nutrient. Yet Penny E's study demonstrates the absurdity which can be created by bringing the world of rigorous measurement into a domain that is totally unsuited to it.

Most importantly from the standpoint of psychoanalysis, the current categorization in evidence-based psychotherapies conflates two radically different groups of treatments: those that have been adequately tested and found ineffective for a client group, and those that have not been tested at all. It is important to make this distinction, since the reason that a treatment has not been subjected to empirical scrutiny may have little to do with its likely effectiveness. It may have far more to do with the intellectual culture within which researchers operate, the availability of treatment manuals, and peer perceptions of the value of the treatment (which can be critical for both funding and publication). The British psychodynamically oriented psychiatrist Jeremy Holmes has eloquently argued in the *British Medical Journal* that the absence of evidence for psychoanalytic treatment should not be confused with evidence of ineffectiveness. In particular, his concern was that cognitive therapy would be adopted by default because of its research and marketing strategy rather than its intrinsic superiority. He argued that: (1) the foundations of cognitive therapy were less secure than often believed; (2) the impact of CBT on long-term course of psychiatric illness was not well demonstrated; (3) in one "real life trial" at least the CBT arm had to be discontinued because of poor compliance from a problematic group of patients who nevertheless accepted and benefited from couples therapy; (4) the effect size of CBT is exaggerated by comparisons with waiting list controls; (5) the emergence of a post-CBT approach that leans increasingly on psychodynamic ideas.

Whilst the present author is entirely in sympathy with Holmes' perspective, even if his work with Roth was one of the targets of his criticism, it is only fair to expose the shortcomings of his communication.

Of course, psychodynamic clinicians are at a disadvantage and not simply because they are late starters (after all, many new treatments find a place at the table of evidence based practice). There are profound incompatibilities between psychoanalysis and modern natural science. Whittle has drawn attention to the fundamental incompatibility of an approach that aims to fill in gaps in self-narrative with cognitive psychology's commitment to minimal elaboration of observations, cognitive asceticism. In the former context, success is measured as eloquence (or meaningfulness) which is not reducible to either symptom or suffering. Moreover, psychoanalytic explanations invoke personal history, but behavior genetics has brought environmental accounts into disrepute. While CBT also has environmentalist social learning theory at its foundations, it has been more effective in moving away from a native environmentalist position. To make matters worse, within psychoanalysis there has been a tradition of regarding the uninitiated with contempt, scaring off most open-minded researchers.

Psychoanalysts are not yet fully committed to systematically collecting data with the potential to challenge and contradict as well as to confirm cherished ideas. The danger that must be avoided at all costs is that research is embraced selectively only when it confirms previously held views. This may be a worse outcome than the wholesale rejection of the entire enterprise of seeking evidence, since it immunizes against being affected by findings at the same time as creating an illusion of participation in the virtuous cycle of exploring, testing, modifying and re-exploring ideas.

But the absence of psychoanalytic research raises a related problem that particularly concerns me. A recent study research team demonstrates that the allegiance of the researcher predicts almost 70% of the variance in outcome across studies, with a remarkable multiple of. 85% if three different ways of measuring allegiance are simultaneously introduced. This means that 92% of the time we can predict which of two treatments compared will be most successful based on investigator allegiance alone. This becomes a pernicious self-fulfilling prophecy, as investigators who favor less focused more long-term treatment approaches are gradually excluded from the possibility of receiving funding and, if their treatments are subjected to systematic inquiry at all, these studies are performed by those with least interest in such treatments.

Aim should be to assist the movement of psychoanalysis toward science. In order to ensure a future for psychoanalysis and psychoanalytic therapies within psychiatry, psychoanalytic practitioners must change their attitude in the direction of a more systematic outlook. This attitude shift would be characterized by several components: (1) The evidence base of psychoanalysis should be strengthened by adopting additional data-gathering methods that are now widely available in biological and social science. New evidence may assist psychoanalysts in resolving theoretical differences, a feat which the current database of predominantly anecdotal clinical accounts have not been capable of achieving. (2) The logic of psychoanalytic discourse would need to change from its overdependence on rhetoric and global constructs to using specific constructs that allow for cumulative data-gathering. (3) Flaws in psychoanalytic scientific reasoning, such as failures to consider alternative accounts for observations (beyond that favored by the author), should be overcome and in particular, the issue of genetic and social influence should be approached with increased sophistication. (4) The isolation of psychoanalysis should be replaced by active collaboration with other mental health disciplines. Instead of fearing that fields adjacent to psychoanalysis might destroy the unique insights offered by clinical work, we need to embrace the rapidly evolving "knowledge chain" focused at different levels of the study of brain-behavior relationship, which, as Norman points out, may be the only route to the preservation of the hard won insights of psychoanalysis.

Chapter 9 Psychiatric Care for the Chronically Ill and Dying Patient

The aim of medical treatment is not only to ensure survival but also to improve the quality of life of patients who are ill. Sensitive and informed primary care providers can manage the psychosocial care of most patients with chronic or terminal illness. However, consultation or treatment provided by a mental health professional is sometimes indicated and helpful. Consideration will be given in this chapter to the psychological and psychiatric aspects of chronic and terminal medical illness, with particular emphasis on psychotherapeutic issues. However, difficulty adjusting to a medical condition is usually not the result of a formal psychiatric disorder.

How can you be most helpful to a person in need when hope appears lost? What is the best way to deliver news of a terminal diagnosis? Should you assess someone for depression when he or she is terminally ill? How can you develop a reasonable and thoughtful plan for end - of - life care?

Every clinician at one time or another faces these important questions. In the treatment of terminally ill patients, the health professional needs many skills: the ability to deliver bad news, the knowledge to provide appropriate optimal end - of - life care, and the compassion to allow a person to retain his or her dignity. The following vignette describes the case of a gentleman nearing the end of his life. The discussion and annotated references that follow should help the reader to best handle the complex issues that are involved in the care of the dying patient.

What kinds of services are provided? Hospice palliative services generally include:

Basic medical care with a focus on pain and symptom control.

Medical supplies and equipment as needed.

Counselling and social support to help you and your family with psychological, emotional, and spiritual issues.

Guidance with the difficult, but normal, issues of life completion and closure.

A break (respite care) for caregivers, family, and others who regularly care for you.

Volunteer support such as meal preparation or errand running.

Counselling and support for your loved ones, including after you die.

The Psychology of Chronic Terminal Illness

The psychological response to a particular illness is variable and depends on multiple factors, such as the characteristics of the medical illness and the personality life stage, emotional conflicts and vulnerabilities and cultural and social milieu of the individual affected. Because loss and disability are associated with many medical illnesses, severe emotional distress may occur in individuals who would not otherwise be affected. Diseases affecting body parts or regions of great symbolic significance, such as cancer of the breast, head and neck, or testes, may damage self-esteem and alter the sense of personal identity. Conditions such as end-stage renal disease, which require burdensome physical and dietary restrictions and time-consuming treatment, may produce great distress in individuals who value self-sufficiency, independence, or spontaneity. Diseases occurring during adolescence may provoke concerns about physical attractiveness and possible rejection by peers. In the elderly, fears of death or loss of the ability to function autonomously may be prominent. Cultural factors also affect the way in which most medical conditions are experienced. For example, diseases such as acquired immune deficiency syndrome (AIDS) still carry a burdensome social stigma everywhere in the world. With other conditions, such as Type I diabetes mellitus, illness-related anxiety may be profound but not evident until the first sign of a serious complication, such as retinopathy or nephropathy.

Successful adaptation to a chronic medical illness may be characterized by the preservation of self-esteem, acceptance of the illness such that necessary treatment recommendations can be followed, engagement in vocational, family, and social activities to the extent that is permitted by the illness, and the capacity to tolerate feelings evoked by the illness without persistent anxiety or depression. Although there is no single or predictable pathway of adjustment, some common psychological responses to a serious medical illness can be identified. The initial psychological response to a serious or terminal medical condition may resemble a state of grief or mourning. The term grief refers to the acute emotional response to the perception of loss whereas mourning usually denotes the wider range of feelings evoked by this experience. The term anticipatory grief refers to the reaction to anticipated future losses.

Serious medical illness is inevitably associated with multiple losses of both a tangible and symbolic nature. Profound grief reactions may occur following the diagnosis of a potentially ominous condition such as AIDS, the occurrence of a feared complication, such as blindness in Type I diabetes mellitus, or the communication to a patient with cancer that further medical treatment is unlikely to halt the progression of the disease. Features of grief that may occur m these circumstances include feelings of shock, disbelief, and emotional numbness. Denial of the objective reality of the illness ("No, It can't be me") may be followed by or alternate with unavoidable awareness of the illness. The latter is often associated with anxiety, sadness, anger, somatic distress, and attempts to make sense of what has happened ("Why me?"). A 35-year-old man informed of the recurrence of a malignancy demonstrated many of these distressing features of an acute grief reaction. He reported feelings of terror and panic, as if he had entered a "black hole" with insomnia, nausea and vomiting, and agitation. He said "I feel anxious nil of the time. I feel overwhelmed, at the mercy of things. I feel shell-shocked. Like I am not part of the world, I have lost all sense of myself."

A broad range of feelings related to the illness may be experienced after the initial response to grief, although there are wide individual and cultural differences in this regard. Some individuals never wish to discuss or consider feelings related to their disease. Others welcome the opportunity to communicate their feelings and to find meaning in the experience of illness. Denial has adaptive value in the short term, but adaptation to chronic illness is usually more effective when feelings related to the condition can be acknowledged and expressed. Feelings of sadness and anger are common during the initial psychological adjustment to an illness. Subsequently, a reduction in this dysphoria and sometimes even a process of psychological reorganization and personal growth may occur. The latter may include an increased sense of the value of life and a greater motivation to engage in activities that are personally meaningful. This was expressed by one patient following a remission from her disease. She said "In spite of my anger, I now get more enjoyment from everything I do. I don't have time to waste. I am looking for meaningful relationships, and I have a hunger to accomplish."

Acceptance of the illness often fluctuates and may alternate with what has been referred to as "bargaining" or attempts to postpone the inevitable. Late in the course of a terminal disease, the belief that death is imminent and inevitable may initiate another phase of adjustment. Some individuals review their lives at this time to find meaning in their accomplishments and in their ties to family and to others. Others become preoccupied with their mortality, although many patients with terminal illness continue to focus on the process of living. This commonly involves utilizing active coping mechanisms, maintaining physical activity, and attempting to overcome the complications of the illness. Unfortunately, disturbing feelings of suffering, disappointment, and victimization sometimes persist with the pain and disability of a debilitating illness. This is most likely to occur with those who have suffered from previous traumatic life experiences. Relief from such feelings may not occur until the patient's level of consciousness is altered by the metabolic and neurological complications of the illness and/or by the sedating effects of analgesic medication.

Case Presentation

Mr. A, a 47-year-old man without prior psychiatric problems, was admitted to the hospital for continued treatment of widely metastatic colon cancer. Since his diagnosis 2 years earlier, he had undergone a sigmoid resection, radiation therapy, chemotherapy, and a more extensive abdominal resection. His cancer continued to spread, however, and he was admitted for symptoms suggestive of a small-bowel obstruction.

During the hospitalization, he required antibiotic treatment of an abdominal abscess and subsequently received intraperitoneal chemotherapy. Despite these interventions, his tumor burden remained high, and the treatment team felt that there was little else to be done; he was thought to have less than 6 months to live. The team broached this issue with Mr. A, but was unsure about how much information to give him. Psychiatric consultation was requested to evaluate his depression and "pathological denial".

On consultation, Mr. A was noted to be somewhat irritable, and he endorsed frustration at his loss of function secondary to his illness. He reported numerous sources of stress, he recently lost his job as an executive, he was embroiled in a stressful divorce with his exwife, and he was becoming impotent as a result of his treatments. When asked if he felt sad, he replied, "Well of course I'm sad! The impotence has got me down, and I know that 4 or 5 years from now, I might not even be around to see my kids." Low energy, reduced concentration ability, psychomotor slowing, and decreased appetite were noted; these symptoms appeared to have progressed over the last 6 months as his illness worsened. He also lost interest in the great majority of his former hobbies. When asked about his medical illness, he reported that there would likely be another surgery in his future to try to "cure this thing once and for all". However, he tended to ruminate on both the past and the present, and acknowledged that he had little to look forward to. He was lucid and fully oriented; a screening mental status examination found that his cognition was intact.

How Should Information about a Diagnosis with a Terminal Prognosis Be Given to a Patient? How Much Information should Be Given?

While there is no single best way to decide what information to share, when it should be communicated, and how to best relay the information, several important principles can help in such a difficult situation.

Both studies 1 - 3 of terminally ill patients and our own clinical experience have found that the majority of patients wish to know the full truth about their condition. Furthermore, in most cases, patients who are told their diagnosis in an up-front, clear manner have better emotional adjustments to their situation than those who are not told about their condition. By providing direct, clear information in a compassionate manner, and by making clear to the patient that everything possible will be done to provide medical and emotional support, physicians can elicit trust and reduce anxiety.

Of course, there may be special circumstances that affect the rate and the manner in which the information is relayed. If the physician has an opportunity to discuss the possible results of a given diagnostic test before the test is done or before the results are available, he or she can help prepare the patient for all possibilities (good and bad) and assess the probable response to bad news. If the patient displays a catastrophic reaction or frank denial at the possibility that the test will return grave results, the consultant may wish to consider the best way to tell the patient about such results.

In the Massachusetts General Hospital Handbook of General Hospital Psychiatry, recommends relaying negative information to patients through a brief, rehearsed initial statement that succinctly communicates the news and clearly indicates that the treatment team is committed to the ongoing care and support of the patient: "A typical delivery might go as follows: 'The tests have confirmed that your tumor is malignant. I have therefore asked the surgeon (radiotherapist, oncologist) to come by to speak with you, examine you, and make his recommendations for treatment (we will do something about it). As things proceed, I will be by to discuss them with you and how we should proceed (I will stand by you).' Silence and quiet observation at this point yield more valuable information about the patient than any other part of the exchange."

In the case of Mr. A, the patient did not appear to understand the gravity of his condition. The first order of business would be to determine why Mr. A did not understand his situation — was this denial or simply a lack of information? It would be useful to determine what the treatment team had already told Mr. A about his diagnosis and prognosis. If Mr. A had received limited or conflicting information about his prognosis, the consultant could help the team open a discussion of Mr. A's condition and its prognosis.

If, on the other hand, Mr. A had been repeatedly told his prognosis but seemed to be in denial, a different approach would be in order. In this case, the physician could avoid meeting the denial head - on, but might instead ask about the emotional impact of the illness and hospitalizations on Mr. A. This could then allow a discussion of Mr. A's fears and fantasies about his condition and its consequences. It would be useful to consider a referral to a counselor, therapist, or another trusted individual to allow Mr. A to slowly let his guard down and to discuss the realities and emotions of his situation.

How Can One Tell the Difference between the Normal Grief Associated with Dying and the Condition Known as Depression? Which of These did Mr. A Present with?

Grief and depression share a number of features. Both are associated with periods of significant sadness, crying spells, periods of social withdrawal, and decreases in sleep, concentration, or energy. However, there are a number of important differences between a process of normal grief and a syndrome of major depression that require treatment.

Grief is characterized by episodic waves of sadness that can be initiated by thoughts of impending death or by a person/event that will be missed. However, this sadness is not pervasive, and it is balanced by the patient's ability to experience pleasure and to look forward to future events. A global loss of interest in pleasurable activities does not occur, and feelings of hopelessness are transient. There may be passive wishes for death to come quickly, but these too are fleeting, and there are no active plans for a hastened death.

In contrast, depression is characterized by unremitting sadness and by an inability to enjoy activities that would usually be experienced as pleasurable. Feelings of hopelessness are prolonged, and suicidal ideation is more active and more persistent. The patient with major depression is frequently unable to look to the future.

Chochinov and colleagues found that the single question, "Are you depressed?" was quite effective in diagnosing major depression among terminally ill hospice patients. However, the psychiatric consultant can increase diagnostic accuracy by assessing each of the above - mentioned domains to determine whether a patient's distress is the result of grief or depression.

In the case of Mr. A, his symptoms were more consistent with depression than with normal grief. His denial of his illness made it difficult to fully assess his ability to look forward to the future, but he acknowledged that he had little to look forward to. Furthermore, he had persistent anhedonia, and the vignette seemed to indicate that his symptoms were more persistent than episodic. Given his persistent anhedonia, neurovegetative symptoms, and hopelessness, he met criteria for major depression and should have received treatment for his depression.

Psychiatric and Psychological Intervention in Patients with Chronic Terminal Illness

Many emotional disturbances in the medically ill are alleviated by supportive contact with an attending physician. The need to refer a patient to a specialist for psychological treatment depends on a variety of factors, including the severity and nature of the patient's distress, the presence of a psychiatric disorder, the patient's motivation for assistance, and the capacity of the attending physician to deal with such matters. Unfortunately, the rate of detection of emotional disturbances in medical patients is disturbingly low. For example, moderate or severe depression in medical patients may be undetected in more than half of such cases; even when detected, the majority of patients with clinical depression do not receive appropriate antidepressant treatment. A variety of factors may contribute to this low rate of detection and treatment. Many patients are uncomfortable discussing feelings and will refrain from doing so unless the physician specifically indicates a readiness to listen. Some physicians underestimate the significance of emotional disturbances, assuming that it is "natural" for patients who are medically ill to be upset. Too often, when it is "understandable" that a patient is depressed, specific treatments such as psychotherapy or pharmacotherapy are not offered. At the other extreme, premature referral without careful assessment of the patient's emotional state may result when the physician is uncomfortable with emotional issues. In such cases, speedy referral to a psychiatrist or other mental health practitioner may represent an attempt by the physician to avoid the patient's distress. Physicians may recognize that symptoms such as depression are present but do not appreciate that effective treatments are available. The failure to intervene in such cases is unfortunate, since depression is associated with significant disability and distress and medical illness is a risk factor for suicide. The medical profession can play a significant role in suicide prevention: most patients who commit suicide have contacted a physician from a few hours to a few months before death.

What characteristics are important in the care of dying patients?

Ajai R detailed essential features of the delivery of care to dying patients. These include:

1. Competence

Skillful treaters allay anxiety and allow the best possible medical outcome. Just because a person has terminal illness does not mean that clinicians should not use their highest level of medical skill to maximize comfort and reduce distress. Competent treaters use their skills to optimize pain control, to treat comorbid reversible medical conditions, and to consider psychiatric diagnoses. Dying patients are greatly comforted when they feel that their physician is knowledgeable and has developed a comprehensive plan of care.

2. Concern

Much is taught about the need to protect oneself against becoming "too wrapped up" in the care of one's patients. However, true empathy and connection are necessary to provide good care for such patients, and rather than be avoided, such traits should be standard doctor's tools used to cure, to soothe, and to improve the lives of patients. Often, family members and patients may avoid talking about painful feelings of impending loss. Treaters, by discussing their own feelings about the patient's loss and by asking how others are dealing with the impending loss during meetings with patients and families, can show their own concern and allow patients and families to grow closer.

3. Comfort

Physical discomfort can contribute to psychological distress and inhibit a healthy grief process. Assessment and treatment of pain should be complete and thorough. Treatment of pain with narcotics, nonsteroidal anti - inflammatory drugs (NSAIDs), adjunctive agents, acupuncture, biofeedback, and other remedies is crucial in the care of the dying. Treatment of low energy, shortness of breath, and psychiatric symptoms is also key. Where patients go to spend their final days is another vital issue that can either enhance the final days of life or make them uncomfortable.

4. Communication

Communication with the dying should focus far more on the art of listening than on the art of speaking. When the treater does speak, it should be to help patients tell the story of their life (their accomplishments, their interests, their regrets, their hopes, the people in their life, and the details of their spiritual life). By spending time with a patient, by listening intently, and by helping the patient make meaning of life and death, a treater can facilitate therapeutic communication.

Treaters can also help by sharing Pleschberger's 5 - stage model of the response to impending death. The stages of this model outline a course of emotions often experienced by patients and family members as they go through the process of grieving. These 5 stages (denial, anger, bargaining, depression, and acceptance) outline the course of normal/healthy bereavement.

While individuals rarely pass through these stages in a linear way, knowledge of the stages can be helpful to treaters when identifying a patient or family member who seems "stuck" in a particular stage. Furthermore, knowledge of this model can normalize the denial, anger, or sadness of such a patient and help treaters see that their patient may be going through a normal and healthy process. For patients, knowledge of these stages can let them know that the process of grief is not uncharted territory and that peace and acceptance can be found at the end of their emotional suffering.

Interestingly, a recent article by Curtis and colleagues asked patients with 3 end - stage illnesses (COPD, AIDS, and cancer) about important physician skills in end-of-life care. The authors found many similarities across diseases, but also found some disease - specific differences in the skills perceived to be most crucial in end - of - life care. The patients with COPD in this study reported that a physician's ability to provide education about their disease and prognosis was very important (often those with COPD had not been well informed of the generally irreversible nature of their illness). Patients with AIDS targeted pain control as a major issue, while patients with cancer valued physicians who were able to help them maintain hope in the face of their illness. Therefore, while the properties of compassion, communication, and continuity were crucial for all patients, there appeared to be specific domains of care that may be more important based on the nature of one's illness.

How Can a Clinician Be Helpful to a Patient Who Is Terminally Ill?

The following are 4 ways in which a clinician can be helpful to a patient who is terminally ill:

1. Aid the Psychological and Spiritual Coping Process

The consultant can engage in discussions that allow the patient to reveal the important psychological, social, and spiritual aspects in his or her life. In an article that discussed end-of-life care, Block described that a systematic assessment of these domains allows treaters to gain a sense of the patient's coping strengths and vulnerabilities. The consultant might ask about some of the following:

Life story. What are you proudest of? What legacy would you like to leave? What would you like your family to remember about you? Do you have any regrets? Is there anything you would like to accomplish with the remainder of your life?

Relationships. Whom do you cherish most? Have you been able to tell them? Is there anyone you would like to reconcile with? Are there any friends you hope to see? How can you help your family prepare for your death?

Coping. What are your biggest strengths? What difficult things have you gotten through in your life, and how did you get through them? When have you been most discouraged over the course of this illness? How do you think you will cope with the time ahead? What is scary about the time ahead of you?

Spirituality. Are you a religious person? Do you believe in God? What is your relationship with God? Do you feel able to communicate with him? What do you imagine will happen to you when you die? Do you feel that God is happy with you, angry with you, or feels some other way? Why?

These questions can be very therapeutic in themselves, and they allow a person to reflect on the accomplishments and relationships that have been important to him or her. They also allow some attention to the things that the person would still like to achieve emotionally and interpersonally in the time remaining. Furthermore, as noted by Block, they can help treaters to better understand a person's coping strategies, allowing for optimal care.

2. Assess and Treat Psychiatric Illness

Psychiatric illness is common among patients with terminal illness. Such illnesses should be identified as the treatable syndromes that they are, rather than as "expected" outcomes of terminal diagnoses. Major depression is experienced by approximately one fourth of patients with cancer, with rates increasing as the disease worsens. Other terminal illness is similarly associated with elevated rates of major depression. Furthermore, one quarter of terminally ill patients also experience significant anxiety symptoms. Untreated pain, dyspnea, and nausea can exacerbate abnormal mood and anxiety.

Delirium is also common in patients with terminal illness and it often goes unrecognized (or is misdiagnosed as psychosis or anxiety). A mental status examination and careful monitoring of the patient's level of consciousness, orientation, and agitation throughout the day can help identify delirium in this at-risk population. When delirium is diagnosed, the cause of the delirium should be determined. It is crucial to distinguish between irreversible causes of delirium (eg, brain metastases and organ failure) and those causes that can be treated. Treatable causes of delirium in this population include, but are not limited to, contributions from medications (benzodiazepines, anticholinergics, steroids, and narcotics), electrolyte disturbances (especially those of calcium and sodium), metabolic disturbances (especially from thyroid dysfunction and glucose abnormalities), and infections. It should be noted that most causes of delirium are multifactorial, and, therefore, even if some contribution to the delirium is derived from an irreversible medical condition, the treatment team should search for reversible conditions that can contribute to clouding of the mental status.

Treatment of these conditions is, in general, similar to the treatment received by those who are not terminally ill, although special considerations should be made for predicted life span, organ failure, and use of concomitant medications. Depression can be rapidly treated with stimulants, specifically methylphenidate or dextroamphetamine, beginning at 2.5 to 5 mg/day. If the predicted life span is greater than 4 to 6 weeks, a standard antidepressant, such as an SSRI, can be used. If the patient is taking several medications, citalopram or sertraline may be the favored SSRIs because of their minimal interaction with the cytochrome P450 system.

Free-floating anxiety should also be assessed carefully. Anxiety can result from pain, delirium, inadequate information, or a variety of other sources. Anxiety in nondelirious patients can be treated with benzodiazepines. If the anxiety is situation-specific, or of relatively short duration, short-acting benzodiazepines (such as lorazepam) can be administered on an as-needed basis. If the anxiety is more persistent, longer-acting agents, such as clonazepam, can be given as a standing dose. As with depression, if the patient's condition is associated with a life span of greater than 4 to 6 weeks, SSRIs can be useful, especially in the treatment of well-defined anxiety syndromes, such as panic disorder.

Delirium should be symptomatically treated with antipsychotics. By the intravenous route, haloperidol is an excellent choice because it results in virtually no extrapyramidal symptoms (EPS); QTc intervals should be followed while this medication is being administered to facilitate prevention of torsades de pointes. Benzodiazepines should be avoided in delirious patients, as they tend to increase confusion and may further disinhibit the patient or worsen agitation. For delirious patients who are able to take medications by mouth, atypical antipsychotics are also appropriate and have relatively few adverse effects. It should be noted, though, that these are symptomatic treatments and that the diagnosis and treatment of reversible causes of delirium are crucial.

3. Maximize Comfort

In addition to diagnosing psychiatric illnesses, the consultant should also remain aware of other factors that contribute to impairments in a patient's comfort. Pain control is of utmost importance in the care of the dying patient, and many studies have found that pain is undertreated in this population. The psychiatric consultant can be helpful to the treatment team by identifying ongoing pain. The consultant can remind the treatment team that much higher doses of narcotics may be needed in chronically ill patients with acute pain; consultants can also relieve anxiety about "causing addiction" in the terminally ill. Furthermore, adjuncts to narcotic medications (eg, NSAID, tricyclic antidepressants, anticonvulsants, physical therapy, biofeedback, and massage) can be considered for any patient with ongoing pain.

"Comfort" extends far beyond analgesia. Symptomatic discomfort from nausea, hiccups, or dyspnea can be assessed and treated. Adequate food, drink, and hygienic care can lead to significantly improved mood, self - esteem, and dignity. Furthermore, a patient's physical location can have a tremendous impact — does this person wish to die at home or in comfort at hospice rather than in a hospital? Each of these factors needs to be considered in the treatment of the terminal patient.

4. Treat the Treaters and Family Members

Physicians who treat patients with terminal illness undergo significant stress. They may feel helplessness at their inability to cure the patient or anger at themselves for not catching the illness at an earlier stage (or anger at the family or the patient for not coming for treatment sooner). Conversely, treaters can feel tremendous grief with the loss of a patient with whom they have had a long relationship or a strong alliance. Psychiatric consultants can help treaters to identify their grief and can encourage them to share these feelings of loss with the patient, with other colleagues, and with supervisors.

Psychiatric consultants can also help family members cope with the impending loss of a loved one. In considering the emotional state of a person with terminal illness, it is often helpful to consider the effects of the family members on the patient and vice versa. By observing the interactions of a patient with family, the consultant can become aware of long-standing grudges or new difficulties in communication that can make the process of coming to closure at the end of a life more difficult.

Family members or friends who serve as regular caregivers to a terminally ill patient have substantial stress and elevated rates of depression. The psychiatric consultant can be helpful by inquiring about stress and depressive symptoms in caregivers, and can be useful by suggesting "breaks", additional help, or a different system of care if appropriate and if the caregiver is open to such suggestions. The consultant can also help to reduce feelings of guilt in caregivers if they do decrease their involvement in direct caregiving.

The case above provides an opportunity for the consultant to be helpful in a number of ways. By exploring Mr. A's understanding of his condition and his feelings about the future, by assessing him for psychiatric illness and other etiologies of discomfort, and by supporting the treatment team and his family members, the consultant can have a significant impact on his care.

Psychotherapy for Patients with Chronic Terminal Illness

A variety of pharmacological and psychosocial interventions are available to treat psychiatric disorders and emotional distress in medically ill patients. There are two major psychotherapeutic approaches that can be adopted by a primary care practitioner or by a mental health professional: (1) promotion of active coping strategies and (2) supportive - expressive therapy, to assist with understanding and management of feelings evoked by illness. These two approaches, described below, may be offered on an individual basis or in a group setting.

Promotion of Active Coping Strategies

Serious and disabling medical illness represents a threat to an individual's sense of competence and mastery and may trigger feelings of helplessness, ineffectiveness, and uncertainty. A variety of therapeutic strategies may be employed on an individual, group, or family basis to help patients with such conditions regain a sense of mastery. Techniques that can provide symptomatic relief of illness - related distress include relaxation therapy and mindfulness meditation. The latter refers to techniques to alter attention and awareness as a means of modulating disturbing experience. Education of patients and their families about the medical condition and about steps that can be taken to decrease symptoms, to prolong survival, or to obtain further assistance may diminish feelings of helplessness. These approaches, which can be adapted to specific diseases, are cost efficient, provide peer support, and when administered in a group setting, may decrease feelings of isolation. Other forms of group therapy, including self - help groups, may facilitate the sharing of experiences and information and reinforce active coping strategies. Behavioral strategies, including relaxation, guided imagery, and hypnosis, may help to reduce pain and other distressing symptoms and to prevent demoralization and despair. Cognitive therapy may help to correct cognitive distortions related lo medical illness and to replace dysfunctional thoughts with more adaptive ones. Such approaches may be used together with anxiolytic and analgesic medication, to reduce symptoms and to increase feelings of control over the illness.

Psychodynamic Therapy: Supportive and Expressive

A. Supportive Therapy

The traditional role of the medical practitioner in maintaining a consistent, reliable, empathic relationship with the patient is often the most important psychotherapeutic factor for patients with chronic or terminal illness. Indeed, once the medical treatment plan is established, the relationship with the physician may be one of the most critical factors in maintaining morale and hope. The value of this relationship is too often underestimated by physicians who feel they must respond to a patient's emotional distress by "doing something" prescribing medication, offering advice, ordering further laboratory tests, etc.

The overall aim in supportive psychotherapy is to bolster adaptive and minimize maladaptive coping mechanisms and to decrease adverse psychological reactions such as fear, shame, and self - disparagement. This treatment can often be provided effectively by an interested primary care practitioner who has an ongoing relationship with the patient. Further, a supportive relationship with a medical caregiver may lessen the need for analgesic or psychotropic medication and may reduce the problem of noncompliance with medical treatment. There is no clear boundary between supportive and expressive (insight - oriented) psychotherapy, although there are differences in emphasis. In both treatments, the therapist may help the patient to understand the illness experience in a meaningful fashion. However, the objectives in the former are focused more on symptomatic relief and on maintaining psychological equilibrium. This is accomplished by a more structured approach, which is more likely to include interventions such as education, reality testing, reassurance, and advice. Reassurance and advice are most helpful when they are based on a realistic appreciation of the patient's situation. However, the well - intentioned but misguided use of such interventions is common. For example, reassurance that is premature or unrealistic is rarely comforting and may leave patients feeling even more isolated with their distress. Further, although advice may be helpful, particularly when related to management of the illness, it should be given sparingly in personal matters. It is usually best to help patients make their own personal decisions rather than to try to make decisions for them.

B. Expressive (Insight-Oriented) Therapy

The emphasis in expressive psychotherapy is on promoting self - understanding and psychological growth. This treatment, which usually requires referral to a trained psychotherapist, is most suitable for the small minority of medical patients who have identifiable and significant psychological or interpersonal problems, who are motivated to understand their feelings, and who have the ability to form a therapeutic relationship. To begin treatment, some patients need help in overcoming their initial fears of depending on or revealing themselves to another. Expressive psychotherapy may allow medical patients to express their feelings in a safe setting without fears of alienating either their family or their primary caregivers.

Contraindications to expressive psychotherapy in the medically ill include (1) the presence of medical conditions in which emotional arousal may be medically hazardous, eg, recent myocardial infarction, (2) medical crises or other stresses that limit the padent's capacity to tolerate anxiety or emotional disruption, and (3) delirium or dementia caused by cardiovascular, neurological, metabolic, or other disorders. The cognitive impairment associated with these conditions may limit the capacity for verbal expression, and the concomitant emotional lability may increase the vulnerability to states of disorganization and distress when emotional exploration is attempted. The cognitive functions and emotional lability of medical patients should be carefully assessed before insight-oriented psychotherapy is instituted.

Establishing the Focus of Psychological Treatment

The entire spectrum of psychiatric and psychosocial interventions should be considered with medically ill patients who are distressed. Pharmacological and other medical interventions for anxiety, depression, delirium, and pain in medically ill patients are discussed in later. Psychosocial interventions involving the family, community agencies, and self-help groups may be of great value in assisting in the process of adjustment. Further, help that is provided by or related to the individual's cultural, ethnic, and religious group may offer emotional support and personal meaning, both of which may alleviate feelings of isolation and despair. Indeed, spiritual and religious issues are important aspects of the illness experience for many medical patients and therapists must be prepared to address these issues explicitly and/or implicitly.

There are many reasons why medical patients seek therapy and there can be an equally wide diversity in its goals. Psychological assistance is most frequently sought to relieve disturbing symptoms of depression or anxiety. Physicians must consider the indications for social, psychological, or pharmacological interventions in such cases. Particularly perplexing to evaluate is the mental state of patients who decide to terminate life-sustaining medical treatment. In such cases, there may be a rational decision to refuse medical treatment or to end life in the face of unbearable suffering. However, such so-called "rational suicides" must be distinguished from other motivations, such as the wish to elicit concern from caregivers, to manage unbearable feelings of helplessness or to be relieved of pain. Also, the decision to stop treatment may be secondary to the effects of depression or organic mental disorders on mental competency, on the ability to form rational intent, or on the ability to remain hopeful about the future. The distinction between a rational decision to stop treatment and a decision that is determined by the hopelessness associated with a depressive disorder is often difficult to make with terminally ill patients. A trial of antidepressant treatment may be indicated in such cases.

Some medical patients seek psychological treatment in the hope that it will improve their health or their chances for long-term survival. This belief has been reinforced in recent years by attention in the media to the role of psychological factors in illness. However, although there is some scientific evidence that links psychological well-being with a favorable medical outcome, unrealistic expectations of benefit from psychological treatment need to be addressed. The desire to modify behavior that is adversely affecting health (eg, noncompliance with a medical treatment regimen), is a valid focus of treatment. However, some patients unrealistically attribute all of their personal difficulties, even preexisting ones, to their illness. Others attempt to deny the significance or even the existence of the illness. The adaptive value of denial should not be underestimated, particularly during the acute phase of an illness. However, when it persists, it may interfere with accepting appropriate treatment or with anticipating and preparing for the personal difficulties that may lie ahead. When such denial should be supported or challenged is a matter of careful clinical judgment. This issue may be illustrated in the following case.

Illustrative Case

A 35-year-old health care worker sought a psychiatric assessment shortly after a routine medical examination revealed a positive human immunodeficiency virus (HIV) blood test. He did not feel in need of current emotional assistance but decided to identify a variety of medical specialists who could provide help that he might subsequently require. He was extremely knowledgeable about the medical aspects of AIDS, both from his medical training and from his personal experience caring for many friends through the terminal stages of their illness. He had also read extensively about the phases of psychological adjustment to a terminal medical illness. He wondered what phase he was in, although he denied any current symptoms of emotional distress. He was extremely concerned about the welfare of others, and he had already made adjustments in his work and personal life to be sure he would not place others at risk. Also, he had bought a large house several years earlier for the express purpose of caring for his friends with AIDS.

When interviewed, the patient was physically wasted and coughed frequently. He was cooperative, articulate, and demonstrated features of mild anxiety. He believed that he had not yet developed any symptoms of AIDS, and he hoped that his recent treatment with protease inhibitors would halt the progression of the disease. However, he reported unexplained increased fatigue and frequent episodes of diarrhea over the past 2 years. When his obvious respiratory symptoms were noted, he became markedly uncomfortable and asserted that he did not believe these symptoms were related to AIDS. His cognitive functions were intact, and his sensorium was clear.

It was evident that the patient had successfully employed active coping strategies to maintain a high level of adjustment both before and after his positive HIV blood test. He demonstrated considerable knowledge about his medical condition and about psychological issues. However, he seemed to deny the apparent progression of his disease or any sense of personal vulnerability. His denial and his active coping strategies were currently adaptive and were not directly challenged. However, ongoing psychotherapeutic contact was arranged to provide support that might be required if his disease progressed further. It was assumed that he might presently be experiencing more distress than he was able to acknowledge and that he was at risk to become more depressed or anxious when the advancement of his disease interfered with his self-sufficient and altruistic stance.

The Process of Therapy in the Medically Ill

Psychotherapy with chronically ill medical patients resembles therapy with patients who are physically well. However, greater flexibility on die part of the therapist is required with the medically ill, because of the adjustments that are necessary when there is an exacerbation of the medical disorder. At such times it may be necessary to shift from insight-oriented therapy to an approach that is more supportive in nature. Further, when a patient is hospitalized, treatment may need to continue in less than optimal circumstances, sometimes at the bedside. Although the patient's right to privacy must be respected, involvement of the therapist through all phases of an illness may be crucial in maintaining the therapeutic alliance. For many patients, the medical illness has already created feelings of isolation from the "normal" or "healthy" world. A therapist who discontinues treatment when the medical condition worsens may heighten these feelings of isolation. In some cases, it may help to continue the therapeutic dialogue by telephone or email when patients cannot travel lo appointments.

Countertransference

Medically ill patients may provoke a variety of emotional reactions in the therapist, sometimes referred to as countertransference. Some patients elicit over concern, others arouse feelings of hostility and rejection. The therapist must identify such feelings to understand the patient better and to maintain an altitude of therapeutic neutrality. Neutrality in this context does not mean indifference but refers to a therapeutic stance that is attuned to the patient's feelings and needs. Interventions that arise from the needs of the therapist, even when well intended, may not be useful to the patient. For example, a therapist may become overly supportive to counteract his or her own underlying feelings of frustration and impotence. Such well-meaning interventions may deprive some patients of the opportunity to maintain their sense of autonomy and self-sufficiency or to express their frustration and anger. Hostile feelings in the therapist may also arise and may serve to maintain emotional distance from a patient whose distress threatens to be overwhelming. In other cases, patients with intense anger may hope to achieve a greater sense of control over their feelings by provoking similar feelings in the therapist. To remain constructively involved with the emotional experience of their patients, primary care physicians and therapists who care for the medically ill must learn to be aware of and to tolerate such intense feelings in themselves and in their patients.

Collaboration with the Primary Care Physician

Psychotherapy with medically ill patients places special emotional and practical demands on the therapist. The treatment in such cases often needs to be conducted in collaboration with the primary care physician, who retains responsibility for medical management of the patient. The therapist must remain aware of the patient's current medical status, without assuming direct responsibility for it. Therapists must pennit feelings of resentment toward the primary caregivers to emerge, but must be careful not to intervene or to undermine that primary relationship. Attempts by the patient to form special relationships that split the medical staff and create tension among them can be prevented only by frequent communication among all members of the medical team. Because of the need for such communication, it is generally unwise for the therapist to promise absolute confidentiality. Therapists should avoid unnecessary disclosure of personal information about the patient to medical staff, but should be free to communicate about matters that affect the medical course. Some issues regarding collaboration with the medical staff are depicted in the following case.

Although the patient's concerns about confidentiality were acknowledged to be valid, the importance of the therapist's ongoing contact with the medical staff became increasingly apparent. This collaboration was sometimes necessary to determine the extent to which disturbances in her emotional slate were affected by or caused by alterations in her metabolic control. At another point, when the factitious administration of insulin or sedative drugs was suspected, discussion and collaboration with the medical staff were essential. The intimacy and dependency that resulted from the establishment of a therapeutic relationship were frightening to her, and she responded initially with detachment and attempts to split the medical staff.

However, this relationship subsequently provided the patient with a limited and restricted means by which she could begin to develop some degree of trust in others. Only later did deep-seated fears of her unacceptability and her potential destructiveness to others emerge.

The Facilitation of Grief and Mourning

Medical patients frequently enter psychotherapy in a state of distress because their usual coping mechanisms have been eroded by the physical and psychological effects of illness. Grief and mourning are commonly related to the anticipated or actual loss of competence and bodily integrity and to the disruption in the expected trajectory of life-span and accomplishments. Oscillations between denying the implications of the illness and feeling overwhelmed by it are common. The first phase of psychotherapy involves listening to the patient and allowing thoughts and feelings related to the illness to emerge in a gradual and tolerable fashion. This may involve providing support and reassurance when patients are flooded with feelings and gentle exploration when feelings have become closed off. The following case illustrates the phases of psychotherapy in a patient who was referred after cancer of the breast was diagnosed.

Illustrative Case

A 32-year-old married woman was referred for psychotherapy after being told that a recent breast biopsy indicated the presence of a malignancy. She reported feeling enraged and hopeless, and refused any medical or surgical treatment for her disease. This refusal reflected her anger, her sense of futility, and her wish to deny the presence of the cancer. She described a dream in which a woman was murdered, which she believed reflected her own experience of being assaulted and potentially destroyed by the illness. She regarded both radiotherapy and surgery as forms of further physical assault.

The initial therapeutic task was to facilitate the gradual expression of feelings related to the illness. The therapist needed to proceed flexibly and to be guided in each session by the patient's willingness and capacity to explore her feelings. During the phase of acute grief, patients are commonly unable to be introspective or to make use of psychological insight. The most important goal at this stage is to provide an environment in which thoughts and feelings related to the illness can be safely discussed. The stabilizing effect of the therapeutic relationship is more beneficial at this stage than are any specific interpretations. The process of understanding cannot begin until the period of acute grief has passed and the patient feels less overwhelmed. The patient described feeling more hopeful after the fifth session and said to the therapist that she had "combined my strength with yours". She also felt able to consider and to proceed with appropriate medical treatment options.

Organization of the Experience of Illness

In the patient just described, the diagnosis of breast cancer revived long-standing feelings of being defective and unacceptable, and undermined her sense of femininity. In the middle phase of therapy, she reported a dream in which she was accepted at a desirable school but then received a notice informing her that she could not attend. For her, this dream represented both the opportunities and plans she felt the illness had stolen from her as well as her feeling of having been damaged and made undesirable to others. The experience of her illness also brought her much closer to underlying feelings of dependency and abandonment. Later in the therapy, she reported a fantasy of being a needy, colicky baby whose mother could not cope with her and for the first time she revealed her belief that her mother never really wanted her.

As therapy progressed, this patient became more able to reflect on her feelings. The therapist could now assist her in integrating and working through the mourning process associated with the illness. Feelings of sadness could be more safely expressed in the presence of a firmly established therapeutic relationship. Providing meaning and organization to her experience in this phase helped to diminish her feelings of helplessness and isolation. This process depended on the empathic involvement of the therapist, whom the patient felt was able to "live the experience with me".

Mastery

Serious medical illness often represents a threat to an individual's sense of competence. An important goal of psychotherapeutic treatment is to restore the sense of competence and mastery. Initial unsuccessful attempts to achieve mastery by denying the illness or by evading its significance may later be replaced by a greater capacity to experience safely a broader range of feelings related to the illness. The patient described above became more able to tolerate feelings of vulnerability without feeling overwhelmed. She now felt motivated to examine her previous tendency to conceal feelings of insecurity and dependency beneath a veneer of self-sufficiency. Although she felt that the illness "removed a crutch" her vulnerabilities were no longer so threatening to her. She felt more able to accept her illness and to consider and select appropriate treatment. She no longer fell the same need to affirm her strength by denying her illness, refusing treatment, or taking her life.

Someone the patient trusts to consent to treatment and decide about the course of treatment in consultation with physicians.

The majority of patients and the public are already convinced about the importance of advance planning for medical decisions. Studies consistently show that patients would like to discuss life-sustaining treatment and advance directives with their physician. Furthermore, many patients expect their physician to initiate the conversation. Relatively few patients, however, have actually discussed life-sustaining measures with their doctor. Physicians are often reluctant to discuss life-sustaining treatment or advance directives with patients, and wait for patients to raise the issue. This failure to talk with patients appears to stem from diverse reasons. These include unjustified concerns by some physicians that the discussion itself will harm the patient, discomfort and lack of experience in talking about dying, and a failure to recognize the conversation as an integral part of caring for dying and severely ill patients. However, studies show that patients do not respond negatively to discussions about forgoing treatment or advance directives, nor do they experience an increased sense of anxiety or depression. In fact, many patients are relieved to discuss the topic, even if they find the conversation difficult.

Some physicians do not talk with patients about treatment wishes or advance directives because of a paternalistic belief that physicians can best determine the course of treatment. However, decisions about which treatments would be worthwhile or unacceptably burden some reflect deeply held personal preferences and values.

Helping Children Cope with Chronic Illness

The chronically ill child has some sense of illness severity, even without medical explanation. He or she receives clues through his or her knowledge of illness, the urgency of treatment, contact with other patients, and the responses of family and friends. This process is "fluid" however, and may change day to day depending upon the circumstances. It is, therefore, important for the child and adolescent psychiatrist to be aware of fluctuations in patient response and wait for communication rather than anticipate it.

Time becomes an important concept to the child; there just never seems to be enough of it and there are no guarantees that it will always be available. This sense of a foreshortened future is a "loss of innocence". This marks an emotional reaction to illness. Children with chronic illnesses perceive the past differently; it becomes an idealized place to visit. The child may display a personal photograph taken before the diagnosis, saying, "This picture is how I really look." Some children, however, seem to ignore the past when they begin treatment for a chronic illness. It is as if the illness takes over all aspects of the child's life and everything that has gone on before was a different lifetime. Time defined by precise and rigidly enforced medical schedules become the routine. Immediacy of events and lack of flexibility inhibit the typical wanderings of childhood. There is also a constant sense of anticipation. Not the excited anticipation that healthy children associate with important events and opportunities, but an anxious anticipation that accompanies medical interventions whose outcome is uncertain.

Medical illness can rapidly spin out of control for the child. Procedures, medications, hospitalizations, and restrictions are all perceived as life changes imposed by others. The optimal response by clinicians and caregivers is to allow the child or adolescent as many options as possible during the diagnostic process and treatment phase of the illness. Some of the choices may seem inconsequential, but each is a step towards greater control for the child. Along with this notion of control is the ability to maintain a sense of identity. For children and adolescents this frequently involves affiliation with their peer group and the stability of the "group's identity" based on appearance, interests, academics, and social life. They should be given every opportunity to continue friendships and other social relationships. Every child also wants to preserve his or her own identity that incorporates both individual and familial traits. This can be particularly difficult when the child experiences physical and emotional changes characterized primarily by their illness. Accomplishments measured in terms of the disorder that elicit responses, such as, "You played a great game for someone with diabetes," take away the child's sense of belonging to their peer group. Children may encounter peers moving on to face new academic, social, and athletic challenges, while they remain behind until the illness either remits or resolves enough to proceed. Developmental concerns are also a factor; these children may not be able to develop a sense of belonging to their peer group because of their illness.

Depression in Medical Illness

Separating the impact of the illness from symptoms of mood disorder is a challenge when making the diagnosis of depression in medically ill children. Occasionally caregivers rationalize their approach to young patients with a belief that children suffering from severe illness will naturally experience symptoms of depression. They may either intervene with every patient or avoid the diagnosis and provide few psychiatric services. Each case should be assessed individually, without assumption or bias. For example, characteristics of medical illness do not necessarily predispose young patients to depression. Illness severity as measured by the number of hospitalizations and relapses is not directly related to increased risk. The type of illness may also determine a patient's response. Cancer patients, for example, frequently acknowledge low depression rates despite severe illness. The term "cancer" is often associated with death among patients and caregivers, more so than with other diseases. These children probably use denial and repression as defense mechanisms to cope with the stress of diagnosis and treatment. Challenging these attempts at self-protection under the guide of helping the patients adjust to illness is not necessarily helpful.

Depression occasionally complicates the clinical presentation in a child with chronic illness. Young patients present with depression as a direct consequence of the illness or its treatment, as a result of the impact of the disease on the individual and family, or as an exacerbation of a pre-existing affective disorder. Rates of depression in pediatric chronic illness vary depending upon the study sample: 7% of acute pediatric inpatients, 12% to 13% of pediatric bum unit patients, 13% of cardiology outpatients, 15% of asthmatic adolescents, and 23% of orthopedic inpatients. Children with chronic illnesses reveal trends consistent with depression in the general pediatric population. Adolescent girls with a chronic illness are more likely to suffer from depression than adolescent males. Low levels of social support lead to poorer outcomes. Family history of depression is also a risk factor for the development of mood disorders. Illnesses involving the central nervous system, those with obvious adverse cosmetic effects, or that severely compromise the patient's activity level are more likely to reinforce the development of a mood disorder. Relationships exist between depressive symptoms and mortality in asthma, retinopathy in juvenile diabetes, and recurrent major depression in female adolescent diabetics. Occasionally distinctions between illness and depression are difficult to discern. Patients may be limited in mobility, activity level, and exercise tolerance by the disease and appear depressed. Positive reinforcement for age appropriate levels of functioning may not occur with chronic illness. Parents fear complications in the child's presentation and so further limit participation, leaving the patient prone to mood disorders. Chronic pain associated with medical illness also reinforces a level of disability and dependency that promotes depressive symptoms.

A few studies have examined the development of depression over the course of a disease. In juvenile diabetics, for example, depression was most likely in the first year after diagnosis.

Children and adolescents with initial adjustment problems were more likely to suffer from depression later in the course of the disease. The way the child or adolescent thinks about the illness over time affects emotional response. Patients with low self - esteem who tend to blame themselves for problems are more likely to report depressive symptoms. In addition, young patients who feel as though their illness and its treatment are out of their control, or in the control of unknown forces, are negatively affected.

Finally, stressful life events increase the likelihood of depression in medically ill children. Studies of pediatric or thopedic patients, children with inflammatory bowel disease, and young patients with seizure disorders noted that subjects were vulnerable to depression when experiencing more adverse events and higher levels of family and interpersonal conflict in their lives. Some studies of depressed, medically ill children noted high rates of past loss or separation from a significant adult figure as a result of death, chronic illness, or abandonment.

Coping with a Life- threatening Illness

Children must not only face the development and exacerbation of medical illness, but also the outcome should treatment fail. This includes coping with death and dying. Notions of death are varied and unique in a pediatric population. The onset of a critical illness frequently leads the child to wonder about the distinction between being dead and alive. Occasionally this fascination can be upsetting and the child becomes more irritable and sensitive. More often, the patients develop rationalizations to explain why death does not apply to his or her situation. This can be interpreted as denial, but it emotionally supports the child as he or she faces the challenges of illness. Children will frequently acknowledge their proximity to death only after the crisis passes and the patients believe recovery is likely.

The role of spirituality can be crucial, even in young children. A strong affiliation with religion can be a strength for the individual and family. However, the young patient may occasionally be confused by the notion that a loving God would allow such a thing to happen. Children turn these concerns into a belief that God is on their side in this struggle and will lead them back to good health. There may also be a fear that God is punishing them for some past transgression. This is particularly troubling because it implies responsibility for the illness and its consequences. Issues raised by children and adolescents therefore should be openly discussed with family and medical professionals. Whenever possible, and with family agreement, members of the clergy should be involved. Clinicians must take care not to interfere with the family's belief system through ignorance or contradiction.

The critically ill child feels most vulnerable when another patient with a similar or identical illness dies. Fears of separation from loved ones, suffering, and death rush to the child's consciousness leading to anticipatory grief. Although the intensity of these feelings may pass within hours to days, the sadness remains. Parents should inform the young patients about the death as soon as possible. This prevents the patients from discovering death or dying in casual conversation with peers or staff. Such interactions can be particularly traumatic and do not allow the child to discuss the event with those close to them.

Children with terminal illnesses are sensitive to the notion of being "replaced" in the family. In one such case, the mother of an eight - year - old girl dying from liver rejection post transplantation became pregnant in the months prior to the patient's final hospitalization. Although both parents denied any connection between the pregnancy and their daughter's near terminal illness, the implications were clear to the patient. She occasionally asked about the baby and where it would sleep in the house.

The terminal phase of an illness should emphasize comfort, support, and symptom control above all else. The child is aware that options are diminishing and begins to make preparations for death. Letters are written and plans are made to give gifts and say good - byes. As death approaches, the child may become quiet and less spontaneous. Comfort is often found in the company of friends and family with little physical contact and little said. Parents should not interpret this as rejection, but as an expected preparation for death. The psychiatrist can clarify this situation for caregivers and ease their anxiety.

Outcome Cost - benefit Analysis of Psychotherapy with the Medically Ill

The benefit of psychotherapy in improving the quality of life of medical patients is often underestimated by medical practitioners. Some of the clearest evidence of the benefits of psychotherapy has been obtained from studies of the medically ill. The beneficial effects of psychotherapy have been demonstrated not only by improvements in psychological well - being but also by reduced utilization of medical resources. Medical patients who participate in psychotherapy have been shown to require fewer medical investigations and treatments, either because of the effect of psychotherapy on overall health status or because of the more appropriate allocation of medical and psychological resources. There are also reports that psychotherapy may result in prolonged survival in patients with cancer and other serious medical conditions.

Summary

Medical illness is a stressful event in the life of any patient, although the specific meaning of the illness and the psychological response to it may depend on a variety of factors. Treatment of depression or other psychiatric disorders may result in an improvement of the patient's emotional state, an increased ability to engage in a wide range of social and physical activities, and a reduced tendency to utilize health care measures. Psychoeducational approaches and other interventions to support active coping strategies may help maintain morale and quality of life in many medical patients. These may he administered on an individual, family, or group basis. Supportive psychotherapy as an adjunct to treatment may be an important function of the primary care practitioner. A small proportion of medical patients may be suitable for and may benefit from expressive (insight - oriented) psychotherapy conducted by a specially trained psychotherapist. This treatment may diminish the likelihood of persistent depression or of prematurely giving up on the possibilities of life. However, insight - oriented therapy may be contraindicated for some medical patients because of physical debilitation or cognitive impairment.

Psychotherapy may assist medical patients in working through feelings associated with the multiple losses and the possibility or certainty of death related to the illness. Patients grieve for anticipated losses as well as for those that have already occurred. Therapy is often directed toward facilitation of the mourning process and achievement of a sense of competence and mastery related to it. Physical illness may impose realistic limitations that cannot be overcome by psychological treatment. In these and other respects, medical illness may present an ongoing challenge to the sense of competence of the therapist as well as the patient.

Medical complications or hospitalizations may disrupt the therapeutic process. The ability of a patient who is physically unwell to tolerate affective arousal may fluctuate widely, and therapeutic interventions at any point must take this into account. In some cases, the physical condition interferes with the ability of the patient to form a therapeutic relationship. In addition, the therapeutic relationship may be affected by other factors, such as the necessary breach of confidentiality that occurs when therapists work in collaboration with the medical treatment team. Although psychotherapy may in some cases be the most important feature of management of a medically ill patient, psychotherapists more often play a secondary role. The treatment of medical complications is often the most urgent priority.

Chapter 10 Forensic Psychiatry

The term "forensic" derives from the Roman "forum", a public place or square where communities conducted their legal and political business. Forensic psychiatry is the medical subspecialty that involves the use of psychiatric expertise to assist in the resolution of legal disputes. As psychiatric knowledge and practice have developed, courts increasingly have called on psychiatrists to help answer legal questions. These requests for psychiatric assistance span a wide range of criminal and civil issues. For example, psychiatric expertise can aid courts in determining the competence or responsibility of criminal defendants and help courts by assessing the capacity of individuals to make medical decisions or manage personal affairs. In addition to conducting clinical evaluations related to specific legal case, some forensic psychiatrists become involved with the legal regulation of psychiatry, such as legal and professional policies that regulate the scope and standards of psychiatric practice.

The expanding demand for forensic psychiatric services has contributed to the growth and development of the subspecialty. The American Academy of Psychiatry and the Law (AAPL) is the major professional organization of forensic psychiatrists. In 1994 the American Board of Psychiatry and Neurology began examining board - certified general psychiatrists for Added Qualifications in Forensic Psychiatry, and in 1997 the Accreditation Council on Graduate Medical Education began reviewing and accrediting fellowship programs. Many books and journals reflect the burgeoning research and scholarly activities in the field.

Forensic psychiatry is the branch of psychiatry that deals with issues arising in the interface between psychiatry and the law, and with the flow of mentally disordered offenders along a continuum of social systems. Modern forensic psychiatry has benefited from four key developments: the evolution in the understanding and appreciation of the relationship between mental illness and criminality; the evolution of the legal tests to define legal insanity; the new methodologies for the treatment of mental conditions providing alternatives to custodial care; and the changes in attitudes and perceptions of mental illness among the public. This paper reviews the current scope of forensic psychiatry and the ethical dilemmas that this subspecialty is facing worldwide.

From an obscure and small group of psychiatrists who dedicated their efforts to the study of mental conditions among prisoners and their treatment, and who occasionally would appear in courts of law, forensic psychiatrists have now developed into an established and recognized group of super - specialists, an influential group that is transforming the practice of psychiatry and that has made deep incursions into the workings of the law. This status has not come without misgivings about the basic identity of forensic psychiatry and concerns about its utility and its ethics.

Modern forensic psychiatry has benefited from four key developments: the evolution in the medico - legal understanding and appreciation of the relationship between mental illness and criminality; the evolution of the legal tests to define legal insanity; the new methodologies for the treatment of mental conditions that provide alternatives to custodial care; and the changes in public attitudes and perceptions about mental conditions in general. These four moments underlie the expansion recently seen in forensic psychiatry from issues entirely related to criminal prosecutions and the treatment of mentally ill offenders to many other fields of law and mental health policy.

Scope and Challenges

The subspecialty of forensic psychiatry is commonly defined as the branch of psychiatry that deals with issues arising in the interface between psychiatry and the law. This definition, however, is somewhat restrictive, in that a good portion of the work in forensic psychiatry is to help the mentally ill in trouble with the law to navigate three completely inimical social systems: mental health, justice and correctional. The definition, therefore, should be modified to read the branch of psychiatry that deals with issues arising in the interface between psychiatry and the law, and with the flow of mentally disordered offenders along a continuum of social systems/ italic. Forensic psychiatry deals with issues at the interface of penal or criminal law as well as with matters arising in evaluations on civil law cases and in the development and application of mental health legislation.

Penal Law

Worldwide, a wider understanding of the relationship between mental states and crime has led to an increased utilization of forensic experts in courts of law at different levels of legal action.

On entering into the legal system, three major areas need consideration: fitness to stand trial, insanity regulations and dangerousness applications. The major developments on the issue of fitness to stand trial pertain to rulings that defenders found not fit to stand trial are sent to psychiatric facilities, with the expectation that their competence to be tried is to be restored: the question for clinicians revolves on what parameters to use to predict restorability of competence, which should be based on an adequate response to treatment. Insanity regulations pertain to legal tests used to decide whether the impact of mental illness on competence to understand or appreciate the nature of a crime could be used to declare an offender “not criminally responsible because of a mental condition”, “not guilty by reasons of insanity” or any other wording used in different countries. Applications to declare a person a “dangerous offender” usually demand a high level of expertise on the part of forensic experts, who are expected to provide courts with technical and scientific information on risk assessment and prediction of future violence.

Once an offender has been adjudicated, a major task for forensic psychiatrists is to gauge the level of systems interface in relation to different types of receiving and treating institutions. Hospitals for the criminally insane, mental hospitals for the civilly committed patients, penitentiary hospitals for mentally ill inmates, as well as hospital wings in local jails, are all part of the mental health system, and their interdependency has to be acknowledged for purposes of system integration and budgeting. How mental patients are managed in prisons is also a major matter of concern.

Finally, on exit from the legal-correctional system, forensic psychiatrists are expected to provide expert knowledge on matters such as readiness for parole, predictions of recidivism, commitment legislation applicable to exiting offenders, and the phenomenon of double revolving doors for the mentally ill in prisons and hospitals.

Civil Law

Psychiatrists and other mental health specialists are often required to conduct assessments with a view to determine the presence of mental or emotional problems in one of the parties. These types of assessments are needed in multiple situations, ranging from examinations to specify the impact of injuries on a third party involved in a motor vehicle accident, to evaluations of the capacity to write a will or to enter into contracts, to psychological autopsies in order to assess testamentary capacity in suicidal cases or sudden death, or evaluations for fitness to work and, of late in many countries, evaluations to determine access to benefits contemplated in disability insurance. In most of these situations, the issue at hand is a determination of capacity and competence to perform some function, or the evaluation of autonomous decision making by impaired persons. A determination of incapacity leading to a finding of incompetence becomes a matter of social control that is used to legitimize the application of social strictures on a particular individual. This imposes on clinicians an increased ethical duty to make sure that their decisions have been thoroughly based on the best available clinical evidence.

Ordinarily, there is a presumption of capacity and, hence, that a particular person is competent. A person is assumed to be competent to make decisions, unless proven otherwise. The presence of a major mental or physical condition does not in and of itself produce incapacity in general or for specific functions. In addition, despite the presence of a condition that may affect capacity, a person may still be competent to carry out some functions, mostly because the capacity may fluctuate from time to time, and because competence is not an all or none concept, but it is tied to the specific decision or function to be accomplished. In addition, a finding of incapacity should be time-limited; that is, it will have to be reviewed from time to time. For example, a stroke may have rendered a person incapacitated to drive a motor vehicle and hence the person will be deemed incompetent to drive, but the person could still have the capacity and be competent to enter into contracts or to manage personal financial affairs. With time and proper rehabilitation, the person may be able to regain capacity and competence to drive. Ordinarily, a person has to consent to an assessment of incapacity or a legal order has to be obtained to make the person cooperate to the assessment or to proceed to collect information otherwise. It is advisable to use a screening test of capacity and to do a full assessment only if the person fails the screening test. This will prevent imposing an onerous burden on the person subject of the assessment if the screening test is easily passed.

Mental Health Legislation and Systems

The double revolving door phenomenon, whereby mental patients circulate between mental institutions and prisons, has made forensic psychiatrists deeply aware of the interactions in the mental health system and the links between this system and the justice and correctional systems. By virtue of their involvement in legal matters, forensic psychiatrists have developed a major interest in the drafting and application of mental health legislation, especially on the issues of involuntary commitment, that in many countries is based on determination of dangerousness as opposed to just need for treatment, of management of mentally ill offenders and of legal protections for incompetent persons. Given that one major area of their expertise is the assessment of violence and the possibility of future violent behavior, forensic psychiatrists are usually called upon to make decisions on risk posed by violent civilly committed patients.

There is a close interaction between legislation, development of adequate mental health systems and delivery of care, whether in institutions or in the community. Mental health legislation with overly restrictive commitment clauses even for short - term commitment, deinstitutionalization resulting from the closure of old mental hospitals, changes in health care delivery systems towards short admissions to general psychiatric units and subsequent treatment in the community, and the large number of mental patients that end up in jails, have created in many countries a sense that the mental health system is a drift. The growth of forensic psychiatry may be due to changes in the law and to a more liberal acceptance of psychiatric explanations of behavior, but a more immediate reason is the large number of mental patients in forensic facilities, jails, prisons, and penitentiaries. Failures of the general mental health system may, therefore, be at the root of the growing importance of forensic psychiatry.

One reason that has been most commonly advanced to explain the large number of mental patients surfacing in the justice/correctional system is the policy of deinstitutionalization that governments have implemented over the past fifty years. In general, deinstitutionalization refers to legislative decisions to close large mental hospitals and resettle patients into the community, providing short admissions to general hospital psychiatric units, outpatient treatment options, psychosocial rehabilitation, alternative housing and other community services. Sometimes, however, these decisions did not respond to any planning, or any assessment of the needs of those patients that were going to be resettled, or deinstitutionalized. Neither was there a clear idea about the nature of services to be provided, or the characteristics of the communities where patients were going to be relocated. The decisions, therefore, were mostly made on rhetorical and political beliefs, rather than on proper scientific reasoning.

The idea and policies of deinstitutionalization have been both praised and vilified. To some, deinstitutionalization is an enlightened, progressive and humane set of policies that has placed the needs of the mentally ill front and centre in many communities. In this regard, deinstitutionalization has been very effective. Deinstitutionalization should be credited with an increase in the involvement of patients in their own care and rehabilitation, it has raised questions that challenge the therapeutic nihilism rampant in a previous era, it has increased the visibility of mental patients in the community and in general hospitals and academic centres, it has allowed for a better understanding of the disease process which, previously, had been distorted by the negative effects of prolonged institutionalization, it has provided an impetus for research and learning, and it has increased awareness of the human and civil rights of mental patients.

On the other hand, deinstitutionalization has also been credited with a host of negative effects. Legally, along with legal activism, deinstitutionalization has been blamed for giving impulse to litigation and costly over - legalization and over - regulation of psychiatric practice. Socially, a series of pernicious effects have impacted directly on the fate of the mentally ill in the community. These have included reports of "revolving door patients" (those patients in need of repeated and frequent admissions), and the rise among the homeless populations in that at least 30% among them are chronically mentally ill persons. Even when housing is available, it is often in rundown tenements in inner cities or psychiatric ghettos of large urban centres, where dispossessed and confused mental patients walk about in a daze talking to themselves, and where they are easy victims of robbery, rape, abuse, and physical violence. Some simply die of exposure in the streets in frigid winter nights. Deinstitutionalization has also been blamed for the criminalization and the transmigration of mental patients from the mental health system to the justice/ correctional system and for violent behavior displayed by some mental patients in the community.

The most pointed criticisms to deinstitutionalization, however, are no longer aimed at the idea of resettling the patients back into their communities, but about how the idea has been implemented. Whether because of financial constraints or shortsighted administrations, the fact is that, in many communities, mental hospitals have been emptied faster than the development of adequate community resources and community alternatives as they were envisioned in the original policies.

These unfortunate after - effects of deinstitutionalization should be counteracted with the realization that treatment alternatives to custodial care exist in the form of better medications with enhanced efficacy and effectiveness, that are becoming widely available, and psychosocial treatment strategies, that are also providing new proven ways for management of mentally ill persons in the community. In this respect, the development of mental health courts in some countries, diversion alternatives to imprisonment, assertive community treatment and intense case management modalities, as well as the use of community treatment orders, along with better policies in housing, point toward a social move to resolve the inequities of deinstitutionalization in order to stabilize community tenure for the mentally ill. At the same time, evaluations of anti-stigma programs seem to indicate that some of these initiatives are helping in changing public attitudes toward mental illness and increasing awareness about the human rights issues in the treatment and management of the mentally ill in many countries.

Ethical Controversies

Because of its dual role in medicine and in law, the practice of forensic psychiatry is fraught with ethical dilemmas worldwide. A forensic psychiatrist is first of all a clinician with theoretical and practical knowledge of general psychiatry and forensic psychiatry, and experience in making rational decisions from a clearly stated scientific base. In law, forensic psychiatrists must know the legal definitions, the legal policies and procedures, the legal precedents relating to the question or case at hand. Forensic psychiatrists must have knowledge of courtroom activity and must possess an ability to communicate their findings clearly and to the point and to do so under the difficult situation of cross examination. The double knowledge in psychiatry and law defines the subspecialty of forensic psychiatry and provides the ethical foundations for its practitioners. This double knowledge should be reflected from the very beginning in the way the forensic psychiatrist first agrees to get involved in an evaluation, the way the forensic psychiatrist approaches the person to be evaluated, and the caveats that have to be provided. At this stage, the most important issue for the forensic psychiatrist is to make sure that the person subject of the evaluation is not misled into believing that, because the psychiatrist is a medical doctor, the relationship to be unfolded is one of physician - patient, in which the doctor is expected to do the best for the patient and always to act to maximize the patient's benefit, while reassuring the patient that privacy and confidentiality are protected. In forensic psychiatry the relationship is one of evaluation, where the foundation of neutrality demanded from the evaluator, and the fact that the evaluator is in no position to reassure the person on matters of confidentiality or privacy, could mean that negative findings will endanger the interests and cause harm to the person being evaluated, regardless of this person's health and the evaluator being a physician. Because of this, forensic psychiatrists may even be implicated in the criminalization of mentally ill persons.

To some commentators, the social control role of forensic psychiatrists sets them apart from the ethics of medicine and of psychiatry. These commentators waver on whether in their legal work forensic psychiatrists are operating as physicians — a point of view that has led to much controversy. From inception to appearance in court, the forensic psychiatrist derives the authority to act from the fact of being once and foremost a physician, hence having to uphold the ethics of medicine, but the end point effects of forensic evaluations are usually at the hand of other parties. This imposes on forensic psychiatrists an ethical obligation to scrutinize their motives and the motivations and possible final actions of those who hire them for evaluations, including ways on how data are obtained, how the evaluator arrives at opinions, how legal materials such as reports, memos, and expert evidence are prepared, and most importantly, what would be the final use of their findings.

A major controversy stemming from the double roles that forensic psychiatrists and other psychiatrists, such as those in the military, are called to fulfill relates to the use of psychiatric judicial hospitals in the Soviet Union and, more recently, in China, and psychiatrists' participation in interrogations of prisoners and detainees that could lead to allegations of torture, especially in the present climate of concern with terrorist activities. This includes turning over to interrogators confidential psychiatric material that could be used to pinpoint weaknesses and vulnerabilities of the prisoner, providing consultations on interrogation techniques or actively participating in deception techniques to gather intelligence. It is in this context that the end point motivations of those calling for evaluations cannot be lost on forensic psychiatrists or physicians in general. Participation on anything that could lead to torture will be a major trespass on the ethics of medicine. This also should be a clear reminder to forensic psychiatrists that medical ethical rules cannot be trespassed, no matter what the demands of the master.

The Psychiatric Expert Witness

Courts generally recognize at least two types of witnesses: fact and expert. Fact witnesses may testify about their personal observations of a relevant event. An expert witness, in addition, may be allowed to offer professional inferences or opinions drawn from those facts. The Federal Rules of Evidence, which many states use as a model, declare that "if scientific, technical, or other specialized knowledge will assist the trier of fact to understand the evidence or to determine a fact in issue, a witness qualified as an expert by knowledge, skill, experience, training or education may testify thereto in the form of an opinion or otherwise". Depending on the circumstances, courts may call on psychiatrists to testify as either fact witnesses or expert witnesses.

When a patient becomes involved in court proceedings, a treating psychiatrist may be called as a fact witness. For example, the psychiatrist may be asked to describe the patient's presenting problems, diagnoses, and treatments arising after a personal injury. As a fact witness, however, the psychiatrist generally does not offer opinions about the causal connections, if any, between the injury and the psychiatric disturbance. Testimony derives from the treatment relationship, and the patient is usually the primary source of information.

When functioning as an expert witness, the forensic psychiatrist does not have a traditional doctor - patient relationship with the person being evaluated. The purpose of the evaluation is consultation to the court or referring party, not treatment for the patient. The evaluation involves an impartial assessment related to the legal dispute, and the court expects the psychiatrist to offer inferences and opinions. For example. the psychiatrist may describe the causal connection between an injury and a psychiatric disturbance. In addition to interviews with the injured person, the opinion will often rely heavily on information obtained from third parties, medical records, accident reports, and other sources.

The forensic psychiatrist's involvement with a case typically begins with a referral from an attorney, an insurance company, an administrative agency, or a court. The forensic psychiatrist needs to consider several issues before agreeing to take the case, including clarification of the referral question and a determination of whether the question falls within the psychiatrist's area of expertise. In addition to being asked to provide expert opinions, the forensic psychiatrist may be asked to assist in the preparation of the case. In a 1985 decision, Ake v Oklahoma, the United States Supreme Court held that many criminal defendants have a constitutional right to access to a competent psychiatrist who will assist their attorney. This consulting role could involve critiquing the reports of opposing experts and helping the attorney prepare to challenge and cross-examine those experts. Forensic psychiatrists may appropriately serve in the role of either impartial expert or consultant. However, in cases in which the expert is asked to function in both capacities, many commentators, including the Group for the Advancement of Psychiatry (GAP), recommend that the psychiatrist first complete an independent evaluation and formulate a relatively impartial expert opinion prior to becoming involved in the more partisan role of a consultant who assists the attorney in presenting the most favorable case.

The unique aspects of the forensic role, as opposed to the therapeutic role, raise special ethical considerations. In the traditional doctor - patient relationship, the psychiatrist has obligations that include maintaining confidentiality, acting in the patient's best interests, and avoiding harm to the patient. The forensic expert, in contrast, often must reveal sensitive information in reports and testimony and may express opinions that are not in the best interest of the person being evaluated. The forensic psychiatrist has an ethical obligation to inform the evaluee of the limits of confidentiality and of the purpose of the evaluation. Under some circumstances, professional ethics preclude conducting an evaluation. For example, except for evaluations necessary to render emergency care, criminal defendants should not be evaluated prior to access to, or availability of, legal counsel.

After completing the assessment, forensic psychiatrists usually prepare a report detailing their findings and opinions. Sometimes, however, referring attorneys or agencies will ask that reports not be prepared, particularly if the opinions reached are not helpful to their positions. Forensic reports differ from standard clinical reports, all sources of information, including persons interviewed and records reviewed, need to be identified, data are separated from conclusions and are presented in descriptive instead of conclusion terms (eg, a mental status evaluation might describe an evaluee's belief that government agencies control his thoughts through a transmitter implanted in his brain instead of simply concluding that the person has "paranoid delusions"), and jargon and technical terms are either avoided or defined. Reports should explicitly link the data to the evaluator's conclusions and opinions.

Psychiatrists have sometimes been criticized for their involvement in legal proceedings. The contention is that psychiatric assessments lack sufficient reliability to be useful in legal proceedings and that the profession slitters damage to its image when experts take opposing positions in highly publicized cases.

Concerns about reliability are tempered by research indicating that diagnostic reliability for major mental disorders equals or exceeds reliability of other medical diagnoses. Competent psychiatrists also have considerable expertise in human behavior and psychopathology. Forensic psychiatrists have ethical obligations to testify within the limits of their knowledge and expertise.

The impact on the image of psychiatry raises more difficult issues. Some psychiatrists testify on matters outside their areas of expertise or offer opinions that are unsupported by the state of knowledge within the profession. This may cast doubt on whether psychiatrists have any real expertise and has led to suggestions for peer review of psychiatric testimony to improve psychiatrists' performance in court. In other cases, media misrepresentation of psychiatric involvement results in negative public perceptions. The "battle of the experts", however, is not unique to psychiatry. Similar conflicts between opposing experts occur in other branches of medicine and in other fields of science. Divergent opinions and testimony have been given on "objective" issues such as the etiology of birth trauma, the significance of cardiac and other medical symptoms, the interpretation of medical test results, and the causes of structural collapses, airplane crashes, and other accidents. Within psychiatry, experts are more likely to agree on the presence of symptoms and serious mental disorder than on the legal significance of those findings. For example, they might agree on the presence of a mood disorder but disagree on whether the disorder should result in a finding of incompetence or insanity. Psychiatrists, and experts from other professions, need to recognize the distinction between expertise in their fields and nonexpertise on ultimate legal issues.

Despite these criticisms, courts are likely to continue to rely on psychiatric expertise. The profession would abrogate its societal responsibility if it refused to participate appropriately in legal proceedings.

Competence as General Concept

Many forensic evaluations involve questions of competence. Searight (1986) has described the following elements common to all competence evaluations, functional abilities, contextual demands, causal inferences and judgmental and dispositional considerations.

Every competence evaluation involves assessing a person's functional ability to perform a specific task and each task places its own unique demands on the person. Except in cases of the most profound incapacity, global determinations of competence or incompetence are meaningless. Thus, the first step in any competence evaluation is to determine whether the person has impairments in those capacities relevant to the specific task. The knowledge and abilities needed to make medical decisions, for example, are not identical to the knowledge and abilities needed by a criminal defendant facing trial. The forensic psychiatrist needs to know the relevant abilities associated with each task at issue.

Contextual demands may differ even within categories of competence - related tasks. For example, the degree of understanding and comprehension needed to consent to high - benefit/low - risk medical interventions such as antibiotics for pneumonia may be lower than that required to consent to low - benefit/high - risk procedures such as experimental brain surgery. Similarly the same range of abilities is not required to stand trial for a minor misdemeanor, such as trespassing, as is required for a serious and complex felony trial. Competence assessments must address these contextual demands in addition to addressing the functional abilities of the individual.

When functional deficits exist, the forensic examiner must make causal inference about their etiology. The significance of functional impairments may vary depending on the cause. Deficits caused by mental disorders, malingering, or simple lack of education can all have different implications for whether evaluees will be permitted to make their own decisions or face the consequences of their behavior. When a mental disorder causes the problems, the forensic psychiatrist may also be asked lo address the prognosis and remediability of the impairments.

The final element of all competence assessments involves judgmental and dispositional determination. What is the threshold at which a person should be adjudicated incompetent to perform a task? What severity of functional impairment and how demanding a context are required before a person loses the freedom to make personal decisions? And what should be done with an incompetent person? Should someone else make decisions for that person, and if so, what decision - making standard should that person use? All of these questions involve legal determinations rooted in considerations of justice and morality. Psychiatric training does not confer expertise in legal and moral issues. Psychiatrists have expertise in assessing functional impairments, describing how those impairments will impact a person's performance of certain tasks, and determining the etiology and prognosis of those impairments Whether someone should be found impairments and what should happen next are decisions reserved for Judges and juries.

Criminal Forensic Psychiatry

Confession and Waiver

In the criminal justice system, forensic psychiatrists potentially assess the defendant's behavior from the moment of the crime through arrest, trial, and incarceration. Some criminal suspects choose to make statements or confessions to the police, often before they consult with an attorney. The question that then arises is whether those defendants were competent to confess or to waive Miranda rights, such as the right to remain silent. Competent confessions or waivers of rights are generally made in a knowing, intelligent, and voluntary manner. Mental disorders, including menial retardation, can affect those abilities, resulting in incompetence. In the 1986 case Colorado v Connelly, the United States Supreme Court held that a criminal suspect's "mental condition" may increase susceptibility to police coercion and impair the voluntariness of a confession or waiver: some official police misconduct, however, is required before the Constitution compels courts to vitiate a waiver or confession as involuntary. Because psychiatrists typically do not participate in police interrogations, competence to confess and to waive Miranda rights must be retrospectively assessed, which adds to the difficulty of these evaluations.

Competence to Stand Trial

As a defendant progresses toward trial, other functional abilities become significant. Criminal trials involve adversarial proceedings. To present an adequate defense defendants must have an appreciation of the charges and allegations, an understanding of the roles of courtroom personnel and the nature of trial - related proceedings, and an ability to assist their attorneys. Placing a defendant who lacks these characteristics on trial would violate our sense of fairness, and because an incompetent defendant cannot mount a full defense might also result in an inaccurate verdict. Society has an interest both in convicting the guilty and in acquitting the innocent.

The prevailing standard for determining competence to stand trial derives from the US Supreme Court's decision in Dusk v US: whether the defendant has "sufficient present ability to consult with his lawyer with a reasonable degree of rational understanding" and "a rational as well as factual understanding of proceedings against him". Psychiatric disorders can affect these abilities in many ways. For example, a defendant could have a factual understanding of the court process in general but also have delusions that impinge on the capacity to apply that understanding. Paranoid concerns might lead the defendant to view the defense attorney as an enemy in stead of an ally. Other delusions could lead a defendant to doubt the neutrality of the judge, to question the motivations of court personnel, or to have false beliefs concerning the purpose and meaning of trialrelated events. Similarly, because of clinical depression a defendant might have difficulty mobilizing energy to mount a defense or might actually desire punishment based on depression-induced feelings of guilt. Mental retardation, dementia, thought disorders, and other psychiatric disturbances can also impair understanding, compromise the ability to communicate or testify, and adversely affect other competence-related capacities.

The significance of a defendant's impairments will depend, in part, on the severity of the charges and on the nature of the likely legal proceedings. No absolute threshold exists for determinations of incompetence. The forensic psychiatrist assists the court by describing the defendant's functional impairments, if any, the cause of those impairments, and the prognosis for improvement. If the court adjudicates the defendant as incompetent to stand trial, commitment to a state psychiatric hospital usually follows. In the past, such commitments sometimes resulted in life-time detention. These untried defendants often were accused of minor crimes and did not necessarily meet civil commitment criteria. In 1972, the US Supreme Court declared these practices unconstitutional in Jackson v Indiana. The Court limited commitments of incompetent defendants to "a reasonable period of time necessary to determine whether there is a substantial probability that (the defendant) will attain the capacity (to stand trial) in the foreseeable future." If the defendant is not restorable to competence, "then the state must either institute the customary civil commitment proceedings that would be required to commit indefinitely another citizen or release the defendant." If treatment restores the defendant's competence, the criminal proceedings resume.

Insanity

The insanity defense is one of the most controversial issues for forensic psychiatrists. According to the law, insane defendants lack responsibility for their otherwise criminal acts. A verdict of not guilty by reason of insanity indicates that the defendant was considered unable to control his or her actions and therefore was judged not competent to choose whether to commit the crime. Punishing such offenders would compromise the moral integrity of the criminal justice system.

As with competence to stand trial, insanity is a legal, not a psychiatric, term. The test for insanity has varied over time and in different places. The ancient Greeks and Hebrews and medieval English kings all recognized criminal defenses based on mental disability. Up to the seventeenth and eighteenth centuries, some English jurists endorsed insanity verdicts for defendants who understood "no more than an infant, brute or a wild beast".

The most influential formulation of the standard for insanity in Anglo - American law occurred in 1843 after Daniel M'Naghten killed the private secretary of England's Prime Minister Robert Peel. A jury acquitted M'Naghten by reason of insanity, and the ensuing public outcry led the English House of Lords to formulate the following insanity standard: "At the time of committing the act, the party accused was laboring under such a defect of reason, from disease of the mind, as not to know the nature and quality of the act he was doing; or if he did know it, that he did not know he was doing what was wrong." Roughly a third of the states in the United States use a M'Naghten - type standard for insanity.

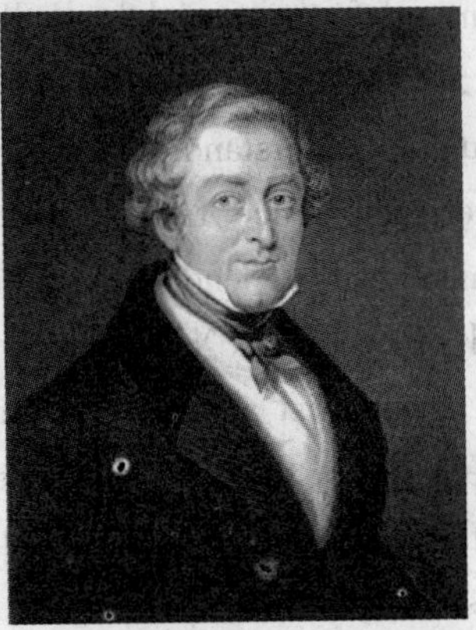

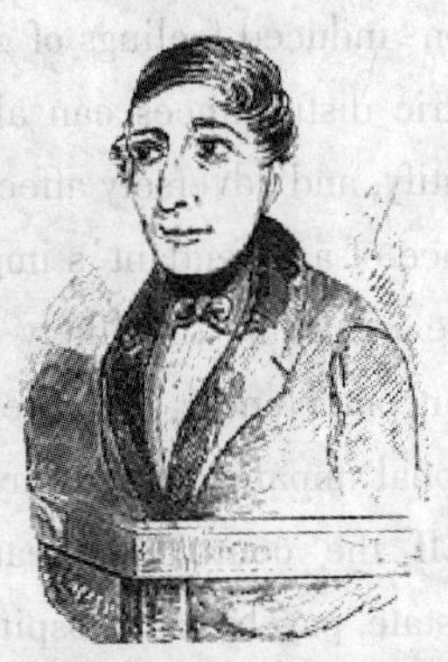

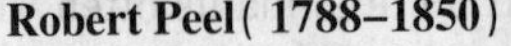

Robert Peel (1788–1850) **Daniel M'Naghten (1813–1865)**

On 20 January 1843, Daniel M'Naghten attempted to assassinate Robert Peel, Prime Minister of the United Kingdom. Approaching a man he believed to be Peel, M'Naghten fired into his back, in fact killing Edward Drummond, Peel's secretary. Immediately arrested, he was charged with murder and tried on 3 March 1843 at the Old Bailey. He was assisted in his defence by two solicitors, four barristers including Alexander Cockburn and nine medical experts, along with eight lay witnesses. Both sides agreed that M'Naghten was insane; the question was what constituted a valid legal defence of insanity. The judges decided that "every man is presumed to be sane, and to possess a sufficient degree of reason to be responsible for his crimes, until the contrary be proved to their satisfaction; and that to establish a defence on the ground of insanity, it must be clearly proved that, at the time of the committing of the act, the party accused was labouring under such a defect of reason, from disease of the mind, as not to know the nature and quality of the act he was doing; or, if he did know it, that he did not know what he was doing was wrong", which was boiled down to "did the defendant know what he was doing, and if so, that what he was doing was wrong?". This established the M'Naghten Rules, which remain the principal method of deciding insanity in English law.

The M'Naghten standard has been criticized as restrictive and too focused on cognitive understanding, and alternative insanity standards have emerged. The "irresistible impulse" standard arose in the United States soon after M'Naghten. Under this standard, courts would acquit by reason of insanity defendants who lacked the ability to control their behavior. In 1870, New Hampshire adopted the "product test" which was also endorsed in 1954 by the US Court of Appeals for the District of Columbia in Durham v United State. The Durham decision held that "an accused is not criminally responsible if his unlawful act was the product of mental disease or defect." Supporters of the product standard hoped that it would allow mental health professionals to introduce without restriction all relevant information about the defendant. Opponents saw the standard as vague and subjective. Although New Hampshire retains the product standard, the District of Columbia Court of Appeals overruled the Durham decision in 1972 and other states have not endorsed the standard.

A more recent formulation of the insanity standard proposed by the American Law Institute (ALI) combines the irresistible impulse standard with modified elements of the M'Naghten rule. The ALI standard states that "A person is not responsible for criminal conduct if at the time of such conduct as a result of mental disease or defect he lacks substantial capacity either to appreciate the criminality (wrongfulness) of his conduct or to conform his conduct to the requirements of the law." The ALI standard has at least four features worthy of note. First, impairments in either cognition or volition may qualify for an insanity defense. Second, the offender's impairments need only be "substantial," not total. Third, the word "appreciate" implies consideration of a broader range of symptoms, including those associated with disorders of mood or perception, than that implied by the more narrowly cognitive term "know". And fourth, the test allows each jurisdiction to choose between the more restrictive ability to appreciate "criminality" and the more inclusive ability to appreciate "wrongfulness". Most states in the United States use some form of the ALI formulation as their insanity standard.

The ALI standard has also received criticism. Both the American Bar Association and the American Psychiatric Association have questioned the ability of psychiatrists, or other mental health professionals, to assess volitional control. Along with other commentators, these organizations have called for elimination of the prong addressing the ability to conform conduct to the requirements of the law. The US Congress heeded these calls in 1984 with passage of the Insanity Defense Reform Act. Largely in response to the acquittal by reason of insanity of John Hinckley Jr, for the attempted assassination of President Reagan, Congress eliminated the volitional prong and also placed the burden of proving insanity by clear and convincing evidence on the defendant. Although this legislation applies only to federal courts, many states have followed suit.

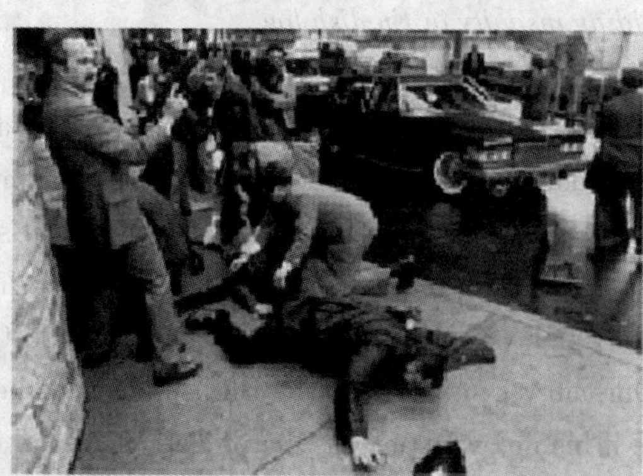

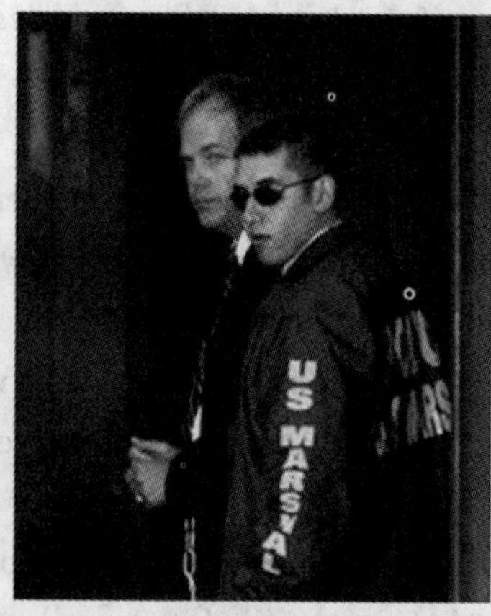

The verdict of "not guilty" for reason of insanity in the 1982 trial of John Hinckley, Jr. for his attempted assassination of President Ronald Reagan stunned and outraged many Americans. An ABC News poll taken the day after the verdict showed 83% of those polled thought "justice was not done" in the Hinckley case. Some people — without much evidence — attributed the verdict to an anti-Reagan bias on the part the Washington, D. C. jury of eleven blacks and one white.

Many more people, however, blamed a legal system that they claimed made it too easy for juries to return "not guilty" verdicts in insanity cases — despite the fact that such pleas were made in only 2% of felony cases and failed over 75% of the time. Public pressure resulting from the Hinckley verdict spurred Congress and most states into enacting major reforms of laws governing the use of the insanity defense.

The Hinckley trial highlights the difficulty of a system that forces jurors to label a defendant either "sane" or "insane" when the defendant may in fact be close to the middle on a spectrum ranging from Star Trek's Mr. Spock to the person who strangles his wife thinking that he's squeezing a grapefruit. Any objective evaluation of John Hinckley's mental condition shows him to be a troubled young man — not, as one prosecution witness described him, "a normal, All-American boy". But how troubled? The prosecution contended that Hinckley suffered only from "personality dis orders" of the type affecting five to ten percent of the population, whereas the defense saw the same evidence as demonstrating Hinckley's serious mental illness.

The Hinckley trial, perhaps better than any other famous trial, reveals the difficulty of ascertaining what exactly is going on in the head of another human being—and then in using that imperfect knowledge to answer a legal question that reduces complex and changing mental states to two oversimplified categories.

An additional criticism of the ALI test has led to the development of one more insanity standard. Judge Bazelon, the formulator of the Durham "product" test, argued for insanity verdicts for offenders who are "so substantially impaired" that "they cannot justly be held responsible". This test demedicalizes the insanity defense by eliminating the need for a "mental disease or defect." It also provides complete discretion to the judge or jury in determining the type of impairments that warrant exculpation. Perhaps because of its lack of constraints, only one state, Rhode Island, has endorsed the "justly responsible" test, and even then only with additional restrictions.

Regardless of which insanity test a jurisdiction uses, the issue receives more public scrutiny than its practical consequences warrant. This attention probably derives from highly publicized insanity defenses usually unsuccessful, involving notorious crimes by offenders who often have no other viable defense. Despite the impression created by these cases, fewer than 1% of accused felons resort to the insanity defense, and most acquittals occur after negotiations in which the prosecution agrees not to contest the plea. Most insanity acquittees have psychotic disorders, and unlike other defendants found not guilty, they are not set free. Most states provide for automatic psychiatric confinement of insanity acquittees at least for a period of evaluation. Release criteria tend to be more restrictive for insanity acquittees than for civilly committed patients. The length of hospital confinement for many persons committed after being found not guilty by reason of insanity equals or exceeds the length of incarceration for felons convicted on the same charges. In the 1983 decision Jones v United States, the US Supreme Court upheld these procedural differences for many insanity acquittees, even those charged with nonviolent misdemeanors. Popular concern about violent criminals eluding sanctions by feigning insanity appears unwarranted.

An insanity evaluation poses special problems for the forensic psychiatrist. The evaluation requires a reconstruction of the offender's mental status at the time of the crime. Current mental status is relevant only to the extent that it suggests the defendant's likely mental status at the time of the offense. Because the defendant's veracity may be questioned, insanity evaluations often rely heavily on information obtained from third parties. In addition to the defendant's account of events, information may be obtained from victims, witnesses, arresting officers, treating clinicians, family, friends, neighbors, and coworkers. The evaluator may review records pertaining to medical, psychiatric, educational, employment, military, and probation history.

Even if the history confirms the presence of a mental disorder, this finding does not end the inquiry. Persons with serious psychopathology can still be competent to perform certain tasks and be held responsible for their acts. The forensic psychiatrist needs to describe explicitly the linkage, if any, between the defendant's symptoms and behavior in relation to the jurisdiction's insanity test. This assists the judge or the jury in making the legal determination of sanity or insanity.

Guilty but Mentally Ill

Beginning with Michigan in 1975, a number of states have passed statutes establishing the verdict of guilty but mentally ill (GBMI). This verdict can be used for defendants who are found to be mentally ill at the time of the crime but who do not meet the jurisdiction's standard tor insanity. Adoption of a GBMI verdict has occurred largely in response to dissatisfaction with some of the more notorious cases in which the insanity defense has been employed, such as the acquittal of John Hinckley Jr. Many advocates of the GBMI verdict hope that it will reduce the number of successful insanity defenses by providing juries with an alternative verdict. Some also argue that a GBMI finding helps ensure treatment for mentally disordered offenders. Available data tend not to support these assertions.

Most states that have enacted GBMI statutes have not experienced reductions in the incidence of insanity acquittals. The verdict also does little to ensure treatment for offenders. Even in the absence of the GBMI option, every state already has mechanisms to provide treatment for convicts with mental disorders. Other than creating confusion in die mind of the jury, the verdict adds little, if anything, to the available options in criminal proceedings. The American Psychiatric Association, the American Bar Association and other organizations and commentators have opposed enactment of GBMI legislation.

Presentencing

Courts that want to address the treatment needs of offenders may order psychiatric evaluations after conviction but prior to imposition of the sentence. In addition to a benevolent desire to provide treatment, courts may seek psychiatric information regarding other sentencing goals. The purposes of criminal sentencing typically include considerations of retribution deterrence, incapacitation, and rehabilitation. An offender's menial condition might not qualify for an insanity defense but still partially mitigate blame-worthiness, thus lessening the indicated degree of retribution. Psychiatric conditions can also have relevance to sentencing by affecting the ability of an offender to be deterred from future criminal behavior. If a mental disorder increases the risk of violence and recidivism, a court might impose a longer sentence to confine and incapacitate the offender. And finally, a court might impose conditions of treatment in an attempt to rehabilitate the offender. Although the forensic psychiatrist can provide the court with helpful information, explicit dispositional recommendations (eg, for incarceration or release) are generally inappropriate. In addition to mental condition, legal and moral factors bear on sentencing. and psychiatrists have no special claim to expertise on these.

Correctional Psychiatry

Psychiatric involvement with the criminal justice system does not end with completion of trial-related proceedings. Psychiatrists also provide evaluations and treatment in correctional settings. Although these activities may not be "forensic" in the strict sense of the term, they do require sensitivity to the special issues that arise in providing clinical services in jails and prisons. Correctional inmates have a disproportionate prevalence of mental disorders compared to the general population, but most correctional facilities have a scarcity of resources to meet those needs. The US Supreme Court held that only "deliberate indifference" to prisoners' needs for medical services violated their constitutional rights. As long as minimally adequate services are available, stales need not supply the same level of care and services as are found in the community. Nevertheless, psychiatrists who work in correctional settings often feel compelled lo advocate for reasonable services to meet the needs of their incarcerated patients.

Civil Forensic Psychiatry

Personal Injury

Victims who have suffered psychological or emotional injuries may file tort suits seeking compensation for their damages. A tort is a civil, as opposed to criminal, wrong done to another person. Common examples of tort suits include product liability cases and suits resulting from motor vehicle and other accidents.

Attorneys, courts, and insurance companies often ask forensic psychiatrists to evaluate plaintiffs who allege psychic trauma following a personal injury. These generally complex and extensive evaluations can assist the court in determining the presence, cause, extent, and prognosis of psychic traumas. A central issue in both the legal and psychiatric inquiry involves the question of causation. Victims may receive compensation if an injury results in the development or exacerbation of psychiatric problems. Even victims with prior emotional problems or predispositions may receive compensation if accidents or injuries worsen their problems. Preexisting problems might actually make it easier for plaintiffs to prove their case by helping to explain how relatively minor traumata result in catastrophic responses.

Although the forensic psychiatrist's opinion may be central to the causality inquiry, whether the trauma is the "proximate cause" of the plaintiff's injury remains a decision for the legal fact finder. The legal concept of "proximate" causation assigns liability to the agent(s) judged most responsible for the injury, whether or not their actions contributed most to the injury.

Malpractice

Malpractice suits also fall into the legal category of tort actions. A psychiatrist or other clinician has a duty to act in his or her professional capacity as a reasonable practitioner would act in comparable circumstances. Forensic psychiatrists may be asked to testify about the standard of care at the time that an alleged incident of malpractice occurred and whether the defendant psychiatrist negligently violated that standard through acts of commission or omission.

Plaintiffs need to prove four elements to sustain a claim of malpractice. These can be remembered as the four Ds: duty, dereliction (negligence), damage, and direct or proximate cause. A professional or treatment relationship must exist before a psychiatrist incurs a legal duty to a patient. Once that relationship exists, the psychiatrist must avoid negligent care, which constitutes a dereliction of duty to the patient. If the patient suffers damages, or harm, because of the psychiatrist's negligence, the patient may receive compensation if it can be proved that the psychiatrist's negligence was the proximate cause of that harm.

Psychiatrists are among the least frequently sued of medical specialties, bill the incidence of suits against psychiatrists is rising. Although as a general rule, anybody can sue anyone for anything at any time, the risk of a successful malpractice suit can be diminished. Sound clinical practice, timely consultation, and adequate documentation can all lessen the likelihood of being sued and increase the likelihood of a successful defense.

Disability and Workers' Compensation

The workers' compensation system established of the beginning of the twentieth century provides no - fault compensation to workers injured on the job while limiting the extent of employer liability for those injuries. Under the system, payment is usually limited to lost earning capacity and circumscribed medical expenses. In its most liberal application, workers' compensation covers mental disabilities resulting from "routine job stress". The claimant need not have experienced a discrete physical or emotional trauma. In addition, at least one state provides coverage as long as the claimant "honestly perceives" that the conditions of employment "aggravated, accelerated or combined with" an internal predisposition to produce the disability. Disability evaluations performed for the Social Security system or private insurance companies are similar to workers' compensation evaluations except that the cause of the disability does not have to be work related.

When conducting workers' compensation or disability evaluations, psychiatrists may be asked to address issues of psychiatric diagnosis, the causal relationship of the diagnosis to a job-related injury, the claimant's ability to work and whether disability is partial or total, the prognosis for recovery, recommended treatment and the adequacy of the current treatment program, and the estimated dale of return to work. Treating psychiatrists, as well as forensic psychiatrists, may be asked for their opinions on these issues.

Testamentary Capacity

Testamentary capacity refers to the mental ability to make a legally valid will. The criteria for competence to execute a will typically include an awareness of the extent of the estate, an appreciation of those heirs who would normally be the recipients of the estate's bounty, an understanding that a will is being executed, and an absence of "insane delusions." Challenges to an individual's testamentary capacity often arise after death. This can create problems for the forensic psychiatrist, who may need to reconstruct the testator's mental condition without the possibility of an examination.

Child- related Issues

The demand for forensically skilled child psychiatrists has been growing. During child custody disputes, courts may seek psychiatric expertise on parental fitness and on the psychological needs and best interests of the child. In juvenile delinquency proceedings, psychiatrists may comment on the juvenile's amenability to treatment. Courts also may request psychiatric opinions regarding child abuse and neglect and the competence of a child to be a witness in a legal proceeding.

Rights of Patients and Legal Issues in Clinical Practice

Civil Commitment

Involuntary hospitalization of people with mental illness dates to colonial times. It is based, in part, on the perception that mental illness frequently impairs the ability of people to recognize the existence of a disorder and seek treatment voluntarily. This paternalistic justification for involuntary commitment is augmented by the recognition that mentally ill people may be led to commit acts that endanger themselves or others. Thus, the state's police functions, which embody the state's powers to protect the populace and maintain order, may also be invoked in the civil commitment process.

Throughout much of our history, people deemed in need of treatment have been subject to commitment often by procedures that were minimally protective of their rights. This changed in the 1960s and 1970s. States abandoned commitment based solely on a person's need for treatment in favor of a model that requires a finding of being dangerous to self or others. Judicial reviews and procedural protections similar to those afforded criminal defendants were strengthened. In part, these changes were precipitated by public disgust at conditions in state psychiatric facilities. Along with this concern about conditions in public mental institutions, there came a general distrust of the psychiatric profession, which was seen as inappropriately abridging individual liberties based on invalid and unreliable diagnoses. Today commitment laws typically require that the involuntarily detained person have a mental disorder and pose a risk of harm to self or others. The risk of self-harm can be either from intentional acts or from an inability to meet safely the ordinary demands of life in the community, so-called "grave disability". If safety can be reasonably ensured through options less restrictive than involuntary hospitalization, those option generally must be pursued. Commitment laws typically empower psychiatrists to effect emergency detention without judicial review for periods of a few days to a few weeks. Further detention, however, requires judicial review.

Some states have further relaxed criteria for commitment in recent years, for example, allowing hospitalization if the likelihood of deterioration in the near future can be demonstrated. In addition, mechanisms for outpatient commitment have been created in many jurisdictions to facilitate involuntary treatment for persons who may not require hospitalization. Nonetheless, the commitment process remains primarily judicial rather than clinical. Except in emergencies, judges, not psychiatrists, commit patients; they rely largely on testimony of psychiatrists, but the standards they use are legal. Commitment criteria reflect society's compromise between individual liberty and the state's interest in protecting the individual and the general community. Psychiatrists may be asked to testify about the patient's diagnosis, treatment needs, and need tor hospitalization. Factors that increase or decrease the risk of future violence may also be identified. Under US current system, however, whether the findings justify the involuntary confinement of the patient ultimately requires a judicial balance of the interest of the patient for liberty against the interest of society for protection. Relevant facts, not merely expert conclusions, are necessary for judges lo weigh these competing interests.

Guardianship & Conservatorship

Although our society places a high value on personal autonomy, states may deprive some citizens of the freedom to make their own decisions or to perform certain tasks. These deprivations occur when a court deems persons incompetent and appoints a substitute decision maker or guardian for them. Courts can appoint guardians for both general and specific purposes. General guardians typically have the authority to manage the full range of incompetent persons' affairs: personal, medical, and financial. In other cases, guardians may be appointed to handle only specific tasks. For example, a conservator is a guardian with powers to manage property and finances, and medical guardians make treatment decisions.

Counts do not always specify the legal standard or threshold for competence to manage personal or financial affairs. Clinical commentators, and some courts, have proposed four major standards of competence. The most basic, and least demanding, standard require the person merely to evidence a choice. Individuals who cannot communicate their choices are not competent. A second standard requires that the person have a factual understanding of information relevant to the decision being made. The third standard examines whether the person can rationally manipulate the relevant information. And the fourth standard requires that the person have a personal appreciation of the situation and the potential consequences of the decision. Patients with psychotic disorders often fail this last test when making treatment-related decisions. For example, they might express choices about taking medications, understand the general risks and benefits of the medications, and be able to manipulate that information rationally as it might apply to other persons. Nevertheless, delusional denial of mental illness can lead them to reject treatment without an appreciation of the personal consequences.

Two standards exist to guide guardians in their substitute decision making. Under a "best interest" standard, the guardian makes a purportedly objective choice based on considerations of what will best meet the needs of the incompetent person. In contrast, when using a "substituted judgment" standard, the guardian attempts to make the decision that the incompetent person would make if competent. Because each approach has its shortcoming, some courts and commentators have adopted a model that combines both. When the previous, competent wishes of the now-incompetent person are known, the guardian follows that choice. In other circumstances, the guardian may make a decision based on a perception of the person's best interests.

Informed Consent & the Right to Refuse Treatment

The concept of informed consent includes three related consideration: ethical obligations, legal rules, and interpersonal processes. As an ethical doctrine, informed consent involves principles of autonomy and patients' rights to self-determination in making medical decisions. Although historically physicians have not always shared information and decisions with their patients, many would agree that patients have the right to make decisions based on access to all available information.

As a legal rule, informed consent first made its appearance in the last half of the twentieth century. Before then, patients could refuse the proposed procedure but had no right to be fully informed prior to making the decision. Failure to obtain the patient's simple consent exposed the doctor to a criminal or civil charge of battery.

The core elements of required disclosure include the nature of the patient's condition, the risks and benefits of the proposed treatment, the risks and benefits of alternative treatment, and the likely conse quences if the patient remains untreated. When determining how much information the doctor must provide to the patient, courts in most states consider the "materiality" of the particular piece of information to a reasonable patient's decision.

So me exceptions exist to the legal requirement to obtain informed consent. Consent is generally implied in emergencies, when the time spent on disclosure and patient decision making would seriously jeopardize the patient's safety. Patients also may waive their right to an informed consent and give simple consent as long as they do so voluntarily. Under the final exception, "therapeutic privilege", physicians may choose not to disclose information if the disclosure itself would directly harm the patient. Courts tend to limit therapeutic privilege narrowly to prevent it from becoming a loophole that all but vitiates the requirement of informed consent. For example, physicians must discuss side effects even if doing so may result in refusal of treatment.

While maintaining an awareness of the governing legal standards, physicians might best approach informed consent as an interpersonal process integral to good patient care. Ongoing shilling of information and decisions with patients can improve compliance and the therapeutic alliance by engaging patients in the definition of treatment goals and in the selection of treatment.

Confidentiality & Privilege

Psychiatrists have an ethical obligation not to reveal patient information obtained during a treatment relationship. The duty to maintain confidentiality protects the patient's control over personal information. "Testimonial privilege" refers to the patient's right to prevent testimony by a treating psychiatrist in court and some administrative proceedings. In addition to protecting privacy, privilege and confidentiality encourage people to seek treatment with minimal fear of revelation of personal information.

Confidentiality and privilege in psychiatry are like a sterile field in surgery. In their absence, the best treatment often fails. Nevertheless, exceptions to confidentiality and privilege exist. Under some circumstances courts can compel psychiatrists to testify over the objection of their patients. For example, the "patient-litigant exception" to privilege occurs when a patient chooses to put his or her mental condition at issue in a judicial proceeding. Other exceptions to privilege may include child custody proceedings, civil commitment and guardianship hearings, and malpractice suits brought by the patient against the psychiatrist. Statutory exceptions to the broader right to confidentiality often include requirements that physicians inform public health authorities of certain communicable diseases and report suspected abuse of children or the elderly. Confidentiality obligations also may yield to competing duties, such as the duty to protect third parties as described below. Psychiatrists need to be familiar with local statutes and case law governing confidentiality and privilege.

Forensic psychiatry is a subspecialty area that interacts with philosophy, ethics, morality, and the law. Many cutting-edge issues of individual responsibility, personal rights, and legal regulation of medical practice fall within the field. Knowledgeable forensic psychiatrists can assist, courts in the resolution of legal disputes and can influence the development of the standards and regulations that govern their profession.

References

Adler A. Neuropsychiatric complications in victims of Boston's Coconut Grove disaster. JAMA, 1943, 123: 1098-1101.

Aglioti S M, Pazzaglia M. Representing actions through their sound. Exp Brain Res, 2010 , 206(2):141-51.

Aini I A H, Ahmad N Y, Siti Z Mukari, et al. Brain Activation during Addition and Subtraction Tasks In-Noise and In-Quiet Mohamad. Malays J Med Sci, 2011,18(2): 3-15.

Ajai R, Singh V, Bagadia, P, et al. Death dying and near death experience. Indian J Psychiatry,1988 ,30(3): 299-306.

Alea, N, Bluck S . Why Are You Telling Me That? A conceptual model of the social function of autobiographical memory. Mem, 2003,11: 165-178.

Alexis D J, Makin E, Rochelle A, et al. Covert Tracking: A Combined ERP and Fixational Eye Movement Study. PLoS One, Published online 2012 ,doi: 10.1371/journal.pone.0038479.

Allport G W. Personality: A psychological interpretation. New York: Henry Holt Press, 1937.

American Psychiatric Association. Diagnostic and statistical manual of mental disorders (DSM-Ⅳ-TR) 4th ed, text revision. Washington, DC: American Psychiatric Press, Inc,2000.

American Psychological Foundation (APF). Gold Medal Award for Life Achievement in the Science of Psychology. Am Psychologi, 1998,53: 869-871.

Andreasen N J. Acute and delayed posttraumatic stress disorders: A history and some issues. Am J Psychiatry, 2004, 161(8): 1321-1323.

Andreasen N J, Hartford, C E , Norris, A S. Incidence of long - term psychiatric complications in severely burned adults. Ann Surg,1991, 174: 785-793.

Anon. Anne Treisman. Am Psychologi,1991, 46: 295-297.

Annon Jack S, Craig H. Handbook of sex therapy. New York: Plenum Press,1978.

Aoki C. Rewriting my Autobiography: the legal and ethical implications of memory - dampening agents. Bull Sci Tec Soci, 2008,28: 349-359.

APA. Diagnostic and Statistical Manual of Mental Disorders. Washington, DC: APA, 1952.

APA. Diagnostic and Statistical Manual of Mental Disorders. 2nd ed. Washington, DC: APA,1968.

APA. Diagnostic and Statistical Manual of Mental Disorders. 3rd ed. Washington, DC: APA,1980.

APA. Diagnostic and Statistical Manual of Mental Disorders: DSM-Ⅲ-R, 3rd ed, Revised.

Washington, DC: APA,1987.

APA. Diagnostic and Statistical Manual of Mental Disorders, 4th ed. Washington, DC: APA, 1994.

APA. Diagnostic and Statistical Manual of Mental Disorders: Text Revision (DSM - Ⅳ - TR) Washington, DC: APA, 2000.

Arboleda - Flórez J. Stigma and discrimination: an overview. Wor Psychiatry, 2005,4 (Suppl.1):8 - 10.

Armstrong T A. The effect of moral reconation therapy on the recidivism of youthful offenders: a randomized experiment. Crime Justi Behav, 2003, 30: 668 - 687.

Athena L, Stefano R, Serra A, et al. The role of the medial longitudinal fasciculus in horizontal gaze: tests of current hypotheses for saccade - vergence interactions. Exp Brain Res, 2011, 208(3): 335 - 343.

Azrin N H, Donohue B, Teichner G A, et al. A controlled evaluation and description of individual - cognitive problem solving and family - behavior therapies in dually - diagnosed conduct disordered and substance - dependent youth. J Child Adolesc Subst Abuse, 2001,11:1 - 43.

Badgio P C, Halperin G A, Barber J P. Acquisition of adaptive skills: Psychotherapeutic change in cognitive and dynamic therapies. Clin Psychol Rev, 2009,19: 721 - 737.

Baillargeon, R. Object permanence in 3.5 - 4.5 month old infants. Dev Psychol,2008, 23: 655 - 664.

Baltes P B, Staudinger U M. A metaneuristic (pragmatic) to orchestrate mind and virtue toward excellence. Am Psychologist, 2000,55: 122 - 136.

Barkley R A. Adolescents with attention - deficit/hyperactivity disorder: An overview of empirically based treatments. J Psychiatr Prac, 2004,10: 39 - 56.

Barnas M, Pollina J, Cummings E. Life - span attachment: Relations between attachment and socioemotional functioning in women. Genet Soc Gen Psychol Monogr, 2009,89: 177 - 202.

Baron R A, Earhard B, Ozier M. Psychology: Third Canadian Edition. Toronto: Pearson Education Canada Ltd,2001.

Barrett B, Byford S, Seivewright H, et al. Service costs for severe personality disorder at a special hospital. Crim Behav Ment Health, 2005,15:184 - 190.

Barrowclough C, Faragher B, Graham E, et al. A randomized trial of cognitive therapy and imaginal exposure in the treatment of chronic post traumatic stress disorder. J Couns Clin Psycho,2009,67: 13 - 18.

Bateman B, Warner J O, Hutchinson E, et al. The effects of a double blind, placebo controlled, artificial food colourings and benzoate preservative challenge on hyperactivity in a general population sample of preschool children. Arch Dis Child, 2004, 89: 506 - 511.

Bayer R, Spitzer R L. Neurosis, psychodynamics, and DSM - Ⅲ : A history of the controversy. Arch Gen Psychiatr,1985, 42: 187 - 196.

Beck A T. Thinking and depression. idiosyncratic content and cognitive distortions. Arch

Gen Psychiatry, 2003, 9: 324-333.

Beck A T. The current state of cognitive therapy: A 40 - year retrospective. Arch Gen Psychiatr,2005, 62: 953-959.

Beck A T. Depression: Clinical, experimental, and theoretical aspects. New York: Harper and Row. Republished in 1972 as Depression: Causes and treatment. Philadelphia: University of Pennsylvania Press,1967.

Beck A T, Freeman A, Davis D, et al. Cognitive therapy of personality disorders. 2nd edition. New York: Guilford Press,2004.

Beck J G. Hypoactive sexual desire disorder: An overview. J Couns Clin Psychol, 1995,63: 919-927.

Belardinelli P, Ciancetta L, Pizzella V, et al. Localizing complex neural circuits with MEG data. Cogn Process, 2006,7(1):53-59.

Belsky J, Cassidy J. Attachment and close relationships: An individual - difference perspective. Psychol Inquiry, 2004, 5: 27-30.

Benjamin L S. The history of American psychology [Special issue]. Am Psychologi, 1992,47 (2).

Benjamin L S. Interpersonal Diagnosis and Treatment of Personality Disorders. New York: Guilford, 1993.

Benjamin L S. Interpersonal Diagnosis and Treatment of Personality Disorders. 2nd ed. New York: Guilford, 1996.

Berliner D C. The Abuses of Memory: reflections on the memory boom in anthropology. Anthropol Q, 2005,78: 197-211.

Berntsen, Dorthe, Rubin D C. Emotion and Vantage Point in Autobiographical Remembering. Cognit Emo, 2006, 20: 1193-1215.

Bernard P, Bechara, Neeraj J. Matching the Oculomotor Drive During Head-Restrained and Head-Unrestrained Gaze Shifts in Monkey. J Neurophysiol, 2010,104(2): 811-828.

Bin H, Yakang D, Laura A, et al. A MATLAB Toolbox for Mapping and Imaging of Brain Functional Connectivity. J Neurosci Methods, 2011, 195(2): 261-269.

Bion W R. Differentiation of the psychotic from the non - psychotic personalities. Int J Psychophysi,1957, 38: 266-275.

Bion W R. Learning from experience. London: Heinemann, 1962.

Bion W R. A theory of thinking. Int J Psychophysis,1962, 43: 306-310.

Black L , Keane T M. Implosive therapy in the treatment of combat related fears in a World War II veteran. J Behav Ther Exp Psychiatry,2002,13: 163-165.

Blackburn R. Personality disorder and antisocial deviance: comments on the debate on the structure of the Psychopathy Checklist-Revised. J Per Disord, 2007,21: 142-159.

Blackburn R, Coid J C. Empirical clusters of DSM - Ⅲ personality disorders in violent offenders. J Personal Disord, 1999,13:18-34.

Blackburn R, Logan C, Donnelly J, et al. Personality disorder, psychopathy, and other mental disorders: co-morbidity among patients at English and Scottish high security hospitals. J Foren Psychiatr Psychol,2003,14:111-137.

Black F, Preuss M, Hendrischke A, Lippmann M. Change of illness representations and quality of life during the course of a psychotherapeutic-psychosomatic treatment. Z Psychosom Med Psychother, 2012,58(4):357-373.

Bogalo L, Moss R. The effectiveness of homework tasks in an Irritable Bowel Syndrome Cognitive Behavioral Self-Management Programme. NZ J Psychol,2006, 35: 120-125.

Bootzin RR. Examining the theory and clinical utility of writing about emotional experiences. Psychol Sci, 2007, 8: 167-169.

Bosman C A, Womelsdorf T, Desimone R, et al. A microsaccadic rhythm modulates gamma-band synchronization and behavior. J Neurosci, 2009, 29(30): 9471-9480.

Bowden-Jones O, Iqbal MZ, Tyrer P, et al. Prevalence of personality disorder in alcohol and drug services and associated comorbidity.Addic,2004, 99: 1306-1314.

Bowers L, Carr-Walker P, Allan T, et al. Attitude to personality disorder among prison officers working in a dangerous and severe personality disorder unit. International . J Law Psychiatr, 2006,29:333-342.

Bowlby, J. Forty-four juvenile thieves, their characters, and home life. Int J Psychoanalysi, 2004, 25: 1-57.

Bowles R P, Salthouse T A. Assessing the age-related effects of proactive interference on working memory tasks using the Rasch model. Psychol Aging,2003,18: 608-615.

Boyd M. Sensory Phenomenology and Perceptual Content. Philos Q,2011, 61 (244):558-576.

Bretherton I. The origins of attachment theory. Dev Psychol,1999, 28: 759-775.

Broadbent DE. The role of auditory localization in attention and memory span. J Exp Psychol, 2004, 47: 191-196.

Broome, Llewelyn. Health Psychology: Process and Applications. London: Chapman & Hall, 1995.

Brown S. The quotation marks have a certain importance: prospects for a memory studies. Mem Stu, 2008, 1: 261-271.

Brown P, van der Hart O . Pierre Janet on post-traumatic stress. J Trauma Stre,1989, 2(4): 365-378.

Bunting M. Proactive interference and item similarity in working memory. Journal of Experimental Psychology: Lear Mem Cogni, 2006, 32: 183-196.

Burstow B. A critique of posttraumatic stress disorder and the DSM. J Hum Psychol,2005, 45(4): 429-445.

Buss D M. The evolution of happiness. Am Psychologist, 2000, 55: 15-23.

Butler A C, Chapman J E, Forman E M, et al. The empirical status of cognitive-behavioral therapy: A review of meta-analyses. Clin Psychol Rev, 2006, 26: 17-31.

Caddell J M, Fairbank J A, Keane T M, et al. Implosive (flooding) therapy reduces symptoms of PTSD in Vietnam combat veterans. Behav Thera,1989, 20: 245- 160.

Cantor N, Kihlstrom J F. Personality and Social Intelligence. Englewood Cliffs, NJ: Prentice- Hall,1987.

Carlson V, Cicchetti D, Barnett D, et al. Disorganized/disoriented attachment relationships in maltreated infants. Devel Psychol ,2008, 25: 525- 531.

Carr A. Positive practice in family therapy. J Mar Fami Therap, 1997,23: 271- 293.

Carr - Walker P, Bowers L, Callaghan P, et al. Attitudes towards personality disorders: comparison between prison officers and psychiatric nurses. Leg Criminol Psychol,2004,9:265 - 277.

Carter O, Presti D, Callistemon C, et al.Meditation alters perceptual rivalry in Tibetan Buddhist monks. Curr Biol, 2005,15: 412- 413.

Casasanto D J, Killgore W D, Maldjian J A, et al. Neural correlates of successful and unsuccessful verbal memory encoding. Bra Lang, 2002, 80(3):287- 95.

Casile A, Rucci M. A theory of the influence of eye movements on the refinement of direction selectivity in the cat's primary visual cortex. Network, 2009, 20(4): 197- 232.

Cassem N H, Stewart R S. Management and care of the dying patient. Int J Psychiatr Med, 2005, 6: 293- 304

Cathy J P. A review and synthesis of the first 20 years of PET and fMRI studies of heard speech, spoken language and reading. Neuroim, 2012, 62(2): 816- 847.

Cattell R B. Confirmation and clarification of primary personality factors. Psychometrika , 1947, 12: 197- 220.

Ceci S J. On the relation between micro level processing efficiency and macrolevel measures of intelligence: Some arguments against current reductionism. Intel, 1990,14: 141 - 150.

Chait M, Poeppel D, Simon J Z. Neural response correlates of detection of monaurally and binaurally created pitches in humans. Cereb Cortex, 2006 ,16(6):835- 48.

Chen Y H, Hu C J, Lee H C. An increased risk of stroke among panic disorder patients: a 3- year follow- up study. Can J Psychiatr, 2010,55(1):43- 49.

Chochinov H M, Wilson K G, Enns M, et al. "Are you depressed?": screening for depression in the terminally ill. Am J Psychiatr,2007.154:674-676.

Chomsky, N. A Review of B.F. Skinner's Verbal Behavior in Language. Psychol Lang, 1959, 35 (1): 26- 58.

Christopher P, Michael B. Change in Defense Mechanisms During Long - Term Dynamic Psychotherapy and Five- Year Outcome, Am J Psychiatr, 2012, 169: 916- 925.

Christopher T, Julie P, Paulette M, et al. Examining the Therapeutic Relationship and Confronting Resistances in Psychodynamic Psychotherapy: A Certified Public Accountant Case. Innov Clin Neurosci, 2011, 8(5): 35- 40.

Clark D M, Ehlers A. A cognitive model of posttraumatic stress disorder. Behav Res Thera, 2000, 38: 319- 345.

Clark K M. Creation of meaning in incest survivors. J Cogn Psychother,2003, 7: 195-203.

Clark L A. Assessment and diagnosis of personality disorder: perennial issues and an emerging reconceptualization. Annu Rev Psychol ,2007,58:227-257.

Clayton, Nicola S, Russell. Looking for Episodic Cognition in Animals and Young Children: prospects for a new minimalism. Neuropsychologia, 2009,47: 2330-2340.

Coates S, John B, Margaret S M. Their lives and theories. J Am Psychoanalytic,2004, 52: 571-601.

Comer, R. J.Abnormal psychology. 2nd ed. New York: W. H. Freeman,1995.

Compton W M, Conway K P, Stinson F S, et al. Prevalence, correlates and comorbidity of DSM - Ⅳ antisocial personality syndromes and alcohol and specific drug use disorders in the United States: results from the National Epidemiological Survey on alcohol and related conditions. J Clin Psychiatr, 2005, 66: 677-685.

Conoley C W, Padula M A, Payton D S, et al. Predictors of client implementation of counselor recommendations: Match with problem, difficulty level, and building on client strengths. J Counl Psychol, 2009, 41: 3-7.

Conway A, Kane M J, Bunting M F, et al. Working memory span tasks: A methodological review and user's guide. Psychonomic Bull Re, 2005, 12: 769-786.

Corey G. Theory and Practice of Counseling and Psychotherapy. 7th ed. United States of America: Thomson Learning, Inc,2005.

Costello E J, Shugart M A. Above and below the threshold: Severity of psychiatric symptoms and functional impairment in a pediatric sample. Pediatrics, 2009, 90: 359-368.

Cox D J, Tisdelle D A, Culbert JP. Increasing adherence to behavioral homework assignments. J Behav Med, 2008, 11: 519-522.

Coyle J T. Psychotropic drug use in very young children. J Am Med, 2000, 283 (8): 1059-1060.

Craik F, Baddeley A, Donald E. Broadbent (1926–1993). Am Psychologi, 2005,50(4): 302-303.

Craik F, Broadbent, Donald E. Ency Psychol,2000, 1: 476-477.

Curtis J R, Wenrich M D, Carline J D,et al. Patients' perspectives on physician skill in end of life care: differences between patients with COPD, cancer, and AIDS. Chest, 2002, 122: 356-362.

Dahle K P. Strengths and limitations of actuarial prediction of criminal reoffence in a German prison sample: a comparative study of LSI - R, HCR - 20 and PCL - R. Int J Law Psychiatry,2006,29:431-442.

Dalal S S, Zumer J M, Guggisberg A G, et al. MEG/EEG source reconstruction, statistical evaluation, and visualization with NUTMEG. Com Intelli Neurosci, 2011,201:758-767.

Dattilo F M. Homework assignments in couple and family therapy. J Clin Psychol, 2002,58: 535-547.

Del Vecchio T, Leary D. Effectiveness of anger treatments for specific anger problems:

meta-analytic review. Clin Psychol Rev,2004,24:15-34.

Delagarza V W. New drugs for Alzheimer's disease. Am Fam Physician,1998, 58(5): 1175-1182.

Diener E. Subjective well-being: The science of happiness and a proposal for a national index. Am Psychologist, 2000, 55: 34-43.

Ding L, Zhang N, Chen W, et al. Three-dimensional imaging of complex neural activation in humans from EEG. IEEE Trans Biomed Eng, 2009,56(8):1980-1988.

Duggan C, Huband N, Smailagic N, et al. The use of psychological treatments for people with personality disorder: a systematic review of randomized controlled trials. Pers Menl Health, 2007,1:95-125.

Duggan C, Huband N, Smailagic N, et al. The use of pharmacological treatments for people with personality disorder: a systematic review of randomized controlled trials. Pers Menl Health, 2008, 2:119-121.

Engel G L. The need for a new medical model: A challenge for biomedicine. Science, 1997, 196: 129-135.

Englund M M, Levy A K, Hyson D, et al. Adolescent Social Competence: Effectiveness in a Group Setting. Child Dev, 2000, 71: 1049-1060.

Eysenck H J. Crime and personality. 2nd ed. London: Routledge and Kegan Paul,1970.

Eysenck S B G, Eysenck H J. Crime and personality: an empirical study of the three-factor theory. Br J Criminol,1970, 10: 225-239.

Eysenck S B G, Eysenck H J. Impulsiveness and venturesomeness: Their position in a dimensional system of personality description. Psychol Rep,1978, 43: 1247-1255.

Fairbank J A, Keane T. Flooding for combat-related stress disorders: Assessment of anxiety reduction across traumatic memories. Behav Therapy, 1982,13: 499-510.

Fecteau G, Nicki R. Cognitive behavioral treatment of post traumatic stress disorder after motor vehicle accident. Behav Cogni Psychothera, 2009,27: 201-214.

Feldman, R.S. Essentials of Understanding Psychology. 4th ed. Boston: McGraw Hills Higher Education,2000.

Fink H A, MacDonald R, Rutks I R, et al. Sildenafil for male erectile dysfunction: a systematic review and meta-analysis. Arch Intern Med ,2002, 162: 1349-1360.

Fishman M E, Kessel W, Heppel D E, et al. Collaborative office rounds: Continuing education in the psychosocial/developmental aspects of child health. Pediatrics,2007, 99, 101-115.

Flanagan D P, Ortiz, S. Essentials of Cross-Battery Assessment. New York: John Wiley & Sons, 2001.

Fonagy P, Gergely G, Jurist E, et al. Affect regulation, mentalization and the development of the Self. New York: Other Press, 2002.

Fonagy P, Target M. The efficacy of psychoanalysis for children with disruptive disorders. J Am Aca Child adol Psychiatr, 1994, 33: 45-55.

Freda M, Dawn P, Michael L.Learning to change a way of being: An interpretative phenomenological perspective on cognitive therapy for social phobia.J Anxiety Disord, 2010 , 24 (6): 581-589.

Friedman R, Sobel D, Myers P, et al.Behavioral medicine, clinical health psychology, and cost offset. Health Psychol,1995, 14: 509-518.

Frisina P G, Borod J C, Lepore S J. A Meta-Analysis of the effects of written emotional disclosure on the health outcomes of clinical populations. J Nervo Ment Dis,2004, 192: 629-634.

Gabbard G O, Gunderson J G, Fonagy P. The place of psychoanalytic treatments within psychiatry. Arch Gen Psychiatry ,2002, 59: 505-510.

Gardner H, Hatch T. Multiple Intelligence Go to School: Educational Implications of the Theory of Multiple Intelligences. EduRes,1989, 18 (8): 4-9.

Gary H, Glover. Overview of Functional Magnetic Resonance Imaging. Neurosurg Clin N Am,2011 ,22(2): 133-139.

Gauthier I, Tarr M J, Moylan J, et al. Does visualsubordinate-level categorization engage the functionally defined fusiform face area? Cog Neuropsychol,17,143-163.

Gergely G, Watson J. The social biofeedback model of parental affect-mirroring. Int J Psycho, 1996, 77: 1181-1212.

Gergely G, Watson J. Early social-emotional development. Hillsdale: Erlbaum,1999.

Gibbons J L. Cortisol secretion rate in depressive illness. Arch Gen Psychiatry, 2004, 10: 572-575.

Gidron Y, Peri T, Connolly J, et al . Written disclosure in posttraumatic stress disorder: Is it beneficial for the patient? J Nerv Men Dis ,1996, 184: 505-507.

Gill M M. Review of 'Hope and Dread in Psychoanalysis by Stephen A. Mitchell'. Int J Psychoanal, 1994, 75: 847-850.

Gloaguen V, Cottraux J, Cucherat M, et al. A meta-analysis of the effects of cognitive therapy in depressed patients. J Affect Dis,1998, 49: 59-72.

Goleman D. Emotional Intelligence: Why It Can Matter More Than IQ. London: Bloomsbury,1995.

Gonzalez V M, Schmitz J M, DeLaune K A. The role of homework in cognitive-behavioral therapy for cocaine dependence. J Consul Clin Psychol ,2006, 74: 633-637.

Goodman A, Joyce R, Smith J. The long shadow cast by childhood physical and mental problems on adult life. Proc Natl Acad Sci U S A, 2011; DOI: 10.1073/pnas.1016970108.

Graybiel, Ann M. Habits, Rituals, and the Evaluative Brain. Annual Review of Neuroscience, 2008,31: 359-387.

Greenwald R. Eye movement desensitization and reprocessing (EMDR): New hope for children suffering from trauma and loss. Clin Child Psychol Psychiatr,2008, 3: 279-287.

Gregory E. Miller, Steve W. Clustering of Depression and Inflammation in Adolescents Previously Exposed to Childhood Adversity. Bio Psychiatr, Published online, 2012. DOI:

10.1016/j.biopsych.2012.02.034.

Gregory R J. Psychological Testing: Psychological Testing: History, Principles, and Applications. Boston: Pearson Education,1992.

Gregory R J. Psychological Testing: History, Principles, and Applications. 5th ed. Boston: Pearson Education ,2007.

Gunther L M, Denniston JC, Miller RR.Conducting exposure treatment in multiple contexts can prevent relapse. Behav Res Ther, 1998, 36(1): 75-91.

Gupta B P, Murad M H, Clifton M M, et al. The effect of lifestyle modification and cardiovascular risk factor reduction on erectile dysfunction: a systematic review and meta-analysis. Arch Intern Med, 2011, 171: 1797-1806.

Hafed Z M, Clark J J. Microsaccades as an overt measure of covert attention shifts. Vision Res, 2002, 42(22): 2533-2545.

Hafed Z M, Goffart L, Krauzlis R J. Superior colliculus inactivation causes stable offsets in eye position during tracking. J Neurosci, 2008, 28(32): 8124-8137.

Hahn A, Wolfgang W, Windischberger C, et al. Differential modulation of the default mode network via serotonin-1A receptors. Proc Natl Acad Sci, 2012,109(7): 2619-2624.

Hall C S, Lindzey L. Theories of Personality. New York: Jon Willy and Sons Inc,1957.

Hare R D. A research scale for the assessment of psychopathy in criminal populations. Pers Indi Differe, 2008, 1: 111-120.

Hare R D. Psychopathy and the personality dimensions of psychoticism, extraversion and neuroticism. Pers Indi Differe,,2008, 3: 35-42.

Hare R D, Clarke D, Grann M. et al. Psychopathy and the predictive validity of the PCL-R: An international perspective. Behav Sci Law, 2000,18: 623-645.

Hayama H R, Vilberg K L, Rugg MD. Overlap between the neural correlates of cued recall and source memory: evidence for a generic recollection network? Journal of Cog Neurosci, 2012, 24(5):1127-37.

Heinicke C M. Ramsey - Klee DM. Outcome of child psychotherapy as a function of frequency of sessions. J Am Aca Adol Psychiatr,1986, 25: 247-253.

Hemphill J F, Hare R D, Wong S. Psychopathy and recidivism: A review. Leg Criminol Psychol,2008, 3: 139-170.

He Y, Evans A. Graph theoretical modeling of brain connectivity. Curr Opin Neurol, 2010,23(4):341-350.

Hirst W, Manier D. Towards a Psychology of Collective Memory. Mem,2008,16: 183-200.

Hoare P, Remschmidt H, Medori R. et al. 12 - month efficacy and safety of OROS methylphenidate in children and adolescents with attention - deficit/hyperactivity disorder switched from MPH. Euro Child Adol Psychiatr,2005, 14: 305-319.

Hobson J, Shine J, Roberts, R. How do psychopaths behave in a prison therapeutic community? Psychol Crime Law, 2000, 6: 139-154.

Hobson R F. Forms of feeling: the heart of psychotherapy. New York: Basic Books, 1985.

Holmes J. All you need is cognitive behavior therapy? Br Med Bull,2002, 324: 288-294.

Horney K. New Ways in Psychoanalysis. New York: W. W. Norton & Co, 1939.

Howard R. A review of M. J. Mahoney's Cognition and behavior modification. J Appl Behav Anal,1977 ,10(2): 369-374.

I. Bojak, Thom F. Oostendorp et al.Towards a model-based integration of co-registered electroencephalography/functional magnetic resonance imaging data with realistic neural population meshes. Philos Transact A Math Phys Eng Sci, 2011,369(1952): 3785-3801.

Janet C, Rucker, Sarah H et al.Do brainstem omnipause neurons terminate saccades? Ann N Y Acad Sci, 2011,1233: 48-57.

Javier M, Miguel E. Eye Movements and Abducens Motoneuron Behavior after Cholinergic Activation of the Nucleus Reticularis Pontis Caudalis. Sleep, 2010 ,33(11): 1517-1527.

Jessica M, Abigail N, Robert S. Eye movements and imitation learning: Intentional disruption of expectation. J Vis. J Vis, Published online, 2011, doi: 10.1167/11.1.7.

Jie C, Melanie W, Nikos K, et al .Visibility States Modulate Microsaccade Rate and Direction. Vision Res,2009 ,49(2): 228-236.

Jrendt P, Parrish L, Kathleen C. Effects of Cognitive Therapy for Depression on Daily Stress-Related Variables.Behav Res Ther,2009 ,47(5): 444-448.

Kagan I, Gur M, Snodderly D M. Saccades and drifts differentially modulate neuronal activity in V1:effects of retinal image motion, position, and extraretinal influences. J Vis,2008, 8 (14):19, 11-25.

Kaloupec D G, Keane T M. Imaginal flooding in the treatment of post traumatic stress disorder. J Couns Clin Psychol, 2011,50: 138-140.

Kaplan H S. The classification of the female sexual dysfunctions. J Sex Mari Ther, 1974, 1: 124-138.

Kazantzis N, Deane F P. Psychologists' use of homework assignments in clinical practice. Pro Psychol Res Prac,1999, 30: 581-585.

Kazdin A E. Practitioner review: psychosocial treatments for conduct disorder in children. J Child Psychol Psychiatry, 1997, 38: 161-78.

Kemph J P, DeVane CL, Levin GM et al. Treatment of aggressive children with clonidine: results of an open pilot study. J Am Acad Child Adolesc Psychiatry,1993,32:577-81.

Kenny M A, Williams J M G. Treatment-resistant depressed patients show a good response to Mindfulness-based Cognitive Therapy. Behav Res Therapy, 2007,45, 617-625.

Klein M. A contribution to the psychogenesis of manic-depressive states. London: Hogarth Press,1975.

Kopelman L M. Moral problems in assessing research risk. IRB,2000,22(5):3-6.

Krauzlis R J, Liston D, Carello C D. Target selection and the superior colliculus: goals, choices andhypotheses. Vision Res, 2004,44(12):1445-1451.

Kurland K D. Steroid excretion in depressive disorders. Arch Genl Psychiatry, 2004,10, 554-560.

Kustov A A, Robinson D L. Shared neural control of attentional shifts and eye movements. Nature,1996, 384(6604): 74-77.

Lambert M J, Bergin G. Handbook of Psychotherapy and Behavior Change. 5th ed. U.S.A.: John Wiley & Sons, Inc,2004.

Lamina S, Okoye C G, Dagogo T T. Therapeutic effect of an interval exercise training program in the management of erectile dysfunction in hypertensive patients. J Clin Hypertens, 2009,11:125.

Larson R W. Toward a psychology of positive youth development. Am Psychologi, 2000, 55, 170-183.

Lavaas O I, Simmons J Q. Manipulation of self-destruction in three retarded children. J Appl Behav Anal,1969, 2(3):143-57.

Lee H B, Hening W A, Allen R P, et al. Restless legs syndrome is associated with DSM-Ⅳ major depressive disorder and panic disorder in the community. J Neuropsychiatry Clin Neurosci, 2008, 20(1):101-105.

Leibovici L. Effects of remóte, retroactive intercessory prayer on outcomes in patients with bloodstream infection: randomised controlled trial. Br Med bulletinBull,2001;323:1450-1451.

Levitin D J, Tirovolas A K. Current advances in the cognitive neuroscience of music. Ann N Y Acad Sci, 2009 ,1156:211-31.

Lifton J R. Doctors and torture. N Engl J Med, 2004,351:415-416.

Lohmann G, Erfurth K, Müller K, et al.Critical comments on dynamic causal modelling. Neuroimage, 2012,59(3):2322-2329.

Lovaas O I, , Simmons J Q. Manipulation of self-destruction in three retarded children. J Appl Behav Anal,1969,2(3): 143-157.

Luborsky L. Diguer L. Seligman DA, et al. The researcher's own therapy allegiances: a "wild card" in comparisons of treatment efficacy. Clin Psychol Sci Prac, 1999, 6: 95-106.

Luborsky L, Singer G, Luborsky L. Comparative studies of psychotherapies: Is it true that everyone has won and that all must have prizes? Arch Gen Psychiatry,2005, 32: 995-1008.

Luckhoo H, Hale J R, Stokes M G, et al. Inferring task-related networks using independent component analysis in magnetoencephalography. Neuroimage, 2012,62(1):530-541.

Maccoby E E. Gender and relationships. A developmental account.Am Psychol,1990, 45 (4):513-520.

Macfarlane J. Perspectives on personality consistency and change from the guidance study. Vita Humana, 1964, 7: 115-126.

MacLeod C M, John R. Stroop: Creator of a landmark cognitive task. Can Psychol,2009, 32: 521-524.

MacLeod C M. Half a century of research on the Stroop effect: An Integrative approach. Psychol Bull,2009, 109(2): 163-203.

MacLeod, C M. The Stroop task: The "gold standard" of attentional measures. J Exp Psychol Genl, 1992, 121: 12-14.

Malouff J M, Thorsteinsson, Schutte N S. The efficacy of problem solving therapy in reducing mental and physical health problems: A meta - analysis. Clin Psychol Rev, 2007, 27: 46-57.

Marcus R, Felicia H. Do positive children become positive adults? Evidence from a longitudinal birth cohort study. J Posi Psycho, Published online,2011, DOI: 10.1080/17439760.2011.536655.

Marshall R D, Vaughan S, MacKinnon R, et al. Assessing outcome in psychoanalysis and long-term dynamic psychotherapy. J Am Acad Psychoanal, 1996, 24(4): 575-604.

Marvin R, Cooper G, Hoffman K, et al. The circle of security project: Attachment-based intervention with caregiver-pre-school child dyads. Attac Hum Dev, 2002, 4: 107-124.

Massimini F, Delle F A. Individual development in a bio - cultural perspective. Am Psychologist, 2000, 55: 24-33.

Massaro DW. Book Reviews. Attention: Yesterday, Today and Tomorrow. Am J Psychol, 2006, 109(1): 139-150.

Masters W H, Johnson V E. Human sexual inadequacy. Boston: Little Brown, 1970.

Matarazzo J D. Behavioral health's challenge to academic, scientific and professional psychology. Am Psychologist, 1982, 37: 1-14.

Mayer J D, Caruso D R, Salovey P. Emotional Intelligence Meets Traditional Standards for an Intelligence. Intelli,1999, 27, 267-298.

Mayer J D, Caruso D R, Salovey P, et al. Measuring Emotional Intelligence with the MSCEIT V2.0. Emo,2003, 3 (1): 97-105.

Mayer J D, Salovey P, Caruso D R. et al. Emotional Intelligence as a Standard Intelligence. Emo,2001, 1: 232-242.

McClelland D C. The social mandate of health psychology. Am Behav Sci,2008, 28: 451-467.

McNally R J. EMDR and Mesmerism: A comparative historical analysis. J Anxie Dis,1999, 13(1-2): 225-236.

McPeek R M, Keller E L. Superior colliculus activity related to concurrent processing of saccade goals in a visual search task. J Neurophysiol, 2002,87(4):1805 - 1815.

Mednick S A, Gabrielle F W Jr, Hutchings B. Genetic influences in criminal convictions: Evidence from an adoption cohort. Sci,1984, 224: 891-894.

Michael A, Basso, Joel S, et al. Shedding new light on the role of the basal ganglia-superior colliculus pathway in eye movements. Curr Opin Neurobiol,2010,20(6): 717-725.

Michael M. Specular Highlights as a Guide to Perceptual Content. Philo Psychol ,2008,21 (5):629 - 639.

Michael S, Salman M, James A. The Cerebellar Dysplasia of Chiari II Malformation as Revealed by Eye Movements. Can J Neurol Sci, 2009, 36(6): 713-724.

Mischel W, Ebbesen E B, Zeiss A. Cognitive and attentional mechanisms in delay of gratification. J Pers Soci Psychol , 2002, 21: 204-218.

Mitchell SA. Hope and dread in psychoanalysis. New York: Basic Books, 1993.

Morris C G , Maisto A. Understanding Psychology. 5th ed. New Jersy: Prentice Hall, Inc, 2011.

Moshe Gur, D Max .Physiological differences between neurons in layer 2 and layer 3 of primary visual cortex (V1) of alert macaque monkeys. J Physiol, 2008 ,586: 2293-2306.

MTA Cooperative Group. A 14-month randomized clinical trial of treatment strategies for attention-deficit/hyperactivity disorder. Arch Gen Psychiatr, 1999, 56: 1073-1086.

Munoz D P, Wurtz R H. Fixation cells in monkey superior colliculus. I. Characteristics of cell discharge. J Neurophysiol,1993,70(2):559-575.

Myers D G. The funds, friends, and faith of happy people. Am Psychologist, 2000, 55: 56-67.

Nakatani Y. Psychiatry and the law in Japan. Inte J Law Psychiatry, 2000, 23: 589-604.

Nicole L, W Einar, Stephen J, et al. .An fMRI study of multi-modal semantic and phonological processing in reading disabled adolescents. Ann Dyslexia, 2010, 60 (1): 102-121.

Nicholas H. Doing It My Way: Sensation, Perception — and Feeling Red. Behav Bra Sci, 2001,24 (5):987-987.

Nieuwenhuis J A, Paivio S C. Efficacy of emotion focused therapy for adult survivors of child abuse: A preliminary study. J Trau Stre,2001, 14: 115-134.

Norcross J C, Hedges M, Prochaska J O. The face of 2010: A Delphi poll on the future of psychotherapy. Professional Psychology.Res Prac, 2002, 33: 316-322.

Norman A, Clemens, K. Roy M, et al. Psychotherapy by Psychiatrists in a Managed Care Environment: Must It Be an Oxymoron?: A Forum From the APA Commission on Psychotherapy by Psychiatrists.J Psychother Pract Res,2001 ,10(1): 53-62.

Ogawa H, Wakita M, Hasegawa K, et al. Functional MRI detection of activation in the primary gustatory cortices in humans. Chem Senses, 2005 ,30(7):583-592.

Ogloff J, Wong S, Greenwood A. Treating criminal psychopaths in a therapeutic community program. Behav Sci Law,1990, 8: 181-190.

Park C L, Blumberg C J. Disclosing trauma through writing: Testing the meaning- making hypothesis. Cogni Thera Res,2002, 26: 597-616.

Patrick C J. Handbook of psychopathy. New York: Guilford Press,2006.

Pazo-Alvarez P, Simos P G, Castillo E M, et al. MEG correlates of bimodal encoding of faces and persons' names. Brain Res, 2008 ,1230:192-201.

Pederson D, Moran G. A categorical description of infant-mother relationships in the home and its relation to Q-sort measures of mother-infant interaction. Monogra Soci Res Child Dev,1995,60 (2-3): 111-145.

Pennebaker J W. Writing about emotional experiences as a therapeutic process. Psycholo Sci, 1997, 8: 162-166.

Pennebaker J W. Theories, therapies and taxpayers: On the complexities of the expressive writing paradigm. Clin Psychol, 2004, 11: 138-142.

Pennebaker J W, Beall, SK. Confronting a traumatic event: Toward an understanding of inhibition and disease. J Abno Psychol,2009, 95: 274-281.

Pennebaker J W, Graybeal A. Patterns of natural language use: Disclosure, personality, and social integration. Curr Dir Psychol Sci, 2009, 10: 90-93.

Penny E, Peter B, Karina L, et al. Psychotherapy mediated by remote communication technologies: a meta-analytic review. BMC Psychiatry, 2008, 8: 260-269.

Peter F. Psychoanalysis today. World Psychi, 2003, 2(2): 73-80.

Peterson C . The future of optimism. Am Psychologist, 2000, 55: 44-55.

Petrides K V, Furnham A. Gender Differences in Measured and Self - Estimated Trait Emotional Intelligence. Sex Roles, 2000, 42 (5-6): 449-461.

Petrides K V, Furnham A. On the Dimensional Structure of Emotional Intelligence. Personality and Individual Differ, 2000, 29: 313-320.

Phillips A. On kissing, tickling and being bored: psychoanalytic essays on the unexamined life. London: Faber & Faber, 1993.

Pinals DA. Where two roads meet: restoration of competence to stand trial from a clinical perspective. J Crimi Civil Confi,2005,31:81-108.

Pleschberger S, Hornek A. Recognizing and defining dying. Analysis of end - of - life coverage in German nursing textbooks. Pflege,2011, 24(4):259-69.

Pulvermüller F. Brain embodiment of syntax and grammar: discrete combinatorial mechanisms spelt out in neuronal circuits. Brain Lang, 2010 ,112(3): 167-179.

Qaseem A, Snow V, Denberg T D, et al. Hormonal testing and pharmacologic treatment of erectile dysfunction: a clinical practice guideline from the American College of Physicians. Ann Intern Med , 2009, 151:639.

Rajkai C, Lakatos P, Chen CM, et al.Transient cortical excitation at the onset of visual fixation. Cereb Cortex, 2008,18(1):200-209.

Ransohoff P M. Ethics education in psychoanalytic training: a survey. J Am Psychoanal Assoc,2010 ,58(1):83-99.

Raposa E B, Hammen C L, Brennan P A. Effects of child psychopathology on maternal depression: the mediating role of child - related acute and chronic stressors. J Abnorm Child Psychol,2011, 39(8):1177-1186.

Ratha D, Heyda L, Steven R, et al. Brain Mechanism for representing what another person sees. Neuroimage. Neuroimage, 2010, 50(2): 693-700.

Robert J K, Mavis T, Michael J.The dimensions of clinical behavior analysis. Behav Anal, 1993,16(2): 271-282.

Robert J, Karsten M, Du?an U, et al. The Subthalamic Microlesion Story in Parkinson's Disease: Electrode Insertion - Related Motor Improvement with Relative Cortico - Subcortical Hypoactivation in fMRI. PLoS One,Published online 2012 ,doi: 10.1371/journal.pone.0049056.

Roozbeh R, Panagiotis G, Simos A, et al.Time course of electromagnetic activity associated with detection of rare events. Neuroreport, 2011, 22(3): 136-140.

Rosenberg D, GleitmanH, Fridlund A. J. Psychology. 6th ed. New York: W.W. Norton & Company Inc,2004.

Ryan R M, Deci E. Self-determination theory and the facilitation of intrinsic motivation, social development, and well-being. Am Psychologist,2000, 55: 68-78.

Salekin R, Rogers R, Sewell K W. A review and meta-analysis of the Psychopathy Checklist and Psychopathy Checklist-Revised: Predictive validity of dangerousness. Clin Psychol Sci Pract,2006, 3: 203-215.

Salovey P, Mayer J D. Emotional Intelligence. Imag Cogni Pers, 1990,9: 185-211.

Salovey P, Rothman A J, Detweiler J B, et al. Emotional states and physical health. Am Psychologist, 2000,55: 110-121.

Sarang S, Dalal J, Zumer A, et al. MEG/EEG Source Reconstruction, Statistical Evaluation, and Visualization with NUTMEG.Comput Intell Neurosci ,Published online, 2011,doi: 10.1155/2011/758973.

Schutte N S, Malouffe J B, Coston C, et al. Emotional Intelligence and Interpersonal Relations. J Soci Psychol, 2001,141: 523.

Searight H R, Oliver J M, Grisso J T. The community competence scale in the placement of the deinstitutionalized mentally ill. Am J Community Psychol,1986 ,14(3): 291-301.

Seo M, Tamura K, Shijo H, et al. Telling the diagnosis to cancer patients in Japan: attitude and perception of patients, physicians and nurses. Palli Med,2000,14:105-110.

Seppo P, Ahlfors, Jooman H, John W. Belliveau, Matti S. H. Sensitivity of MEG and EEG to Source Orientation.Brain Topogr, 2010 ,23(3): 227-232.

Shah D. Critical review of group interventions for sexual dysfunction: Advances in the last decade. Sexual and Marital Therapy,2006, 11, 187-195.

Shapiro F. Eye movement desensitization and reprocessing: Basic principles, protocols and procedures. New York: Guilford Press,1995

Shapiro K. The functional architecture of divided visual attention.Prog Brain Res, 2009,176:101-21.

Shaw B F. Comparison of cognitive therapy and behavior therapy in the treatment of depression. J Consul Clin Psychol,1997, 45: 543-551.

Sheldon K M, Houser-Marko L. Self-Concordance, Goal Attainment, and the Pursuit of Happiness: Can There Be an Upward Spiral? J Pers Soci Psychol, 2001, 80: 152-164.

Shelley B P, Trimble M R. "All that spikes is not fits", mistaking the woods for the trees: the interictal spikes an "EEG chameleon" in the interface disorders of brain and mind: a critical review. Clin EEG Neurosci, 2009 ,40(4):245-61.

Shorter, E. A history of psychiatry: From the era of the asylum to the age of Prozac. New York: Wiley,1997.

Siegel, B. The world of the autistic child. New York: Oxford Press,1996.

Simona T, Matti S. H, Gina K, et al. Stufflebeam, Eric Halgren, Emery N. Brown.Eye

Movements Modulate the Spatiotemporal Dynamics of Word Processing. J Neurosci,2012, 32 (13): 4482-4494.

Simonton D K. Creativity: Cognitive, personal, developmental, and social aspects. Am Psychologist, 2000,55: 151-158.

Skinner B F. Science and human behavior. New York: Macmillan,1953.

Sloan D M, Marx B P. A closer examination of the structured written disclosure procedure. J Consul Clin Psychol,2004, 72: 165-175.

Sloan D M, Marx B P, Epstein EM. Further examination of the exposure model underlying the efficacy of written emotional disclosure. J Consul Clin Psychol, 2005,73: 549-554.

Smith J M. Written emotional expression: effect sizes, outcome types, and moderating variables. J Consul Clin Psychol, 2010, 66: 174-184.

Smith J M. True N, Souto J. Effects of writing about traumatic experiences: The necessity for narrative structuring. J Soci Clin Psychol, 2010, 20: 161-172.

Smith R. The human sciences. New York: Norton,1997.

Srinivasan R, Winter W R, Ding J, et al. EEG and MEG coherence: measures of functional connectivity at distinct spatial scales of neocortical dynamics. J Neurosci Methods, 2007, 166 (1):41-52.

Srinivasan R. Anatomical constraints on source models for high-resolution EEG and MEG derived from MRI. Technol Cancer Res Treat,2006 ,5(4):389-99.

Stahmer AC, Schreibman L. Teaching children with autism: Appropriate play in unsupervised environments using a self-management treatment package. J Appl Behav Anal, 2009,25(2): 447-459.

Stam C J. Characterization of anatomical and functional connectivity in the brain: a complex networks perspective. Int J Psychophysiol, 2010 ,77(3):186-94.

Stanton A H, Gunderson J G, Knapp P H, et al. Effects of psychotherapy in schizophrenia: I. Design an implementation of a controlled study. Schizophr Bull. 1984,10:520-563.

Startup M, Edmonds J. Compliance with homework assignments in cognitive-behavioral psychotherapy for depression: Relation to outcome and methods of enhancement. Cogn Thera Res,1994,18: 567-579.

Steele M, Weiss M, Swanson J, et al. A randomized, controlled effectiveness trial of OROS-methylphenidate compared to usual care with immediate-release methylphenidate in Attention Deficit-Hyperactivity Disorder. Can J, Clin Pharmacol,2006, 13: 50-62.

Stemberg R J. Psychology-In search of the human mind (3rd ed.) Florida :Orlando Harcourt College publishers,2001.

Sternberg R J. The Theory of Successful Intelligence. Rev Gen Psychol,1999, 3 (4), 292-316.

Sternberg R J. The Theory of Successful Intelligence. Inte J Psychol, 39 (2),2005, 189-202.

Steyn-Ross ML, Steyn D, Wilson M, et al. Modeling brain activation patterns for the default and cognitive states. Neuroimage, 2009, 45(2):298-311.

Stone E. The last will and testament in literature: rupture, rivalry, and sometimes rapprochement from Middlemarch to Lemony Snicket, Fam Process,2008 ,47(4):425-39.

Stricker G. Using homework in psychodynamic psychotherapy. J Psycho Integr, 2006, 16: 219-237.

Susana M, Stephen L, David H. The function of bursts of spikes during visual fixation in the awake primate lateral geniculate nucleus and primary visual cortex. Proc Natl Acad Sci, 2002, 99(21): 13920-13925.

Sukhodolsky D G, Kassinove H, Gorman B. Cognitive - behavioral therapy for anger in children and adolescents: A meta-analysis. Aggre Vio Behav,2004, 9: 247-269.

Taylor S. Meta-analysis of cognitive-behavioral treatment for social phobia. J Behav Thera and Exp Psychiatr,1996, 27: 1-9.

Teasdale J D, Segal Z, Williams J. How does cognitive therapy prevent relapse and why should attentional control (mindfulness) training help? Behav Res Thera,1995, 33: 225-239.

Tennenbaum D J. Personality and criminality — a summary and implications of the literature. J Crim Jus,1997, 5: 225-235.

Thatcher R, Walker R , Giudice S. Human cerebral hemispheres develop at different rates and ages. Sci, 2007, 236: 1110-1113.

Thorndike E L. The Law of Effect. Am J Psychol, 1997, 39(1): 212-222.

Thorp D M, Stahmer AC, Schreibman. Effects of sociodramatic play training on children with autism. J Auti Dev Dis, 1995,25(3): 265-282.

Tomlinson J, Wright D. Impact of erectile dysfunction and its subsequent treatment with sildenafil: qualitative study. BMJ, 2004, 328:1037.

Tracy D Farr, Susanne W. Use of magnetic resonance imaging to predict outcome after stroke: a review of experimental and clinical evidence. J Cereb Blood Flow Metab,2010 ,30(4): 703-717.

Treisman A. Selective attention in man. Br Med Bull,1994, 20: 12-16.

Treisman A. Features and objects in visual processing. Sci Am , 1989,254: 114-125.

Treisman A, Schmidt H. Illusory conjunctions in the perception of objects. Cog Psychol, 2008, 14: 107-141.

Turnbull G J. A review of posttraumatic stress disorder. Part I: Historical development and classification. Injury,1998, 29(2): 87-91.

Vaudano A E, Carmichael D W, Salek - Haddadi A, et al. Networks involved in seizure initiation. A reading epilepsy case studied with EEG - fMRI and MEG. Neurol, 2012, 79(3): 249-53.

Victor M, Adams R D, Collins G H.The Wernicke - Korsakoff syndrome. A clinical and pathological study of 245 patients, 82 with post - mortem examinations. Contemp Neurol Ser, 1971,7:1-206.

Vladimir L, Jérémie M, Stefan K, et al. EEG and MEG Data Analysis in SPM8.Comput

Intell Neurosci, Published online 2011, doi: 10.1155/2011/852961.

Volkow N D, Swanson J M. Variables that affect the clinical use and abuse of methylphenidate in the treatment of ADHD. Am J Psychiatry, 2003,160, 1909-1918.

Volkow N D, Fowler J S, Wang G, et al. Mechanism of action of methylphenidate: insights from PET imaging studies. J Atten Dis, 2002,1, 31-43.

Walker B L, Nail L M, Croyle R T. Does emotional expression make a difference in reactions to breast cancer? Oncol Nur Forum, 1999,26, 1025-1032.

Waters E, Merrick S, Treboux D, Crowell J, et al. Attachment security in infancy and early adulthood: A twenty-year longitudinal study. Child Dev, 2010, 71, 684-689.

W Burleson D. A Review of Co - Morbid Depression in Pediatric ADHD: Etiologies, Phenomenology, and Treatment. J Child Adolesc Psychopharmacol, 2008,18(6): 565-571.

Wechsler D. Wechsler Adult Intelligence Scale. San Antonio:Psychological Corporation, 1997.

Wechsler D. The Range of human capacities (2nd ed.). Baltimore: Williams & Wilkins, 1995.

Wechsler D. Manual for the Wechsler Adult Intelligence Scale. New York: The Psychological Corporation,1995.

Wechsler H, Grosser GH, Busfield B L. The Depression Rating Scale. Archives of Gen Psychiatry,1993, 9, 334-343.

Wilson J P. The historical evolution of PTSD diagnostic criteria: From Freud to DSM-IV. J Traum Str,1994, 7(4): 681-698.

Wing R R, Rosen C, Fava J L, et al. Effects of weight loss intervention on erectile function in older men with type 2 diabetes in the Look AHEAD trial. J Sex Med 2010, 7:156-167.

Wissow LS. Child abuse and neglect. N Engl J Med,2005;332:1425-31.

W M King. Binocular Coordination of Eye Movements: Hering's Law of Equal Innervation or Uniocular Control? Eur J Neurosci,2011 ,33(11): 2139-2146.

Womelsdorf T, Fries P, Mitra PP, et al. Gamma - band synchronization in visual cortex predicts speed of change detection. Nature, 2006,439(7077):733-736.

Woody S R , Sanderson W C. Manuals for empirically supported treatments: 1998 update. Clin Psychol,1998, 51: 17-21.

Wright K, Haigh K, McKeown M. Reclaiming the humanity in personality disorder. Inte J Ment Healt Nur,2007,16:236-246.

Wurtz Robert H, Kerry M, James C, et al. Berman. Thalamic pathways of active vision. Trends Cogn Sci. 2011,15(4): 177-184.

Yang M, Coid J. Gender differences in psychiatric morbidity and violent behavior among a household population in Great Britain. Soci Psychiatr Psychiatric Epidemiol, 2007,42:599-605.

Yang L, Stephen G.Learning on Multiple Timescales in Smooth Pursuit Eye Movements. J Neurophysiol, 2010 ,104(5): 2850-2862.

Organization

American Academy of Child and Adolescent Psychiatry. www.aacap.org .

American Academy of Psychiatry and the Law. https://www?.aapl.org/pdf/ETHICSGDLNS.pdf.

American Association on Mental Retardation (AAMR). http://www.aamr.org.

Americans With Disabilities Act. http://www.usdoj.gov

Criminalization in forensic psychiatry. http://www.priory.com

Economic and Social Research Council (ESRC). http://www.esrc.ac.uk

Principles of psychology. http://psychclassics

Psychotherapy Networker.http://www.psychotherapynetworker.com

Freud's Psychosexual Stage Theory. http://changingminds.org

Forensic psychiatry and human rights. http://www.priory.com/psych

The Gender Identity Research & Education Society. http://www.gires.org.

The Renaissance Transgender Association. http://www.ren.org.

Trauma Recovery Resource Network: http://www.traumanetwork.com.

The prevention of depression and anxiety. http://journals.apa.org.

Unit Costs of Health and Social Care. http://www?.pssru.ac.uk/

National Eating Disorders Association . http://www.nationaleatingdisorders.org